Cardiopulmonary Anatomy & Physiology

Essentials for Respiratory Care

Fifth Edition

LIBRARY USE
TEXAS HEART INSTITUTE

To
Katherine, Alexander, Destinee, and Ashley
The Next Generation

Grandpa T

Cardiopulmonary
Anatomy & Physiology

Essentials for Respiratory Care

Fifth Edition

Terry Des Jardins, MEd, RRT

Professor Emeritus
Director
Department of Respiratory Care
Parkland College
Champaign, Illinois

THOMSON

DELMAR LEARNING

Australia   Brazil   Canada   Mexico   Singapore   Spain   United Kingdom   United States

THOMSON

DELMAR LEARNING

Cardiopulmonary Anatomy & Physiology: Essentials for Respiratory Care, Fifth Edition
by Terry Des Jardins

Vice President, Health Care Business Unit:
William Brottmiller

Director of Learning Solutions:
Matthew Kane

Senior Acquisitions Editor:
Rhonda Dearborn

Product Manager:
Sarah Prime

Marketing Director:
Jennifer McAvey

Marketing Coordinator:
Andrea Eobstel

Technology Product Manager:
Mary Colleen Liburdi

Technology Project Manager:
Carolyn Fox

Production Director:
Carolyn Miller

Senior Content Project Manager:
James Zayicek

Senior Art Director:
Jack Pendleton

COPYRIGHT © 2008 Thomson Delmar Learning, a division of Thomson Learning Inc. Thomson, the Star logo, and Delmar Learning are trademarks used herein under license.

Printed in the Canada
2 3 4 5 6 7 XXX 10 09 08 07

For more information, contact Thomson Delmar Learning, 5 Maxwell Drive, Clifton Park, NY 12065

Or find us on the World Wide Web at
http://www.delmarlearning.com

ALL RIGHTS RESERVED. No part of this work covered by the copyright hereon may be reproduced or used in any form or by any means—graphic, electronic, or mechanical, including photocopying, recording, taping, Web distribution or information storage and retrieval systems—without the written permission of the publisher.

For permission to use material from this text or product, contact us by
Tel (800) 730-2214
Fax (800) 730-2215
www.thomsonrights.com

Library of Congress Cataloging-in-Publication Data

Des Jardins, Terry R.
  Cardiopulmonary anatomy & physiology : essentials for respiratory care /
Terry Des Jardins.—5th ed. p. ; cm.
  Includes bibliographical references and index.
ISBN 978-1-4180-4278-3
1. Cardiopulmonary system—Physiology.
2. Cardiopulmonary system—Anatomy.
3. Respiratory therapy. I. Title. II. Title:
Cardiopulmonary anatomy and physiology.
  [DNLM: 1. Respiratory Physiology.
2. Respiratory System—anatomy & histology. 3. Cardiovascular Physiology.
4. Cardiovascular System—anatomy & histology. WF 101 D441c 2008]

QP121.D47 2008

612.1—dc22   2007017383

NOTICE TO THE READER

Publisher does not warrant or guarantee any of the products described herein or perform any independent analysis in connection with any of the product information contained herein. Publisher does not assume, and expressly disclaims, any obligation to obtain and include information other than that provided to it by the manufacturer.

The reader is expressly warned to consider and adopt all safety precautions that might be indicated by the activities described herein and to avoid all potential hazards. By following the instructions contained herein, the reader willingly assumes all risks in connection with such instructions.

The publisher makes no representations or warranties of any kind, including but not limited to, the warranties of fitness for particular purpose or merchantability, nor are any such representations implied with respect to the material set forth herein, and the publisher takes no responsibility with respect to such material. The publisher shall not be liable for any special, consequential, or exemplary damages resulting, in whole or part, from the reader's use of, or reliance upon, this material.

CONTENTS

SECTION ONE   1

The Cardiopulmonary System—The Essentials

CHAPTER 1
The Anatomy and Physiology of the Respiratory System   3

CHAPTER 2
Ventilation   67

CHAPTER 3

The Diffusion of Pulmonary Gases

CHAPTER 4

Pulmonary Function Measurements

CHAPTER 5

The Anatomy and Physiology of the Circulatory System

SECTION TWO 395

**Advanced Cardiopulmonary Concepts and
Related Areas—The Essentials**

LIST OF TABLES

FOREWORD
TO THE FIFTH EDITION

As I sit down to pen a few lines for the foreword to this edition, and after reviewing the significant new additions to this work, I am taken back many years (50!!) to the time when I first had classroom contact with the teachers of basic anatomy and physiology in medical school.

The memories are not altogether happy ones! Right out of a liberal arts education in college, I was dumped into the world of pure science in first-year medical school coursework in anatomy, physiology and biochemistry. What a cold water bath *that* was.

I still recall, all these years later, that my reflexive way to get through this data onset was to **memorize, memorize, memorize.** Flash cards tumbled out of every freshman medical student's lab coat, and now, as I reminisce, I wonder how much of it really stuck. Part I of the National Board of Medical Examiner's test (at least then) was a test of one's memory, and little else; for instance, "Which vessels drain into the right atrium?"

Things have changed in medical education, praise be, in that now clinical subjects are integrated into the curriculum in the first year. The questions now read, "What happens to the pulmonary artery pressure in congestive (left) heart failure?" Just in the nick of time, say I!

In a two- to four-year long respiratory education program there is now a more compact curriculum that starts out with a consideration of **functional** cardiopulmonary anatomy, with clinical-based case examples right from the start. I applaud Mr. Des Jardins for his efforts in this fifth edition of his widely accepted and useful textbook. Each chapter is crisply written, and the student is but a few pages away from the illustrations of normal cardiopulmonary anatomy and physiology and how it presents to the examiner.

I also applaud Mr. Des Jardins in his attempt to update the material that has served so well in the previous editions of this textbook. I especially like the new chapter on sleep physiology. The writing style is crisp, and the illustrative material is beautifully presented and comprehensive. It goes to show that it *is* possible to present complicated, advanced-level material in an easily read, integrated format.

If anything at all, I would have devoured this textbook 50 years ago; but alas, that will never be. I wish the ready respiratory care student a good journey in my place.

George G. Burton, MD, FACP, FAARC
Clinical Professor of Medicine
Writer State University School of Medicine
Dayton, Ohio

PREFACE

OVERVIEW

It is important to emphasize that knowledge of an anatomic *structure* is essential to the understanding of the *function* of that structure. It therefore makes little sense to present students with physiologic details without first establishing a solid foundation in anatomy. Because most college-level anatomy courses spend only a limited amount of time on the cardiopulmonary system, respiratory care educators generally need to cover this subject themselves. With regard to a textbook, however, educators usually find the cardiopulmonary section of college-level anatomy and physiology texts too introductory in nature. On the other hand, textbooks concentrating solely on the respiratory system are too complex or esoteric.

As a solution to this problem, the fifth edition of this book is designed to provide students of cardiopulmonary anatomy and physiology with accurate and complete information essential for respiratory care. It is assumed that the student has no previous knowledge of respiratory anatomy or physiology. Great efforts have been made to present a comprehensive overview of the subject matter in an organized, interesting, and readable manner. The organization of this book is based on my experiences as an educator of respiratory anatomy and physiology since 1973 and the many things I have learned from my students. In response to these personal experiences and helpful suggestions, the following pedagogic approach is used in this book.

ORGANIZATION

The fifth edition of this book is divided into three major sections. Section I, *The Cardiopulmonary System—The Essentials,* consists of Chapters 1 through 11. Chapter 1 provides the student with a thorough discussion of anatomic structures associated with the respiratory system. This chapter also features a large number of colorful illustrations. The visual impact of this chapter is intended to (1) stimulate interest in the subject under discussion,

(2) facilitate the rapid visualization of anatomic structures, and (3) help the student relate classroom knowledge to clinical experiences. Chapters 2 through 9 cover the major concepts and mechanisms of respiratory physiology. The discussions are comprehensive, logically organized, and, most importantly, presented at a level suitable for the average college student. When appropriate, anatomic and physiologic principles are applied to common clinical situations to enhance understanding and retention (e.g., the gas transport calculations and their clinical application to the patient's hemodynamic status). In addition, a large number of colorful line drawings and tables appear throughout these chapters to assist in the understanding of various concepts and principles.

Chapters 2, 3, and 6 through 8 feature several unique line drawings that relate familiar visual concepts to standard graphs and nomograms. While I have found that the types of graphs and nomograms presented in this book are often (at first) difficult for students to understand, it is important to stress that the "physiology literature" uses these items extensively. *The student must understand how to read every graph and nomogram in this book to comprehend its contents fully.*

Chapter 10 covers the major anatomic structures and physiologic mechanisms associated with fetal and newborn gas exchange and circulation. It presents the basic cardiopulmonary foundation required to understand fetal and neonatal respiratory disorders. Chapter 11 describes changes that occur in the cardiopulmonary system with age. Because the older age groups are expected to increase each year until about the year 2050, basic knowledge of this material will become increasingly important to respiratory care practitioners.

Section II, *Advanced Cardiopulmonary Concepts and Related Areas— The Essentials,* consists of Chapters 12 through 17. Chapter 12 covers the essential electrophysiology of the heart required for ECG interpretation, Chapter 13 presents the major components of the standard 12-ECG system, and Chapter 14 provides a systematic approach to ECG interpretation and the major cardiac dysrhythmias seen by the respiratory care practitioner. Chapter 15 gives the reader the essential knowledge foundation required for hemodynamic measurements and interpretations. Chapter 16 presents the structure and function of the renal system and the major cardiopulmonary problems that develop when the renal system fails. This chapter is particularly important for respiratory care practitioners working with patients in the critical care unit. Chapter 17, which is new to this edition, presents sleep physiology and its relationship to the cardiopulmonary system. During the past few years, there has been a tremendous increase in the demand for sleep medicine care services. Many of these sleep care centers are staffed with respiratory care practitioners who work routinely with patients who have various sleep-related disorders that adversely impact the cardiopulmonary system, such as obstructive sleep apnea.

Section III, *The Cardiopulmonary System During Unusual Environmental Conditions,* consists of Chapters 18 through 20. Chapter 18 presents the effects of exercise on the cardiopulmonary system. During heavy exercise, the components of the cardiopulmonary system may be stressed to their limits. Cardiac patients involved in exercise training after myocardial infarction demonstrate a significant reduction in mortality and major cardiac mishaps. As our older population increases, cardiovascular rehabilitation programs will become increasingly more important to respiratory care practitioners. Chapter 19 describes the effects of high altitude on the cardiopulmonary system. It provides a better understanding of chronic oxygen deprivation, which can then be applied to the treatment of chronic hypoxia caused by lung disease. Chapter 20 provides an overview of high-pressure environments and their profound effect on the cardiopulmonary system. The therapeutic administration of oxygen at increased ambient pressures (hyperbaric medicine) is now being used to treat a number of pathologic conditions.

Finally, at the end of each chapter there is a set of review questions designed to facilitate learning and retention. In addition, at the end of Chapters 2 through 10 and 15 and 16, the reader is provided with a clinical application section. In this part of the chapters, two clinical scenarios are presented that apply several of the concepts, principles, or formulas that are presented in the chapter to actual clinical situations. These items are flagged throughout the chapters with an icon to direct the reader's attention to important points as they appear in the chapter. This feature nicely facilitates the transfer of classroom material to the clinical setting. Following the clinical applications are related questions to facilitate the development of critical thinking skills.

A glossary is included at the end of the text, followed by appendices that cover symbols, abbreviations, and units of measurement commonly used in respiratory physiology. Also included is a nomogram that can be copied and laminated for use as a handy clinical reference tool in the interpretation of specific arterial blood gas abnormalities. Finally, the answers to the chapter review questions appear in the last appendix.

NEW TO THE FIFTH EDITION

The following changes and features are new to this edition:

Chapter 1: The Anatomy and Physiology of the Respiratory System

- New figures illustrating the excessive bronchial secretions associated with cystic fibrosis, Croup syndrome, and acute epiglottitis
- Eight new and revised figures in this chapter!

Chapter 2: Ventilation

- Clarified and updated content covering ventilation and the pressure differences across the lung
- Simplified and updated discussion of the elastic properties of the lungs and chest wall
- Updated discussion of airway resistance and types of bronchial gas flow
- New figures illustrating driving pressure, positive and negative transmural pressure, tension pneumothorax, and excessive bronchial secretions associated with chronic bronchitis
- Twelve new and revised figures in this chapter!

Chapter 3: The Diffusion of Pulmonary Gases

- New figure showing a cross-sectional view of alveoli with pulmonary edema in Clinical Application 1.
- Eight revised figures in this chapter!

Chapter 4: Pulmonary Function Measurements

- Restructured discussion of the dynamic compression mechanism
- Six revised figures in this chapter!

Chapter 5: The Anatomy and Physiology of the Circulatory System

- New discussion covering mean arterial blood pressure and formula
- New figures of the anterior and posterior view of the heart, the relationship of the heart to the sternum, ribs, and diaphragm, and mean intraluminal blood pressure at various point in the pulmonary and systemic vascular systems
- Six new and revised figures in this chapter!

Chapter 6: Oxygen Transport

- Updated and restructured presentation of Table 6–10, showing clinical factors affecting various oxygen transport calculation values
- New section covering the differences between hypoxemia and hypoxia
- Revised section clarifying and updating the types of hypoxia
- Clarified and updated content covering pulmonary shunting and venous admixture
- Two new tables showing the hypoxemia classification and an overview of the types of hypoxia
- New figure illustrating asthma in Clinical Application 1

Chapter 7: Carbon Dioxide Transport and Acid-Base Balance

- New and extensive content covering the basic principles of acid-base reactions and pH

- New and extensively revised section, covering acid-base disturbances, including the discussion and identification of the acid-base disturbances on the $P_{CO_2}/HCO_3^-/pH$ nomogram
- Eleven new and user-friendly colored $P_{CO_2}/HCO_3^-/pH$ nomograms showing the reader how to identify the various types of acid-base disturbances
- Revised and simplified discussion on base excess/deficit
- New self-assessment questions
- Fourteen new and revised figures in this chapter!

Chapter 8: Ventilation-Perfusion Relationships

- Revised and simplified discussion on how the ventilation-perfusion ratio affects the alveolar gases
- Three new and revised figures in this chapter!

Chapter 9: Control of Ventilation

- Updated discussion of the respiratory components of the medulla oblongata—the respiratory centers
- Updated content covering the pneumotaxic center
- Revised content covering reflexes that influence ventilation

Chapter 10: Fetal Development and the Cardiopulmonary System

- Updated discussion covering circulatory changes at birth

Chapter 11: Aging and the Cardiopulmonary System

- Updated content covering dynamic maneuvers of ventilation
- Updated content covering pulmonary diffusing capacity
- Updated content covering alveolar dead space ventilation
- New content covering arterial blood gases
- Updated content covering the control of ventilation
- New content covering the defense mechanisms
- New content covering aerobic capacity

Chapter 12: Electrophysiology of the Heart

- Updated and simplified content discussion covering the conductive system
- New figure illustrating the conductive system of the heart

Chapter 15: Hemodynamic Measurements

- New figure showing the insertion of the pulmonary catheter

NEW Chapter 17: Sleep Physiology and Its Relationship to the Cardiopulmonary System

- Ten new user-friendly illustrations provided to enhance the understanding of the material presented in the chapter
- Two new tables showing the common EEC waveforms, and the types of sleep observed during stages of sleep
- The differentiation of sleep from a coma
- A discussion of polysomnography
- The description of the purpose for the electroencephalogram (EEG), electrooculogram (EOG), and electromyogram (EMG)
- The differentiation between various EEG waveforms
- A discussion and identification of the major epoch physiologic components
- A discussion of the normal sleep cycle.
- A description of the two most widely accepted theories regarding the purpose of sleep: restoration and energy conservation
- Descriptions of circadian rhythms
- The description of the normal sleep patterns for newborns, toddlers, children, young adults, and older adults
- A list of factors that affect sleep
- Descriptions of six common sleep disorders
- Descriptions of the physiologic changes that occur during sleep

Chapter 18: Exercise and Its Effects on the Cardiopulmonary System

- Updated discussion covering the relationship between oxygen consumption and alveolar ventilation
- Revised and simplified discussion covering cardiovascular rehabilitation

Chapter 19: High Altitude and Its Effects on the Cardiopulmonary System

- Updated discussion of oxygen diffusion capacity

Chapter 20: High-Pressure Environments and Their Effects on the Cardiopulmonary System

- New figure showing how pressure increases linearly with depth
- New content covering the mammalian diving reflex

NEW RESOURCES FOR STUDENTS

StudyWARE software on CD-ROM includes helpful activities for each chapter:

- Multiple-choice quizzes
- Case study presentations and questions
- Labeling exercises
- Hangman game
- Championship ("Jeopardy-like") game
- Flash cards

In the **Student Workbook** (ISBN 1-4180-4282-X), additional exercises/questions are organized by major topic headings. This organization allows students to concentrate on specific topics, if necessary. Includes:

- Written exercise(s) and problems that parallel the content presented in the textbook
- Designed to enhance learning, understanding, retention, and clinical application of the content presented in the textbook
- Completed sections provide an excellent study resource quiz and test preparations

NEW RESOURCES FOR INSTRUCTORS

The **Instructor's Manual** (ISBN 1-4180-4279-X) is a testbank organized by chapter. Each chapter begins with a listing of the text objectives. Questions are then organized by major topic headings and numbered objectives. Instructors can devise tests to cover specific topics only or can use all questions for a comprehensive test. Answers to questions are given at the end of each chapter.

An **Electronic Classroom Manager** (ISBN 1-4180-4283-8) provides instructors with complete support in the classroom, including **Power-Point** presentations with animations, a **Computerized Test Bank**, and an **Image Library** of many of the illustrations from the text.

Web Tutor Advantage (ISBN 1-4180-4281-1 on Blackboard; ISBN 1-4180-4280-3 on WebCT) is a combination of course management tools and additional content for students and instructors. Each chapter includes quizzes, exams, interactive activities and animations, flash cards, and more. Instructors have access to PowerPoint presentations, the Computerized Test Bank, and tools including a course calendar, chat, e-mail, threaded discussions, Web links, and a white board.

Terry Des Jardins, MEd, RRT

ACKNOWLEDGMENTS

A number of people have provided important contributions to the development of the fifth edition of this textbook. First, I extend a very special thank-you to Wenda Speers for all the new and revised artwork she provided for this book. Especially striking is the new art Ms. Speers rendered for Chapter 7, Carbon Dioxide Transport and Acid-Base Balance, and Chapter 17, Sleep Physiology and Its Relationship to the Cardiopulmonary System. For all the new and revised anatomy, physiology, and pathology artwork generated for this book, an extended thank-you to Joe Chovan. The colored illustrations provided by these two talented individuals continue to enhance the visualization—and, importantly, the understanding—of the material presented throughout the textbook.

For his outstanding work in writing all of the activities for the student StudyWARE software package on CD-ROM, my gratitude goes out to Jim Sills, MEd, CPFT, RRT. I am also grateful to Dr. George Burton for his close attention and editing of the many drafts of Chapter 17, Sleep Physiology and Its Relationship to the Cardiopulmonary System. Dr. Burton's edits and suggestions were very helpful. For his close review of the revised and updated chemistry section in Chapter 7, my gratitude goes out to Ed O'Sullivan, MS, MEd.

For their extensive and comprehensive reviews and suggestions regarding the depth, breadth, and accuracy of the material presented in this textbook, I offer my most sincere thank-you to the following outstanding respiratory care educators:

Becki L. Evans, MS, RRT
Coordinator Allied Health Services
Tulsa Community College
Tulsa, Oklahoma

Diane Flatland, MS, RRT-NPS, CPFT
Division Chair, Allied Health
Program Director, Respiratory Care and Polysomnography
Alvin Community College
Alvin, Texas

Robert R. Fluck, Jr., MS, RRT
Associate Professor
Department of Respiratory Therapy Education
SUNY Upstate Medical University
Syracuse, New York

Tad M. Hunt, MS, RRT
Instructor
Southeast Community College
Lincoln, Nebraska

Joel S. Livesay, BA, RRT, RVT
Director of Clinical Education
Spartanburg Technical College
Spartanburg, South Carolina

Esther L. Seligman, BA, RRT
Clinical Coordinator/Faculty
Respiratory Care Program
School of Health
Springfield Technical Community College
Springfield, Massachusetts

Perry W. Sheppard, MEd, RRT-NPS, RPFT, RCP
Program Coordinator, Respiratory Therapy (Advanced Practitioner)
Forsyth Technical Community College
Winston-Salem, North Carolina

Thomas Smalling, MS, RRT, RPFT, RPSGT
Clinical Assistant Professor
Health, Technology and Management
Stony Brook University
Stony Brook, New York

Helen M. Sorenson, MA, RRT
Assistant Professor, Department of Respiratory Care
University of Texas Health Science Center at San Antonio
San Antonio, Texas

Robert D. Tarkowski, Jr., RRT, RPFT, NPS
Assistant Professor
Director of Clinical Education
Respiratory Care Program
Gannon University
Erie, Pennsylvania

David N. Yonutas, PhD
Coordinator, Educational Technologies
Santa Fe Community College
Gainesville, Florida

Finally, I am very grateful to Sarah Prime, Jim Zayicek, Lorretta Palagi, Susan Fitzgerald, and Gunjan Chandola. Their work and helpful coordination during the development of this textbook, and the supplemental student and instructor packages associated with this book, has been most appreciated.

Terry Des Jardins, MEd, RRT

HOW TO USE THE TEXT

Objectives at the beginning of each chapter lists in detail the theoretical and practical goals of the chapter.

By the end of this chapter, the student should be able to:

1. List the abbreviations and normal ranges of the following hemodynamic values *directly* measured by means of the pulmonary artery catheter:
   —Central venous pressure
   —Right atrial pressure
   —Mean pulmonary artery pressure
   —Pulmonary capillary wedge pressure
   —Cardiac output
2. List the abbreviations and normal ranges of the following *computed* hemodynamic values:
   —Stroke volume
   —Stroke volume index
   —Cardiac index
   —Right ventricular stroke work index
   —Left ventricular stroke work index

—Pulmonary vascular resistance
—Systematic vascular resistance
3. List factors that increase and decrease the following:
   —Stroke volume
   —Stroke volume index
   —Cardiac output
   —Cardiac index
   —Right ventricular stroke work index
   —Left ventricular stroke work index
4. List the factors that increase and decrease the *pulmonary vascular resistance.*
5. List the factors that increase and decrease the *systematic vascular resistance.*
6. Complete the review questions at the end of this chapter.

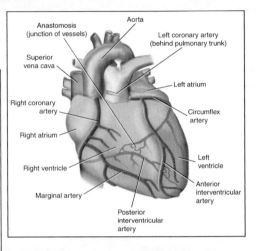

Over **65 new and revised figures** assist in understanding the various concepts and principles of anatomy, physiology, and pathophysiology.

A new chapter on **Sleep Physiology** and its relation to the cardiopulmonary system, including 10 user-friendly illustrations, has been provided to enhance the understanding of the material.

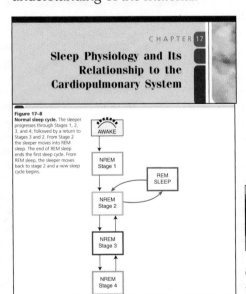

Figure 17–8
Normal sleep cycle. The sleeper progresses through Stages 1, 2, 3, and 4; followed by a return to Stages 3 and 2. From Stage 2 the sleeper moves into REM sleep. The end of REM sleep ends the first sleep cycle. From REM sleep, the sleeper moves back to stage 2 and a new sleep cycle begins.

1 CLINICAL APPLICATION CASE

A 34-year-old male construction worker fell from a second-story platform and was impaled by a steel enforcement rod that was protruding vertically about 3 feet from a cement structure. The steel rod entered the side of his lower right abdomen and exited from the left side of the abdomen, about 2 cm below the twelfth rib (see x-ray below). Although the steel rod pierced the side of the descending aorta, no other major organs were seriously damaged.

The man was still conscious when workers cut through the steel rod to free him from the cement structure. While he was being cut free, an emergency medical team (EMT) inserted an intravenous infusion line, placed a nonrebreathing mask over his face, and worked to stop the bleeding as

best they could. When the man was finally cut free, he was immediately transported to the trauma center. It was later estimated that he had lost about half of his blood volume at the accident site.

A full trauma team was assembled in the emergency department when the patient arrived. The patient was unconscious and very cyanotic. Even though he still had spontaneous breaths, he had an oral airway in place and was being manually ventilated with an inspired oxygen concentration ($F_{I_{O_2}}$) of 1.0. His blood pressure was 65/40 mm Hg and heart rate was 120 beats/min. The respiratory therapist intubated the patient and continued manual ventilation with an $F_{I_{O_2}}$ of 1.0.

Almost simultaneously a portable x-ray film was taken STAT to aid the trauma surgeons in the removal of the steel rod. A blood specimen was obtained for the following laboratory assays: glucose, BUN (blood urea nitrogen), creatinine, electrolytes, CBC (complete blood cell) count, and a type and screen and blood gas analysis. The emergency department physician called the laboratory to alert lab staff that 10 units of uncrossmatched

CLINICAL APPLICATION CASE
1
See page 331

An increased $\dot{V}/\dot{Q}$ ratio can develop from either (1) an increase in ventilation or (2) a decrease in perfusion. When the $\dot{V}/\dot{Q}$ ratio increases, the $P_{A_{O_2}}$ rises and the $P_{A_{CO_2}}$ falls. The $P_{A_{CO_2}}$ decreases because it is washed out of the alveoli faster than it is replaced by the venous blood. The $P_{A_{O_2}}$ increases because it does not diffuse into the blood* as fast as it enters (or is ventilated into) the alveolus (Figure 8–3). The $P_{A_{O_2}}$ also increases

Clinical Application Cases provide opportunities to use critical thinking skills to reflect on the material and relate the concepts to real-life situations. **Icons** signal the relation of specific text content to the clinical application case studies.

AND SOFTWARE

CHAPTER SUMMARY

REVIEW QUESTIONS

CLINICAL APPLICATION QUESTIONS

At the end of each chapter, reinforce your understanding of the concepts covered through the **Chapter Summary, Review Questions,** and **Clinical Application Questions.**

StudyWARE™

StudyWARE™ is interactive software with learning activities and quizzes to help you study key concepts and test your comprehension. The activities and quiz content correspond with each chapter of the book.

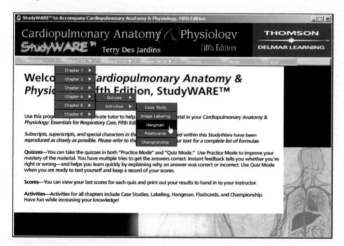

Each unit contains **Quizzes** that can be taken in practice mode, which provides immediate feedback after each question, or in quiz mode, which allows your score for each quiz to be stored or printed.

The activities include **Flash Cards, Hangman, Labeling Questions,** and **Championship Games.**

SECTION ONE

THE CARDIOPULMONARY SYSTEM—THE ESSENTIALS

CHAPTER 1

The Anatomy and Physiology of the Respiratory System

O B J E C T I V E S

By the end of this chapter, the student should be able to:

1. List the following three major components of the upper airway:
   —Nose
   —Oral cavity
   —Pharynx

2. List the primary functions of the upper airway:
   —Conductor of air
   —Humidify air
   —Prevent aspiration
   —Area for speech and smell

3. List the following three primary functions of the nose:
   —Filter
   —Humidify
   —Warm

4. Identify the following structures that form the outer portion of the nose:
   —Nasal bones
   —Frontal process of the maxilla
   —Lateral nasal cartilage
   —Greater alar cartilage
   —Lesser alar cartilages
   —Septal cartilage
   —Fibrous fatty tissue

5. Identify the following structures that form the internal portion of the nose:
   —Nasal septum
   • Perpendicular plate of the ethmoid

   • Vomer
   • Septal cartilage
   —Nasal bones
   —Frontal process of the maxilla
   —Cribriform plate of the ethmoid
   —Palatine process of the maxilla
   —Palatine bones
   —Soft palate
   —Nares
   —Vestibule
   —Vibrissae
   —Stratified squamous epithelium
   —Pseudostratified ciliated columnar epithelium
   —Turbinates (conchae)
   • Superior
   • Middle
   • Inferior
   —Paranasal sinuses
   • Maxillary
   • Frontal
   • Ethmoid
   • Sphenoid
   —Olfactory region
   —Choanae

6. Identify the following structures of the oral cavity:
   —Vestibule

(continues)

—Hard palate
- Palatine process of the maxilla
- Palatine bones

—Soft palate

—Uvula

—Levator veli palatinum muscle

—Palatopharyngeal muscles

—Stratified squamous epithelium

—Palatine arches
- Palatoglossal arch
- Palatopharyngeal arch

—Palatine tonsils

7. Identify the location and structure of the following:
—Nasopharynx
- Pseudostratified ciliated columnar epithelium
- Pharyngeal tonsils (adenoids)
- Eustachian tubes

—Oropharynx
- Lingual tonsil
- Stratified squamous epithelium
- Vallecula epiglottica

—Laryngopharynx
- Esophagus
- Epiglottis
- Aryepiglottic folds
- Stratified squamous epithelium

8. Identify the following cartilages of the larynx:
—Thyroid cartilage
—Cricoid cartilage
—Epiglottis
—Arytenoid cartilages
—Corniculate cartilages
—Cuneiform cartilages

9. Identify the structure and function of the following components of the interior portion of the larynx:
—False vocal folds
—True vocal folds
—Vocal ligament
—Glottis (rima glottidis)

—Epithelial lining above and below the vocal cords

10. Identify the structure and function of the following laryngeal muscles:
—Extrinsic muscles
- Infrahyoid group
  - Sternohyoid
  - Sternothyroid
  - Thyrohyoid
  - Omohyoid
- Suprahyoid group
  - Stylohyoid
  - Mylohyoid
  - Digastric
  - Geniohyoid
  - Stylopharyngeus

—Intrinsic muscles
- Posterior cricoarytenoid
- Lateral cricoarytenoid
- Transverse arytenoid
- Thyroarytenoid
- Cricothyroid

11. Describe the following ventilatory functions of the larynx:
—Primary function: Free flow of air
—Secondary function: Valsalva's maneuver

12. Describe the histology of the tracheobronchial tree, including the following components:
—Components of the epithelial lining (upper and lower airways)
- Pseudostratified ciliated columnar epithelium
- Basement membrane
- Basal cells
- Mucous blanket
  - Sol layer
  - Gel layer
- Goblet cells
- Bronchial glands (submucosal glands)
- Mucociliary transport mechanism

—Components of the lamina propria
- Blood vessels
- Lymphatic vessels
- Branches of the vagus nerve

(continues)

- Smooth-muscle fibers
- Peribronchial sheath
- Mast cells
  - Immunologic mechanism
—Cartilaginous layer

13. Identify the location (generation) and structure of the following *cartilaginous* airways:
—Trachea
—Carina
—Main stem bronchi
—Lobar bronchi
—Segmental bronchi
—Subsegmental bronchi

14. Identify the location (generation) and structure of the following *noncartilaginous* airways:
—Bronchioles
—Terminal bronchioles
  - Canals of Lambert
  - Clara cells

15. Describe how the cross-sectional area of the tracheobronchial tree changes from the trachea to the terminal bronchioles.

16. Describe the structure and function of the following components of the bronchial blood supply:
—Bronchial arteries
—Azygos veins
—Hemiazygos veins
—Intercostal veins

17. Describe the structure and function of the following sites of gas exchange:
—Respiratory bronchioles
—Alveolar ducts
—Alveolar sacs
—Primary lobule
  - Acinus
  - Terminal respiratory unit
  - Lung parenchyma
  - Functional units

18. Discuss the structure and function of the following components of the alveolar epithelium:

—Alveolar cell types
  - Type I cell (squamous pneumocyte)
  - Type II cell (granular pneumocyte)
—Pulmonary surfactant
—Pores of Kohn
—Alveolar macrophages (Type III alveolar cells)

19. Describe the structure and function of the interstitium, including the:
—Tight space
—Loose space

20. Describe the structure and function of the following components of the pulmonary vascular system:
—Arteries
  - Tunica intima
  - Tunica media
  - Tunica adventitia
—Arterioles (resistance vessels)
  - Endothelial layer
  - Elastic layer
  - Smooth-muscle fibers
—Capillaries
  - Single squamous epithelial layer
—Venules and veins (capacitance vessels)

21. Describe the structure and function of the following components of the lymphatic system:
—Lymphatic vessels
—Lymphatic nodes
—Juxta-alveolar lymphatic vessels

22. Describe how the following components of the autonomic nervous system relate to the neural control of the lungs:
—Sympathetic nervous system
  - Neural transmitters
  - Epinephrine
  - Norepinephrine
  - Receptors
    - Beta$_2$ receptors
    - Alpha receptors
—Parasympathetic nervous system
  - Neural transmitters
    - Acetylcholine

(continues)

23. Identify the effects the sympathetic and parasympathetic nervous systems have on the following:
    —Heart
    —Bronchial smooth muscle
    —Bronchial glands
    —Salivary glands
    —Stomach
    —Intestines
    —Eye
24. Identify the following structures of the lungs:
    —Apex
    —Base
    —Mediastinal border
    —Hilum
    —Specific right lung structures
      • Upper lobe
      • Middle lobe
      • Lower lobe
      • Oblique fissure
      • Horizontal fissure
    —Specific left lung structures
      • Upper lobe
      • Lower lobe
      • Oblique fissure
25. Identify the following lung segments from the anterior, posterior, lateral, and medial views:
    —Right lung segments
      • Upper lobe
        ○ Apical
        ○ Posterior
        ○ Anterior
      • Middle lobe
        ○ Lateral
        ○ Medial
      • Lower lobe
        ○ Superior
        ○ Medial basal
        ○ Anterior basal
        ○ Lateral basal
        ○ Posterior basal
    —Left lung segments
      • Upper lobe
        ○ Upper division

        1) Apical-posterior
        2) Anterior
        ○ Lower division (lingular)
        1) Superior lingula
        2) Inferior lingula
      • Lower lobe
        ○ Superior
        ○ Anterior medial basal
        ○ Lateral basal
        ○ Posterior basal
26. Identify the following components of the mediastinum:
    —Trachea
    —Heart
    —Major blood vessels
    —Nerves
    —Esophagus
    —Thymus gland
    —Lymph nodes
27. Identify the following components of the pleural membranes:
    —Parietal pleurae
    —Visceral pleurae
    —Pleural cavity
28. Identify the following components of the bony thorax:
    —Thoracic vertebrae
    —Sternum
      • Manubrium
      • Body
      • Xiphoid process
    —True ribs
    —False ribs
    —Floating ribs
29. Describe the structure and function of the diaphragm and include the following:
    —Hemidiaphragms
    —Central tendon
    —Phrenic nerves
    —Lower thoracic nerves
30. Describe the structure and function of the following accessory muscles of inspiration:
    —Scalene muscles
    —Sternocleidomastoid muscles

—Pectoralis major muscles
—Trapezius muscles
—External intercostal muscles
31. Describe the structure and function of the
following accessory muscles of expiration:
—Rectus abdominis muscles

—External abdominis obliquus muscles
—Internal abdominis obliquus muscles
—Transversus abdominis muscles
—Internal intercostal muscles
32. Complete the review questions at the end of
this chapter.

THE AIRWAYS

The passageways between the ambient environment and the gas exchange units of the lungs (the alveoli) are called the **conducting airways**. Although no gas exchange occurs in the conducting airways, they are, nevertheless, important to the overall process of ventilation. The conducting airways are divided into the **upper airway** and the **lower airways**.

THE UPPER AIRWAY

The upper airway consists of the **nose**, **oral cavity**, **pharynx**, and **larynx** (Figure 1–1). The primary functions of the upper airway are (1) to act as a conductor of air, (2) to humidify and warm the inspired air, (3) to prevent foreign materials from entering the tracheobronchial tree, and (4) to serve as an important area involved in speech and smell.

The Nose

The primary functions of the nose are to *filter, humidify*, and *warm* inspired air. The nose is also important as the site for the sense of smell and to generate resonance in phonation.

The outer portion of the nose is composed of bone and cartilage. The upper third of the nose (the bridge) is formed by the **nasal bones** and the **frontal process of the maxilla**. The lower two-thirds consist of the **lateral nasal cartilage**, the **greater alar cartilage**, the **lesser alar cartilages**, the **septal cartilage**, and some **fibrous fatty tissue** (Figure 1–2).

In the internal portion of the nose a partition, the **nasal septum**, separates the nasal cavity into two approximately equal chambers. Posteriorly, the nasal septum is formed by the **perpendicular plate of the ethmoid bone** and by the **vomer**. Anteriorly, the septum is formed by the **septal cartilage**. The roof of the nasal cavity is formed by the **nasal bones**, the **frontal process of the maxilla**, and the **cribriform plate of the ethmoid bone**. The floor is formed by the **palatine process of the**

Figure 1–1
Sagittal section of human head, showing the upper airway.

Figure 1–2
Structure of the nose.

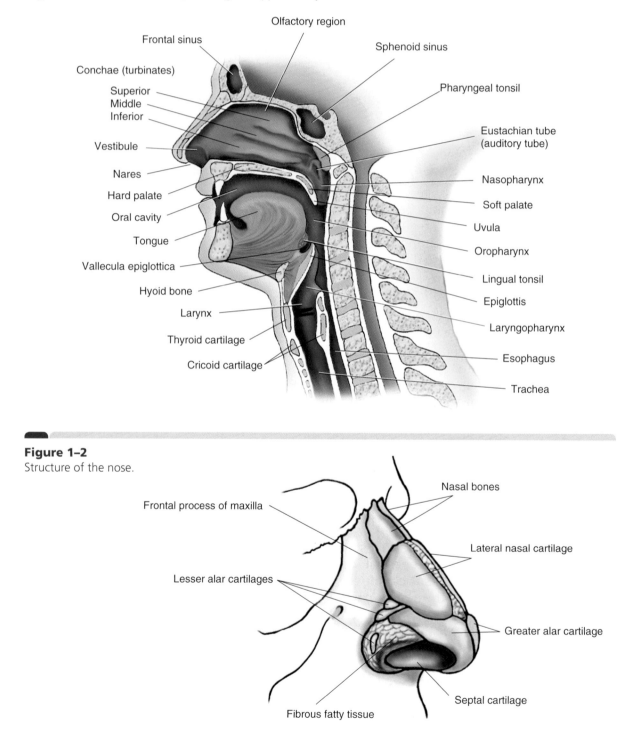

Figure 1–3
Sagittal section through the nose, showing the parts of the nasal septum.

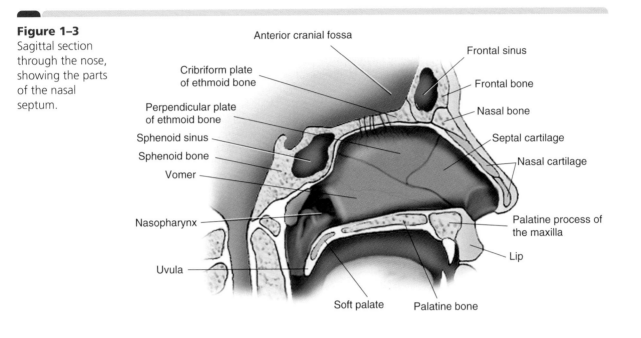

maxilla and by the **palatine bones**—the same bones that form the hard palate of the roof of the mouth. The posterior section of the nasal cavity floor is formed by the superior portion of the **soft palate** of the oral cavity, which consists of a flexible mass of densely packed collagen fibers (Figure 1–3).

Air enters the nasal cavity through the two openings formed by the septal cartilage and the alae nasi, called the **nares**, or **nostrils**. Initially, the air passes through a slightly dilated area called the **vestibule** (see Figure 1–1), which contains hair follicles called **vibrissae**. The vibrissae function as a filter and are the tracheobronchial tree's first line of defense. **Stratified squamous epithelium** (nonciliated) lines the anterior one-third of the nasal cavity (Figure 1–4A). The posterior two-thirds of the nasal cavity are lined with **pseudostratified ciliated columnar epithelium** (Figure 1–4B). The cilia propel mucus toward the nasopharynx.

There are three bony protrusions on the lateral walls of the nasal cavity called the **superior**, **middle**, and **inferior nasal turbinates**, or **conchae**. The turbinates separate inspired gas into several different airstreams. This action, in turn, increases the contact area between the inspired air and the warm, moist surface of the nasal mucosa. The turbinates play a major role in the humidification and warming of inspired air (see Figure 1–1).

Immediately below the superior and middle turbinates are the openings of the **paranasal sinuses**, which are air-filled cavities in the bones of the skull that communicate with the nasal cavity. The paranasal sinuses

Figure 1–4

A. Stratified squamous epithelium consists of several layers of cells. This tissue is found in the anterior portion of the nasal cavity, oral cavity, oropharynx, and laryngopharynx. **B. Pseudostratified columnar ciliated epithelium** appears stratified because the nuclei of the cells are located at different levels. These cells have microscopic hairlike projections called cilia that extend from the outer surface. Mucous-producing goblet cells are also found throughout this tissue. Pseudostratified columnar ciliated epithelium lines the posterior two-thirds of the nasal cavity and the tracheobronchial tree. **C. Simple cuboidal epithelium** consists of a single layer of cube-shaped cells. These cells are found in the bronchioles. **D. Simple squamous epithelium** consists of a single layer of thin, flattened cells with broad and thin nuclei. Substances such as oxygen and carbon dioxide readily pass through this type of tissue. These cells form the walls of the alveoli and the pulmonary capillaries that surround the alveoli.

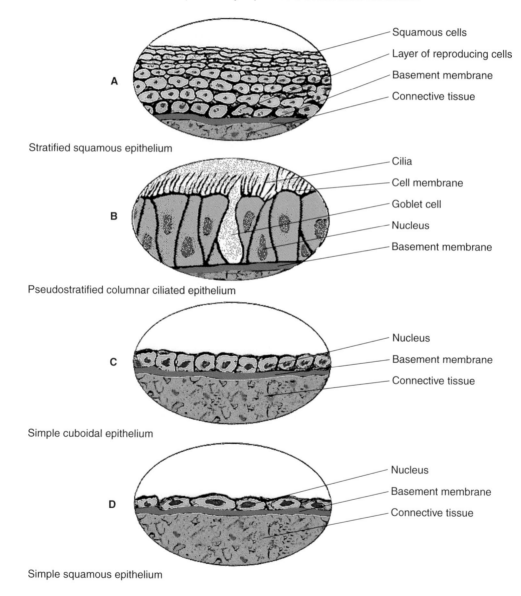

A — Squamous cells
— Layer of reproducing cells
— Basement membrane
— Connective tissue

Stratified squamous epithelium

B — Cilia
— Cell membrane
— Goblet cell
— Nucleus
— Basement membrane

Pseudostratified columnar ciliated epithelium

C — Nucleus
— Basement membrane
— Connective tissue

Simple cuboidal epithelium

D — Nucleus
— Basement membrane
— Connective tissue

Simple squamous epithelium

Figure 1–5
Lateral view of the head, showing sinuses.

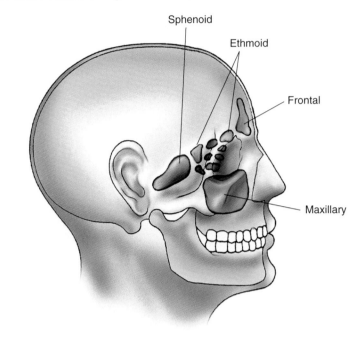

include the **maxillary**, **frontal**, **ethmoid**, and **sphenoid sinuses** (Figure 1–5). The paranasal sinuses produce mucus for the nasal cavity and act as resonating chambers for the production of sound. The receptors for the sense of smell are located in the **olfactory region**, which is near the superior and middle turbinates (see Figure 1–1). The two nasal passageways between the nares and the nasopharynx are also called the **choanae**.

Oral Cavity

The **oral cavity** is considered an accessory respiratory passage. It consists of the **vestibule**, which is the small outer portion between the teeth (and gums) and lips, and a larger section behind the teeth and gums that extends back to the oropharynx (Figure 1–6). The oral cavity houses the anterior two-thirds of the tongue. The posterior one-third of the tongue is attached to the hyoid bone and the mandible in the pharynx.

The roof of the mouth is formed by the **hard** and **soft palate**. The hard palate is composed of the **palatine process of the maxilla** and the **palatine bones** (see Figure 1–3). The soft palate consists of a flexible mass of densely packed collagen fiber that projects backward and downward, ending in the soft, fleshy structure called the **uvula** (see Figure 1–6). The soft palate closes off the opening between the nasal and oral pharynx by moving upward and backward during swallowing, sucking, and blowing

Figure 1–6
Oral cavity.

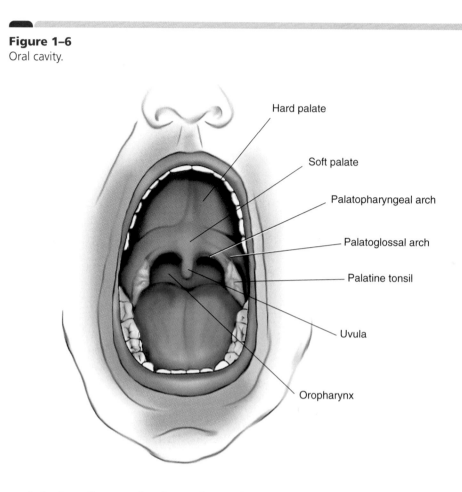

Hard palate

Soft palate

Palatopharyngeal arch

Palatoglossal arch

Palatine tonsil

Uvula

Oropharynx

and during the production of certain speech sounds. The **levator veli palatinum muscle** elevates the soft palate, and the **palatopharyngeal muscles** draw the soft palate forward and downward. The oral cavity is lined with nonciliated **stratified squamous epithelium** (see Figure 1–4A).

Two folds of mucous membrane pass along the lateral borders of the posterior portion of the oral cavity. These folds form the **palatoglossal arch** and the **palatopharyngeal arch**, named for the muscles they cover. Collectively, these arches are called the **palatine arches**. The **palatine tonsils** (faucial) are located between the palatine arches on each side of the oral cavity (see Figure 1–6). The palatine tonsils, like the pharyngeal tonsils or nasopharynx adenoids, are lymphoid tissues and are believed to serve certain immunologic defense functions.

The Pharynx

After the inspired air passes through the nasal cavity, it enters the **pharynx**. The pharynx is divided into three parts: nasopharynx, oropharynx, and laryngopharynx (see Figure 1–1).

Nasopharynx

The **nasopharynx** is located between the posterior portion of the nasal cavity (posterior nares) and the superior portion of the soft palate. The nasopharynx is lined with pseudostratified ciliated columnar epithelium (see Figure 1–4B). Lymphoid tissues called **pharyngeal tonsils**, or **adenoids**, are located on the surface of the posterior nasopharynx (see Figure 1–1). When the pharyngeal tonsils are inflamed and swollen, they may completely block the passage of air between the nose and throat. The openings of the **eustachian tubes** (auditory tubes) are located on the lateral surface of the nasopharynx. The eustachian tubes connect the nasopharynx to the middle ears and serve to equalize the pressure in the middle ear. Inflammation and excessive mucous production in the eustachian tubes may disrupt the pressure-equalizing process and impair hearing.

Oropharynx

The **oropharynx** lies between the soft palate superiorly and the base of the tongue inferiorly (at the level of the hyoid bone) (see Figure 1–1). Two masses of lymphoid tissue are located in the oropharynx: the **lingual tonsil**, located near the base of the tongue; and the **palatine tonsil**, located between the palatopharyngeal arch and the palatoglossal arch (see Figure 1–6). The mucosa of the oropharynx is composed of nonciliated stratified squamous epithelium (see Figure 1–4A). The **vallecula epiglottica** is located between the glossoepiglottic folds on each side of the posterior oropharynx. It appears as a depression or crevice that runs from the base of the tongue to the epiglottis (Figure 1–7). The vallecula epiglottica is an important anatomic landmark during the insertion of an endotracheal tube into the trachea (see next section for more information about endotracheal tubes).

Laryngopharynx

The **laryngopharynx** (also called hypopharynx) lies between the base of the tongue and the entrance of the **esophagus**. The laryngopharynx is lined with nonciliated stratified squamous epithelium (see Figure 1–4A). The **epiglottis**, the upper part of the larynx, is positioned directly anterior to the laryngopharynx (see Figure 1–1). The **aryepiglottic folds** are mucous membrane folds that extend around the margins of the larynx from the epiglottis. They function as a sphincter during swallowing. Clinically, the major structures associated with the laryngopharynx are often viewed from above using a laryngoscope while the patient is supine (see Figure 1–7).

The laryngopharyngeal musculature receives its sensory innervation from the ninth cranial (glossopharyngeal) nerve and its motor innervation from the tenth cranial (vagus) nerve. When stimulated, these muscles and nerves work together to produce the **pharyngeal reflex** (also called the "gag" or "swallowing" reflex), which helps to prevent the aspiration of

Figure 1–7
View of the base of the tongue, vallecula epiglottica epiglottis, and vocal cords.

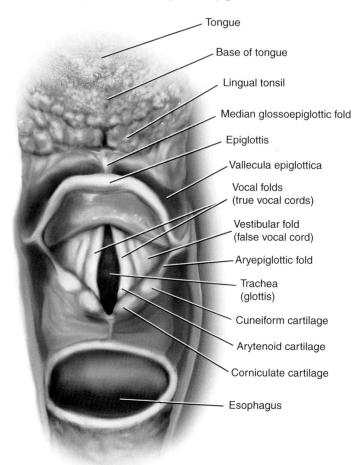

Tongue

Base of tongue

Lingual tonsil

Median glossoepiglottic fold

Epiglottis

Vallecula epiglottica

Vocal folds
(true vocal cords)

Vestibular fold
(false vocal cord)

Aryepiglottic fold

Trachea
(glottis)

Cuneiform cartilage

Arytenoid cartilage

Corniculate cartilage

Esophagus

foods and liquids. It also helps to prevent the base of the tongue from falling back and obstructing the laryngopharynx, even in the person who is asleep in the supine position.

In the clinical setting, the entire upper airway is often bypassed to better *ventilate* and *oxygenate* the patient. A nasal or oral **endotracheal tube** is used to by-pass the patient's upper airway (Figure 1–8). When an endotracheal tube is in place, the gas being delivered to the patient must be appropriately *warmed* and *humidified.* Failure to do so dehydrates the mucous layer of the tracheobronchial tree, which in turn causes the mucous layer to become thick and immobile. As shown in Figure 1–9, thick and immobile secretions lead to (1) excessive accumulation, (2) partial airway obstruction and air-trapping, or (3) complete airway obstruction and airway collapse.

Finally, it should be emphasized that the respiratory care practitioner must learn—and differentiate—the major anatomic landmarks of the

Figure 1–8

An oral endotracheal tube placed in proper position in the trachea. The inflated cuff at the tip of the tube separates the lower airways from the upper airway.

laryngopharynx and larynx (e.g., vallecula, epiglottis, esophagus, vocal folds, and trachea), especially when inserting an endotracheal tube. For example, an endotracheal tube can easily be inserted into the patient's esophagus rather than into the trachea, especially during an emergency situation. When this occurs, the patient's stomach is ventilated. A misplaced endotracheal tube in the esophagus can be fatal (Figure 1–10).

The Larynx

The **larynx**, or voice box, is located between the base of the tongue and the upper end of the trachea (see Figure 1–1). The larynx is commonly described as a vestibule opening into the trachea from the pharynx. The larynx serves three functions: (1) it acts as a passageway of air between the pharynx and the trachea, (2) it serves as a protective mechanism against the aspiration of solids and liquids, and (3) it generates sounds for speech.

Cartilages of the Larynx

The larynx consists of a framework of nine cartilages (Figure 1–11). Three are single cartilages: **thyroid cartilage**, **cricoid cartilage**, and the epiglottis. Three are paired cartilages: **arytenoid**, **corniculate**, and **cuneiform cartilages** (see Figure 1–11A, B). The cartilages of the larynx

Figure 1–9
Cystic fibrosis. Pathology includes (1) excessive production and accumulation of thick bronchial secretions, (2) partial bronchial obstruction and air trapping, and (3) alveolar hyperinflation.

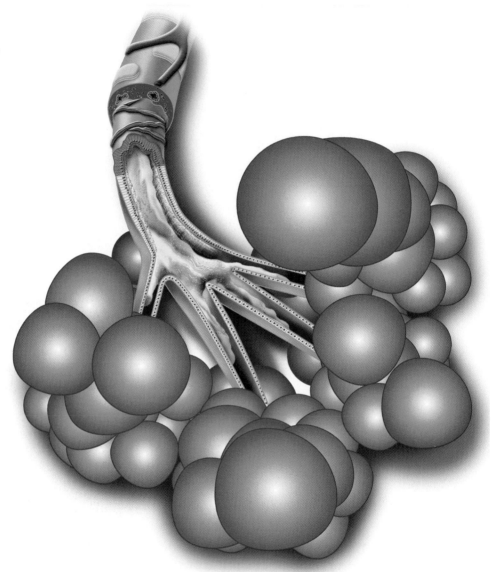

are held in position by ligaments, membranes, and **intrinsic** and **extrinsic muscles**. The interior of the larynx is lined with mucous membrane.

The thyroid cartilage (commonly called the Adam's apple) is the largest cartilage of the larynx. It is a double-winged structure that spreads over the anterior portion of the larynx. Along its superior border is a V-shaped notch, the **thyroid notch**. The upper portion of the thyroid cartilage is suspended from the horseshoe-shaped **hyoid bone** by the **thyrohyoid membrane**. Technically, the hyoid bone is not a part of the larynx.

Figure 1–10
A. An endotracheal tube misplaced in patient's esophagus. Note that the endotracheal tube is positioned to the right (patient's left) of the spinal column. Clinically, this is an excellent sign that the tube is in the esophagus. **B.** Stomach inflated with air.

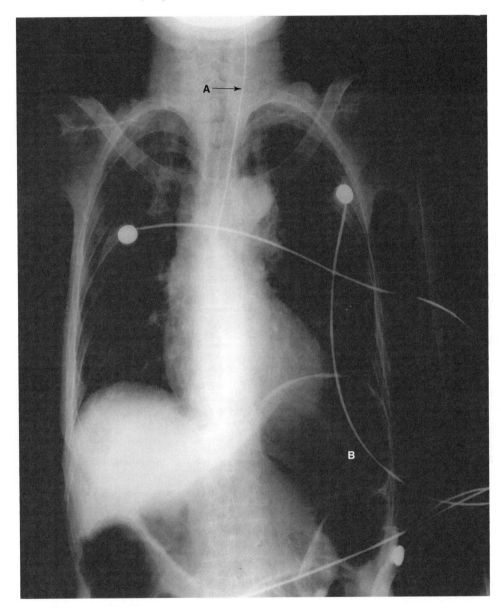

The epiglottis is a broad, spoon-shaped fibrocartilaginous structure. Normally, it prevents the aspiration of foods and liquids by covering the opening of the larynx during swallowing. The epiglottis and the base of the tongue are connected by folds of mucous membranes, which form a

Figure 1–11
Cartilages and intrinsic muscles of the larynx.

Epiglottis

Hyoid bone

Thyrohyoid membrane

Cuneiform cartilage

Corniculate cartilage

Thyroid cartilage

Arytenoid cartilage

Vocal process

Cricothyroid ligament

Vocal ligament

Cricoid cartilage

Trachea

Anterior view
A

LARYNGEAL CARTILAGES

Posterior view
B

Epiglottis

Aryepiglottic fold

Cuneiform tubercle
(cartilage)

Corniculate tubercle
(cartilage)

Aryepiglottic
muscle

Oblique
arytenoid muscle

Transverse
arytenoid muscle

Thyroarytenoid
muscle

Lateral
cricoarytenoid
muscle

Posterior
cricoarytenoid
muscle

Cricoid
cartilage

Cricothyroid muscle
(cut away)

Lateral view
C

Posterior view
D

INTRINSIC MUSCLES OF THE LARYNX

small space (the vallecula) between the epiglottis and the base of the tongue. Clinically, the vallecula serves as an important anatomic landmark when inserting an endotracheal tube (see Figure 1–7).

The cricoid cartilage is shaped like a signet ring. It is located inferior to the thyroid cartilage and forms a large portion of the posterior wall of the larynx. The inferior border of the cricoid cartilage is attached to the first C-shaped cartilage of the trachea (see Figure 1–11).

The paired arytenoid cartilages are shaped like a three-sided pyramid. The base of each arytenoid cartilage rests on the superior surface of the posterior portion of the cricoid cartilage. The apex of each arytenoid cartilage curves posteriorly and medially and flattens for articulation with the corniculate cartilages. At the base of each arytenoid cartilage is a projection called the **vocal process**. The **vocal ligaments**, which form the medial portion of the vocal folds, attach to the vocal process.

The paired cuneiform cartilages and corniculate cartilages are small accessory cartilages that are closely associated with the arytenoid cartilages. The cuneiform cartilages are embedded within the aryepiglottic folds that extend from the apices of the arytenoid cartilages to the epiglottis. They probably act to stiffen the folds. The two corniculate cartilages lie superior to the arytenoid cartilages.

Interior of the Larynx

The interior portion of the larynx is lined by a mucous membrane that forms two pairs of folds that protrude inward. The upper pair are called the **false vocal folds**, because they play no role in vocalization. The lower pair functions as the **true vocal folds** (vocal cords). The medial border of each vocal fold is composed of a strong band of elastic tissue called the **vocal ligament**. Anteriorly, the vocal cords attach to the posterior surface of the thyroid cartilage. Posteriorly, the vocal folds attach to the vocal process of the arytenoid cartilage. The arytenoid cartilages can rotate about a vertical axis through the cricoarytenoid joint, allowing the medial border to move anteriorly or posteriorly. This action, in turn, loosens or tightens the true vocal cords.

The space between the true vocal cords is termed the **rima glottidis** or, for ease of reference, the **glottis** (see Figure 1–7). In the adult, the glottis is the narrowest point in the larynx. In the infant, the cricoid cartilage is the narrowest point. Glottic and subglottic swelling (edema) secondary to viral or bacterial infection are commonly seen in infants and young children. This is known as the *croup syndrome* (laryngotracheobronchitis and acute epiglottitis) and is characterized by a high-pitched crowing sound (called **stridor**) during *inspiration* (Figure 1–12).

Above the vocal cords, the laryngeal mucosa is composed of (nonciliated) stratified squamous epithelium (see Figure 1–4A). Below the vocal cords, the laryngeal mucosa is covered by pseudostratified ciliated columnar epithelium (see Figure 1–4B).

Figure 1–12
Croup syndrome: **(A)** acute epiglottitis (swollen epiglottis); **(B)** laryngotracheobronchitis (swollen trachea tissue below the vocal cords).

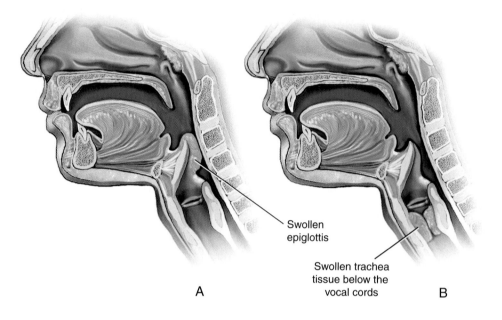

Swollen
epiglottis

Swollen trachea
tissue below the
vocal cords

A   B

Laryngeal Musculature

The muscles of the larynx consist of the **extrinsic** and **intrinsic** muscle groups. The extrinsic muscles are subdivided into an **infrahyoid** and a **suprahyoid** group. The infrahyoid group consists of the **sternohyoid, sternothyroid, thyrohyoid,** and **omohyoid muscles** (Figure 1–13). These muscles pull the larynx and hyoid bone down to a lower position in the neck. The suprahyoid group consists of the **stylohyoid, mylohyoid, digastric, geniohyoid,** and **stylopharyngeus muscles**. These muscles pull the hyoid bone forward, upward, and backward (see Figure 1–13). The major intrinsic muscles that control the movement of the vocal folds are illustrated in Figure 1–11C, D. The action(s) of these muscles are described below.

Posterior Cricoarytenoid Muscles. These muscles pull inferiorly on the lateral angles of the arytenoids, causing the vocal folds to move apart *(abduct)* and thus allowing air to pass through (Figure 1–14A).

Lateral Cricoarytenoid Muscles. The action of these muscles opposes that of the posterior cricoarytenoid muscles. These muscles pull

Figure 1–13
Extrinsic laryngeal muscles.

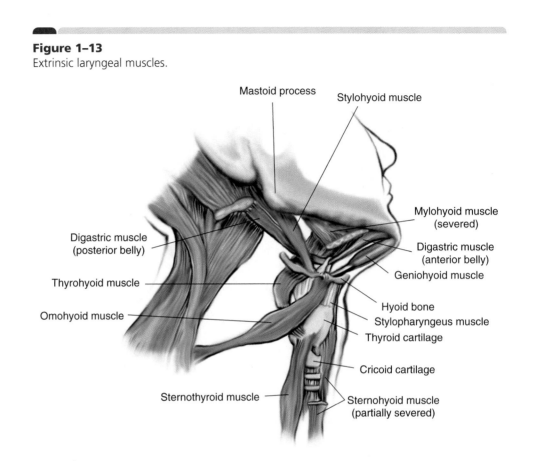

Mastoid process

Stylohyoid muscle

Mylohyoid muscle
(severed)

Digastric muscle
(posterior belly)

Digastric muscle
(anterior belly)

Geniohyoid muscle

Thyrohyoid muscle

Hyoid bone

Stylopharyngeus muscle

Omohyoid muscle

Thyroid cartilage

Cricoid cartilage

Sternothyroid muscle

Sternohyoid muscle
(partially severed)

laterally on the lateral angles of the arytenoids, causing the vocal folds to move together *(adduct)* (Figure 1–14B).

Transverse Arytenoid Muscles. These muscles pull the arytenoid cartilages together and thereby position the two vocal folds so that they vibrate as air passes between them during exhalation, thus generating the sounds for speech or singing (Figure 1–14C).

Thyroarytenoid Muscles. These muscles lie in the vocal folds lateral to the vocal ligaments. Contraction of the thyroarytenoid muscles pulls the arytenoid cartilages forward. This action loosens the vocal ligaments and allows a lower frequency of phonation (Figure 1–14D).

Cricothyroid Muscles. These muscles, which are located on the anterior surface of the larynx, can swing the entire thyroid cartilage anteriorly. This action provides an additional way to tense the vocal folds and thereby change the frequency of phonation (Figure 1–14E).

Figure 1–14
Intrinsic laryngeal muscles.

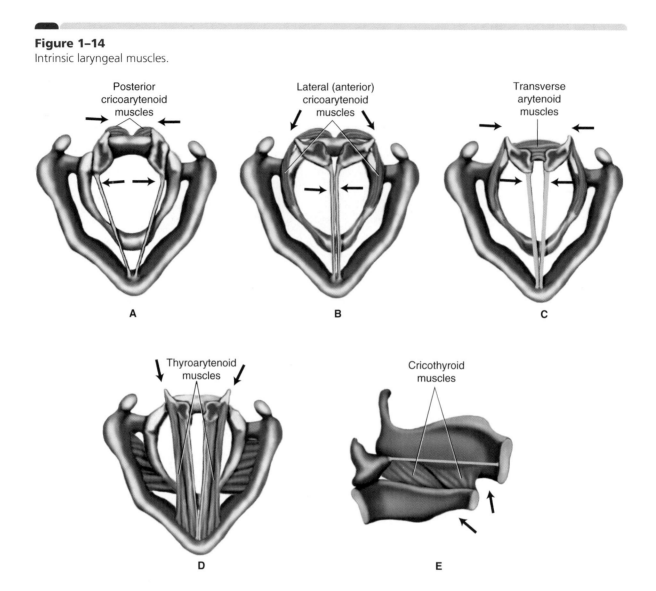

Ventilatory Function of the Larynx

A primary function of the larynx is to ensure a free flow of air to and from the lungs. During a quiet inspiration, the vocal folds move apart (abduct) and widen the glottis. During exhalation, the vocal folds move slightly toward the midline (adduct) but always maintain an open glottal airway.

A second vital function of the larynx is effort closure during exhalation, also known as **Valsalva's maneuver**. During this maneuver, there is a massive undifferentiated adduction of the laryngeal walls, including both the true and false vocal folds. As a result, the lumen of the larynx is tightly sealed, preventing air from escaping during physical work such as lifting, pushing, coughing, throat-clearing, vomiting, urination, defecation, and parturition.

THE LOWER AIRWAYS

The Tracheobronchial Tree

After passing through the larynx, inspired air enters the tracheobronchial tree, which consists of a series of branching airways commonly referred to as *generations,* or *orders.* These airways become progressively narrower, shorter, and more numerous as they branch throughout the lungs (Figure 1–15). Table 1–1 lists the major subdivisions of the tracheobronchial tree.

In general, the airways exist in two major forms: (1) **cartilaginous airways** and (2) **noncartilaginous airways**. (The main structures of these airways are discussed in detail on pages 36–39). The cartilaginous airways serve only to conduct air between the external environment and the sites of gas exchange. The noncartilaginous airways serve both as conductors of air and as sites of gas exchange. These will be discussed in detail below.

Figure 1–15
Tracheobronchial tree.

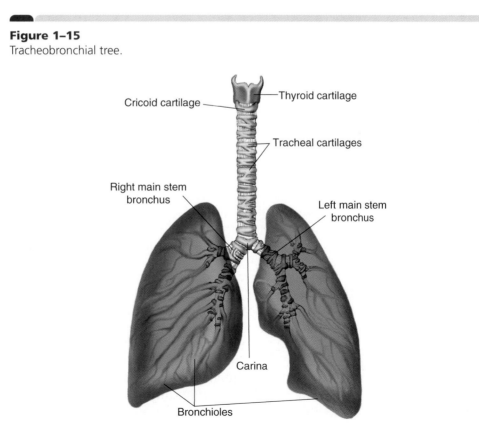

TABLE 1–1

Major Structures and Corresponding Generations of the Tracheobronchial Tree

	Structures of the Lungs	Generations*	
Conducting Zone	Trachea	0	Cartilaginous airways
	Main stem bronchi	1	
	Lobar bronchi	2	
	Segmental bronchi	3	
	Subsegmental bronchi	4–9	
	Bronchioles	10–15	Noncartilaginous airways
	Terminal bronchioles	16–19	
Respiratory Zone	Respiratory bronchioles[†]	20–23	Sites of gas exchange
	Alveolar ducts[†]	24–27	
	Alveolar sacs[†]	28	

* NOTE: The precise number of generations between the subsegmental bronchi and the alveolar sacs is not known.

[†] These structures collectively are referred to as a primary lobule (see pages 36–39) or lung parenchyma; they are also called terminal respiratory units and functional units.

Histology of the Tracheobronchial Tree

The tracheobronchial tree is composed of three layers: an epithelial lining, the lamina propria, and a cartilaginous layer (Figure 1–16).

The Epithelial Lining. The **epithelial lining** is predominantly composed of pseudostratified ciliated columnar epithelium interspersed with numerous mucous glands and separated from the lamina propria by a **basement membrane** (see Figure 1–16). Along the basement membrane of the epithelial lining are oval-shaped **basal cells**. These cells serve as a reserve supply of cells and replenish the superficial ciliated cells and mucous cells as needed.

The pseudostratified ciliated columnar epithelium extends from the trachea to the respiratory bronchioles. There are about 200 cilia per ciliated cell. The length of each cilium is about 5 to 7 μm (microns). As the bronchioles become progressively smaller, the columnar structure of the epithelium decreases in height and appears more cuboidal than columnar (see Figure 1–4C). The cilia progressively disappear in the terminal bronchioles and are completely absent in the respiratory bronchioles.

A mucous layer, commonly referred to as the **mucous blanket**, covers the epithelial lining of the tracheobronchial tree (Figure 1–17).

Figure 1–16
Histology of the tracheobronchial tree.

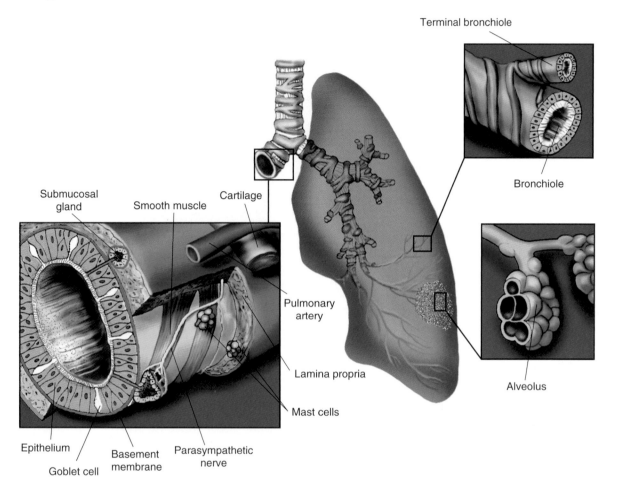

In general, the mucous blanket is composed of 95 percent water, with the remaining 5 percent consisting of glycoproteins, carbohydrates, lipids, DNA, some cellular debris, and foreign particles. The mucous is produced by (1) the **goblet cells**, and (2) the **submucosal**, or **bronchial**, **glands** (see Figure 1–16). The goblet cells are located intermittently between the pseudostratified ciliated columnar cells and have been identified down to, and including, the terminal bronchioles. The submucosal glands, which produce most of the mucous blanket, extend deep into the lamina propria. These glands are innervated by the vagal parasympathetic nerve fibers (the tenth cranial nerve) and produce about 100 mL of bronchial secretions per day. Increased sympathetic activity decreases glandular secretions. The submucosal glands are particularly numerous in the

Figure 1–17
Epithelial lining of the tracheobronchial tree.

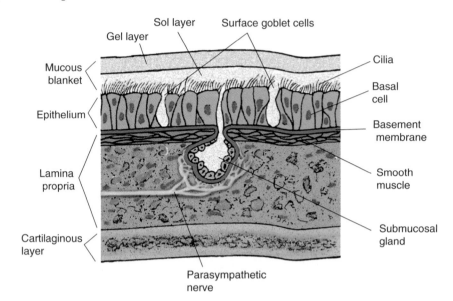

medium-sized bronchi and disappear in the distal terminal bronchioles (see Figure 1–17).

The viscosity of the mucous blanket progressively increases from the epithelial lining to the inner luminal surface. The blanket has two distinct layers: (1) the **sol layer**, which is adjacent to the epithelial lining, and (2) the **gel layer**, which is the more viscous layer adjacent to the inner luminal surface. Under normal circumstances, the cilia move in a wavelike fashion through the less viscous sol layer and continually strike the innermost portion of the gel layer (approximately 1500 times per minute). This action propels the mucous layer, along with any foreign particles stuck to the gel layer, toward the larynx at an estimated average rate of 2 cm per minute. Precisely what causes the cilia to move is unknown. At the larynx, the cough mechanism moves secretions beyond the larynx and into the oropharynx. This process is commonly referred to as the **mucociliary transport mechanism** or the **mucociliary escalator**, and is an important part of the cleansing mechanism of the tracheobronchial tree. Clinically, a number of factors are now known to slow the rate of the mucociliary transport. Some common factors are:

- Cigarette smoke
- Dehydration
- Positive-pressure ventilation
- Endotracheal suctioning
- High inspired oxygen concentrations

- Hypoxia
- Atmospheric pollutants (e.g., sulfur dioxide, nitrogen dioxide, ozone)
- General anesthetics
- Parasympatholytics (e.g., atropine).

The Lamina Propria. The **lamina propria** is the submucosal layer of the tracheobronchial tree. Within the lamina propria there is a loose, fibrous tissue that contains tiny blood vessels, lymphatic vessels, and branches of the vagus nerve. Also found within the lamina propria are two sets of smooth-muscle fibers. These sets of muscles wrap around the tracheobronchial tree in fairly close spirals, one clockwise and the other counterclockwise. The smooth-muscle fibers extend down to, and include, the alveolar ducts (see the section on sites of gas exchange in this chapter). The outer portion of the lamina propria is surrounded by a thin connective tissue layer called the **peribronchial sheath**.

Immune Response. **Mast cells** play an important role in the immunologic mechanism. Mast cells are found in the lamina propria—near the branches of the vagus nerve and blood vessels and scattered throughout the smooth-muscle bundles, in the intra-alveolar septa, and as one of the cell constituents of the submucosal glands (Figure 1–18). Outside of the lungs, mast cells are found in the loose connective tissue of the skin and intestinal submucosa.

Figure 1–18
Cross-section of a bronchus showing the mast cells in the lamina propria.

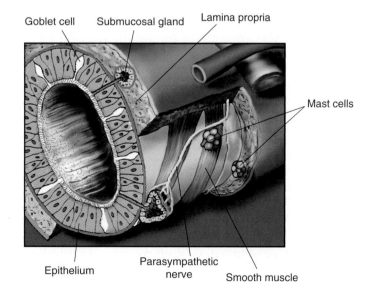

When they are activated, numerous substances are released from the mast cells that can significantly alter the diameter of the bronchial airways. Because of this fact, a basic understanding of how the mast cells function in the immunologic system is essential for the respiratory care practitioner.

There are two major immune responses: **cellular immunity** and **humoral immunity**. The *cellular immune response* involves the sensitized lymphocytes that are responsible for tissue rejection in transplants. This immune response is also termed a type IV, or delayed, type of hypersensitivity.

The *humoral immune response* involves the circulating antibodies that are involved in allergic responses such as allergic asthma. Antibodies (also called immunoglobulins) are serum globulins, or proteins, that defend against invading environmental antigens such as pollen, animal dander, and feathers. Although five different immunoglobulins (IgG, IgA, IgM, IgD, and IgE) have been identified, the IgE (reaginic) antibody is basic to the allergic response. The mechanism of the IgE antibody-antigen reaction is as follows:

1. When a susceptible individual is exposed to a certain antigen, the lymphoid tissues release specific IgE antibodies. The newly formed IgE antibodies travel through the bloodstream and attach to surface receptors on the mast cells. It is estimated that there are between 100,000 and 500,000 IgE receptor sites on the surface of each mast cell. Once the IgE antibodies attach to the mast cell, the individual (or more specifically, the mast cell) is said to be sensitive to the specific antigen (Figure 1–19A).

2. Each mast cell also has about 1000 secretory granules that contain several chemical mediators of inflammation. Continued exposure, or reexposure, to the same antigen creates an IgE antibody-antigen reaction on the surface of the mast cell, which works to destroy or inactivate the antigen. This response, however, causes the mast cell to degranulate (break down) and to release the following chemical mediators (Figure 1–19B):
   a. Histamine
   b. Heparin
   c. Slow-reacting substance of anaphylaxis (SRS-A)
   d. Platelet-activating factor (PAF)
   e. Eosinophilic chemotactic factor of anaphylaxis (ECF-A)
   f. Leukotrienes.

3. The release of these chemical mediators causes increased vascular permeability, smooth-muscle contraction, increased mucous secretion, and vasodilation with edema.

Such a reaction in the lungs can be extremely dangerous and is seen in individuals during an allergic asthmatic episode. The production of IgE antibodies may be 20 times greater than normal in some patients with

Figure 1–19
Immunologic mechanisms.

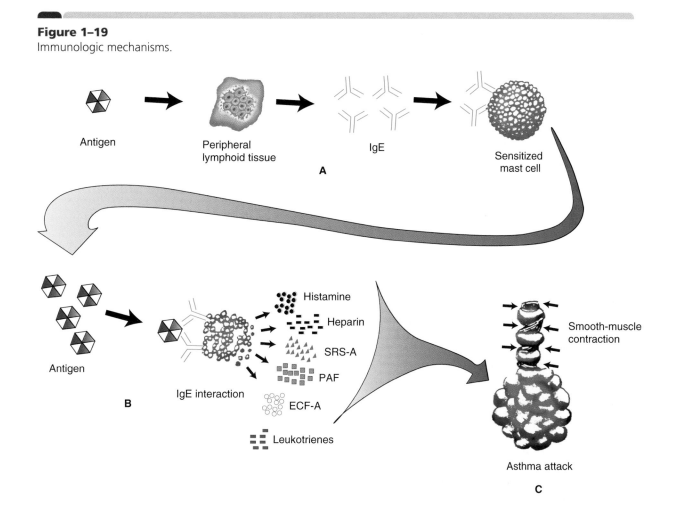

asthma (the normal IgE antibody level in the serum is about 200 ng/mL). During an asthmatic attack, the patient demonstrates bronchial edema, bronchospasms and wheezing, increased mucous production, mucous plugging, air trapping, and lung hyperinflation (Figure 1–19C).

The Cartilaginous Layer. The **cartilaginous layer**, which is the outermost layer of the tracheobronchial tree, progressively diminishes in size as the airways extend into the lungs. Cartilage is completely absent in bronchioles less than 1 mm in diameter (see Figure 1–16).

The Cartilaginous Airways

As shown in Table 1–1, the cartilaginous airways consist of the **trachea**, **main stem bronchi**, **lobar bronchi**, **segmental bronchi**, and **subsegmental bronchi**. Collectively, the cartilaginous airways are referred to as the *conducting zone*.

Trachea. The adult trachea is about 11 to 13 cm long and 1.5 to 2.5 cm in diameter (Figure 1–20). It extends vertically from the cricoid cartilage of the larynx to about the level of the second costal cartilage, or fifth thoracic vertebra. At this point, the trachea divides into the right and left main stem bronchi. The bifurcation of the trachea is known as the **carina**. Approximately 15 to 20 C-shaped cartilages support the trachea. These cartilages are incomplete posteriorly where the trachea and the esophagus share a fibroelastic membrane (Figure 1–21).

Figure 1–20
Tracheobronchial tree.

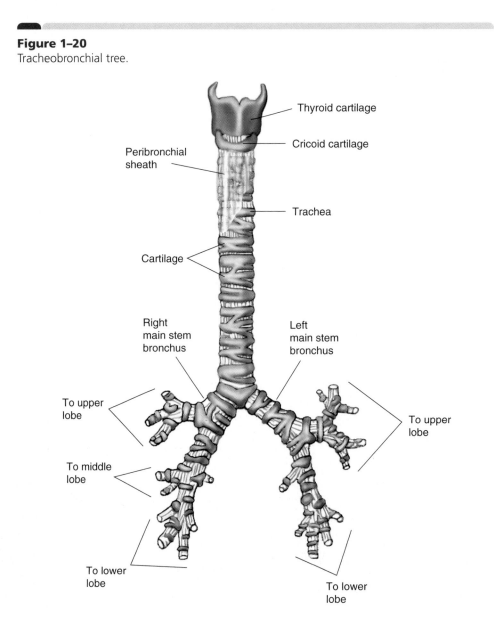

Thyroid cartilage

Cricoid cartilage

Peribronchial sheath

Trachea

Cartilage

Right main stem bronchus

Left main stem bronchus

To upper lobe

To upper lobe

To middle lobe

To lower lobe

To lower lobe

Figure 1–21
Cross-section of trachea.

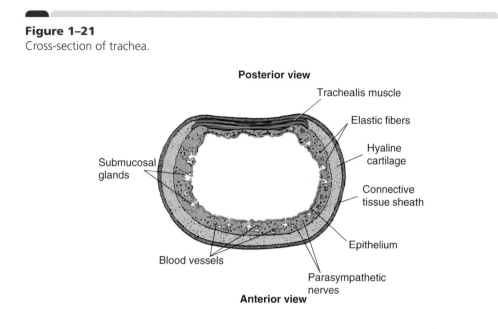

Clinically, the tip of the endotracheal tube should be about 2 cm above the carina. The correct position of the endotracheal tube is verified with a chest radiogram (i.e., the tip of the tube can be seen about 2 cm above the carina). When an endotracheal tube is inserted too deeply (beyond the carina), it most commonly enters the *right main stem bronchus*. When this occurs, the left lung receives little or no ventilation and alveolar collapse (atelectasis) ensues (Figure 1–22A). When this condition is identified (via chest radiogram or absence of breath sounds over the left lung), the endotracheal tube should be pulled back immediately (Figure 1–22B).

Main Stem Bronchi. The right main stem bronchus branches off the trachea at about a 25-degree angle; the left main stem bronchus forms an angle of 40 to 60 degrees with the trachea. The right main stem bronchus is wider, more vertical, and about 5 cm shorter than the left main stem bronchus. Similar to the trachea, the main stem bronchi are supported by C-shaped cartilages. In the newborn, both the right and left main stem bronchi form about a 55-degree angle with the trachea. The main stem bronchi are the tracheobronchial tree's first generation.

Lobar Bronchi. The right main stem bronchus divides into the upper, middle, and lower lobar bronchi. The left main stem bronchus branches into the upper and lower lobar bronchi. The lobar bronchi are the tracheobronchial tree's second generation. The C-shaped cartilages that support

Figure 1–22

Chest radiogram of 86-year-old open-heart patient. **A.** Shows the endotracheal tube tip in the right main stem bronchus (see arrow). Because of the preferential ventilation to the right lung, atelectasis and volume loss are present in the patient's left lung (your right) (i.e., white fluffy areas in left lung). **B.** The same patient 20 minutes after the endotracheal tube was pulled back above the carina (see arrow). Note that the patient's left lung is better ventilated (i.e., more darker areas in the left lung).

A

B

the trachea and the main stem bronchi progressively form cartilaginous plates around the lobar bronchi.

Segmental Bronchi. A third generation of bronchi branch off the lobar bronchi to form the segmental bronchi. There are 10 segmental bronchi in the right lung and 8 in the left lung. Each segmental bronchus is named according to its location within a particular lung lobe.

Subsegmental Bronchi. The tracheobronchial tree continues to subdivide between the fourth and approximately the ninth generation into progressively smaller airways called subsegmental bronchi. These bronchi range in diameter from 1 to 4 mm. Peribronchial connective tissue containing nerves, lymphatics, and bronchial arteries surrounds the subsegmental bronchi to about the 1-mm diameter level. Beyond this point, the connective tissue sheaths disappear.

The Noncartilaginous Airways

The noncartilaginous airways are composed of the bronchioles and the terminal bronchioles.

Bronchioles. When the bronchi decrease to less than 1 mm in diameter and are no longer surrounded by connective tissue sheaths, they are called **bronchioles**. The bronchioles are found between the tenth and fifteenth generations. At this level, cartilage is absent and the lamina propria is directly connected with the lung parenchyma (see lung parenchyma in the section on sites of gas exchange in this chapter). The bronchioles are surrounded by spiral muscle fibers and the epithelial cells are more cuboidal in shape (see Figure 1–16). The rigidity of the bronchioles is very low compared with the cartilaginous airways. Because of this, the airway patency at this level may be substantially affected by intra-alveolar and intrapleural pressures and by alterations in the size of the lungs. This lack of airway support often plays a major role in respiratory disease.

Terminal Bronchioles. The conducting tubes of the tracheobronchial tree end with the **terminal bronchioles** between the sixteenth and nineteenth generations. The average diameter of the terminal bronchioles is about 0.5 mm. At this point, the cilia and the mucous glands progressively disappear, and the epithelium flattens and becomes cuboidal in shape (see Figures 1–4C and 1–16).

As the wall of the terminal bronchioles progressively becomes thinner, small channels, called the **canals of Lambert**, begin to appear between the inner luminal surface of the terminal bronchioles and the adjacent alveoli that surround them (Figure 1–23). Although specific information as to their function is lacking, it is believed that these tiny pathways may be important secondary avenues for collateral ventilation in patients with certain respiratory disorders (e.g., chronic obstructive pulmonary disease [COPD]).

Also unique to the terminal bronchioles is the presence of **Clara cells**. These cells have thick protoplasmic extensions that bulge into the lumen of the terminal bronchioles. The precise function of the Clara cells is not known. They may have secretory functions that contribute to the extracellular liquid lining the bronchioles and alveoli. They may also contain enzymes that work to detoxify inhaled toxic substances.

The structures beyond the terminal bronchioles are the sites of gas exchange and, although directly connected to it, are not considered part of the tracheobronchial tree.

Bronchial Cross-Sectional Area

The total cross-sectional area of the tracheobronchial tree steadily increases from the trachea to the terminal bronchioles. The total cross-sectional area increases significantly beyond the terminal bronchioles

Figure 1–23
Canals of Lambert.

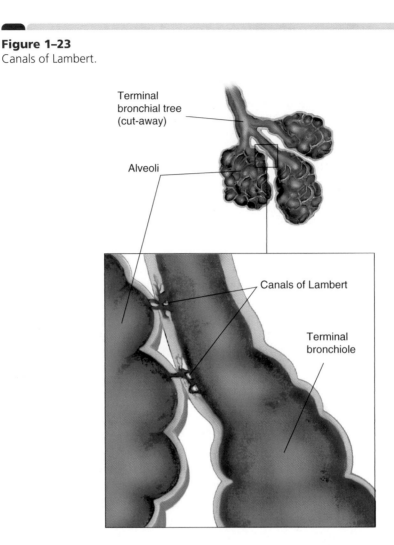

because of the many branches that occur at this level. The structures distal to the terminal bronchioles are collectively referred to as the **respiratory zone** (Figure 1–24).

Air flows down the tracheobronchial tree as a mass to about the level of the terminal bronchioles, like water flowing through a tube. Because the cross-sectional area becomes so great beyond this point, however, the forward motion essentially stops and the molecular movement of gas becomes the dominant mechanism of ventilation.

Bronchial Blood Supply

The **bronchial arteries** nourish the tracheobronchial tree. The arteries arise from the aorta and follow the tracheobronchial tree as far as the terminal bronchioles. Beyond the terminal bronchioles, the bronchial

Figure 1–24

Cross-section of bronchial area. Note the rapid increase in the total cross-sectional area of the airways in the respiratory zone.

arteries lose their identity and merge with the pulmonary arteries and capillaries, which are part of the pulmonary vascular system. The normal bronchial arterial blood flow is about 1 percent of the cardiac output. In addition to the tracheobronchial tree, the bronchial arteries nourish the mediastinal lymph nodes, the pulmonary nerves, a portion of the esophagus, and the visceral pleura.

About one-third of the bronchial venous blood returns to the right atrium by way of the **azygos**, **hemiazygos**, and **intercostal veins**. Most of this blood comes from the first two or three generations of the tracheobronchial tree. The remaining two-thirds of the bronchial venous blood drains into the pulmonary circulation, via **bronchopulmonary anastomoses**, and then flows to the left atrium by way of the pulmonary veins. In effect, the bronchial venous blood, which is low in oxygen and high in carbon dioxide, mixes with blood that has just passed through the alveolar-capillary system, which is high in oxygen and low in carbon dioxide. The mixing of venous blood and freshly oxygenated blood is known as **venous admixture**. (The effects of venous admixture are discussed in greater detail in Chapter 7.)

THE SITES OF GAS EXCHANGE

The structures distal to the terminal bronchioles are the functional units of gas exchange. They are composed of about three generations of **respiratory bronchioles**, followed by about three generations of **alveolar ducts** and, finally, ending in 15 to 20 grapelike clusters, the **alveolar sacs** (Figure 1–25). The respiratory bronchioles are characterized by alveoli budding from their walls. The walls of the alveolar ducts that arise from the respiratory bronchioles are completely composed of alveoli separated by septal walls that contain smooth-muscle fibers. Most gas exchange takes place at the alveolar-capillary membrane (Figure 1–26). In the lungs of the adult male, there are approximately 300 million alveoli between 75 and 300 μm in diameter, and small pulmonary capillaries cover about

Figure 1–25

Schematic drawing of the structures distal to the terminal bronchioles; collectively, these are referred to as the primary lobule.

Figure 1–26
Alveolar-capillary network.

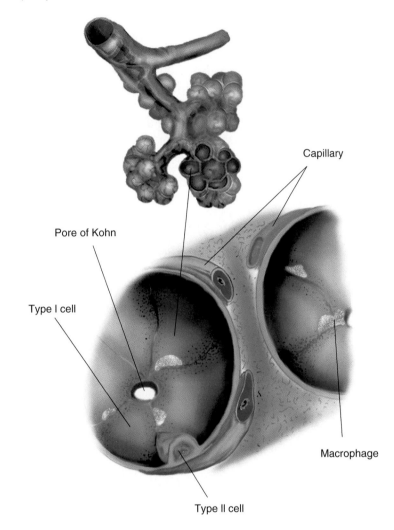

Capillary

Pore of Kohn

Type I cell

Macrophage

Type II cell

85 to 95 percent of the alveoli. This arrangement provides an average surface area of 70 square meters (about the size of a tennis court) available for gas exchange.

Collectively, the respiratory bronchioles, alveolar ducts, and alveolar clusters that originate from a single terminal bronchiole are referred to as a **primary lobule**. Each primary lobule is about 3.5 mm in diameter and contains about 2000 alveoli. It is estimated that there are approximately 130,000 primary lobules in the lung. Synonyms for primary lobule include **acinus**, **terminal respiratory unit**, **lung parenchyma**, and **functional units** (see Table 1–1).

Alveolar Epithelium

The alveolar epithelium is composed of two principal cell types: the **type I cell**, or **squamous pneumocyte**, and the **type II cell**, or **granular pneumocyte**.

Type I cells are primarily composed of a cytoplasmic ground substance. They are broad, thin cells that form about 95 percent of the alveolar surface. They are 0.1 to 0.5 μm thick and are the major sites of alveolar gas exchange.

Type II cells form the remaining 5 percent of the total alveolar surface. They have microvilli and are cuboidal in shape. They are believed to be the primary source of **pulmonary surfactant**. Surfactant molecules are situated at the air–liquid interface of the alveoli and play a major role in decreasing the surface tension of the fluid that lines the alveoli (see Figure 1–26).

Pores of Kohn

The **pores of Kohn** are small holes in the walls of the interalveolar septa (see Figure 1–26). They are 3 to 13 μm in diameter and permit gas to move between adjacent alveoli. The formation of the pores may include one or more of the following processes: (1) the desquamation (i.e., shedding or peeling) of epithelial cells due to disease, (2) the normal degeneration of tissue cells as a result of age, and (3) the movement of macrophages, which may leave holes in the alveolar walls. The formation of alveolar pores is accelerated by diseases involving the lung parenchyma, and the number and size of the pores increase progressively with age.

Alveolar Macrophages

Alveolar macrophages, or type III alveolar cells, play a major role in removing bacteria and other foreign particles that are deposited within the acini. Macrophages are believed to originate from stem cell precursors in the bone marrow. Then, as monocytes, they presumably migrate through the bloodstream to the lungs, where they move about or are embedded in the extracellular lining of the alveolar surface. There is also evidence that the alveolar macrophages reproduce within the lung (see Figure 1–26).

Interstitium

The alveolar-capillary clusters are surrounded, supported, and shaped by the **interstitium** (Figure 1–27). The interstitium is a gel-like substance composed of hyaluronic acid molecules that are held together by a web-like network of collagen fibers. The interstitium has two major compartments: the **tight space** and the **loose space**. The tight space is the area between the alveolar epithelium and the endothelium of the pulmonary capillaries—the area where most gas exchange occurs. The loose space is

Figure 1–27
Interstitium. Most gas exchange occurs in the tight space area. The area around the bronchioles, alveolar ducts, and alveolar sacs is called the loose space.

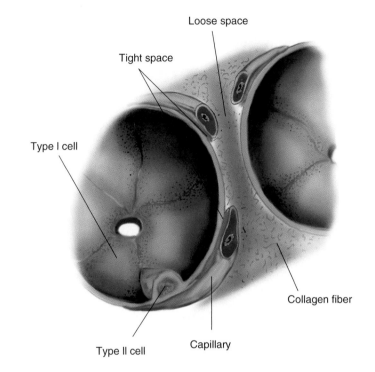

primarily the area that surrounds the bronchioles, respiratory bronchioles, alveolar ducts, and alveolar sacs. Lymphatic vessels and neural fibers are found in this area. Water content in this area can increase more than 30 percent before a significant pressure change develops.

The collagen in the interstitium is believed to limit alveolar distensibility. Expansion of a lung unit beyond the limits of the interstitial collagen can (1) occlude the pulmonary capillaries or (2) damage the structural framework of the collagen fibers and, subsequently, the wall of the alveoli.

THE PULMONARY VASCULAR SYSTEM*

The pulmonary vascular system delivers blood to and from the lungs for gas exchange. In addition to gas exchange, the pulmonary vascular system provides nutritional substances to the structures distal to the terminal bronchioles. Similar to the systemic vascular system, the pulmonary

See Chapter 5 for a more comprehensive presentation of the pulmonary vascular system.

vascular system is composed of arteries, arterioles, capillaries, venules, and veins.

Arteries

The right ventricle of the heart pumps deoxygenated blood into the **pulmonary artery**. Just beneath the aorta the pulmonary artery divides into the right and left branches (Figure 1–28). The branches then penetrate their respective lung through the hilum, which is that part of the lung where the main stem bronchi, vessels, and nerves enter. In general, the pulmonary artery follows the tracheobronchial tree in a posterolateral relationship branching or dividing as the tracheobronchial tree does.

Figure 1–28
Major pulmonary vessels.

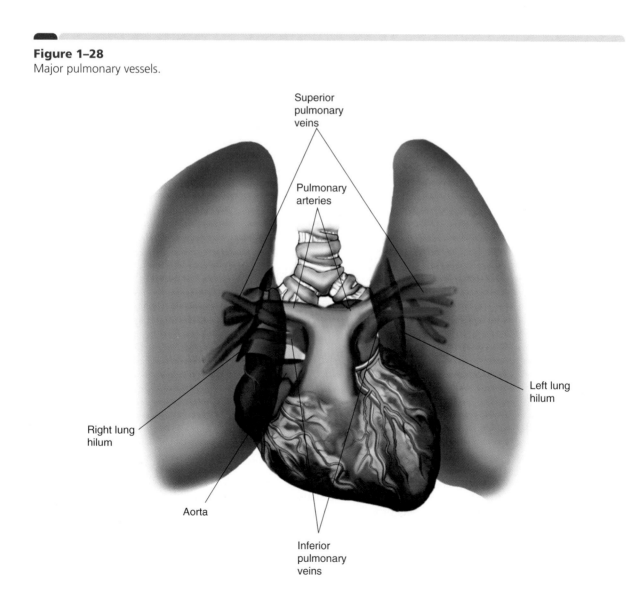

Superior
pulmonary
veins

Pulmonary
arteries

Left lung
hilum

Right lung
hilum

Aorta

Inferior
pulmonary
veins

Figure 1–29
Schematic drawing of the components of the pulmonary blood vessels.

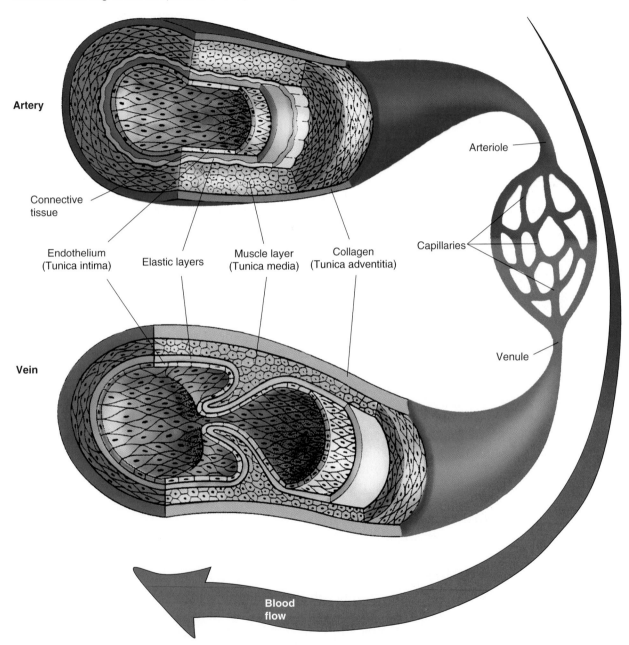

The pulmonary **arteries** have three layers of tissue in their walls (Figure 1–29). The inner layer is called the **tunica intima** and is composed of endothelium and a thin layer of connective and elastic tissue. The middle layer is called the **tunica media** and consists primarily of elastic connective tissue in large arteries and smooth muscle in medium-sized to small arteries. The tunica media is the thickest layer in the arteries. The outermost layer is called the **tunica adventitia** and is composed of connective tissue. This layer also contains small vessels that nourish all three layers. Because of the different layers, the arteries are relatively stiff vessels that are well suited for carrying blood under high pressures in the systemic system.

Arterioles

The walls of the pulmonary **arterioles** consist of an endothelial layer, an elastic layer, and a layer of smooth-muscle fibers (see Figure 1–29). The elastic and smooth-muscle fibers gradually disappear just before entering the alveolar-capillary system. The pulmonary arterioles supply nutrients to the respiratory bronchioles, alveolar ducts, and alveoli. By virtue of their smooth-muscle fibers, the arterioles play an important role in the distribution and regulation of blood and are called the **resistance vessels**.

Capillaries

The pulmonary arterioles give rise to a complex network of capillaries that surround the alveoli. The **capillaries** are composed of an endothelial layer (a single layer of squamous epithelial cells) (see Figure 1–29). The capillaries are essentially an extension of the inner lining of the larger vessels. The walls of the pulmonary capillaries are less than 0.1 μm thick and the external diameter of each vessel is about 10 μm. The capillaries are where gas exchange occurs. The pulmonary capillary endothelium also has a selective permeability to substances such as water, electrolytes, and sugars.

In addition to gas and fluid exchange, the pulmonary capillaries play an important biochemical role in the production and destruction of a broad range of biologically active substances. For example, serotonin, norepinephrine, and some prostaglandins are destroyed by the pulmonary capillaries. Some prostaglandins are produced and synthesized by the pulmonary capillaries, and some circulating inactive peptides are converted to their active form; for example, the inactive angiotensin I is converted to the active angiotensin II.

Venules and Veins

After blood moves through the pulmonary capillaries, it enters the pulmonary venules, which are actually tiny veins continuous with the capillaries. The **venules** empty into the **veins**, which carry blood back to the heart. Similar to the arteries, the veins usually have three layers of tissue in their walls (see Figure 1–29).

The veins differ from the arteries, however, in that the middle layer is poorly developed. As a result, the veins have thinner walls and contain less smooth muscle and less elastic tissue than the arteries. There are only two layers in the smaller veins, lacking a layer comparable to the tunica adventitia. In the systemic circulation, many medium- and large-sized veins (particularly those in the legs) contain one-way, flaplike valves that aid blood flow back to the heart. The valves open as long as the flow is toward the heart but close if flow moves away from the heart.

The veins also differ from the arteries in that they are capable of collecting a large amount of blood with very little pressure change. Because of this unique feature, the veins are called **capacitance vessels**. Unlike the pulmonary arteries, which generally parallel the airways, the veins move away from the bronchi and take a more direct route out of the lungs. Ultimately, the veins in each lung merge into two large veins and exit through the lung hilum. The four pulmonary veins then empty into the left atrium of the heart (see Figure 1–28).

THE LYMPHATIC SYSTEM

Lymphatic vessels are found superficially around the lungs just beneath the visceral pleura and in the dense connective tissue wrapping of the bronchioles, bronchi, pulmonary arteries, and pulmonary veins. The primary function of the lymphatic vessels is to remove excess fluid and protein molecules that leak out of the pulmonary capillaries.

Deep within the lungs, the lymphatic vessels arise from the loose space of the interstitium. The vessels follow the bronchial airways, pulmonary arteries, and veins to the hilum of the lung (Figure 1–30). Single-leaf, funnel-shaped valves are found in the lymphatic channels. These one-way valves direct fluid toward the hilum. The larger lymphatic channels are surrounded by smooth-muscle bands that actively produce peristaltic movements regulated by the autonomic nervous system. Both the smooth-muscle activity and the normal, cyclic pressure changes generated in the thoracic cavity move lymphatic fluid toward the hilum. The vessels end in the pulmonary and bronchopulmonary **lymph nodes** located just inside and outside the lung parenchyma (Figure 1–31).

The lymph nodes are organized collections of lymphatic tissue interspersed along the course of the lymphatic stream. Lymph nodes produce lymphocytes and monocytes. The nodes act as filters, keeping particulate matter and bacteria from entering the bloodstream.

There are no lymphatic vessels in the walls of the alveoli. Some alveoli, however, are strategically located immediately adjacent to peribronchovascular lymphatic vessels. These vessels are called **juxta-alveolar lymphatics** and are thought to play an active role in the removal of excess fluid and other foreign material that gain entrance into the interstitial space of the lung parenchyma.

There are more lymphatic vessels on the surface of the lower lung lobes than on that of the upper or middle lobes. The lymphatic channels on the left lower lobe are more numerous and larger in diameter than the lymphatic

Figure 1–30
Lymphatic vessels of the bronchial airways, pulmonary arteries, and veins.

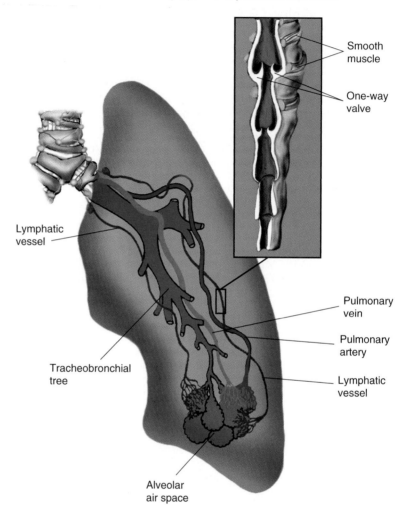

vessels on the surface of the right lower lobe (Figure 1–32). This anatomic difference provides a possible explanation why patients with **bilateral effusion** (i.e., the escape of fluid from the blood vessels from both lungs) commonly have more fluid in the lower right lung than in the lower left.

NEURAL CONTROL OF THE LUNGS

The balance, or tone, of the bronchial and arteriolar smooth muscle of the lungs is controlled by the **autonomic nervous system**. The autonomic nervous system is the part of the nervous system that regulates involuntary vital functions, including the activity of cardiac muscle, smooth muscle, and

Figure 1–31
Lymph nodes associated with the trachea and the right and left main stem bronchi.

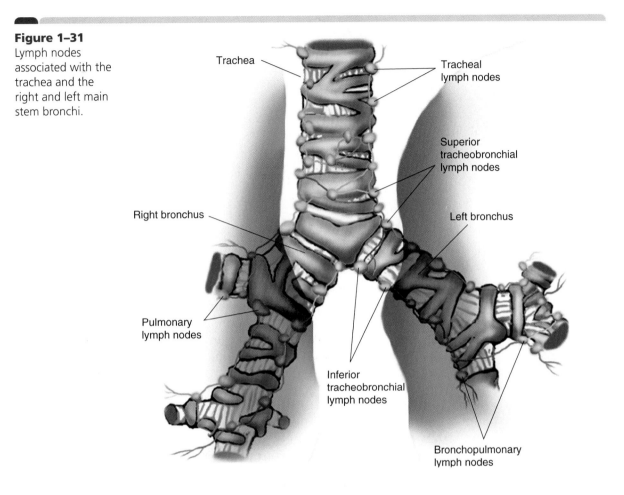

Trachea

Tracheal lymph nodes

Superior tracheobronchial lymph nodes

Right bronchus

Left bronchus

Pulmonary lymph nodes

Inferior tracheobronchial lymph nodes

Bronchopulmonary lymph nodes

Figure 1–32
Lymphatic vessels of the visceral pleura of the lungs.

Superficial lymphatic vessels

TABLE 1–2
Some Effects of Autonomic Nervous System Activity

Effector Site	Sympathetic Nervous System	Parasympathetic Nervous System
Heart	Increases rate	Decreases rate
	Increases strength of contraction	Decreases strength of contraction
Bronchial smooth muscle	Relaxation	Constriction
Bronchial glands	Decreases secretions	Increases secretions
Salivary glands	Decreases secretions	Increases secretions
Stomach	Decreases motility	Increases motility
Intestines	Decreases motility	Increases motility
Eyes	Widens pupils	Constricts pupils

glands. It has two divisions: (1) the **sympathetic nervous system**, which accelerates the heart rate, constricts blood vessels, relaxes bronchial smooth muscles, and raises blood pressure; and (2) the **parasympathetic nervous system**, which slows the heart rate, constricts bronchial smooth muscles, and increases intestinal peristalsis and gland activity. Table 1–2 lists some effects of the two divisions of the autonomic nervous system.

When the sympathetic nervous system is activated, neural transmitters, such as **epinephrine** and **norepinephrine**, are released. These agents stimulate (1) the **beta$_2$ receptors** in the bronchial smooth muscles, causing relaxation of the airway musculature, and (2) the **alpha receptors** of the smooth muscles of the arterioles, causing the pulmonary vascular system to constrict. When the parasympathetic nervous system is activated, the neutral transmitter **acetylcholine** is released, causing constriction of the bronchial smooth muscle.

Inactivity of either the sympathetic or the parasympathetic nervous system allows the action of the other to dominate the bronchial smooth-muscle response. For example, if a beta$_2$-blocking agent such as **propranolol** is administered to a patient, the parasympathetic nervous system becomes dominant and bronchial constriction ensues. In contrast, if a patient receives a parasympathetic blocking agent such as **atropine**, the sympathetic nervous system becomes dominant and bronchial relaxation occurs.

THE LUNGS

The apex of each lung is somewhat pointed and the base is broad and concave to accommodate the convex diaphragm (Figures 1–33 and 1–34). As shown in Figure 1–35, the apices of the lungs rise to about the level of the first rib. The base extends anteriorly to about the level of the sixth rib

Figure 1–33
Anterior view of the lungs.

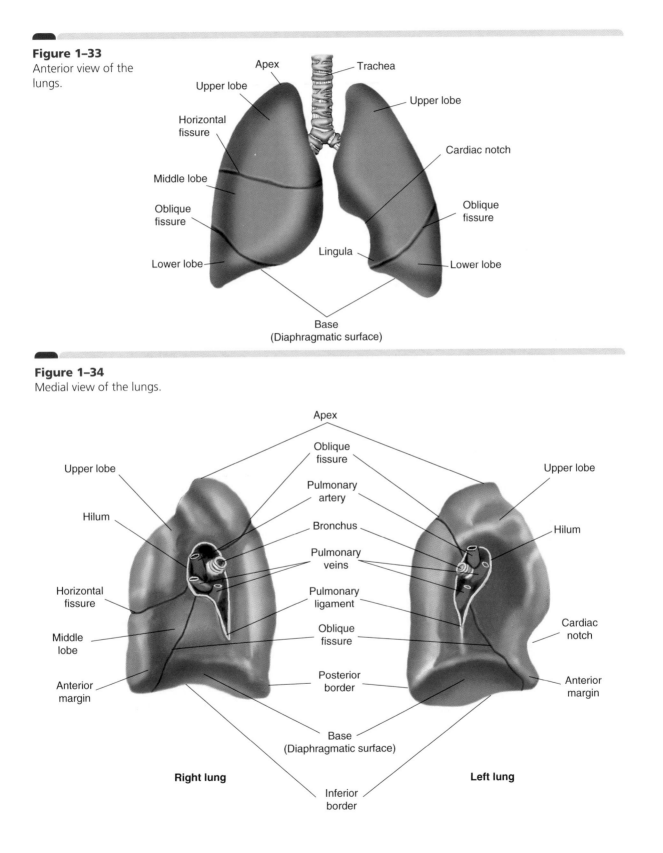

Figure 1–34
Medial view of the lungs.

Figure 1–35
Anatomic relationship of the lungs and the thorax.

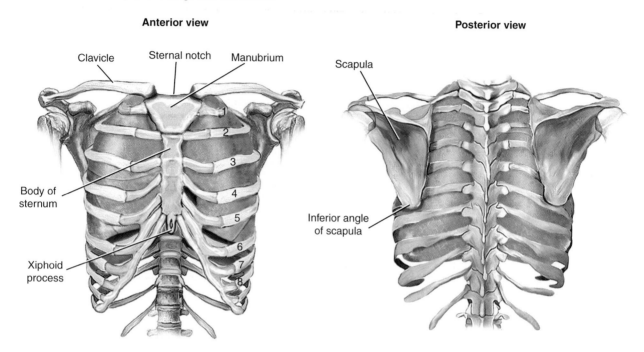

Anterior view   Posterior view

(xiphoid process level), and posteriorly to about the level of the eleventh rib (two ribs below the inferior angle of the scapula). The **mediastinal border** of each lung is concave to fit the heart and other mediastinal structures. At the center of the mediastinal border is the **hilum**, where the main stem bronchi, blood vessels, lymph vessels, and various nerves enter and exit the lungs.

The **right lung** is larger and heavier than the left. It is divided into the **upper**, **middle**, and **lower lobes** by the **oblique** and **horizontal fissures**. The oblique fissure extends from the costal to the mediastinal borders of the lung and separates the upper and middle lobes from the lower lobe. The horizontal fissure extends horizontally from the oblique fissure to about the level of the fourth costal cartilage and separates the middle from the upper lobe.

The **left lung** is divided into only two lobes—the upper and the lower. These two lobes are separated by the **oblique fissure**, which extends from the costal to the mediastinal borders of the lung.

All lobes are further subdivided into **bronchopulmonary segments**. In Figure 1–36, the segments are numbered to demonstrate their relationship.

Figure 1–36
Lung segments. Although the segment subdivisions of the right and left lungs are similar, there are some slight anatomic differences, which are noted by combined names and numbers. Because of these slight variations, some researchers consider that, technically, there are only eight segments in the left lung and that the apical-posterior segment is number 1 and the anteromedial segment is number 6.

Right lung		Left lung	
Upper lobe		Upper lobe	
Apical	1	Upper division	
Posterior	2	Apical/Posterior	1 & 2
Anterior	3	Anterior	3
Middle lobe		Lower division (lingular)	
Lateral	4	Superior lingula	4
Medial	5	Inferior lingula	5
Lower lobe		Lower lobe	
Superior	6	Superior	6
Medial basal	7	Anterior medial basal	7 & 8
Anterior basal	8	Lateral basal	9
Lateral basal	9	Posterior basal	10
Posterior basal	10		

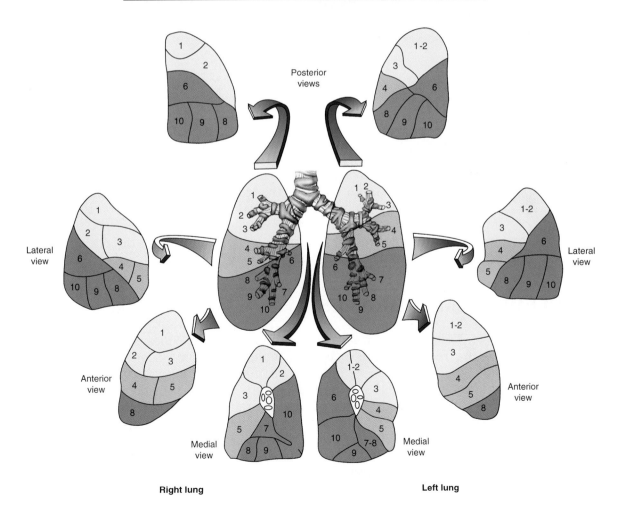

Right lung

Left lung

Figure 1–37
Major structures surrounding the lungs.

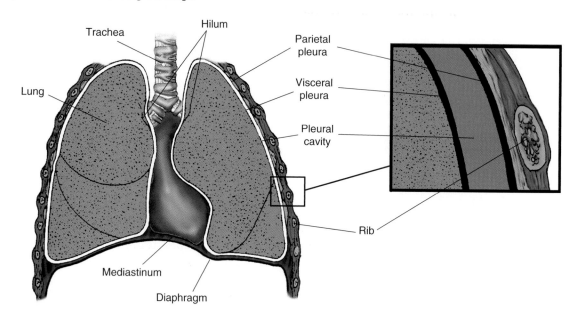

THE MEDIASTINUM

The **mediastinum** is a cavity that contains organs and tissues in the center of the thoracic cage between the right and left lungs (Figure 1–37). It is bordered anteriorly by the sternum and posteriorly by the thoracic vertebrae. The mediastinum contains the trachea, the heart, the major blood vessels (commonly known as the great vessels) that enter and exit the heart, various nerves, portions of the esophagus, the thymus gland, and lymph nodes. If the mediastinum is compressed or distorted, it can severely compromise the cardiopulmonary system.

THE PLEURAL MEMBRANES

Two moist, slick-surfaced membranes called the **visceral** and **parietal pleurae** are closely associated with the lungs. The visceral pleura is firmly attached to the outer surface of each lung and extends into each of the interlobar fissures. The parietal pleura lines the inside of the thoracic walls, the thoracic surface of the diaphragm, and the lateral portion of the mediastinum. The potential space between the visceral and parietal pleurae is called the **pleural cavity** (see Figure 1–37).

The visceral and parietal pleurae are held together by a thin film of serous fluid—somewhat like two flat, moistened pieces of glass. This fluid layer allows the two pleural membranes to glide over each other during inspiration and expiration. Thus, during inspiration the pleural membranes hold the lung tissue to the inner surface of the thorax and diaphragm, causing the lungs to expand.

Because the lungs have a natural tendency to collapse and the chest wall has a natural tendency to expand, a negative or subatmospheric pressure (negative intrapleural pressure) normally exists between the parietal and visceral pleurae. Should air or gas be introduced into the pleural cavity (e.g., as a result of a chest puncture wound), the intrapleural pressure rises to atmospheric pressure and causes the pleural membranes to separate, a condition called **pneumothorax**.

THE THORAX

The **thorax** houses and protects the organs of the cardiopulmonary system. Twelve **thoracic vertebrae** form the posterior midline border of the thoracic cage. The **sternum** forms the anterior border of the chest. The sternum is composed of the **manubrium sterni**, the **body**, and the **xiphoid process** (Figure 1–38).

Figure 1–38
The thorax.

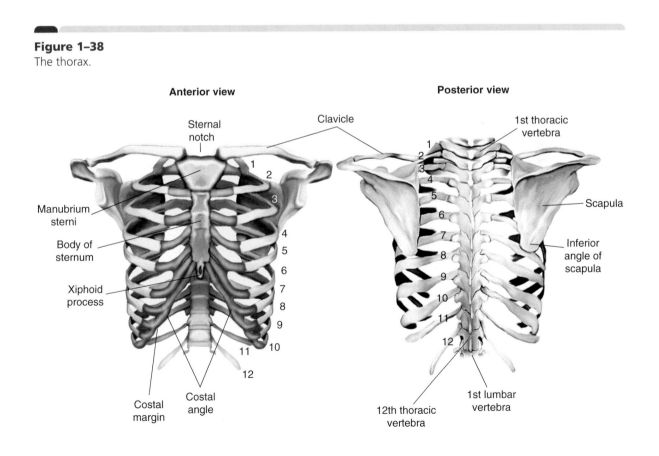

Anterior view

Posterior view

Sternal notch

Clavicle

1st thoracic vertebra

Manubrium sterni

Body of sternum

Xiphoid process

Scapula

Inferior angle of scapula

Costal margin

Costal angle

12th thoracic vertebra

1st lumbar vertebra

Figure 1–39
The intercostal space.

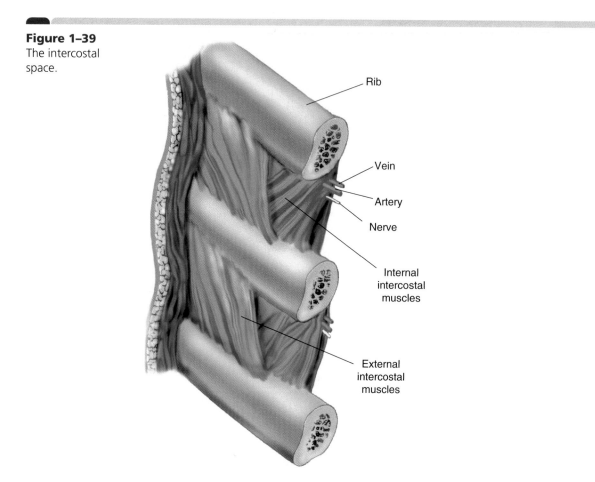

Rib

Vein

Artery

Nerve

Internal intercostal muscles

External intercostal muscles

The 12 pairs of ribs form the lateral boundary of the thorax. The ribs attach directly to the vertebral column posteriorly and indirectly by way of the costal cartilage anteriorly to the sternum. The first seven ribs are referred to as **true ribs**, because they are attached directly to the sternum by way of their costal cartilage. Because the cartilage of the eighth, ninth, and tenth ribs attaches to the cartilage of the ribs above, they are referred to as **false ribs**. Ribs eleven and twelve float freely anteriorly and are called **floating ribs**. There are 11 intercostal spaces between the ribs; these spaces contain blood vessels, intercostal nerves, and the external and internal intercostal muscles (Figure 1–39).

THE DIAPHRAGM

The **diaphragm** is the major muscle of ventilation (Figure 1–40). It is a dome-shaped musculofibrous partition located between the thoracic cavity and the abdominal cavity. Although the diaphragm is generally referred

Figure 1–40
The diaphragm.

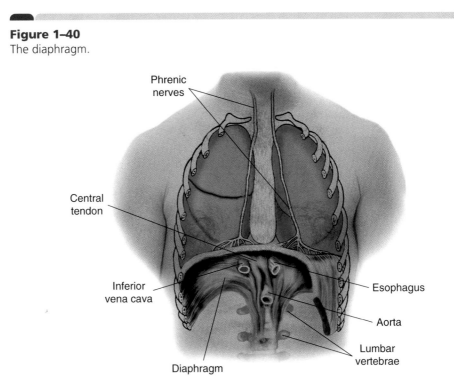

to as one muscle, it is actually composed of two separate muscles known as the **right** and **left hemidiaphragms**. Each hemidiaphragm arises from the lumbar vertebrae, the costal margin, and the xiphoid process. The two muscles then merge at the midline into a broad connective sheet called the **central tendon**. The diaphragm is pierced by the esophagus, the aorta, several nerves, and the inferior vena cava. Terminal branches of the **phrenic nerves**, which leave the spinal cord between the third and fifth cervical segments, supply the primary motor innervation to each hemidiaphragm. The **lower thoracic nerves** also contribute to the motor innervation of each hemidiaphragm.

When stimulated to contract, the diaphragm moves downward and the lower ribs move upward and outward. This action increases the volume of the thoracic cavity which, in turn, lowers the intrapleural and intra-alveolar pressures in the thoracic cavity. As a result, gas from the atmosphere flows into the lungs. During expiration, the diaphragm relaxes and moves upward into the thoracic cavity. This action increases the intra-alveolar and intrapleural pressures, causing gas to flow out of the lungs.

The Accessory Muscles of Ventilation

During normal ventilation by a healthy person, the diaphragm alone can manage the task of moving gas in and out of the lungs. However, during vigorous exercise and the advanced stages of COPD, the accessory muscles of inspiration and expiration are activated to assist the diaphragm.

The Accessory Muscles of Inspiration

The accessory muscles of inspiration are those muscles that are recruited to assist the diaphragm in creating a subatmospheric pressure in the lungs to enable adequate inspiration. The major accessory muscles of inspiration are:

- Scalenus muscles
- Sternocleidomastoid muscles
- Pectoralis major muscles
- Trapezius muscles
- External intercostal muscles.

Scalenus Muscles

The **scalenus muscles** are three separate muscles that function as a unit. They are known as the **anterior**, the **medial**, and the **posterior** scalene muscles. They originate on the transverse processes of the second to the sixth cervical vertebrae and insert into the first and second ribs (Figure 1–41).

Figure 1–41
Scalenus muscles.

The primary function of these muscles is to flex the neck. When used as accessory muscles for inspiration, they elevate the first and second ribs, an action that decreases the intrapleural pressure.

Sternocleidomastoid Muscles

The **sternocleidomastoid muscles** are located on each side of the neck (Figure 1–42). They originate from the sternum and the clavicle and insert into the mastoid process and occipital bone of the skull. Normally, the sternocleidomastoid muscles pull from their sternoclavicular origin and rotate the head to the opposite side and turn it upward. When the sternocleidomastoid muscles function as an accessory muscle of inspiration, the head and neck are fixed by other muscles and the sternocleidomastoid pulls from its insertion on the skull and elevates the sternum. This action increases the anteroposterior diameter of the chest.

Pectoralis Major Muscles

The **pectoralis major muscles** are powerful, fan-shaped muscles located on each side of the upper chest. They originate from the clavicle and the sternum and insert into the upper part of the humerus.

Figure 1–42
Sternocleidomastoid muscles.

Mastoid process

Sternocleidomastoid muscles

Clavicle

Manubrium sterni

Normally, the pectoralis majors pull from their sternoclavicular origin and bring the upper arm to the body in a hugging motion (Figure 1–43). When functioning as accessory muscles of inspiration, they pull from the humeral insertion and elevate the chest, resulting in an increased antero-posterior diameter. Patients with COPD frequently brace their arms against something stationary and use their pectoralis majors to increase the diameter of their chest (Figure 1–44).

Figure 1–43
Pectoralis major muscles.

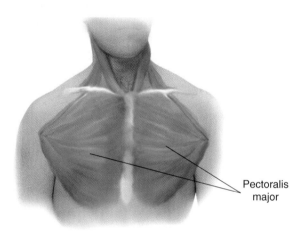

Pectoralis major

Figure 1–44
How an individual may appear when using the pectoralis major muscles for inspiration.

Trapezius Muscles

The **trapezius muscles** are large, flat, triangular muscles that are situated superficially in the upper back and the back of the neck. They originate from the occipital bone, the ligamentum nuchae, and the spinous processes of the seventh cervical vertebra and all the thoracic vertebrae. They insert into the spine of the scapula, the acromion process, and the lateral third of the clavicle (Figure 1–45).

Normally, the trapezius muscles rotate the scapula, raise the shoulders, and abduct and flex the arms. Their action is typified in shrugging of the shoulders (Figure 1–46). When used as accessory muscles of inspiration, the trapezius muscles help to elevate the thoracic cage.

External Intercostal Muscles

The **external intercostal muscles** arise from the lower border of each rib (the upper limit of an intercostal space) and insert into the upper border of the rib below. Anteriorly, the fibers run downward and medially. Posteriorly, the fibers run downward and laterally (Figure 1–47). The external intercostal muscles contract during inspiration and pull the ribs upward and outward, increasing both the lateral and anteroposterior diameter of the thorax (an antagonistic action to the internal intercostal muscles). This action increases lung volume and prevents retraction of the intercostal space during an excessively forceful inspiration.

Figure 1–45
Trapezius muscles.

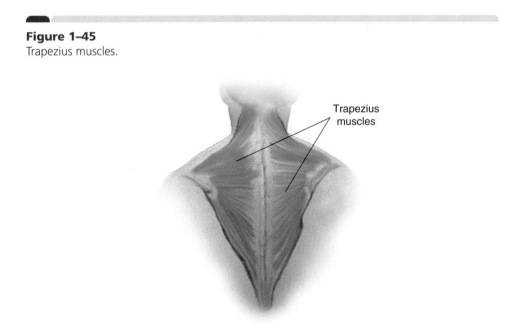

Trapezius
muscles

Figure 1–46
Shrugging of the shoulders typifies the action of the trapezius muscles.

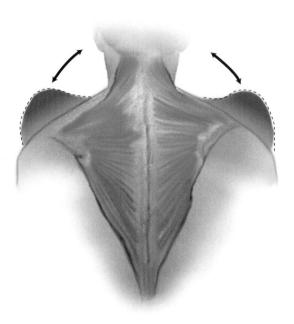

Figure 1–47
Internal and external intercostal muscles.

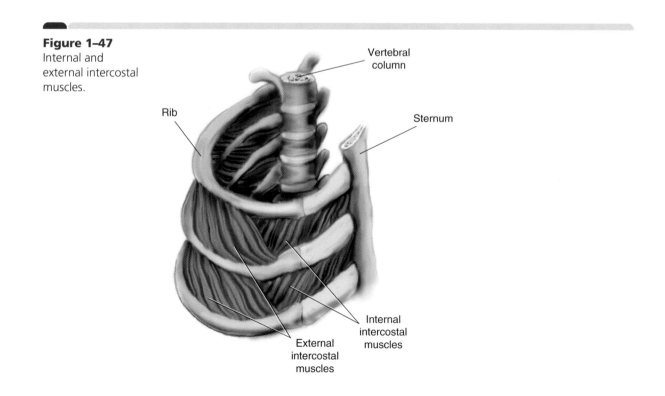

The Accessory Muscles of Expiration

The accessory muscles of expiration are the muscles recruited to assist in exhalation when airway resistance becomes significantly elevated. When these muscles contract, they increase the intrapleural pressure and offset the increased airway resistance. The major accessory muscles of exhalation are:

- Rectus abdominis muscles
- External abdominis obliquus muscles
- Internal abdominis obliquus muscles
- Transversus abdominis muscles
- Internal intercostal muscles.

Rectus Abdominis Muscles

The **rectus abdominis muscles** are a pair of muscles that extend the entire length of the abdomen. Each muscle forms a vertical mass about 10 cm wide and is separated from the other by the **linea alba**. The muscles arise from the iliac crest and pubic symphysis and insert into the xiphoid process and the fifth, sixth, and seventh ribs.

When contracted, the rectus abdominis muscles assist in compressing the abdominal contents. This compression, in turn, pushes the diaphragm into the thoracic cage (Figure 1–48A), thereby assisting in exhalation.

Figure 1–48
Accessory muscles of expiration.

A	B	C	D
Rectus abdominis	External oblique	Internal oblique	Transversus abdominis

External Abdominis Obliquus Muscles

The **external abdominis obliquus** muscles are broad, thin muscles located on the anterolateral sides of the abdomen. They are the longest and the most superficial of all the anterolateral abdominal muscles. They arise by eight digitations from the lower eight ribs and the abdominal aponeurosis and insert into the iliac crest and the linea alba.

When contracted, the external abdominis obliquus muscles assist in compressing the abdominal contents which, in turn, push the diaphragm into the thoracic cage (Figure 1–48B), thereby assisting in exhalation.

Internal Abdominis Obliquus Muscles

Smaller and thinner than the external abdominis obliques, the **internal abdominis obliquus muscles** are located in the lateral and ventral parts of the abdominal wall directly under the external abdominis obliquus muscles. They arise from the inguinal ligament, the iliac crest, and the lower portion of the lumbar aponeurosis. They insert into the last four ribs and into the linea alba.

The internal abdominis obliquus muscles also assist in exhalation by compressing the abdominal contents and in pushing the diaphragm into the thoracic cage (Figure 1–48C).

Transversus Abdominis Muscles

The **transversus abdominis muscles** are found immediately under the internal abdominis obliquus muscles. These muscles arise from the inguinal ligament, the iliac crest, the thoracolumbar fascia, and the lower six ribs and insert into the linea alba. When activated, they also help to constrict the abdominal contents (Figure 1–48D).

When all four pairs of accessory muscles of exhalation contract, the abdominal pressure increases and drives the diaphragm into the thoracic cage. As the diaphragm moves into the thoracic cage during exhalation, the intrapleural pressure increases, thereby enhancing the amount of gas flow (Figure 1–49).

Internal Intercostal Muscles

The **internal intercostal muscles** run between the ribs immediately beneath the external intercostal muscles. The muscles arise from the inferior border of each rib and insert into the superior border of the rib below. Anteriorly, the fibers run in a downward and lateral direction. Posteriorly, the fibers run downward and in a medial direction (see Figure 1–47). The internal intercostal muscles contract during expiration and pull the ribs downward and inward, decreasing both the lateral and anteroposterior diameter of the thorax (an antagonistic action to the external intercostal

Figure 1–49
The collective action of the accessory muscles of expiration causes the intrapleural pressure to increase, the chest to move outward, and bronchial gas flow to increase.

Bronchial
gas flow

Diaphragmatic
pressure

muscles). This action decreases lung volume and offsets intercostal bulging during excessive expiration.

CHAPTER SUMMARY

An essential cornerstone to the understanding of the practice of respiratory care is a strong knowledge base of the anatomy and physiology of the respiratory system. The major anatomic components of the respiratory system include the structures found in the upper airway, including the nose, oral cavity, pharynx, and larynx; the lower airways, including the tracheobronchial tree and its histology; the sites of gas exchange, including the alveolar epithelium, pores of Kohn, alveolar macrophages, and interstitium; the pulmonary vascular system, including the arteries, arterioles, capillaries, venules, and veins; the lymphatic system, including the lymphatic vessels, lymph nodes, and juxta-alveolar lymphatics; the neural control of the lungs, including the autonomic nervous system, sympathetic nervous system, and parasympathetic nervous system; the lungs, including mediastinal border, hilum, right lung (upper, middle, and lower lobes), left lung (upper and lower lobes), and bronchopulmonary segments; the mediastinum, the pleural membranes, the thorax, including the thoracic vertebrae, sternum, manubrium sterni, xyphoid process, true ribs, false ribs, and floating ribs; the diaphragm, including the right and left hemidiaphragms, the central tendon, the phrenic nerve, and the lower thoracic nerves; the accessory muscles of ventilation, including the scalene muscles, sternocleidomastoid muscles, pectoralis major muscles, trapezius muscles, and external intercostal muscles; and the accessory muscles of expiration, including the rectus abdominis muscles, external abdominis obliquus muscles, internal abdominis obliquus muscles, and the internal intercostal muscles.

For the respiratory care practitioner, a strong foundation of the normal anatomy and physiology of the respiratory system is an essential prerequisite to better understand (1) the anatomic alterations of the lungs caused by specific respiratory disorders, (2) the pathophysiologic mechanisms activated throughout the respiratory system as a result of the anatomic alterations, (3) the clinical manifestations that develop as a result of the pathophysiologic mechanisms, and (4) the basic respiratory therapies used to improve the anatomic alterations and pathophysiologic mechanisms caused by the disease. When the anatomic alterations and pathophysiologic mechanisms caused by the disorder are improved, the clinical manifestations also should improve.

REVIEW QUESTIONS

1. Which of the following line the anterior one-third of the nasal cavity?
   A. Stratified squamous epithelium
   B. Simple cuboidal epithelium
   C. Pseudostratified ciliated columnar epithelium
   D. Simple squamous epithelium

2. Which of the following form(s) the nasal septum?
   I. Frontal process of the maxilla bone
   II. Ethmoid bone
   III. Nasal bones
   IV. Vomer
      A. III only
      B. IV only
      C. I and III only
      D. II and IV only

3. Which of the following prevents the aspiration of foods and liquids?
   A. Epiglottis
   B. Cricoid cartilage
   C. Arytenoid cartilages
   D. Thyroid cartilages

4. The canals of Lambert are found in the
   A. trachea
   B. terminal bronchioles
   C. alveoli
   D. main stem bronchi

5. The eustachian tubes are found in the
   A. nasopharynx
   B. oropharynx
   C. laryngopharynx
   D. oral cavity

6. The inferior portion of the larynx is composed of the
   A. thyroid cartilage
   B. hyoid bone
   C. glottis
   D. cricoid cartilage

7. Which of the following has the greatest combined cross-sectional area?
   A. Terminal bronchioles
   B. Lobar bronchi
   C. Trachea
   D. Segmental bronchi

8. The left main stem bronchus angles off from the carina at about
   A. 10–20 degrees from the carina
   B. 20–30 degrees from the carina
   C. 30–40 degrees from the carina
   D. 40–60 degrees from the carina

9. Ninety-five percent of the alveolar surface is composed of which of the following?
   I. Type I cells
   II. Granular pneumocytes
   III. Type II cells
   IV. Squamous pneumocytes
       A. I only
       B. II only
       C. II and III only
       D. I and IV only

10. Which of the following is (are) released when the parasympathetic nerve fibers are stimulated?
    I. Norepinephrine
    II. Atropine
    III. Epinephrine
    IV. Acetylcholine
        A. II only
        B. IV only
        C. I and III only
        D. I, II, and III only

11. Which of the following is (are) released when the sympathetic nerve fibers are stimulated?
    I.   Norepinephrine
    II. Propranolol
    III. Acetylcholine
    IV. Epinephrine
       A. I only
       B. II only
       C. I and IV only
       D. II, III, and IV only

12. Pseudostratified ciliated columnar epithelium lines which of the following?
    I.   Oropharynx
    II. Trachea
    III. Nasopharynx
    IV. Oral cavity
    V.   Laryngopharynx
       A. II only
       B. I and IV only
       C. II and III only
       D. I, II, III, and V only

13. Which of the following is (are) accessory muscles of inspiration?
    I.   Trapezius muscles
    II. Internal abdominis obliquus muscles
    III. Scalene muscles
    IV. Transversus abdominis muscles
       A. I only
       B. II only
       C. I and III only
       D. II and IV only

14. The horizontal fissure separates the
    A.   middle and upper lobes of the right lung
    B.   upper and lower lobes of the left lung
    C.   middle and lower lobes of the right lung
    D.   oblique fissure of the left lung

15. Which of the following supply the motor innervation of each hemidiaphragm?
    I.   Vagus nerve (tenth cranial nerve)
    II. Phrenic nerve
    III. Lower thoracic nerves
    IV. Glossopharyngeal nerve (ninth cranial nerve)
       A. I only
       B. II only
       C. I and IV only
       D. II and III only

16. The lung segment called the superior lingula is found in the
    A. left lung, lower division of the upper lobe
    B. right lung, lower lobe
    C. left lung, upper division of the upper lobe
    D. right lung, upper lobe

17. Cartilage is found in which of the following structures of the tracheobronchial tree?
    I.   Bronchioles
    II. Respiratory bronchioles
    III. Segmental bronchi
    IV. Terminal bronchioles
       A. I only
       B. III only
       C. II and III only
       D. I and IV only

18. The bronchial arteries nourish the tracheobronchial tree down to, and including, which of the following?
    A. Respiratory bronchioles
    B. Segmental bronchi
    C. Terminal bronchioles
    D. Segmental bronchi

19. Which of the following elevates the soft palate?
    A. Palatoglossal muscle
    B. Levator veli palatine muscle
    C. Stylopharyngeus muscles
    D. Palatopharyngeal muscle

20. Which of the following are called the resistance vessels?
    A. Arterioles
    B. Veins
    C. Venules
    D. Arteries

CHAPTER 2

Ventilation

O B J E C T I V E S

By the end of this chapter, the student should be able to:

1. Define ventilation.
2. Differentiate between the following pressure differences across the lungs:
   —Driving pressure
   —Transairway pressure
   —Transmural pressure
   —Transpulmonary pressure
   —Transthoracic pressure
3. Describe the role of the diaphragm in ventilation.
4. Explain how the excursion of the diaphragm affects the intrapleural pressure, intra-alveolar pressure, and bronchial gas flow during
   —inspiration
   —end-inspiration
   —expiration
   —end-expiration
5. Describe the elastic properties of the lung and chest wall.
6. Calculate lung compliance.
7. Explain how Hooke's law can be applied to the elastic properties of the lungs.
8. Define surface tension.
9. Describe Laplace's law.
10. Describe how Laplace's law can be applied to the alveolar fluid lining.
11. Explain how pulmonary surfactant offsets alveolar surface tension.
12. List respiratory disorders that cause a deficiency of pulmonary surfactant.
13. Define the term dynamic.
14. Describe how Poiseuille's law arranged for flow relates to the radius of the bronchial airways.
15. Describe how Poiseuille's law arranged for pressure relates to the radius of the bronchial airways.
16. Describe how Poiseuille's law can be rearranged to simple proportionalities.
17. Define airway resistance and explain how it relates to
   —laminar flow
   —turbulent flow
   —tracheobronchial or transitional flow
18. Calculate airway resistance.
19. Define time constants and explain how they relate to alveolar units with
   —increased airway resistance
   —decreased compliance
20. Define dynamic compliance and explain how it relates to
   —auto PEEP and its relationship to airway resistance
   —frequency dependence
21. Describe how the following relates to the normal ventilatory pattern:
   —Tidal volume (V_T)
   —Ventilatory rate
   —I:E ratio

(continues)

22. Differentiate between alveolar ventilation and dead space ventilation, and explain the following:
    —Anatomic dead space
    —Alveolar dead space
    —Physiologic dead space
23. Describe how the following affect alveolar ventilation:
    —Depth of breathing
    —Rate of breathing
24. Calculate an individual's alveolar ventilation when given the following information:
    —Alveolar ventilation
    —Dead space ventilation
    —Breaths per minute
25. Describe how the normal intrapleural pressure differences cause regional differences in normal lung ventilation.
26. Describe how the following alter the ventilatory pattern (i.e., the respiratory rate and tidal volume):
    —Decreased lung compliance
    —Increased airway resistance

27. Compare and contrast the following types of ventilation:
    —Apnea
    —Eupnea
    —Biot's breathing
    —Hyperpnea
    —Hyperventilation
    —Hypoventilation
    —Tachypnea
    —Cheyne-Stokes breathing
    —Kussmaul's breathing
    —Orthopnea
    —Dyspnea
28. Complete the review questions at the end of this chapter.

The term **ventilation** is defined as the process that moves gases between the external environment and the alveoli. It is the mechanism by which oxygen is carried from the atmosphere to the alveoli and by which carbon dioxide (delivered to the lungs in mixed venous blood) is carried from the alveoli to the atmosphere.

To fully understand the process of ventilation, the respiratory care practitioner must understand (1) the pressure differences across the lungs, (2) the elastic properties of the lungs and chest wall, (3) the dynamic characteristics of the lungs and how they affect ventilation, and (4) the characteristics of normal and abnormal ventilatory patterns.

PRESSURE DIFFERENCES ACROSS THE LUNGS

Understanding the pressure differences across the lungs—relative to the atmospheric pressure—is an essential building block in the study of ventilation and pulmonary mechanics. The difference between two pressures is called a

pressure gradient. Pressure gradients are responsible for (1) moving air in and out of the lungs and (2) for maintaining the lungs in an inflated state.

Gas always flows from high to low pressures. There is no gas flow when the pressure gradient is zero; that is, the pressure between two points is equal. Pressure gradients commonly used in ventilation include driving pressure, transairway pressure, transmural pressure, transpulmonary pressure, and transthoracic pressure. Once these pressure gradients are understood, the differences between spontaneous ventilation, positive pressure ventilation, and negative pressure ventilation become crystal clear.

Driving pressure is the pressure difference between two points in a tube or vessel; it is the force moving gas or fluid through the tube or vessel. For example, if the gas pressure at the beginning of a tube is 20 mm Hg and the pressure at the end of the same tube is 5 mm Hg, then the driving pressure is 15 mm Hg. In other words, the force required to move the gas through the tube is 15 mm Hg (Figure 2–1).

Transairway pressure (P_{ta}) (also called Transrespiratory pressure) is the barometric pressure difference between the mouth pressure (P_m) and the alveolar pressure (P_{alv}).

$$P_{ta} = P_m - P_{alv}$$

For example, if the P_{alv} is 757 mm Hg and the P_m is 760 mm Hg during inspiration, then the P_{ta} is 3 mm Hg (Figure 2–2A).

$$P_{ta} = P_m - P_{alv}$$
$$= 760 \text{ mm Hg} - 757 \text{ mm Hg}$$
$$= 3 \text{ mm Hg}$$

Or, if the P_{alv} is 763 mm Hg and the P_m is 760 mm Hg during expiration, then the P_{ta} is −3 mm Hg. Gas in this example, however, is moving in the opposite direction (Figure 2–2B). The transairway pressure causes airflow in and out of the conducting airways. In essence, the P_{ta} represents the driving pressure (the pressure difference between the mouth and the alveolus) that forces gas in or out of the lungs.

Figure 2–1
Driving pressure. At point A, gas pressure is 20 mm Hg. At point B, gas pressure is 5 mm Hg. Thus, the driving pressure between point A and point B is 15 mm Hg.

Figure 2–2

Transairway pressure: The difference between the pressure at the mouth (P_m) and the alveolar pressure (P_{alv}). Even though gas is moving in opposite directions in A and B, the transairway pressure is 3 mm Hg in both examples. Note: In this illustration, the pressure at the mouth (P_m) is equal to the barometric pressure (P_B).

Transmural pressure (P_{tm}) is the pressure differences that occur across the airway wall. The transmural pressure is calculated by subtracting the intra-airway pressure (P_{iaw}) from the pressure on the outside of the airway (P_{oaw}).

$$P_{tm} = P_{iaw} - P_{oaw}$$

Positive transmural pressure is said to exist when the pressure is greater within the airway than the pressure outside the airway. For example, if the P_{iaw} pressure is 765 mm Hg and the P_{oaw} is 760 mm Hg, there is a positive transmural pressure of 5 mm Hg (Figure 2–3A).

$$P_{tm} = P_{iaw} - P_{oaw}$$
$$= 765 \text{ mm Hg} - 760 \text{ mm Hg}$$
$$= 5 \text{ mm Hg (positive transmural pressure)}$$

Negative transmural pressure is said to exist when the pressure is greater outside the airway than the pressure inside the airway. For example, if the P_{iaw} pressure is 755 mm Hg and the P_{oaw} is 760 mm Hg, there is a negative transmural pressure of 5 mm Hg (Figure 2–3B).

Transpulmonary pressure (P_{tp}) is the difference between the alveolar pressure (P_{alv}) and the pleural pressure (P_{pl}).

$$P_{tp} = P_{alv} - P_{pl}$$

For example, if the P_{pl} is 755 mm Hg and the P_{alv} is 760 mm Hg (e.g., inspiration), then the P_{tp} is 5 mm Hg (Figure 2–4).

$$P_{tp} = P_{alv} - P_{pl}$$
$$= 760 \text{ mm Hg} - 755 \text{ mm Hg}$$
$$= 5 \text{ mm Hg}$$

Figure 2–3

Transmural pressure: the pressure difference that occurs across the wall of the airway. **(A)** Airway with a positive transmural pressure. **(B)** Airway with a negative transmural pressure.

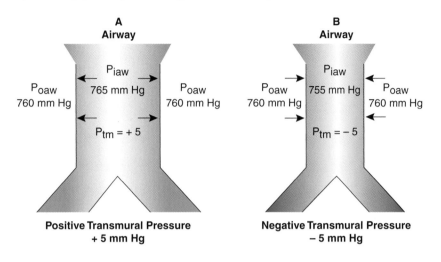

A
Airway

P_{iaw}
765 mm Hg

P_{oaw}
760 mm Hg

P_{oaw}
760 mm Hg

$P_{tm} = +5$

Positive Transmural Pressure
+ 5 mm Hg

B
Airway

P_{iaw}
755 mm Hg

P_{oaw}
760 mm Hg

P_{oaw}
760 mm Hg

$P_{tm} = -5$

Negative Transmural Pressure
– 5 mm Hg

Figure 2–4

Transpulmonary pressure: The difference between the alveolar pressure (P_{alv}) and the pleural pressure (P_{pl}). This illustration assumes a barometric pressure (P_B) of 761 mm Hg.

A

Gas Flow

P_{alv} = 760 mm Hg

P_{pl} = 755 mm Hg

Inspiration

P_B = 761 mm Hg

Transpulmonary Pressure

5 mm Hg

B

Gas Flow

P_{alv} = 763 mm Hg

P_{pl} = 758 mm Hg

Expiration

CLINICAL APPLICATION CASE

2

See page 121

Or, if the P_{alv} is 763 mm Hg and the P_{pl} is 758 mm Hg (e.g., expiration), then the P_{tp} is 5 mm Hg (Figure 2–4B). In the normal lung, the P_{alv} is always greater than the P_{pl}, which, in turn, maintains the lungs in an inflated state.

Transthoracic pressure (P_{tt}) is the difference between the alveolar pressure (P_{alv}) and the body surface pressure (P_{bs}).

$$P_{tt} = P_{alv} - P_{bs}$$

Figure 2–5

Transthoracic pressure: The difference between the alveolar pressure (P_{alv}) and the body surface pressure (P_{bs}). Note: In this illustration, the body surface pressure (P_{bs}) is equal to the barometric pressure (P_B).

For example, if the P_{alv} is 757 mm Hg and the P_{bs} is 760 mm Hg (e.g., inspiration), then the P_{tt} is −3 mm Hg (Figure 2–5A).

$$P_{tt} = P_{alv} - P_{bs}$$

$$= 757 \text{ mm Hg} - 760 \text{ mm Hg}$$

$$= -3 \text{ mm Hg}$$

Or, if the P_{alv} is 763 mm Hg and the P_{bs} is 760 mm Hg (e.g., expiration), then the P_{tt} is 3 mm Hg (Figure 2–5B). The P_{tt} is the pressure responsible for expanding the lungs and chest wall in tandem.

Technically, there is no real difference between the transairway pressure (P_{ta}) and the transthoracic pressure (P_{tt}). The P_{tt} is merely another way to view the pressure differences across the lungs.

ROLE OF THE DIAPHRAGM IN VENTILATION

CLINICAL
APPLICATION
CASE

2

See page 121

The flow of gas in and out of the lungs is caused by the transpulmonary and transairway pressure changes that occur in response to the action of the diaphragm (Figure 2–6). As illustrated in Figure 2–7, when stimulated to contract during inspiration by the phrenic nerves, the diaphragm moves downward, causing the thoracic volume to increase and the intrapleural and intra-alveolar pressures to decrease. Because the intra-alveolar pressure is less than the barometric pressure during this period, gas from the atmosphere moves down the tracheobronchial tree until the intra-alveolar pressure and the barometric pressure are in

Figure 2–6
The diaphragm.

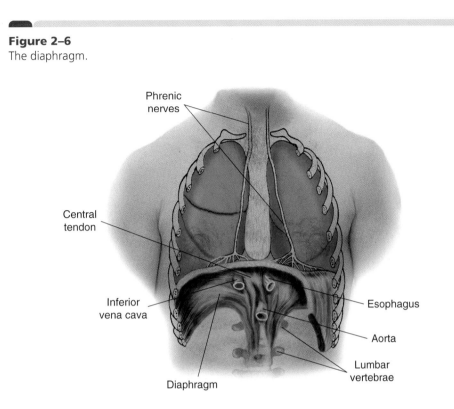

equilibrium. This equilibrium point is known as **end-inspiration** (pre-expiration).

During expiration, the diaphragm relaxes and moves upward, causing the thoracic volume to decrease and the intrapleural and intra-alveolar pressures to increase. During this period, the intra-alveolar pressure is greater than the barometric pressure and gas flows out of the lungs until the intra-alveolar pressure and the barometric pressure are once again in equilibrium. This equilibrium point is known as **end-expiration** (pre-inspiration). The intrapleural pressure during normal inspiration and expiration is always less than the barometric pressure.

At rest, the normal excursion (movement) of the diaphragm is about 1.5 cm, and the normal intrapleural pressure change is about 3 to 6 cm H_2O pressure (2 to 4 mm Hg). During a deep inspiration, however, the diaphragm may move as much as 6 to 10 cm, a fact which can cause the average intrapleural pressure to drop to as low as 50 cm H_2O subatmospheric pressure. During a forced expiration, the intrapleural pressure may climb to between 70 and 100 cm H_2O above atmospheric pressure.

Figure 2–7
How the excursion of the diaphragm affects the intra-pleural pressure, intra-alveolar pressure, and bronchial gas flow during inspiration and expiration.

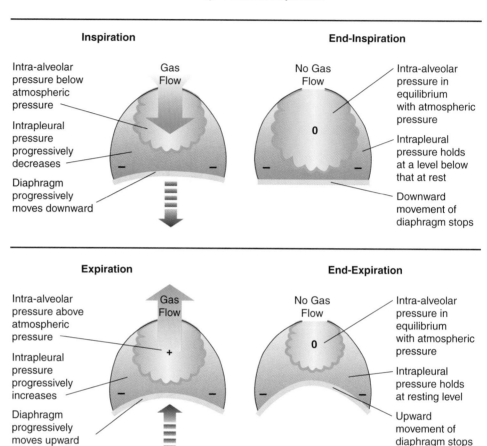

Normal Inspiration and Expiration

Inspiration

Intra-alveolar pressure below atmospheric pressure

Gas Flow

Intrapleural pressure progressively decreases

Diaphragm progressively moves downward

End-Inspiration

No Gas Flow

Intra-alveolar pressure in equilibrium with atmospheric pressure

0

Intrapleural pressure holds at a level below that at rest

Downward movement of diaphragm stops

Expiration

Intra-alveolar pressure above atmospheric pressure

Gas Flow

Intrapleural pressure progressively increases

+

Diaphragm progressively moves upward

End-Expiration

No Gas Flow

Intra-alveolar pressure in equilibrium with atmospheric pressure

0

Intrapleural pressure holds at resting level

Upward movement of diaphragm stops

POSITIVE PRESSURE VENTILATION

Clinically, when the patient is placed on a positive pressure ventilator, the intra-alveolar pressure, intrapleural pressure, and the diaphragmatic movements illustrated in Figure 2–7 will be quite different.

Figure 2–8 shows that when the patient receives a positive pressure breath from a mechanical ventilator, the intra-alveolar pressure progressively rises above atmospheric pressure. For instance, if the mechanical ventilator delivered 30 cm H_2O pressure to the patient's lung during inspiration, the intra-alveolar pressure would increase to about 30 cm H_2O above the atmospheric pressure at the end of inspiration. As the positive pressure progressively increases in the alveoli during inspiration, the intrapleural pressure also increases. As shown in Figure 2–8, the intra-pleural pressure would gradually increase to about 30 cm H_2O above its

Figure 2–8
How a positive pressure breath from a mechanical ventilator affects the intra-alveolar pressure, intrapleural pressure, the excursion of the diaphragm, and gas flow during inspiration and expiration.

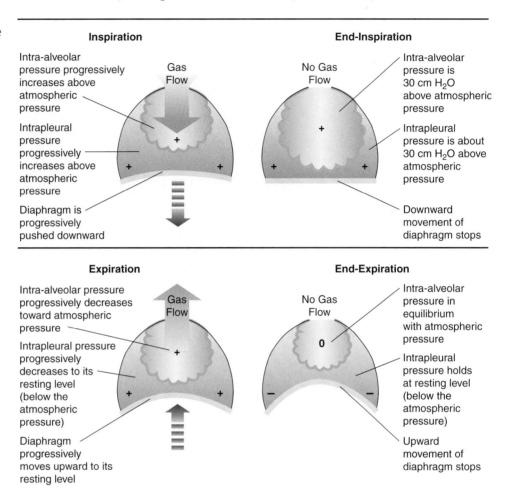

Mechanical Ventilation Positive Pressure Breath
(30 cm H$_2$O Pressure Above Atmospheric Pressure)

Inspiration

Intra-alveolar pressure progressively increases above atmospheric pressure

Gas Flow

Intrapleural pressure progressively increases above atmospheric pressure

Diaphragm is progressively pushed downward

End-Inspiration

No Gas Flow

Intra-alveolar pressure is 30 cm H$_2$O above atmospheric pressure

Intrapleural pressure is about 30 cm H$_2$O above atmospheric pressure

Downward movement of diaphragm stops

Expiration

Intra-alveolar pressure progressively decreases toward atmospheric pressure

Gas Flow

Intrapleural pressure progressively decreases to its resting level (below the atmospheric pressure)

Diaphragm progressively moves upward to its resting level

End-Expiration

No Gas Flow

Intra-alveolar pressure in equilibrium with atmospheric pressure

Intrapleural pressure holds at resting level (below the atmospheric pressure)

Upward movement of diaphragm stops

normal resting level, which, as illustrated in Figure 2–7, is normally below atmospheric pressure. Finally, as the intra-alveolar and intrapleural pressure increase during a positive pressure breath, the lungs expand, pushing the diaphragm downward. This process continues until the positive pressure breath stops.

During exhalation, the intra-alveolar pressure decreases toward atmospheric pressure. This means that the high intra-alveolar pressure moves in the direction of the low atmospheric pressure until the intra-alveolar pressure is in equilibrium with the atmospheric pressure. As the intra-alveolar pressure returns to normal, the intrapleural pressure decreases to its resting level (below the atmospheric pressure), and the diaphragm moves upward to its resting level.

Figure 2–9
Right-side tension pneumothorax. In severe cases, the gas accumulation and subsequent pressure causes the lung to collapse on the affected side, pushes the diaphragm downward, and pushes the heart and mediastinum to the unaffected side.

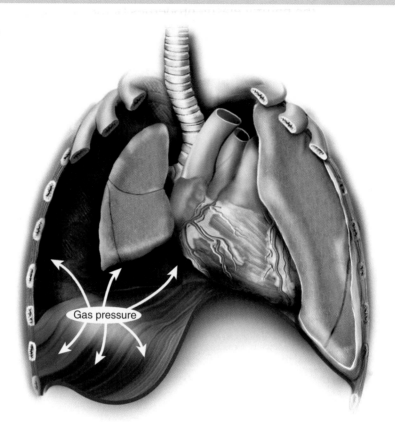

Gas pressure

At end-expiration, the intra-alveolar pressure is in equilibrium with atmospheric pressure. The intrapleural pressure is held at its resting level which, under normal circumstances, is below atmospheric pressure. The upward movement of the diaphragm stops at end-expiration. The administration of positive pressure ventilation may also cause a number of adverse side effects, including lung rupture and gas accumulation between the lungs and chest wall (tension pneumothorax) (Figure 2–9).

ELASTIC PROPERTIES OF THE LUNG AND CHEST WALL

CLINICAL
APPLICATION
CASES
1 & 2
See pages 119–121

Both the lungs and the chest wall each have their own elastic properties—and, under normal conditions, each elastic system works against each other. That is, the chest wall has a natural tendency to move outward or to expand, as a result of the bones of the thorax and surrounding muscles. The lungs have a natural tendency to move inward or collapse, because of the natural elastic properties of the lung tissue. This lung-chest wall relationship is often compared to that of two springs working against each other—that is, the chest wall works to spring outward; the lungs work to recoil inward. Clinically, the elastic forces of the lungs are routinely evaluated by measuring the lung compliance.

Lung Compliance

How readily the elastic force of the lungs accepts a volume of inspired air is known as **lung compliance** (C_L); C_L is defined as the *change in lung volume* (ΔV) per *unit pressure change* (ΔP). Mathematically, C_L is expressed in liters per centimeter of water pressure (L/cm H_2O). In other words, C_L determines how much air, in liters, the lungs will accommodate for each centimeter of water pressure change (e.g., each transpulmonary pressure change).

For example, if an individual generates a negative intrapleural pressure change of 5 cm H_2O during inspiration, and the lungs accept a new volume of 0.75 L of gas, the C_L of the lungs would be expressed as 0.15 L/cm H_2O:

$$C_L = \frac{\Delta V \ (L)}{\Delta P \ (cm \ H_2O)}$$

$$= \frac{0.75 \ L \ of \ gas}{5 \ cm \ H_2O}$$

$$= 0.15 \ L/cm \ H_2O \ (or \ 150 \ mL/cm \ H_2O)$$

It is irrelevant whether the change in driving pressure is in the form of positive or negative pressure. In other words, a negative 5 cm H_2O pressure generated in the intrapleural space, around the lungs, will produce the same volume change as a positive 5 cm H_2O pressure delivered to the tracheobronchial tree (e.g., by means of a mechanical ventilator) (Figure 2–10).

At rest, the average C_L for each breath is about 0.1 L/cm H_2O. In other words, approximately 100 mL of air is delivered into the lungs per 1 cm H_2O pressure change (see Figure 2–10). When lung compliance is increased, the lungs accept a greater volume of gas per unit of pressure change. When C_L is decreased, the lungs accept a smaller volume of gas per unit of pressure change. This relationship is also illustrated by the volume-pressure curve in Figure 2–11.

Note that—both in the normal and abnormal lung—C_L progressively decreases as the alveoli approach their total filling capacity. This occurs because the elastic force of the alveoli steadily increases as the lungs expand, which, in turn, reduces the ability of the lungs to accept an additional volume of gas (see Figure 2–11).

Figure 2–10

Normal volume-pressure curve. The curve shows that lung compliance progressively decreases as lungs expand in response to increased volume. For example, note the greater volume change between 5 and 10 cm H_2O (small/medium alveoli) than between 30 and 35 cm H_2O (large alveoli).

Figure 2–11

How changes in lung compliance affect the volume-pressure curve. When lung compliance decreases, the volume-pressure curve shifts to the right. When lung compliance increases, the volume-pressure curve shifts to the left.

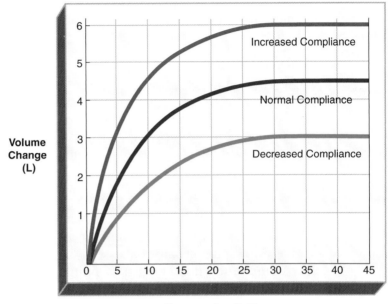

Chest Wall Compliance

As discussed earlier, the chest wall has its own elastic properties, caused by the bones of the thorax and surrounding muscles. As a result, the chest wall works to offset the normal elastic properties of the lungs. If unopposed, the normal compliance of both the lungs and chest wall are about equal at 0.2 L/cm H_2O. However, because the lungs are enclosed within the thorax—and attached to the internal surface of the chest wall—the two elastic systems function as springs that naturally recoil away from each other. This action, in turn, decreases the compliance of each elastic system to about one-half of their individual components—or 0.1 L/cm H_2O. In other words, the normal lung compliance of 0.1 L/H_2O is actually the end result of the "combined" chest wall compliance and lung compliance.

Under normal conditions, the lungs and chest wall recoil to a resting volume, the functional residual capacity (FRC).* When the normal lung-chest wall relationship is disrupted, the chest wall expands to a volume greater than the FRC, and the lungs tend to collapse to a volume less than the FRC. Clinically, this lung-chest wall relationship has many clinical

*See more on the functional residual capacity in Chapter 4.

implications. For example, pulmonary disorders that decrease a patient's lung compliance (e.g., pneumonia, atelectasis, or acute respiratory distress syndrome) not only hinder the patient's lung expansion, but can also significantly decrease the patient's chest wall expansion. On the other hand, a pulmonary disorder that causes the lungs to break away from the chest wall (e.g., pneumothorax) can result in an overexpansion of the chest wall on the affected side (see Figure 2–9).

Hooke's Law

Hooke's law provides another way to explain compliance by describing the physical properties of an elastic substance. **Elastance** is the natural ability of matter to respond directly to force and to return to its original resting position or shape after the external force no longer exists. In pulmonary physiology, elastance is defined as the change in pressure per change in volume:

$$\text{Elastance} = \frac{\Delta P}{\Delta V}$$

Elastance is the reciprocal (opposite) of compliance. Thus, lungs with high compliance (greater ease of filling) have low elastance; lungs with low compliance (lower ease of filling) have high elastance. Note that elastance is the reciprocal of compliance for only a truly elastic body. Because the normal lung-chest wall is not a total, or absolute, elastic mechanism, it functions in a more *sigmoidal* than *linear* manner. Regardless of this point, it is still a satisfactory and practical approximation. Also, because of the viscous nature of the lungs and thorax, a mild degree of *hysteresis* is demonstrated on the volume-pressure curves when comparing inspiration to expiration (see Figure 2–21 later in this chapter).

Hooke's law states that when a truly elastic body, like a spring, is acted on by 1 unit of force, the elastic body will stretch 1 unit of length, and when acted on by 2 units of force it will stretch 2 units of length, and so forth. This phenomenon is only true, however, within the elastic body's normal functional range. When the force exceeds the elastic limits of the substance, the ability of length to increase in response to force rapidly decreases. Should the force continue to rise, the elastic substance will ultimately break (Figure 2–12).

When Hooke's law is applied to the elastic properties of the lungs, *volume* is substituted for *length,* and *pressure* is substituted for *force.* Thus, over the normal physiologic range of the lungs, volume varies directly with pressure. The lungs behave in a manner similar to the spring, and once the elastic limits of the lung unit are reached, little or no volume change occurs in response to pressure changes. Should the change in pressure continue to rise, the elastic limits are exceeded and the lung unit will rupture (Figure 2–13).

Figure 2–12

Hooke's law. When a truly elastic body—such as the spring in this illustration—is acted on by 1 unit of force, the elastic body will stretch 1 unit of length; when acted on by 2 units of force, it will stretch 2 units of length; and so forth. When the force goes beyond the elastic limit of the substance, however, the ability of length to increase in response to force quickly ceases.

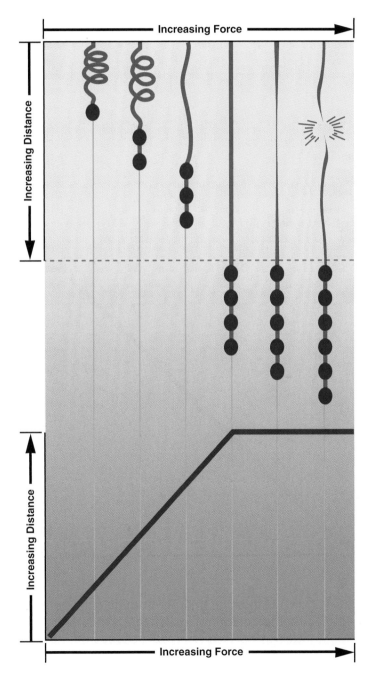

Figure 2–13

Hooke's law applied to the elastic properties of the lungs. Over the physiologic range, volume changes vary directly with pressure changes. Once the elastic limits are reached, however, little or no volume change occurs in response to pressure change.

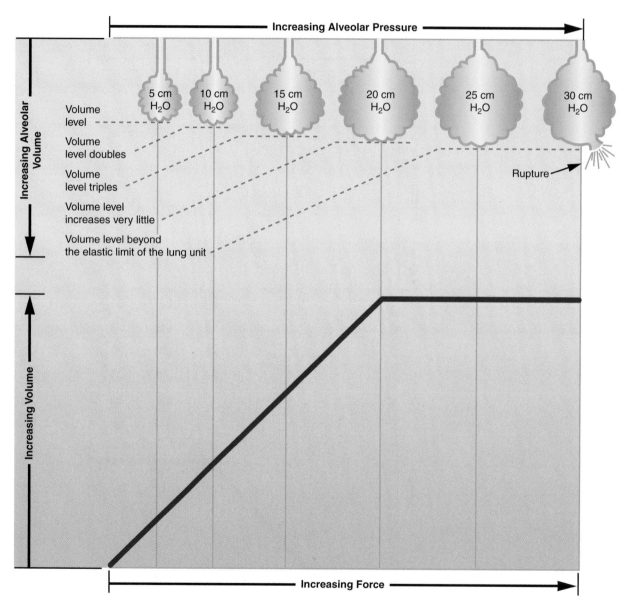

Clinically, this phenomenon explains a hazard associated with mechanical ventilation. That is, if the pressure during mechanical ventilation (positive pressure breath) causes the lung unit to expand beyond its elastic capability, the lung unit could rupture, allowing alveolar gas to move into the intrapleural space, and thus causing the lungs to collapse. This condition is called a **tension pneumothorax** (see Figure 2–9).

Surface Tension and Its Effect on Lung Expansion

In addition to the elastic properties of the lungs, the fluid (primarily H_2O) that lines the inner surface of the alveoli can profoundly resist lung expansion. To understand how the liquid coating the intra-alveolar surface can affect lung expansion, an understanding of the following is essential: (1) surface tension, (2) Laplace's law, and (3) how the substance called pulmonary surfactant offsets alveolar surface tension.

Surface Tension

When liquid molecules are completely surrounded by identical molecules, the molecules are mutually attracted toward one another and, therefore, move freely in all directions (Figure 2–14A). When a liquid–gas interface exists, however, the liquid molecules at the liquid–gas interface are strongly attracted to the liquid molecules within the liquid mass (Figure 2–14B). This molecular, cohesive force at the liquid–gas interface is called *surface tension.* It is the surface tension, for example, that maintains the shape of a water droplet, or makes it possible for an insect to move or stay afloat on the surface of a pond.

Surface tension is measured in dynes per centimeter. One dyne/cm is the force necessary to cause a tear 1 cm long in the surface layer of a liquid. This is similar to using two hands to pull a thin piece of cloth apart until a split 1 cm in length is formed (1 cm H_2O pressure equals 980 dynes/cm). The liquid film that lines the interior surface of the alveoli

Figure 2–14

In model A, the liquid molecules in the middle of the container are mutually attracted toward each other and, therefore, move freely in all directions. In model B, the liquid molecules near the surface (liquid–gas interface) are strongly attracted to the liquid molecules within the liquid mass. This molecular force at the liquid–gas interface is called surface tension.

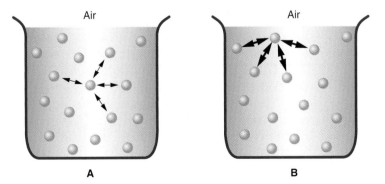

has the potential to exert a force in excess of 70 dynes/cm, a force that can easily cause complete alveolar collapse.

Laplace's Law

Laplace's law describes how the *distending pressure* of a liquid bubble (not an alveolus) is influenced by (1) the surface tension of the bubble and (2) the size of the bubble itself. When Laplace's law is applied to a sphere with one liquid–gas interface (e.g., a bubble completely submerged in a liquid), the equation is written as follows:

$$P = \frac{2\ ST}{r}$$

where P is the pressure difference (dynes/cm^2), ST is surface tension (dynes/cm), and r is the radius of the liquid sphere (cm); the factor 2 is required when the law is applied to a liquid sphere with one liquid–gas interface.

When the law is applied to a bubble with two liquid–gas interfaces (e.g., a soap bubble blown on the end of a tube has a liquid–gas interface both on the inside and on the outside of the bubble), the numerator contains the factor 4 rather than 2:

$$P = \frac{4\ ST}{r}$$

Laplace's law shows that the *distending pressure* of a liquid sphere is (1) directly proportional to the surface tension of the liquid and (2) inversely proportional to the radius of the sphere.

In other words, the numerator of Laplace's law shows that (1) as the surface tension of a liquid bubble increases, the distending pressure necessary to hold the bubble open increases, or (2) the opposite—when the surface tension of a liquid bubble decreases, the distending pressure of the bubble decreases (Figure 2–15). The denominator of Laplace's law shows that (1) when the size of a liquid bubble increases, the distending pressure necessary to hold the bubble open decreases, or (2) the opposite—when the size of the bubble decreases, the distending pressure of the bubble increases (Figure 2–16). Because of this interesting physical phenomenon, when two different size bubbles—having the same surface tension—are in direct communication, the greater pressure in the smaller bubble will cause the smaller bubble to empty into the larger bubble (Figure 2–17).

During the formation of a new bubble (e.g., a soap bubble blown on the end of a tube), the principles of Laplace's law do not come into effect until the distending pressure of the liquid sphere goes beyond what is called the *critical opening pressure*. As shown in Figure 2–18, the critical opening pressure is the high pressure (with little volume change) that is initially required to overcome the liquid molecular force during the formation of a new bubble—similar to the high pressure first required to blow up a new balloon. Figure 2–18 also shows that, prior to the critical

Figure 2–15

Bubbles A and B are the same size. The surface tension (ST) of bubble A is 10 dynes/cm and requires a distending pressure (P) of 5 cm H_2O to maintain its size. The surface tension of bubble B is 20 dynes/cm H_2O (twice that of bubble A) and requires a distending pressure of 10 cm H_2O (twice that of bubble A) to maintain its size (r = radius).

$$P = \frac{4\,ST}{r}$$

ST = 10 dynes/cm

Bubble A
Distending Pressure
5 cm H_2O

ST = 20 dynes/cm

Bubble B
Distending Pressure
10 cm H_2O

Figure 2–16

The surface tension (ST) of bubbles A and B is identical. The radius (r) of bubble A is 2 cm, and it requires a distending pressure (P) of 5 cm H_2O to maintain its size. The radius of bubble B is 1 cm (one-half that of bubble A), and it requires a distending pressure of 10 cm H_2O (twice that of bubble A) to maintain its size.

$$P = \frac{4\,ST}{r}$$

r = 1 cm

r = 2 cm

Bubble A
Distending Pressure
5 cm H_2O

Bubble B
Distending Pressure
10 cm H_2O

opening pressure, the distending pressure must progressively increase to enlarge the size of the bubble. In other words, the distending pressure is *directly proportional* to the radius of the bubble (the opposite of what Laplace's law states).

Once the critical opening pressure is reached, however, the distending pressure progressively decreases as the bubble increases in size—the

Figure 2–17

Bubbles A and B have the same surface tension. When the two bubbles are in direct communication, the higher pressure in the smaller bubble **(A)** causes it to empty into the large bubble **(B).**

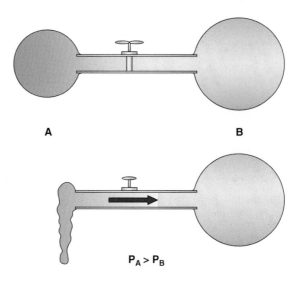

A   B

$P_A > P_B$

Figure 2–18

(A) Model showing the formation of a new liquid bubble at the end of a tube. **(B)** Graph showing the distending pressure required to maintain the bubble's size (volume) at various stages. Initially, a very high pressure, providing little volume change, is required to inflate the bubble. Once the critical opening pressure (same as critical closing pressure) is reached, however, the distending pressure progressively decreases as the size of the bubble increases. Thus, between the critical opening pressure and the point at which the bubble ruptures, the bubble behaves according to Laplace's law. Laplace's law applies to the normal functional size range of the bubble.

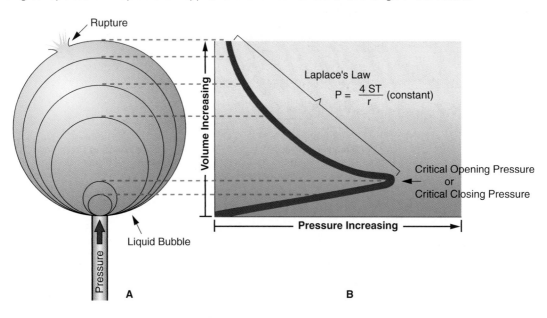

Rupture

Laplace's Law

$$P = \frac{4\,ST}{r} \text{ (constant)}$$

Volume Increasing

Critical Opening Pressure
or
Critical Closing Pressure

Pressure Increasing

Liquid Bubble

Pressure

A   B

distending pressure, as described by Laplace's law, is *inversely proportional* to the radius of the bubble. The distending pressure will continue to decrease until the bubble enlarges to its breaking point and ruptures. It is interesting to note that just before the bubble breaks, the distending pressure is at its lowest level (see Figure 2–18).

Conversely, Laplace's law shows that as an inflated bubble decreases in size, the distending pressure proportionally increases until the pressure reaches what is called the *critical closing pressure* (actually the same pressure as the critical opening pressure). When the size of the bubble decreases beyond this point, the liquid molecular force of the bubble becomes greater than the distending pressure and the bubble collapses (see Figure 2–18).

It should be emphasized that *Laplace's law does not state that the surface tension varies with the size of the bubble.* To the contrary, the law shows that as a liquid bubble changes in size, it is the *distending pressure,* not the *surface tension,* that varies inversely with the radius. In fact, as the radius of the sphere increases, the surface tension remains the same until the size of the bubble goes beyond its natural elastic limit and ruptures.

The fact that the surface tension remains the same while the radius of a liquid sphere changes can be illustrated mathematically by rearranging Laplace's law as follows:

1. Because surface tension is a property of the fluid and is constant for any specific fluid, Laplace's law can be restated as:

$$P = \frac{k}{r}$$

   where k is a constant (in this case, the constant k equals surface tension) and P (pressure) is inversely proportional to r (radius).

2. The equation $P = k \div r$ can be rearranged as follows:

$$Pr = k$$

   The formula now shows that the variable quantities (Pr) are inversely proportional and that their product is a constant (k). Thus, as one variable increases, the other must decrease to maintain a constant product (k).

   To demonstrate this concept, consider taking a 400-mile automobile trip. With the formula distance = rate × time (d = rt), which represents product (d) and variable quantities (rt), we have:

   $$400 = rt \ (d = 400 \text{ miles})$$

   or

   $$\frac{400}{r} = t$$

On such a trip, assume that we travel at 50 miles per hour (mph) and that the trip takes 8 hours (400 ÷ 50 = 8). If we travel by train and

Figure 2–19

Rate and time are inversely proportional (as rate increases, time decreases; and as rate decreases, time increases).

increase the speed to 100 mph, the time of the trip decreases to 4 hours. If, however, we decrease the speed to 25 mph, the time increases to 16 hours (400 ÷ 25 = 16). In other words, as the speed increases the time decreases and vice versa, but the product (d) remains a constant 400 miles, which is determined by the length of the trip.

3. Thus, when two variables are inversely proportional, such as rt = 400 or t = 400 ÷ r, the time increases as the rate decreases, and time decreases as the rate increases (Figure 2–19). Note the similarity of the graph in Figure 2–19 to the portion of the graph that represents Laplace's law in Figure 2–18B.

Laplace's Law Applied to the Alveolar Fluid Lining

Because the liquid film that lines the alveolus resembles a bubble or sphere, according to Laplace's law, when the alveolar fluid is permitted to behave according to its natural tendency, a high transpulmonary pressure must be generated to keep the small alveoli open (see Figure 2–18). Fortunately, in the healthy lung the natural tendency for the smaller alveoli to collapse is offset by a fascinating substance called pulmonary surfactant.

How Pulmonary Surfactant Regulates Alveolar Surface Tension

Pulmonary surfactant is an important and complex substance that is produced and stored in the alveolar type II cells (see Figure 1–26). It is composed of **phospholipids** (about 90 percent) and **protein** (about

10 percent). The primary surface tension-lowering chemical in pulmonary surfactant is the phospholipid **dipalmitoyl phosphatidylcholine (DPPC)**. The DPPC molecule has both a *hydrophobic* (water-insoluble) end and a *hydrophilic* (water-soluble) end. This unique hydrophobic/hydrophilic structure causes the DPPC molecule to position itself at the alveolar gas liquid interface so that the hydrophilic end is toward the liquid phase and the hydrophobic end is toward the gas phase. Pulmonary surfactant at the alveolar liquid–gas interface can profoundly lower alveolar surface tension.

The DPPC molecule at the alveolar gas–liquid interface causes surface tension to decrease in proportion to its ratio to alveolar surface area. That is, when the alveolus decreases in size (exhalation), the proportion of DPPC to the alveolar surface area increases. This, in turn, increases the effect of the DPPC molecules and causes the alveolar surface tension to decrease (Figure 2–20A).

Figure 2–20

In the normal lung, the surface tension is low in the small alveolus **(A)** because the ratio of surfactant to alveolar surface is high. As the alveolus enlarges **(B)**, the surface tension steadily increases because the ratio of surfactant to alveolar surface decreases.

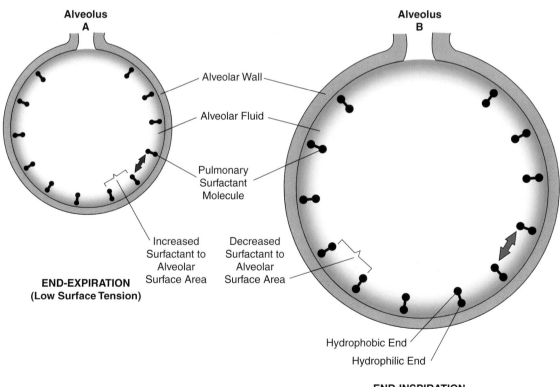

Alveolus
A

Alveolus
B

Alveolar Wall

Alveolar Fluid

Pulmonary
Surfactant
Molecule

Increased
Surfactant to
Alveolar
Surface Area

Decreased
Surfactant to
Alveolar
Surface Area

END-EXPIRATION
(Low Surface Tension)

Hydrophobic End

Hydrophilic End

END-INSPIRATION
(High Surface Tension)

In contrast, when the alveolus increases in size (inhalation), the relative amount of DPPC to the alveolar surface area decreases (because the number of surfactant molecules does not change when the size of the alveolus changes), which decreases the effect of the DPPC molecules and causes the alveolar surface tension to increase (Figure 2–20B). In fact, as the alveolus enlarges, the surface tension will progressively increase to the value it would naturally have in the absence of pulmonary surfactant. Clinically, however, the fact that surface tension increases as the alveolus enlarges is not significant because according to Laplace's law, the distending pressure required to maintain the size of a bubble progressively decreases as the size of the bubble increases (see Figure 2–18).

It is estimated that the surface tension of the average alveolus varies from 5 to 15 dynes/cm (when the alveolus is very small) to about 50 dynes/cm (when the alveolus is fully distended) (Figure 2–21). Because pulmonary surfactant has the ability to reduce the surface tension of the small alveoli, the high distending pressure that would otherwise be required to offset the critical closing pressure of the small alveoli is virtually eliminated.

In the absence of pulmonary surfactant, however, the alveolar surface tension increases to the level it would naturally have (50 dynes/cm), and the distending pressure necessary to overcome the recoil forces of the liquid film coating the small alveoli is very high. In short, the distending pressure required to offset the recoil force of the alveolar fluid behaves according to Laplace's law. As a result, when the distending pressure of the small alveoli falls below the critical closing pressure, the liquid molecular force pulls the alveolar walls together (see Figure 2–18). Once the liquid walls of the alveolus come into contact with one another, a liquid bond develops that strongly resists the re-expansion of the alveolus. Complete alveolar collapse is called **atelectasis**.

Table 2–1 lists some respiratory disorders that cause pulmonary surfactant deficiency.

Summary of the Elastic Properties of the Lungs

There are two major elastic forces in the lungs that cause an inflated lung to recoil inward: (1) the elastic properties of the lungs and (2) the surface tension of the liquid film that lines the alveoli.

In the healthy lung, both the elastic tension and the degree of surface tension are low in the small alveoli. As the alveoli increase in size, both the elastic tension and the degree of surface tension progressively increase. The elastic tension, however, is the predominant force, particularly in the large alveoli (Figure 2–22).

In the absence of pulmonary surfactant, the alveolar fluid lining behaves according to Laplace's law—that is, a high intrapleural pressure must be generated to keep the small alveoli open. When such a condition exists, the surface tension force predominates in the small alveoli (see Figure 2–22).

Figure 2–21

In the normal lung, the surface tension force progressively increases as the alveolar size increases. Similarly, as the alveolar size decreases, the surface tension force progressively decreases. Note that because of the alveolar surface tension, the actual physical change of the alveolus lags behind the pressure applied to it. When such a phenomenon occurs in the field of physics (i.e., a physical manifestation lagging behind a force), a hysteresis is said to exist. When this lung characteristic is plotted on a volume-pressure curve, the alveolus is shown to deflate along a different curve than that inscribed during inspiration and the curve has a looplike appearance. The hysteresis loop shows graphically that at any given pressure the alveolar volume is less during inspiration than it is during expiration. This alveolar hysteresis is virtually eliminated when the lungs are inflated experimentally with saline; such an experimental procedure removes the alveolar liquid–gas interface and, therefore, the alveolar surface tension. Inspiratory capacity is the volume of air that can be inhaled after a normal exhalation. Functional residual capacity is the volume of air remaining in the lungs after a normal exhalation.

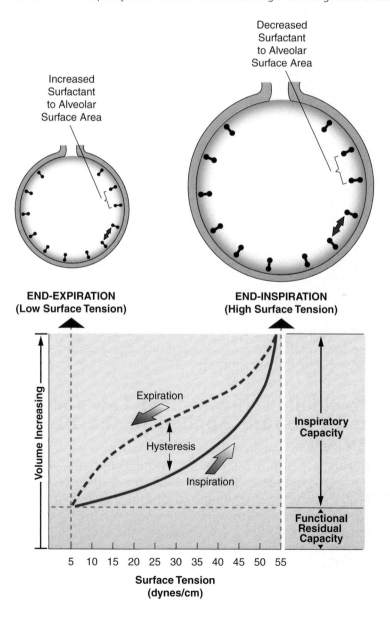

See page 119

TABLE 2–1
Causes of Pulmonary Surfactant Deficiency

General Causes

Acidosis
Hypoxia
Hyperoxia
Atelectasis
Pulmonary vascular congestion

Specific Causes

Acute respiratory distress syndrome (ARDS)
Infant respiratory distress syndrome (IRDS)
Pulmonary edema
Pulmonary embolism
Pneumonia
Excessive pulmonary lavage or hydration
Drowning
Extracorporeal oxygenation

DYNAMIC CHARACTERISTICS OF THE LUNGS

The term **dynamic** refers to the study of forces in action. In the lungs, dynamic refers to the movement of gas in and out of the lungs and the pressure changes required to move the gas. The dynamic features of the lung are best explained by (1) Poiseuille's law for flow and pressure and (2) the airway resistance equation.

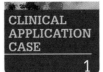

CLINICAL
APPLICATION
CASE

1

Poiseuille's (Pwah-Sōy) Law for Flow and Pressure Applied to the Bronchial Airways

During a normal inspiration, intrapleural pressure decreases from its normal resting level (about −3 to −6 cm H_2O pressure), which causes the bronchial airways to lengthen and to increase in diameter *(passive dilation)*. During expiration, intrapleural pressure increases (or returns to its normal resting state), which causes the bronchial airways to decrease in length and in diameter *(passive constriction)* (Figure 2–23). Under normal circumstances, these anatomic changes of the bronchial airways are not remarkable. In certain respiratory disorders (e.g., emphysema, chronic

Figure 2–22

In the normal lung, both the surface tension force **(A)** and the elastic force **(B)** progressively increase as the alveolus enlarges. The elastic force is the predominant force in both the small and the large alveoli. In the absence of pulmonary surfactant, the surface tension force **(C)** predominates in the small alveoli. The elastic force **(B)** still predominates in the large alveoli. Note that, as the alveolus enlarges, the pressure required to offset the "abnormal" surface tension force **(C)** ultimately decreases to the same pressure required to offset the "normal" surface tension force **(B)**. Thus, it can be seen that when there is a deficiency of pulmonary surfactant, the surface tension of the small alveoli creates a high recoil force. If a high pressure is not generated to offset this surface tension force, the alveoli will collapse.

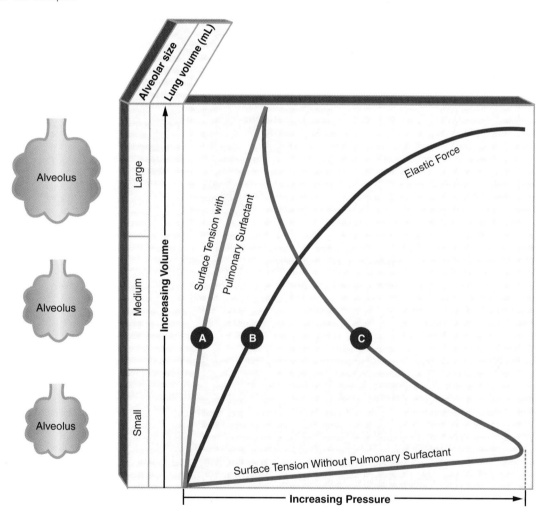

bronchitis), however, bronchial gas flow and intrapleural pressure may change significantly, particularly during expiration, when passive constriction of the tracheobronchial tree occurs. The reason for this is best explained in the relationship of factors described in Poiseuille's law. Poiseuille's law can be arranged for either flow or pressure.

Figure 2–23

During inspiration, the bronchial airways lengthen and increase in diameter. During expiration, the bronchial airways decrease in length and diameter.

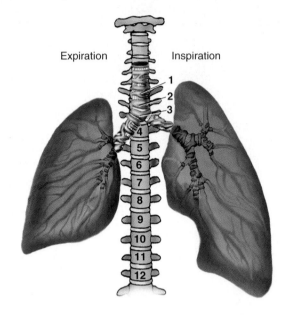

Poiseuille's Law Arranged for Flow

When Poiseuille's law is arranged for flow, it is written as follows:

$$\dot{V} = \frac{\Delta P r^4 \, \pi}{8 l \eta}$$

where η = the viscosity of a gas (or fluid), ΔP = the change of pressure from one end of the tube to the other, r = the radius of the tube, l = the length of the tube, $\dot{V}$ = the gas (or fluid) flowing through the tube; π and 8 = constants, which will be excluded from the discussion.

The equation states that flow is directly proportional to P and r^4 and inversely proportional to l and η. In other words, flow will decrease in response to decreased P and tube radius, and flow will increase in response to decreased tube length and fluid viscosity. Conversely, flow will increase in response to an increased P and tube radius and decrease in response to an increased tube length and fluid viscosity.

It should be emphasized that flow is profoundly affected by the radius of the tube. As Poiseuille's law illustrates, $\dot{V}$ is a function of the fourth power of the radius (r^4). In other words, assuming that pressure (P) remains constant, decreasing the radius of a tube by one-half reduces the gas flow to 1/16 of its original flow.

For example, if the radius of a bronchial tube through which gas flows at a rate of 16 milliliters per second (mL/sec) is reduced to one-half its

Figure 2–24

Poiseuille's law for flow applied to a bronchial airway with its radius reduced 50 percent.

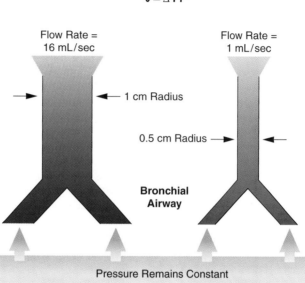

$$\dot{V} \approx \Delta \, Pr^4$$

Flow Rate = 16 mL/sec

Flow Rate = 1 mL/sec

1 cm Radius

0.5 cm Radius

Bronchial Airway

Pressure Remains Constant

original size because of mucosal swelling, the flow rate through the bronchial tube would decrease to 1 mL/sec (1/16 the original flow rate) (Figure 2–24).

Similarly, decreasing a tube radius by 16 percent decreases gas flow to one-half its original rate. For instance, if the radius of a bronchial tube through which gas flows at a rate of 16 mL/sec is decreased by 16 percent (because of mucosal swelling, for example), the flow rate through the bronchial tube would decrease to 8 mL/sec (one-half the original flow rate) (Figure 2–25).

Poiseuille's Law Arranged for Pressure

When Poiseuille's law is arranged for pressure, it is written as follows:

$$P = \frac{\dot{V}8l\eta}{r^4\pi}$$

The equation now states that pressure is directly proportional to $\dot{V}$, l, and η and inversely proportional to r^4. In other words, pressure will increase in response to a decreased tube radius and decrease in response to a decreased flow rate, tube length, or viscosity. The opposite is also true: pressure will decrease in response to an increased tube radius and increase in response to an increased flow rate, tube length, or viscosity.

Pressure is a function of the radius to the fourth power (r^4) and therefore is profoundly affected by the radius of a tube. In other words, if flow ($\dot{V}$) remains constant, then decreasing a tube radius to one-half of its previous size requires an increase in pressure to 16 times its original level.

Figure 2–25
Poiseuille's law for flow applied to a bronchial airway with its radius reduced 16 percent.

$$\dot{V} \approx \Delta Pr^4$$

Flow Rate =
16 mL/sec

Flow Rate =
8 mL/sec

1 cm Radius

0.84 cm Radius

**Bronchial
Airway**

Pressure Remains Constant

If the radius of a bronchial tube with a driving pressure of 1 cm H_2O is reduced to one-half its original size because of mucosal swelling, the driving pressure through the bronchial tube would have to increase to 16 cm H_2O ($16 \times 1 = 16$) to maintain the same flow rate (Figure 2–26).

Similarly, decreasing the bronchial tube radius by 16 percent increases the pressure to twice its original level. For instance, if the radius of a bronchial tube with a driving pressure of 10 cm H_2O is decreased by 16 percent because of mucosal swelling, the driving pressure through the bronchial tube would have to increase to 20 cm H_2O (twice its original pressure) to maintain the same flow (Figure 2–27).

Poiseuille's Law Rearranged to Simple Proportionalities

When Poiseuille's law is applied to the tracheobronchial tree during spontaneous breathing, the two equations can be rewritten as simple proportionalities:

$$\dot{V} \approx Pr^4$$

$$P \approx \frac{\dot{V}}{r^4}$$

Based on the proportionality for flow, it can be stated that because gas flow varies directly with r^4 of the bronchial airway, flow must diminish during exhalation because the radius of the bronchial airways decreases. Stated differently, assuming that the pressure remains constant as the

Figure 2–26

Poiseuille's law for pressure applied to a bronchial airway with its radius reduced 50 percent.

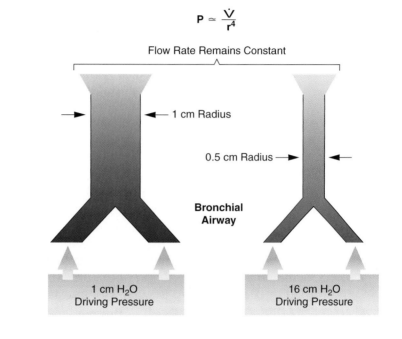

$$P \simeq \frac{\dot{V}}{r^4}$$

Flow Rate Remains Constant

1 cm Radius

0.5 cm Radius

Bronchial
Airway

1 cm H_2O
Driving Pressure

16 cm H_2O
Driving Pressure

Figure 2–27

Poiseuille's law for pressure applied to a bronchial airway with its radius reduced 16 percent.

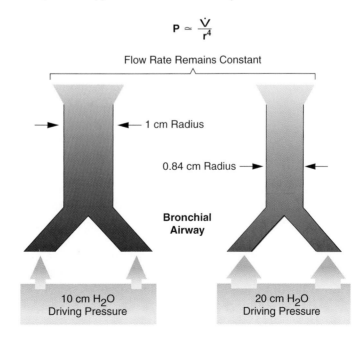

$$P \simeq \frac{\dot{V}}{r^4}$$

Flow Rate Remains Constant

1 cm Radius

0.84 cm Radius

Bronchial
Airway

10 cm H_2O
Driving Pressure

20 cm H_2O
Driving Pressure

radius (r) of the bronchial airways decreases, gas flow ($\dot{V}$) also decreases. During normal spontaneous breathing, however, the reduction in gas flow during exhalation is negligible.

In terms of the proportionality for pressure ($P \approx \dot{V} \div r^4$), if gas flow is to remain constant during exhalation, then the transthoracic pressure must vary inversely with the fourth power of the radius (r^4) of the airway. In other words, as the radius of the bronchial airways decreases during exhalation, the driving pressure must increase to maintain a constant gas flow.*

During normal spontaneous breathing, the need to increase the trans-airway pressure during exhalation in order to maintain a certain gas flow is not significant. However, in certain respiratory disorders (e.g., emphysema, bronchitis, asthma), gas flow reductions and transthoracic pressure increases may be substantial as a result of the bronchial narrowing that develops in such disorders.

Airway Resistance

Airway resistance (R_{aw}) is defined as the pressure difference between the mouth and the alveoli (*transairway pressure*) divided by flow rate. In other words, the rate at which a certain volume of gas flows through the bronchial airways is a function of the pressure gradient and the resistance created by the airways to the flow of gas. Mathematically, R_{aw} is measured in centimeters of water per liter per second (L/sec), according to the following equation:

$$R_{aw} = \frac{\Delta P (\text{cm H}_2\text{O})}{\dot{V}(\text{L/sec})}$$

For example, if an individual produces a flow rate of 4 L/sec during inspiration by generating a transairway pressure of 4 cm H_2O, then R_{aw} would equal 1 cm H_2O/L/sec:

$$R_{aw} = \frac{\Delta P}{\dot{V}}$$

$$= \frac{4 \text{ cm H}_2\text{O}}{4 \text{ L/sec}}$$

$$= 1 \text{ cm H}_2\text{O/L/sec}$$

Normally, the R_{aw} in the tracheobronchial tree is about 0.5 to 1.5 cm H_2O/L/sec in adults. In patients with COPD (e.g., chronic bronchitis), however, R_{aw} may be very high (Figure 2–28). The value of R_{aw} is also much higher in newborn infants than in normal adults (see Chapter 10).

The movement of gas through a tube (or bronchial airway) can be classified as (1) laminar flow, (2) turbulent flow, or (3) a combination of laminar flow and turbulent flow—called tracheobronchial flow or transitional flow (Figure 2–29).

*See mathematical discussion of Poiseuille's law in Appendix III.

Figure 2–28

Chronic bronchitis. Pathology includes (1) inflammation and swelling of the peripheral airways, (2) excessive mucus production and accumulation, and (3) alveolar hyperinflation.

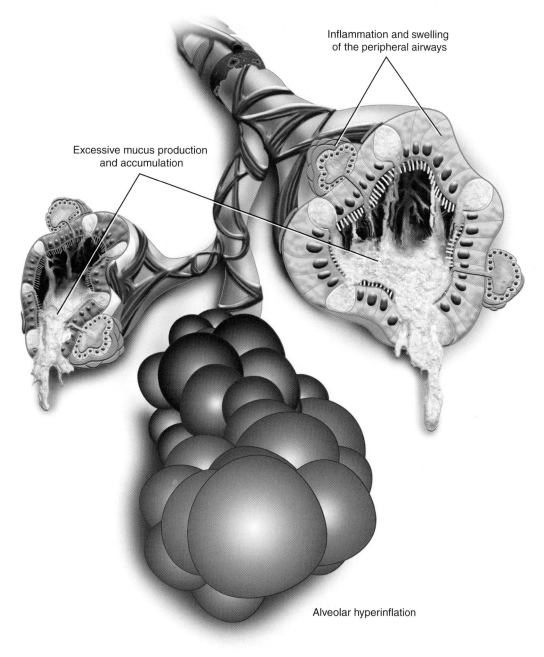

Inflammation and swelling
of the peripheral airways

Excessive mucus production
and accumulation

Alveolar hyperinflation

Figure 2–29
Types of gas flow.

Laminar

Turbulent

Laminar Flow

Laminar gas flow refers to a gas flow that is streamlined. The gas molecules move through the tube in a pattern parallel to the sides of the tube. This flow pattern occurs at low flow rates and at low pressure gradients.

Turbulent Flow

Turbulent gas flow refers to gas molecules that move through a tube in a random manner. Gas flow encounters resistance from both the sides of the tube and from the collision with other gas molecules. This flow pattern occurs at high flow rates and at high pressure gradients.

Tracheobronchial or Transitional Flow

Tracheobronchial gas flow occurs in the areas where the airways branch. Depending on the anatomic structure of the branching airways, and the velocity of gas flow, either laminar flow or turbulent flow may predominate.

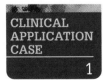

CLINICAL
APPLICATION
CASE

1

See page 119

Time Constants

A product of airway resistance (R_{aw}) and lung compliance (C_L) is a phenomenon called **time constant**. Time constant is defined as the time (in seconds) necessary to inflate a particular lung region to about 60 percent* of its potential filling capacity. Lung regions that have either an increased

Technically, 63 percent.

R_{aw} or an increased C_L require more time to inflate. These alveoli are said to have a *long time constant.* In contrast, lung regions that have either a decreased R_{aw} or a decreased C_L require less time to inflate. These alveoli are said to have a *short time constant.*

Mathematically, the time constant (T_C) is expressed as follows:

$$T_C \text{ (sec)} = \underbrace{\frac{\Delta P(\text{cm } H_2O)}{\dot{V}(\text{L/sec})}}_{(R_{aw})} \times \underbrace{\frac{\Delta V(\text{L})}{\Delta P(\text{cm } H_2O)}}_{(C_L)}$$

$$= \frac{\text{cm } H_2O \times L}{\text{L/sec} \times \text{cm } H_2O}$$

This equation shows that as R_{aw} increases, the value for pressure (P, in cm H_2O) in the numerator increases. Or, when C_L decreases, the value for volume (V) in liters (L) in the numerator decreases.

Thus, assuming that all other variables remain constant, if the R_{aw} of a specific lung region doubles, then the time constant will also double (i.e., the lung unit will take twice as long to inflate). In contrast, if the C_L is reduced by half, then the time constant will also be reduced by half—and, importantly, the potential filling capacity of the lung region is also reduced by half. To help illustrate this concept, consider the time constants illustrated in Figure 2–30.

In Figure 2–30A, two alveolar units have identical R_{aw} and C_L. Thus, the two alveoli require the same amount of time to inflate—they have the same time constants. Figure 2–30B shows two alveolar units with the same R_{aw} but with two different C_L. Because the C_L in unit B is one-half the C_L of unit A, unit B (low compliance) receives one-half the volume of unit A (high compliance). It is important to realize that (1) unit B has a shorter time constant than unit A, and (2) unit B receives only one-half the volume received by unit A.

In Figure 2–30C, the two alveolar units have the same compliance, but two different R_{aw}. Because the R_{aw} leading to unit B is twice the R_{aw} leading to unit A, unit B (high R_{aw}) requires twice the time to fill to the same volume as unit A (low R_{aw}). It is important to note that the two alveolar units do not have the same time constant—the time constant for unit B is twice that of unit A. Thus, it is also important to note that as the breathing frequency increases, the time necessary to fill unit B may not be adequate. Clinically, how readily a lung region fills with gas during a specific time period is called **dynamic compliance**.

Dynamic Compliance

CLINICAL
APPLICATION
CASE

1

See page 119

The measurement called dynamic compliance is a product of the time constants. Dynamic compliance is defined as the change in the volume of the lungs divided by the change in the transpulmonary pressure (obtained via a partially swallowed esophageal pressure balloon) during the time required for one breath. Dynamic compliance is distinctively different from the lung compliance (C_L) defined earlier in this chapter as the change in

Figure 2–30

Time constants for hypothetical alveoli with differing lung compliances (C_L), supplied by airways with differing resistances (R_{aw}).

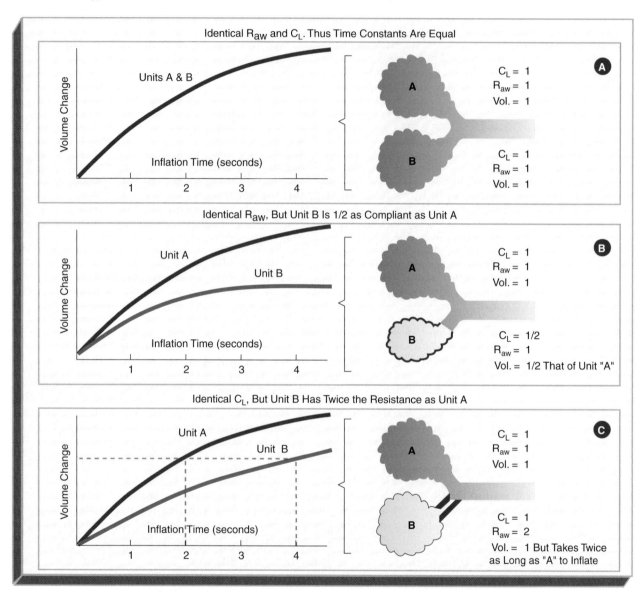

lung volume (ΔV) per unit pressure change (ΔP) (see Figure 2–10). In short, lung compliance is determined during a period of no gas flow, whereas dynamic compliance is measured during a period of gas flow.

In the healthy lung, the dynamic compliance is about equal to lung compliance at all breathing frequencies (the ratio of dynamic compliance to lung compliance is 1:1) (Figure 2–31).

Figure 2–31

Dynamic compliance/lung compliance ratio at different breathing frequencies. In normal individuals there is essentially no ratio change. In individuals with obstructive disorders, however, the ratio decreases dramatically as the respiratory rate increases.

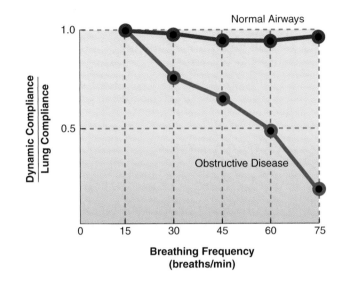

In patients with partially obstructed airways, however, the ratio of dynamic compliance to lung compliance falls significantly as the breathing frequency rises (see Figure 2–31). In other words, the alveoli distal to the obstruction do not have enough time to fill to their potential filling capacity as the breathing frequency increases. The compliance of such alveoli is said to be **frequency dependent**.

Auto PEEP and Its Relationship to R_{aw} During Rapid Ventilatory Rates

During rapid ventilatory rates, small airways with high R_{aw} may not have sufficient time to fully deflate during exhalation. The pressure in the alveoli distal to these airways may still be positive when the next inspiration begins. **Positive end-expiratory pressure** (PEEP) caused by inadequate expiratory time is called **auto-PEEP** (also called air trapping, intrinsic PEEP, occult PEEP, inadvertent PEEP, and covert PEEP). Auto-PEEP increases a patient's *work of breathing* (WOB) in two ways:

1. As a result of auto-PEEP, the patient's *functional residual capacity* (FRC) increases (see Chapter 4). When the FRC increases, the patient is forced to breathe at a higher, less compliant, point on the *volume-pressure curve* (see Figure 2–10). Thus, air trapping and alveolar hyperinflation (auto-PEEP) decrease lung compliance, causing the WOB to increase.

2. When auto-PEEP produces air trapping and alveolar hyperinflation, the patient's diaphragm is pushed downward; this causes the patient's inspiratory efforts to become less efficient, causing WOB to increase. Normally, an individual needs to create an inspiratory effort that causes the alveolar pressure (P_A) to decrease −1 or 2 cm H_2O below the ambient pressure to have air to flow into the alveoli. When auto-PEEP is present, the P_A is higher than the ambient pressure at the beginning of inspiration. For example, if as a result of auto-PEEP the P_A is +4 cm H_2O (above atmospheric pressure), then the inspiratory effort must decrease the P_A more than 4 cm H_2O before gas can start to flow into the lungs, requiring increased WOB.

VENTILATORY PATTERNS

The Normal Ventilatory Pattern

The ventilatory pattern consists of (1) the tidal volume (V_T), (2) the ventilatory rate, and (3) the time relationship between inhalation and exhalation (I:E ratio).

Tidal volume is defined as the volume of air that normally moves into and out of the lungs in one quiet breath. Normally, V_T is about 7 to 9 mL/kg (3 to 4 mL/lb) of ideal body weight. The normal adult ventilatory rate is about 15 breaths per minute. The I:E ratio is usually about 1:2. That is, the time required to inhale a normal breath is about one-half the time required to exhale the same breath.

Technically, however, the time required to inhale and exhale while at rest is about equal (a 1:1 ratio) in terms of "true" gas flow. The reason exhalation is considered twice as long as inhalation in the I:E ratio is that the ratio includes the normal pause, during which there is no gas flow, that typically occurs at end-expiration as part of the exhalation phase (Figure 2–32).

This normal pause that occurs at end-exhalation is usually about equal, in terms of time, to either the inspiratory or expiratory phase. Thus, when an individual is at rest, the time required for a normal ventilatory cycle consists of approximately three equal phases: (1) the inspiratory phase, (2) the expiratory phase, and (3) the pause phase at end-expiration (see Figure 2–32).

Alveolar Ventilation versus Dead space Ventilation

Only the inspired air that reaches the alveoli is effective in terms of gas exchange. This portion of the inspired gas is referred to as **alveolar ventilation**. The volume of inspired air that does not reach the alveoli is not effective. This portion of gas is referred to as **dead space ventilation**

Figure 2–32
Normal, spontaneous breathing (eupnea). The I : E ratio typically is 1 : 2.

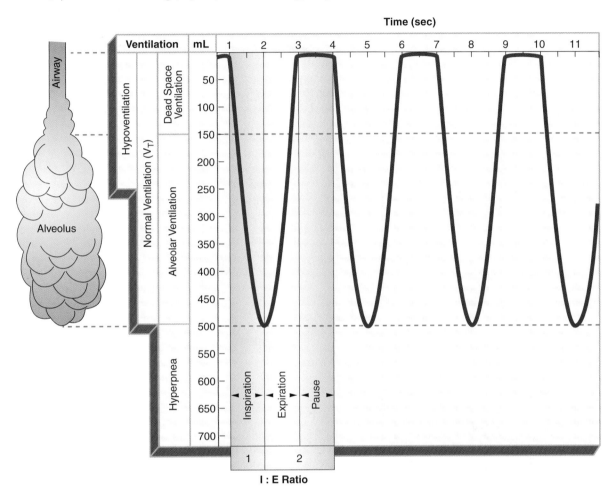

(Figure 2–33). There are three types of dead space: (1) **anatomic**, (2) **alveolar**, and (3) **physiologic**.

Anatomic Dead Space

Anatomic dead space is the volume of gas in the conducting airways: the nose, mouth, pharynx, larynx, and lower airways down to, but not including, the respiratory bronchioles. The volume of anatomic dead space is approximately equal to 1 mL/lb (2.2 mL/kg) of "idea" body weight. Thus, if an individual weighs 150 pounds, approximately 150 mL of inspired gas would be anatomic dead space gas (or physiologically ineffective).

Figure 2–33
Dead space ventilation (V_D).

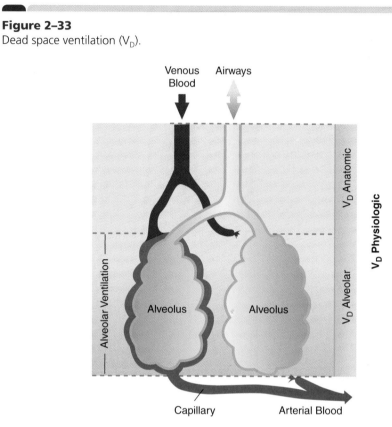

Dead Space Ventilation (V_D)

Moreover, because of the anatomic dead space, the gas that does enter the alveoli during each inspiration (alveolar ventilation) is actually a combination of (1) anatomic dead space gas (non-fresh gas) and (2) gas from the atmosphere (fresh gas). To visualize this, consider the inspiration and expiration of 450 mL (V_T) in an individual with an anatomic dead space of 150 mL (Figure 2–34).

Inspiration. As shown in Figure 2–34A, 150 mL of gas fill the anatomic dead space at pre-inspiration. This gas was the last 150 mL of gas to leave the alveoli during the previous exhalation. Thus, as shown in Figure 2–34B, the first 150 mL of gas to enter the alveoli during inspiration are from the anatomic dead space (non-fresh gas). The next 300 mL of gas to enter the alveoli are from the atmosphere (fresh gas). The last 150 mL of fresh gas inhaled fill the anatomic dead space (see Figure 2–34B). Thus, of the 450 mL of gas that enter the alveoli, 150 mL come from the conducting airways (non-fresh gas) and 300 mL come from the atmosphere (fresh gas).

Figure 2–34
Alveolar ventilation versus dead space ventilation during one ventilatory cycle.

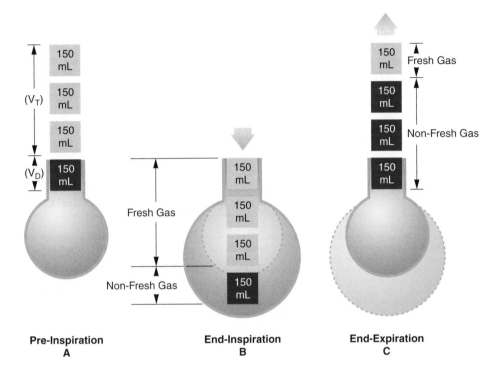

Expiration. As shown in Figure 2–34C, 450 mL of gas are forced out of the alveoli during expiration. The first 150 mL of gas exhaled are from the anatomic dead space. This gas was the last 150 mL that entered the conducting airways during the previous inspiration (see Figure 2–34B). The next 300 mL of gas exhaled come from the alveoli. The last 150 mL of gas to leave the alveoli fill the anatomic dead space. During the next inspiration, the last 150 mL of gas exhaled from the alveoli will, again, reenter the alveoli, thus diluting the oxygen concentration of any atmospheric gas that enters the alveoli (see Figure 2–34A).

Therefore, minute alveolar ventilation (V_A) is equal to the tidal volume (V_T) minus the dead space ventilation (V_D) multiplied by the breaths per minute (frequency):

$$\dot{V}_A = (V_T - V_D) \times \text{breaths/min}$$

For example, if:

$$V_T = 450 \text{ mL}$$

$$V_D = 150 \text{ mL}$$

$$\text{Breaths/min} = 12$$

then minute alveolar ventilation would be computed as follows:

$$\dot{V}_A = V_T - V_D \times \text{breaths/min}$$

$$= 450 \text{ mL} - 150 \text{ mL} \times 12$$

$$= 300 \times 12$$

$$= 3600 \text{ mL}$$

Finally, an individual's breathing pattern (depth and rate of breathing) can profoundly alter the total alveolar ventilation. For example, Table 2–2 shows three different subjects, each having a total minute ventilation (MV) of 6000 mL and each having an anatomic dead space volume of 150 mL. Each subject, however, has a different tidal volume and breathing frequency. Subject A has a tidal volume of 150 mL and a breathing frequency of 40 breaths/min. Even though gas rapidly moves in and out of the lungs, the actual alveolar ventilation is zero. Subject A is merely moving 150 mL of gas in and out of the anatomic dead space at a rate of 40 times per minute. Clinically, this subject would become unconscious in a few minutes.

Subject B has a tidal volume of 500 mL and a breathing frequency of 12 breaths/min. This subject has an alveolar ventilation of 4200 mL. Subject C has a tidal volume of 1000 mL and a frequency of 6 breaths/min. This subject has an alveolar ventilation of 5100 mL.

The important deduction to be drawn from Table 2–2 is that *an increased depth of breathing is far more effective than an equivalent increase in breathing rate in increasing an individual's total alveolar ventilation.* Or, conversely, a decreased depth of breathing can lead to a significant and, perhaps, a critical reduction of alveolar ventilation. This is because the anatomic dead space volume represents a fixed volume (normally about

TABLE 2–2

Effect of Breathing Depth and Frequency on Alveolar Ventilation

Subject	Breathing Depth (V_T) (mL)	Breathing Frequency (breaths/min)	Total MV* (mL/min)	V_D† (mL/min)	V_A‡ (mL/min)
A	150	40	6000	$150 \times 40 = 6000$	0
B	500	12	6000	$150 \times 12 = 1800$	4200
C	1000	6	6000	$150 \times 6 = 900$	5100

* Total alveolar ventilation, or minute ventilation (MV), is the product of breathing depth, or tidal volume (V_T), times breathing frequency, or breaths per minute.
† Total dead space ventilation (V_D) is the product of anatomic dead space volume (150 mL in each subject) times breathing frequency.
‡ V_A = alveolar ventilation.

one-third), and the fixed volume will make up a larger portion of a decreasing tidal volume. This fraction increases as the tidal volume decreases until, as demonstrated by subject A, it represents the entire tidal volume. On the other hand, any increase in the tidal volume beyond the anatomic dead space goes entirely toward increasing alveolar ventilation.

Alveolar Dead Space

Alveolar dead space occurs when an alveolus is ventilated but not perfused with pulmonary blood. Thus, the air that enters the alveolus is not effective in terms of gas exchange, because there is no pulmonary capillary blood flow. The amount of alveolar dead space is unpredictable.

Physiologic Dead Space

Physiologic dead space is the sum of the anatomic dead space and alveolar dead space. Because neither of these two forms of dead space is effective in terms of gas exchange, the two forms are combined and are referred to as physiologic dead space.

HOW NORMAL INTRAPLEURAL PRESSURE DIFFERENCES CAUSE REGIONAL DIFFERENCES IN NORMAL LUNG VENTILATION

As discussed earlier, the diaphragm moves air in and out of the lungs by changing the intrapleural and intra-alveolar pressures. Ordinarily, the intrapleural pressure is always below atmospheric pressure during both inspiration and expiration (see Figure 2–7).

The intrapleural pressure, however, is not evenly distributed within the thorax. In the normal individual in the upright position, there is a natural intrapleural pressure gradient from the upper lung region to the lower. The negative intrapleural pressure at the apex of the lung is normally greater (from −7 to −10 cm H_2O pressure) than at the base (from −2 to −3 cm H_2O pressure). This gradient is gravity dependent and is thought to be due to the normal weight distribution of the lungs above and below the hilum. In other words, because the lung is suspended from the hilum, and because the lung base weighs more than the apex (primarily due to the increased blood flow in the lung base), the lung base requires more pressure for support than does the lung apex. This causes the negative intrapleural pressure around the lung base to be less.

Because of the greater negative intrapleural pressure in the upper lung regions, the alveoli in those regions are expanded more than the alveoli in the lower regions. In fact, many of the alveoli in the upper lung regions may be close to, or at, their total filling capacity. This means, therefore, that the compliance of the alveoli in the upper lung regions is normally less than the compliance of the alveoli in the lower lung regions

Figure 2–35

Intrapleural pressure gradient in the upright position. The negative intrapleural pressure normally is greater in the upper lung regions compared with the lower lung regions. Because of this, the alveoli in the upper lung regions expand more than those in the lower lung regions. This condition causes alveolar compliance to be lower in the upper lung regions and ventilation to be greater in the lower lung regions.

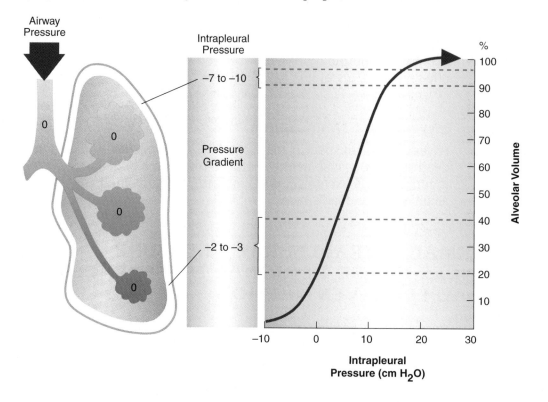

in the normal person in the upright position. As a result, during inspiration the alveoli in the upper lung regions are unable to accommodate as much gas as the alveoli in the lower lung regions. Thus, in the normal individual in the upright position, ventilation is usually much greater and more effective in the lower lung regions (Figure 2–35).

THE EFFECT OF AIRWAY RESISTANCE AND LUNG COMPLIANCE ON VENTILATORY PATTERNS

As already mentioned, the respiratory rate and tidal volume presented by an individual are known as the *ventilatory pattern*. The normal ventilatory pattern is a respiratory rate of about 15 breaths per minute and a tidal volume of about 500 mL. Although the precise mechanism is not clear, it is well documented that these ventilatory patterns frequently develop in response to changes in lung compliance and airway resistance.

When lung compliance decreases, the patient's ventilatory rate generally increases while, at the same time, the tidal volume decreases. When airway resistance increases, the patient's ventilatory frequency usually decreases while, at the same time, the tidal volume increases (Figure 2–36).

The ventilatory pattern is determined by both **ventilatory efficiency** (to minimize dead space ventilation) and **metabolic efficiency** (to minimize the work or oxygen cost of breathing). The body is assumed to adjust both rate and depth of breathing to give the best trade-off between the

Figure 2–36
The effects of increased airway resistance and decreased lung compliance on ventilatory frequency and tidal volume.

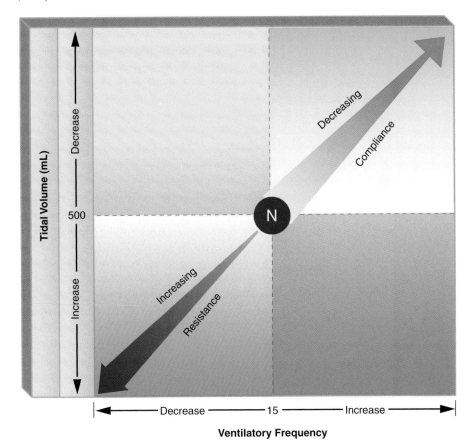

two. In severe cases, an increase in ventilation will ultimately reach a point in which the increase in oxygen delivery is exceeded by the increase in oxygen demanded by the respiratory muscles. In short, the ventilatory pattern adopted by a patient is based on minimum work requirements, rather than ventilatory efficiency.

In physics, work is defined as the force applied multiplied by the distance moved (work = force × distance). In respiratory physiology, the changes in transpulmonary pressure (force) multiplied by the change in lung volume (distance) may be used to quantitate the amount of work required to breathe (work = pressure × volume). Normally, about 5 percent of an individual's total energy output goes to the work of breathing.

Thus, because the patient may adopt a ventilatory pattern based on the **expenditure of energy** rather than the efficiency of ventilation, it cannot be assumed that the ventilatory pattern acquired by the patient in response to a certain respiratory disorder is the most efficient one in terms of physiologic gas exchange. Such ventilatory patterns are usually seen in the more severe pulmonary disorders that cause lung compliance to decrease or airway resistance to increase.

The patient's adopted ventilatory pattern is frequently modified in the clinical setting because of secondary heart or lung problems. For example, a patient with chronic emphysema, who has adopted a decreased ventilatory rate and an increased tidal volume because of increased R_{aw}, may demonstrate an increased ventilatory rate and a decreased tidal volume in response to a lung infection (pneumonia) that causes lung compliance to decrease.

OVERVIEW OF SPECIFIC BREATHING CONDITIONS

The following are types of breathing conditions frequently seen by the respiratory care practitioner in the clinical setting.

Apnea: Complete absence of spontaneous ventilation. This causes the $P_{A_{O_2}}$* and Pa_{O_2}[†] to rapidly decrease and the $P_{A_{CO_2}}$[‡] and Pa_{CO_2}[§] to increase. Death will ensue in minutes.

Eupnea: Normal, spontaneous breathing (see Figure 2–32).

Biot's breathing: Short episodes of rapid, uniformly deep inspirations, followed by 10 to 30 seconds of apnea (Figure 2–37).

*$P_{A_{O_2}}$ = *alveolar oxygen tension.*
[†]Pa_{O_2} = *arterial oxygen tension.*
[‡]$P_{A_{CO_2}}$ = *alveolar carbon dioxide tension.*
[§]Pa_{CO_2} = *arterial carbon dioxide tension.*

Figure 2–37

Biot's breathing: Short episodes of rapid, uniformly deep inspirations, followed by 10 to 30 seconds of apnea.

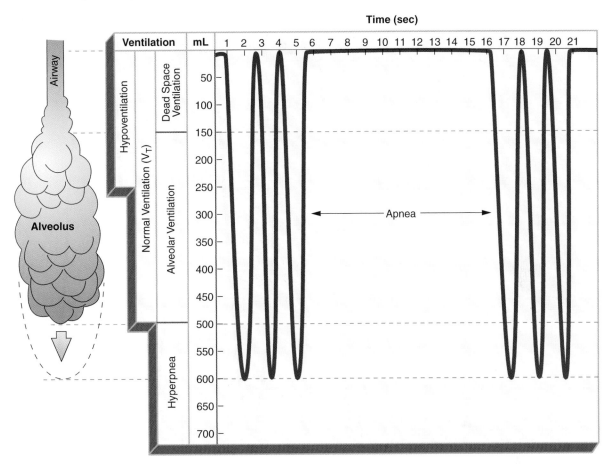

This pattern was first described in patients suffering from meningitis.

Hyperpnea: Increased depth (volume) of breathing with or without an increased frequency (Figure 2–38).

Hyperventilation: Increased alveolar ventilation (produced by any ventilatory pattern that causes an increase in either the ventilatory rate or the depth of breathing) that causes the $P_{A_{CO_2}}$ and, therefore, the Pa_{CO_2} to decrease (Figure 2–39).

Hypoventilation: Decreased alveolar ventilation (produced by any ventilatory pattern that causes a decrease in either the ventilatory

Figure 2–38
Hyperpnea: Increased depth of breathing.

rate or the depth of breathing) that causes the $P_{A_{CO_2}}$ and, therefore, the Pa_{CO_2} to increase (Figure 2–40) (page 116).

Tachypnea: A rapid rate of breathing.

Cheyne-Stokes breathing: Ten to 30 seconds of apnea, followed by a gradual increase in the volume and frequency of breathing, followed by a gradual decrease in the volume of breathing until another period of apnea occurs (Figure 2–41) (page 117). As the depth of breathing increases, the $P_{A_{O_2}}$ and Pa_{O_2} fall and the $P_{A_{CO_2}}$ and Pa_{CO_2} rise. Cheyne-Stokes breathing is associated with cerebral disorders and congested heart failure (CHF).

Figure 2–39

Hyperventilation: Increased rate **(A)** or depth **(B)**, or some combination of these, of breathing that causes the $P_{A_{CO_2}}$ and, therefore, the Pa_{CO_2} to decrease.

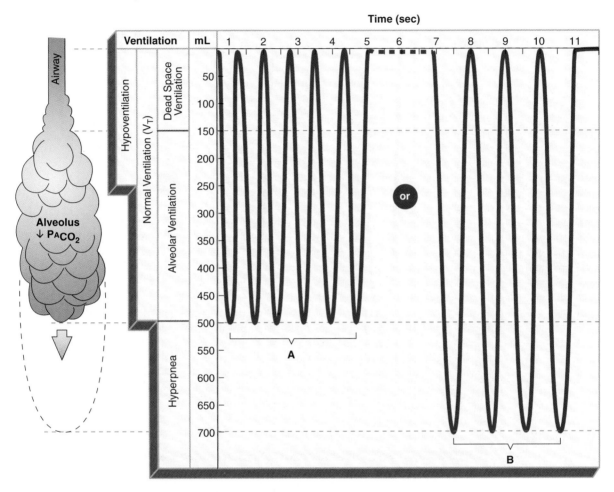

Kussmaul's breathing: Both an increased depth (hyperpnea) and rate of breathing (Figure 2–42) (page 118). This ventilatory pattern causes the $P_{A_{CO_2}}$ and Pa_{CO_2} to decline and the $P_{A_{O_2}}$ and Pa_{O_2} to increase. Kussmaul's breathing is commonly associated with diabetic acidosis (ketoacidosis).

Orthopnea: A condition in which an individual is able to breathe most comfortably only in the upright position.

Dyspnea: Difficulty in breathing, of which the individual is aware.

Figure 2–40

Hypoventilation: Decreased rate **(A)** or depth **(B)**, or some combination of both, of breathing that causes the $P_{A_{CO_2}}$ and, therefore, the Pa_{CO_2} to increase.

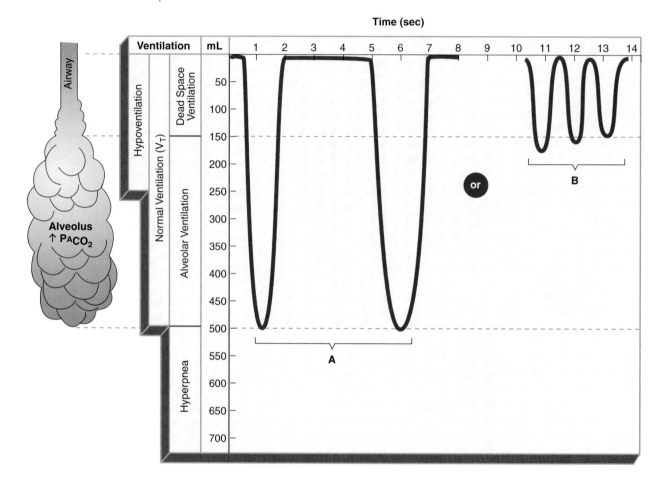

CHAPTER SUMMARY

The essential knowledge base for ventilation consists of four major areas. *First,* the respiratory practitioner must understand how the excursion of the diaphragm changes the intra-alveolar and intrapleural pressures. Important components of this subject are (1) the pressure differences across the lungs, including the driving pressure, transairway pressure, transmural pressure, transpulmonary pressure, and transthoracic pressure; (2) the role of the diaphragm in ventilation, (3) how the excursion of the diaphragm affects the intrapleural pressure, intra-alveolar pressure, and bronchial gas

Figure 2–41

Cheyne-Stokes breathing: A gradual increase and decrease in the volume and rate of breathing, followed by 10 to 30 seconds of apnea.

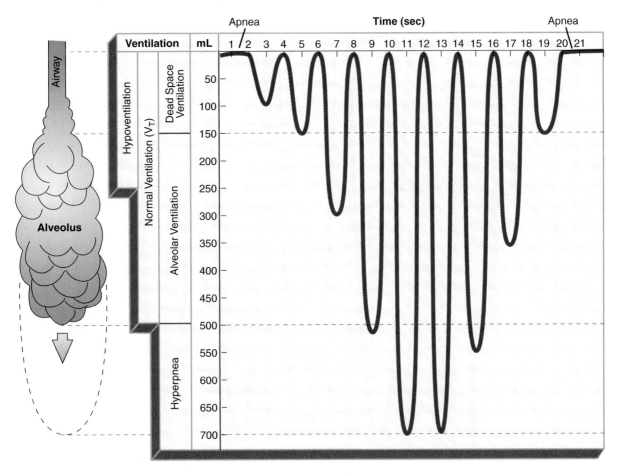

flow during inspiration, end-inspiration, expiration, and end-expiration. *Second,* the respiratory care practitioner must understand the elastic properties of the lungs. Major components of this subject include (1) lung compliance, including the calculation of lung compliance; (2) elastance, including Hooke's law; and (3) surface tension and its relationship to Laplace's law, pulmonary surfactant, and the deficiency of pulmonary surfactant.

Third, the practitioner must have a good understanding of the dynamic characteristics of the lungs. This important subject includes (1) how Poiseuille's law arranged for either flow or pressure relates to the radius of the bronchial airways; (2) airway resistance, including its calculation, and its relationship to laminar and turbulent flow; and (3) dynamic compliance and its relationship to increased airway resistance and frequency dependence. *Finally,* the respiratory care practitioner needs a good

Figure 2–42

Kussmaul's breathing: Increased rate and depth of breathing. This breathing pattern causes the PA_{CO_2} and Pa_{CO_2} to decrease and PA_{O_2} and Pa_{O_2} to increase.

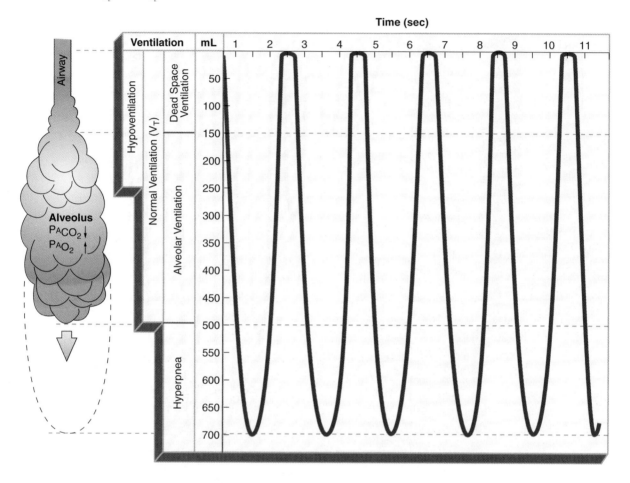

knowledge base of the characteristics of normal and abnormal ventilatory patterns. This subject consists of (1) knowing the meaning of the normal ventilatory pattern, including the tidal volume, ventilatory rate, and I:E ratio; (2) differentiating between alveolar ventilation and dead space ventilation; (3) knowing how the depth and rate of breathing affects alveolar ventilation; (4) being able to calculate an individual's alveolar ventilation; (5) understanding how the normal intrapleural pressure differences cause regional differences in normal lung ventilation; (6) knowing how the respiratory rate and tidal volume change in response to a decreased lung compliance or an increased airway resistance; and (7) the ability to recognize specific breathing conditions, such as Biot's breathing, hypoventilation, tachypnea, Cheyne-Stokes breathing, Kussmaul's breathing, orthopnea, and dyspnea.

1 CLINICAL APPLICATION CASE

This 14-year-old girl with a long history of asthma presented in the emergency department in moderate to severe respiratory distress. She appeared very frightened and tears were running down her face. She was sitting perched forward with her arms braced in a tripod-like position on the side of a gurney, hands clutching the edge of the gurney. She was using her accessory muscles of inspiration. When asked about her condition, she stated, "I can't get enough air." She could only speak two or three words at a time, between each breath.

The patient's skin appeared pale and bluish. She had a frequent and strong cough, productive of large amounts of thick, white secretions. Her vital signs were blood pressure—151/93 mm Hg, heart rate—106 beats/min and strong, and respiratory rate—32 breaths/min. Wheezes were heard over both lung fields. Chest x-ray showed that her lungs were hyperinflated and that her diaphragm was depressed. Her peripheral oxygen saturation level (Sp_{O_2}), measured by pulse oximetry over the skin of her index finger, was 89 percent (normal, 97 percent).

The respiratory therapist working in the emergency department started the patient on oxygen via a 6-liter (6 L/min) nasal cannula, and on a bronchodilator continuously, via a handheld aerosol. The therapist also remained at the patient's bedside to monitor the patient's response to treatment, and to encourage the patient to take slow, deep inspirations.

Forty-five minutes later, the patient had substantially improved. She was sitting up in bed and no longer appeared to be in respiratory distress. She could speak in longer sentences without getting short of breath. Her skin color was normal. Her vital signs were blood pressure—126/83 mm Hg, heart rate—87 beats/min, and respiratory rate—14 breaths/min.

When instructed to cough, she generated a strong, nonproductive cough. Although wheezes could still be heard over the patient's lungs, they were not as severe as they were on admission. A second chest x-ray showed that her lungs were normal and her diaphragm was no longer depressed. Her Sp_{O_2} was 94 percent.

DISCUSSION

This case illustrates (1) an acute decreased lung compliance condition, (2) how *Poiseuille's law* can be used to demonstrate the effects of bronchial constriction and excessive airway secretions on bronchial gas flow and the work of breathing, (3) the effects of an increased *airway resistance* (R_{aw}) on *time constants*, and (4) the *frequency-dependent* effects of a decreased ventilatory rate on the ventilation of alveoli.

As the severity of the tracheobronchial tree constriction progressively increased, the patient's ability to exhale fully declined. This process caused the patient's lungs to hyperinflate (but not with fresh air). As a result of the hyperinflation, the patient's work of breathing increased, because her lungs were functioning at the very top of their volume-pressure curve—the flat portion of the curve (see Figure 2–10). As the volume-pressure curve shows, lung compliance is very low on the upper, flat portion of the volume-pressure curve. Because of this, the patient was working extremely hard to breathe (i.e., generating large intrapleural pressure changes), with little or no change in her alveolar ventilation (volume), as shown in Figure 2–10.

(continues)

In addition, as Poiseuille's law demonstrates, the tracheobronchial tree constriction and excessive airway secretions, both caused by the asthma attack, can have a tremendous impact on gas flow and on the patient's work of breathing. Poiseuille's law shows that gas flow is *directly* related to the fourth power of the radius (r^4) of the tracheobronchial tree, and pressure (e.g., intrapleural pressure changes) is *indirectly* related to the fourth power of the radius of the airways. Thus, if the patient's bronchial constriction and bronchial secretions decreased the radius of the airways by one-half, the flow of gas would decrease to 1/16 of the original flow (see Figure 2–24). Similarly, in order for the patient to maintain the same flow rate, she would have to increase her work of breathing to 16 times her original level (see Figure 2–26).

Airway resistance (R_{aw}) can be defined as the intrapleural pressure difference (ΔP) generated by the patient to move a volume of gas divided by the flow rate ($\dot{V}$). Again, according to Poiseuille's law, it can be seen that as the airways narrow, intrapleural pressure will increase significantly while, at the same time, gas flow through the airways will decrease. Because $R_{aw} = \Delta P \div \dot{V}$, it is easy to see mathematically how quickly airway resistance can increase during an asthmatic episode.

Finally, as the airway resistance (R_{aw}) increased, the alveoli distal to the bronchial constriction required a longer time to inflate. These alveoli are said to have a long *time constant* (see Figure 2–30). A product of the time constants is the measurement called *dynamic compliance,* which is the change in volume of the lungs divided by the change in the transpulmonary pressure during the time required for one breath (i.e., during a period of gas flow).

In the healthy lung, the dynamic compliance is approximately equal to lung compliance at all breathing frequencies. In the patient with partially obstructed airways, however, the ratio of dynamic compliance to lung compliance decreases as the respiratory rate increases. The alveoli distal to the airway obstruction do not have enough time to fully inflate as the breathing frequency rises. The compliance of these alveoli is said to be *frequency dependent.* This is why it was important for the respiratory therapist to remain at the bedside and encourage the patient to take slow, deep breaths.

Because the patient was having trouble inhaling a normal volume of gas and because her oxygen saturation level (Sp_{O_2}) was below normal, oxygen therapy was clearly indicated. The continuous bronchodilator therapy was also indicated and worked to offset the effects of airway constriction (as described by Poiseuille's law), increased airway resistance, air trapping, and hyperinflation. As the lung hyperinflation progressively declined, lung compliance steadily increased, or returned to normal (i.e., returned back to the steep portion of the volume-pressure curve). The patient continued to improve and was discharged from the hospital by the next afternoon.

A 22-year-old male who had been in a motorcycle crash was brought to the emergency department with several facial, neck, and shoulder abrasions and lacerations, and multiple broken ribs. During each breath, the patient's right anterior chest moved inward during inspiration and outward during exhalation (clinically this is called a *flail chest*). The patient was alert, in pain, and stated, "I can't breathe. Am I going to die?"

The patient's skin was pale and blue. His vital signs were blood pressure—166/93 mm Hg, heart rate—135 beats/min, and respiratory rate—26 breaths/min and shallow. While on a simple oxygen mask, the patient's peripheral oxygen saturation level (Sp_{O_2}), measured over the skin of his index finger, was 79 percent (normal, 97 percent). Chest x-ray showed that the third, fourth, fifth, sixth, and seventh ribs were each broken in two or three places on the right anterior chest. The chest x-ray also revealed that his right lung was partially collapsed.

A chest tube was inserted and the patient was immediately transferred to the intensive care unit (ICU), sedated, intubated, and placed on a mechanical ventilator. The mechanical ventilator was set at a ventilatory rate of 12 breaths/minute, an oxygen concentration of 0.5, and a positive end-expiratory pressure (PEEP) of +5 cm H_2O.* No spontaneous breaths were present between the mandatory mechanical breaths.

Four hours later, the patient appeared comfortable and his skin color was normal. The ventilator was set at a rate of 12 breaths/min, an inspired oxygen concentration (FI_{O_2}) of 0.3, and a PEEP of +5 cm H_2O. No spontaneous breaths were generated between each mechanical ventilation. During each mechanical breath, both the right and left side of the patient's chest expanded symmetrically. His blood pressure was 127/83 mm Hg and heart rate was 76 beats/min. A second chest x-ray revealed that his right lung had re-expanded. His peripheral oxygen saturation level (Sp_{O_2}) was 97 percent.

DISCUSSION

This case illustrates (1) the effects on *trans-thoracic pressure* when the thorax is unstable, (2) how the excursions of the diaphragm affect the intrapleural pressure, (3) acute decreased lung compliance, and (4) the therapeutic effects of positive pressure ventilation in flail chest cases.

Under normal conditions, on each inhalation, the diaphragm moves downward and causes the intrapleural pressure and alveolar pressure to decrease (see Figure 2–7). In this case, however, the patient's ribs were broken on the right side and caved in during each inspiration when the intrapleural and alveolar pressure decreased. This caused the right lung to partially collapse—an acute decreased lung compliance condition (see Figure 2–10).

This process was corrected when the patient was ventilated with positive pressure. The patient no longer had to generate negative pressure to inhale. During each positive pressure breath, the chest wall expanded evenly and returned to normal resting level at the end of each expiration. This process allowed the ribs to heal. After 10 days, the patient was weaned from the ventilator; he was discharged 3 days later.

At the end of a normal spontaneous expiration, the pressure in the alveoli is equal to the barometric pressure. A +5 cm H_2O of PEEP means that at the end of each exhalation, the patient's alveoli still had a positive pressure of 5 cm H_2O above atmospheric pressure. Therapeutically, this helps to re-expand collapsed alveoli or to prevent the collapse of alveoli.

REVIEW QUESTIONS

1. The average compliance of the lungs and chest wall combined is
   A. 0.1 L/cm H_2O
   B. 0.2 L/cm H_2O
   C. 0.3 L/cm H_2O
   D. 0.4 L/cm H_2O

2. Normally, the airway resistance in the tracheobronchial tree is about
   A. 0.5–1.5 cm H_2O/L/sec
   B. 1.0–2.0 cm H_2O/L/sec
   C. 2.0–3.0 cm H_2O/L/sec
   D. 3.0–4.0 cm H_2O/L/sec

3. In the normal individual in the upright position
   I. the negative intrapleural pressure is greater (i.e., more negative) in the upper lung regions
   II. the alveoli in the lower lung regions are larger than the alveoli in the upper lung regions
   III. ventilation is more effective in the lower lung regions
   IV. the intrapleural pressure is always below atmospheric pressure during a normal ventilatory cycle
      A. I and II only
      B. II and III only
      C. II, III, and IV only
      D. I, III, and IV only

4. When lung compliance decreases, the patient commonly has
   I. an increased ventilatory rate
   II. a decreased tidal volume
   III. an increased tidal volume
   IV. a decreased ventilatory rate
      A. I only
      B. II only
      C. III only
      D. I and II only

5. When arranged for flow ($\dot{V}$), Poiseuille's law states that $\dot{V}$ is
   I. inversely proportional to r^4
   II. directly proportional to P
   III. inversely proportional to η
   IV. directly proportional to l
      A. I only
      B. II only
      C. II and III only
      D. III and IV only

6. During a normal exhalation, the
   I.   intra-alveolar pressure is greater than the atmospheric pressure
   II. intrapleural pressure is less than the atmospheric pressure
   III. intra-alveolar pressure is in equilibrium with the atmospheric pressure
   IV. intrapleural pressure progressively decreases
   A. I only
   B. IV only
   C. I and II only
   D. III and IV only

7. At rest, the normal intrapleural pressure change during quiet breathing is about
   A.   0–2 mm Hg
   B.   2–4 mm Hg
   C.   4–6 mm Hg
   D.   6–8 mm Hg

8. Normally, an individual's tidal volume is about
   A.   1–2 mL/lb
   B.   3–4 mL/lb
   C.   5–6 mL/lb
   D.   7–8 mL/lb

9. A rapid and shallow ventilatory pattern is called
   A.   hyperpnea
   B.   apnea
   C.   alveolar hyperventilation
   D.   tachypnea

10. Assuming that pressure remains constant, if the radius of a bronchial airway through which gas flows at a rate of 400 L/min is reduced to one-half of its original size, the flow through the bronchial airway would change to
    A.   10 L/min
    B.   25 L/min
    C.   100 L/min
    D.   200 L/min

11. The difference between the alveolar pressure and the pleural pressure is called the
    A.   transpulmonary pressure
    B.   transthoracic pressure
    C.   driving pressure
    D.   transairway pressure

12. According to Laplace's law, if a bubble with a radius of 4 cm and a distending pressure of 10 cm H_2O is reduced to a radius of 2 cm, the new distending pressure of the bubble will be
    A.   5 cm H_2O
    B.   10 cm H_2O
    C.   15 cm H_2O
    D.   20 cm H_2O

13. If alveolar unit A has one-half the compliance of alveolar unit B, then the
    I.   time constant of unit A is essentially the same as that of unit B
    II.   volume in unit B is two times greater than volume in unit A
    III. time constant of unit B is twice as long as that of unit A
    IV.   volume in unit B is essentially the same as the volume of unit A
        A. I only
        B. III only
        C. IV only
        D. II and III only

14. If a patient weighs 175 pounds and has a tidal volume of 550 mL and a respiratory rate of 17 breaths/min, what is the patient's minute alveolar ventilation?

    Answer: _____

15. Lung compliance study

    Part I: If a patient generates a negative intrapleural pressure change of −8 cm H_2O during inspiration, and the lungs accept a new volume of 630 mL, what is the compliance of the lungs?

    Answer: _____

    Part II: If the same patient, 6 hours later, generates an intrapleural pressure of −12 cm H_2O during inspiration, and the lungs accept a new volume of 850 mL, what is the compliance of the lungs?

    Answer: _____

    Part III: In comparing Part II to Part I, the patient's lung compliance is
    A.   increasing
    B.   decreasing

16. If a patient produces a flow rate of 5 L/sec during a forced exhalation by generating a transairway pressure of 20 cm H_2O, what is the patient's R_{aw}?
    A.   1 cm H_2O/L/sec
    B.   2 cm H_2O/L/sec
    C.   3 cm H_2O/L/sec
    D.   4 cm H_2O/L/sec

17. As R_{aw} increases, the patient commonly manifests
   I.   a decreased ventilatory rate
   II. an increased tidal volume
   III. a decreased tidal volume
   IV. an increased ventilatory rate
     A. I only
     B. II only
     C. I and II only
     D. III and IV only

18. If the radius of a bronchial airway, which has a driving pressure of 2 mm Hg, is reduced by 16 percent of its original size, what will be the new driving pressure required to maintain the same gas flow through the bronchial airway?
     A.   4 mm Hg
     B.   8 mm Hg
     C.   12 mm Hg
     D.   16 mm Hg

19. In the healthy lung, when the alveolus decreases in size during a normal exhalation, the
   I.   surface tension decreases
   II. surfactant to alveolar surface area increases
   III. surface tension increases
   IV. surfactant to alveolar surface area decreases
     A. I only
     B. III only
     C. IV only
     D. I and II only

20. At end-expiration, P_{ta} is:
     A.   0 mm Hg
     B.   2 mm Hg
     C.   4 mm Hg
     D.   6 mm Hg

CLINICAL APPLICATION QUESTIONS

CASE 1

1. As a result of the hyperinflation, the patient's work of breathing increased because her lungs were inflated to the very top of their volume-pressure curve. As the volume-pressure curve illustrates, lung compliance is very (high _____; low _____) on the upper, flat portion of the volume-pressure curve.

2. Because of the lung hyperinflation described in question 1, the patient was generating (small _____; large _____) intrapleural pressure changes with (little or no _____; moderate to large _____) volume changes.

3. What two major tracheobronchial tree changes occurred during the asthma attack that caused gas flow to significantly decrease, as described by Poiseuille's law?

   _____

   _____

4. As the airway resistance increased in this case, the alveoli distal to the bronchial constriction required (shorter _____; longer _____) time to inflate. These alveoli are said to have a (short _____; long _____) time constant.

5. A product of the time constants is the measurement called dynamic compliance, which is the change in volume of the lungs divided by the change in the transpulmonary pressure during the time for one breath. During an asthmatic episode, the patient's dynamic compliance (increases _____; decreases _____; remains the same _____).

CASE 2

1. Because this patient's ribs were broken on the right side, his right chest (bulged outward _____; caved inward _____) during each inspiration.

2. As a result of the condition described above, the patient's right lung _____, which in turn caused an acute (decreased _____; increased _____) lung compliance condition.

3. The pathophysiologic process that developed in this case was corrected with _____. During each breath, the patient's chest wall (caved inward _____; moved outward _____) and then returned to normal _____ at the end of each expiration.

CHAPTER 3

The Diffusion of Pulmonary Gases

OBJECTIVES

By the end of this chapter, the student should be able to:

1. Define *diffusion.*
2. State the following gas laws:
   —Ideal gas law
   —Boyle's law
   —Charles' law
   —Gay-Lussac's law
   —Dalton's law
3. Identify the percentage and partial pressure of the gases that compose the *barometric pressure:*
   —Nitrogen
   —Oxygen
   —Argon
   —Carbon dioxide
4. Identify the partial pressure of the gases in the *air, alveoli,* and *blood:*
   —Oxygen (P_{O_2})
   —Carbon dioxide (P_{CO_2})
   —Water (P_{H_2O})
   —Nitrogen (P_{N_2})
5. Calculate the *ideal alveolar gas equation.*
6. Name the nine major structures of the *alveolar-capillary membrane* through which a gas molecule must diffuse.
7. Describe how oxygen and carbon dioxide normally diffuse across the alveolar-capillary membrane.
8. Explain how *Fick's law* relates to gas diffusion.
9. Describe how the following relate to the *diffusion constants* in Fick's law:
   —Henry's law
   —Graham's law
10. Describe how Fick's law can be applied to certain clinical conditions.
11. Define *perfusion limited,* and explain how it relates to a gas such as nitrous oxide.
12. Define *diffusion limited,* and explain how it relates to a gas such as carbon monoxide.
13. Describe how oxygen can be classified as perfusion or diffusion limited.
14. Complete the review questions at the end of this chapter.

As discussed in Chapter 2, the mass movement of air in and out of the lungs occurs because of transpulmonary and transairway pressure changes generated by the action of the diaphragm. This mechanism carries oxygen from the atmosphere to the alveoli and carbon dioxide from the alveoli to the external environment. The process of ventilation, however, merely moves gases from one point to another (e.g., from the atmosphere to the alveoli); it does not move gas molecules across the alveolar-capillary membrane. This process occurs by **passive diffusion**.

Diffusion is defined as the movement of gas molecules from an area of relatively high concentration of gas to one of low concentration. Different gases each move according to their own individual partial pressure gradients. Diffusion continues until all the gases in the two areas are in equilibrium.

To understand how gases transfer (diffuse) across the alveolar-capillary membrane, a brief review of the physical principles governing the behavior of gases (gas laws) and the partial pressures of the atmospheric gases is appropriate.

GAS LAWS—REVIEW

Ideal Gas Law

The behavior of gases surrounding the earth is described in a mathematical relationship known as the *ideal gas law:*

$$PV = nRT$$

where P is pressure, V is volume, T is temperature on the Kelvin (K) scale,* n is the number of moles of gas molecules present, and R is the gas constant, which has a fixed value of 0.0821.

Assuming that the amount of gas remains constant (i.e., n remains unchanged), the ideal gas law can be used to predict specific changes of temperature, pressure, and volume under different conditions. In other words, if nR remains constant, then:

$$\frac{P_1 \times V_1}{T_1} = \frac{P_2 \times V_2}{T_2}$$

Thus, when any one of the above variables (P, V, T) is held constant while one of the others changes in value, the new value of the third variable can be calculated. The following laws illustrate the interrelationship of P, V, and T.

Boyle's Law

Boyle's law ($P_1 \times V_1 = P_2 \times V_2$) states that if temperature remains constant, pressure will vary inversely to volume. For example, if an airtight container, which has a volume of 200 mL and a pressure of 10 cm H_2O,

Whenever the temperature of gases is involved in calculations, all temperatures must be converted to the Kelvin scale. Fahrenheit (°F) is converted first to Celsius (°C) as follows: 5 ÷ 9 (F − 32). Celsius is converted to Kelvin (K) by adding 273 to the Celsius temperature (e.g., 37°C + 273 = 310 K).

has its volume reduced 50 percent (100 mL), the new pressure in the container can be computed as follows:

$$P_2 = \frac{P_1 \times V_1}{V_2}$$

$$= \frac{10 \text{ cm H}_2\text{O} \times 200 \text{ mL}}{100 \text{ mL}}$$

$$= 20 \text{ cm H}_2\text{O}$$

Charles' Law

Charles' law ($V_1 \div T_1 = V_2 \div T_2$) states that if pressure remains constant, volume and temperature will vary directly. That is, if the temperature of the gas in a 3-liter balloon is increased from 250 to 300 K, the resulting volume of the balloon can be calculated as follows:

$$V_2 = \frac{V_1 \times T_2}{T_1}$$

$$= \frac{3 \text{ L} \times 300 \text{ K}}{250 \text{ K}}$$

$$= 3.6 \text{ L}$$

Gay-Lussac's Law

Gay-Lussac's law ($P_1 \div T_1 = P_2 \div T_2$) states that if the volume remains constant, pressure and temperature will vary directly. For instance, if the temperature of the gas in a closed container, having a pressure of 50 cm H_2O, is increased from 275 to 375 K, the resulting pressure in the container can be calculated as follows:

$$P_2 = \frac{P_1 \times T_2}{T_1}$$

$$= \frac{50 \text{ cm H}_2\text{O} \times 375 \text{ K}}{275 \text{ K}}$$

$$= \frac{18,750}{275}$$

$$= 68 \text{ cm H}_2\text{O}$$

Dalton's Law

Because the earth's atmosphere consists of several kinds of gases, it is essential to understand how these gases behave when they are mixed together. This is described by Dalton's law, which states that in a mixture of gases, the total pressure is equal to the sum of the partial pressures of

Figure 3–1
Dalton's law.

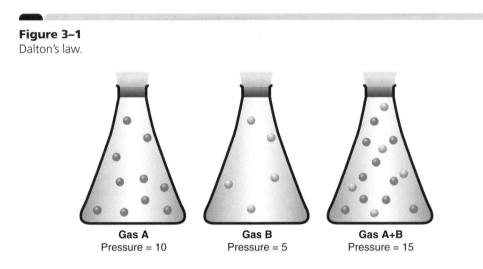

Gas A
Pressure = 10

Gas B
Pressure = 5

Gas A+B
Pressure = 15

each separate gas. In other words, if 10 molecules of gas are enclosed in a container, the total pressure may be expressed as 10; if 5 molecules of a different gas are enclosed in another container of equal volume, the total pressure may be expressed as 5; if both these gases are enclosed in a container of equal volume, the total pressure may be expressed as 15 (Figure 3–1).

It should be stressed that the pressure produced by a particular gas is completely unaffected by the presence of another gas. Each gas in a mixture will individually contribute to the total pressure created by the mixture of gases.

THE PARTIAL PRESSURES OF ATMOSPHERIC GASES

The atmospheric gases that surround the earth exert a force on the earth's surface called the *barometric pressure.* At sea level the barometric pressure is about 760 mm Hg and is a function of Dalton's law. The barometric pressure is primarily derived from the gases listed in Table 3–1.

The pressure between the external atmosphere and the alveoli is in equilibrium, except for slight changes (3–6 cm H_2O) that take place during inspiration or expiration. Within the circulatory system, however, the sum of the partial pressures is reduced, because the venous blood, which has a reduced P_{O_2} owing to cellular metabolism, is not in equilibrium with the atmosphere.

Note also that the barometric pressure decreases with an increase in altitude. For example, as one ascends a mountain, the barometric pressure steadily decreases, because the density of the different gases surrounding the earth decreases with increased altitude. As the density of the

TABLE 3–1

Gases That Compose the Barometric Pressure

Gas	% of Atmosphere	Partial Pressure (mm Hg)
Nitrogen (N_2)	78.08	593
Oxygen (O_2)	20.95	159
Argon (Ar)	0.93	7
Carbon dioxide (CO_2)	0.03	0.2

various gases decreases, the partial pressure exerted by each gas also decreases. Also, even though the barometric pressure varies with the altitude, the percent concentration of the atmospheric gases (see Table 3–1) is the same at both high and low elevations. (For further discussion of pressure at high altitude, see the section titled "Alveolar-Arterial P_{O_2} Difference" in Chapter 19.)

Partial Pressures of Oxygen and Carbon Dioxide

Table 3–2 shows the partial pressure of gases in dry air, alveolar gas, arterial blood, and venous blood. Note that even though the total barometric pressure is the same in the atmosphere and in the alveoli, the partial pressure of oxygen in the atmosphere (159 mm Hg) is significantly higher than the partial pressure of oxygen in the alveoli (100 mm Hg). This is because

TABLE 3–2

Partial Pressure (in mm Hg) of Gases in the Air, Alveoli, and Blood*

Gases	Dry Air	Alveolar Gas	Arterial Blood	Venous Blood
P_{O_2}	159.0	100.0	95.0	40.0
P_{CO_2}	0.2	40.0	40.0	46.0
P_{H_2O} (water vapor)	0.0	47.0	47.0	47.0
P_{N_2} (and other gases in minute quantities)	600.8	573.0	573.0	573.0
Total	760.0	760.0	755.0	706.0

* The values shown are based on standard pressure and temperature.

TABLE 3–3
Relationship Between Temperature, Absolute Humidity, and Water Vapor Pressure*

Temperature (Celsius)	Absolute (Maximum) Humidity (mg/L)	Water Vapor Pressure (mm Hg)
37°	44.0	47.0
35°	39.6	42.2
30°	30.4	31.8
27°	25.8	26.7
25°	23.0	23.8
20°	17.3	17.5

* At sea level (760 mm Hg).

alveolar oxygen must mix—or compete, in terms of partial pressures—with alveolar CO_2 pressure ($P_{A_{CO_2}}$ = 40 mm Hg) and alveolar water vapor pressure (P_{H_2O} = 47 mm Hg), which are not nearly as high in the atmosphere. In short, by the time the oxygen molecules reach the alveoli, they are diluted by the addition of CO_2 and H_2O molecules. This leads to a decrease in the partial pressure of oxygen in the alveoli ($P_{A_{O_2}}$).

Water Vapor Pressure

Depending on the surrounding temperature and pressure, water can exist as a liquid, gas, or solid. Water in the gaseous form is called *water vapor,* or *molecular water.* When water vapor is present in a volume of gas, it behaves according to the gas laws and exerts a partial pressure. Because alveolar gas is 100 percent humidified (saturated) at body temperature, the alveolar gas is assumed to have an *absolute humidity* of 44 mg/L, and a *water vapor pressure* (P_{H_2O}) of 47 mm Hg—regardless of the humidity of the inspired air (Table 3–3).

THE IDEAL ALVEOLAR GAS EQUATION

Clinically, the alveolar oxygen tension $P_{A_{O_2}}$ can be computed from the **ideal alveolar gas equation**. A useful clinical approximation of the ideal alveolar gas equation is as follows:

$$P_{A_{O_2}} = [P_B - P_{H_2O}]F_{I_{O_2}} - Pa_{CO_2}(1.25)$$

where $P_{A_{O_2}}$ is the partial pressure of oxygen in the alveoli, P_B is the barometric pressure, P_{H_2O} is the partial pressure of water vapor in the alveoli ($P_{H_2O} = 47$ mm Hg), $F_{I_{O_2}}$ is the fractional concentration of inspired oxygen, and Pa_{CO_2} is the partial pressure of arterial carbon dioxide. The number 1.25 is a factor that adjusts for alterations in oxygen tension due to variations in the *respiratory exchange ratio* (RR), which is the ratio of the amount of oxygen that moves into the pulmonary capillary blood to the amount of carbon dioxide that moves out of the pulmonary blood and into the alveoli. Normally, about 200 mL/minute of carbon dioxide move into the alveoli while about 250 mL/minute of oxygen move into the pulmonary capillary blood, making the respiratory exchange ratio about 0.8.

Thus, if a patient is receiving an $F_{I_{O_2}}$ of 0.40 on a day when the barometric pressure is 755 mm Hg, and if the Pa_{CO_2} is 55 mm Hg, then the patient's alveolar oxygen tension ($P_{A_{O_2}}$) can be calculated as follows:

$$P_{A_{O_2}} = [P_B - P_{H_2O}]F_{I_{O_2}} - Pa_{CO_2}(1.25)$$

$$= [755 - 47]0.40 - 55(1.25)$$

$$= [708]0.40 - 68.75$$

$$= [283.2] - 68.75$$

$$= 214.45$$

Clinically, when the Pa_{CO_2} is less than 60 mm Hg, and when the patient is receiving oxygen therapy greater than 0.6, the following simplified version of the alveolar gas equation may be used:

$$P_{A_{O_2}} = [P_B - P_{H_2O}]F_{I_{O_2}} - Pa_{CO_2}$$

THE DIFFUSION OF PULMONARY GASES

The process of diffusion is the passive movement of gas molecules from an area of high partial pressure to an area of low partial pressure until both areas are equal in pressure. Once equilibrium occurs, diffusion ceases.

In the lungs, a gas molecule must diffuse through the alveolar-capillary membrane (Figure 3–2), which is composed of (1) the liquid lining the intra-alveolar membrane, (2) the alveolar epithelial cell, (3) the basement membrane of the alveolar epithelial cell, (4) loose connective tissue (the interstitial space), (5) the basement membrane of the capillary endothelium, (6) the capillary endothelium, (7) the plasma in the capillary blood, (8) the erythrocyte membrane, and (9) the intracellular fluid in the erythrocyte until a hemoglobin molecule is encountered. The thickness of these physical barriers is between 0.36 and 2.5 μm. Under normal circumstances, this is a negligible barrier to the diffusion of oxygen and carbon dioxide.

Figure 3–2
The major barriers of the alveolar-capillary membrane through which a gas molecule must diffuse.

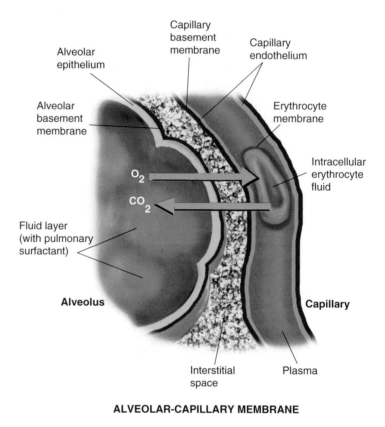

ALVEOLAR-CAPILLARY MEMBRANE

OXYGEN AND CARBON DIOXIDE DIFFUSION ACROSS THE ALVEOLAR-CAPILLARY MEMBRANE

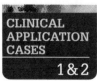

CLINICAL APPLICATION CASES

1 & 2

See pages 147–150

In the healthy resting individual, venous blood entering the alveolar-capillary system has an average oxygen tension ($P\bar{v}_{O_2}$) of 40 mm Hg, and an average carbon dioxide tension ($P\bar{v}_{CO_2}$) of 46 mm Hg. As blood passes through the capillary, the average alveolar oxygen tension (PA_{O_2}) is about 100 mm Hg, and the average alveolar carbon dioxide tension (PA_{CO_2}) is about 40 mm Hg (see Table 3–2).

Thus, when venous blood enters the alveolar-capillary system, there is an oxygen pressure gradient of about 60 mm Hg and a carbon dioxide pressure gradient of about 6 mm Hg. As a result, oxygen molecules

Figure 3–3

Normal gas pressures for oxygen (O_2) and carbon dioxide (CO_2) as blood moves through the alveolar-capillary membrane. $P\bar{v}_{O_2}$ = partial pressure of oxygen in mixed venous blood; $P\bar{v}_{CO_2}$ = partial pressure of carbon dioxide in mixed venous blood; PA_{O_2} = partial pressure of oxygen in alveolar gas; PA_{CO_2} = partial pressure of carbon dioxide in alveolar gas; Pa_{O_2} = partial pressure of oxygen in arterial blood; Pa_{CO_2} = partial pressure of carbon dioxide in arterial blood.

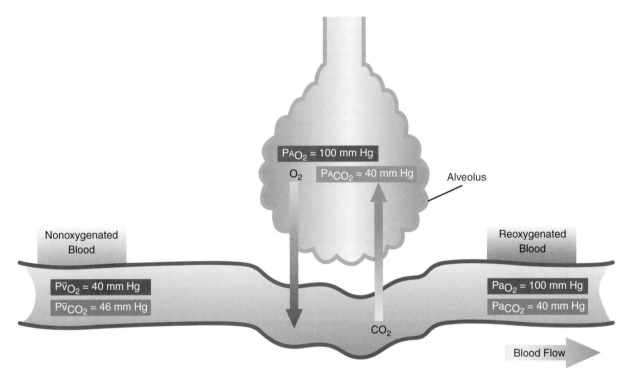

diffuse across the alveolar-capillary membrane into the blood while, at the same time, carbon dioxide molecules diffuse out of the capillary blood and into the alveoli (Figure 3–3).

The diffusion of oxygen and carbon dioxide will continue until equilibrium is reached; this is usually accomplished in about 0.25 second. Under normal resting conditions, the total transit time for blood to move through the alveolar-capillary system is about 0.75 second. Thus, the diffusion of oxygen and carbon dioxide is completed in about one-third of the time available (Figure 3–4).

In exercise, however, blood passes through the alveolar-capillary system at a much faster rate and, therefore, the time for gas diffusion decreases (i.e., the time available for gas diffusion is <0.75 second). In the

Figure 3–4

Under normal resting conditions, blood moves through the alveolar-capillary membrane in about 0.75 second. The oxygen pressure (P_{O_2}) and carbon dioxide pressure (P_{CO_2}) reach equilibrium in about 0.25 second—one-third of the time available. $P\bar{v}_{O_2}$ = partial pressure of oxygen in mixed venous blood; $P\bar{v}_{CO_2}$ = partial pressure of carbon dioxide in mixed venous blood; $P_{A_{O_2}}$ = partial pressure of oxygen in alveolar gas; $P_{A_{CO_2}}$ = partial pressure of carbon dioxide in alveolar gas; Pa_{O_2} = partial pressure of oxygen in arterial blood; Pa_{CO_2} = partial pressure of carbon dioxide in arterial blood.

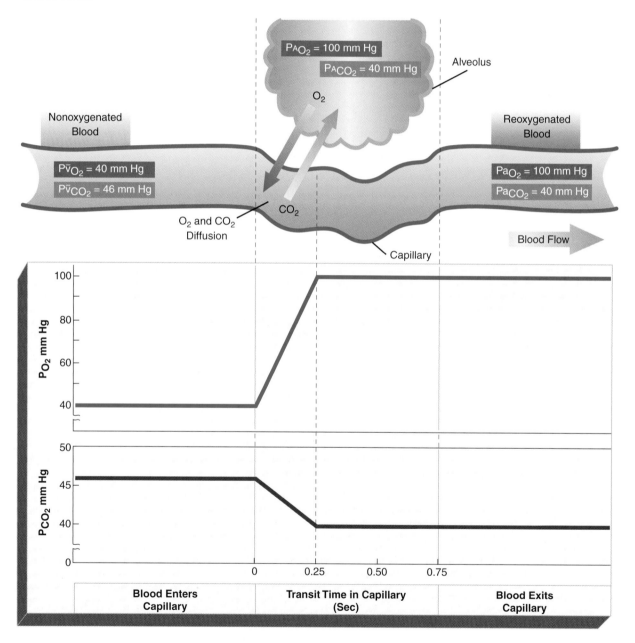

Figure 3–5
During exercise or stress, the total transit time for blood through the alveolar-capillary membrane is less than normal (normal = 0.75 second). In the healthy individual, however, oxygen equilibrium usually occurs. $P\bar{v}_{O_2}$ = partial pressure of oxygen in mixed venous blood; PA_{O_2} = partial pressure of oxygen in alveolar gas; Pa_{O_2} = partial pressure of oxygen in arterial blood.

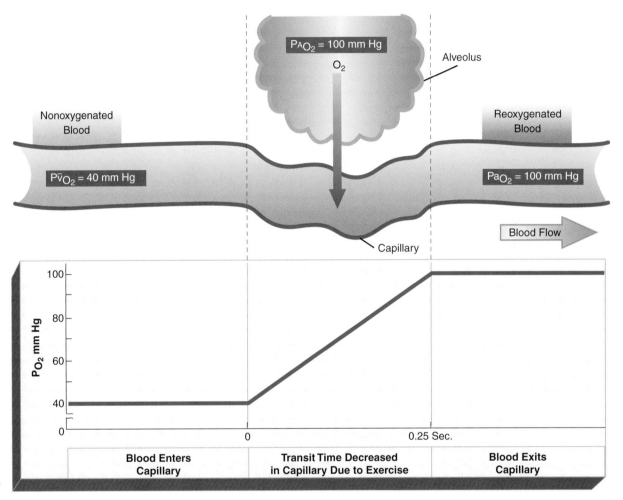

healthy lung, oxygen equilibrium usually occurs in the alveolar-capillary system during exercise—in spite of the shortened transit time (Figure 3–5). In the presence of certain pulmonary diseases, however, the time available to achieve oxygen equilibrium in the alveolar-capillary system may not be adequate. Such diseases include alveolar fibrosis, alveolar consolidation, and pulmonary edema (Figure 3–6).

Figure 3–6

When the rate of diffusion is decreased because of alveolar thickening, oxygen equilibrium will likely not occur when the total transit time is decreased as a result of exercise or stress. $P\bar{v}_{O_2}$ = partial pressure of oxygen in mixed venous blood; Pa_{O_2} = partial pressure of oxygen in alveolar gas; Pa_{O_2} = partial pressure of oxygen in arterial blood.

GAS DIFFUSION

**CLINICAL
APPLICATION
CASES**

1 & 2

See pages 147–150

Fick's Law

The diffusion of gas takes place according to Fick's law, which is written as follows:

$$\dot{V} \, \text{gas} \approx \frac{AD(P_1 - P_2)}{T}$$

Figure 3–7
Fick's law.

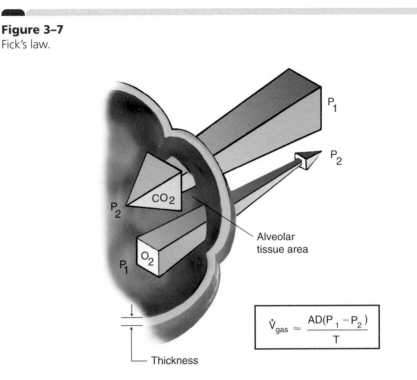

where $\dot{V}$ gas is the amount of gas that diffuses from one point to another, A is surface area, D is diffusion constant, $P_1 - P_2$ is the difference in partial pressure between two points, and T is thickness.

The law states that the rate of gas transfer across a sheet of tissue is directly proportional to the surface area of the tissue, to the diffusion constants, and to the difference in partial pressure of the gas between the two sides of the tissue, and is inversely proportional to the thickness of the tissue (Figure 3–7).

The diffusion constant (D) noted in Fick's law is determined by Henry's law and Graham's law.

Henry's Law

Henry's law states that the amount of a gas that dissolves in a liquid at a given temperature is proportional to the partial pressure of the gas. The amount of gas that can be dissolved by 1 mL of a given liquid at standard pressure (760 mm Hg) and specified temperature is known as the *solubility coefficient* of the liquid. At 37°C and 760 mm Hg pressure, the solubility coefficient of oxygen is 0.0244 mL/mm Hg/mL H_2O. The solubility coefficient of carbon dioxide is 0.592 mL/mm Hg/mL H_2O. The solubility coefficient varies inversely with temperature (i.e., if the temperature rises, the solubility coefficient decreases in value).

On the basis of the solubility coefficients of oxygen and carbon dioxide, it can be seen that in a liquid medium (e.g., alveolar-capillary membrane) carbon dioxide is more soluble than oxygen:

$$\frac{\text{Solubility } CO_2}{\text{Solubility } O_2} = \frac{0.592}{0.0244} = \frac{24}{1}$$

Graham's Law

Graham's law states that the rate of diffusion of a gas through a liquid is (1) directly proportional to the solubility coefficient of the gas and (2) inversely proportional to the square root of the gram-molecular weight (GMW) of the gas. In comparing the relative rates of diffusion to oxygen (GMW = 32) and carbon dioxide (GMW = 44), it can be seen that, because oxygen is the lighter gas, it moves faster than carbon dioxide:

$$\frac{\text{Diffusion rate for } CO_2}{\text{Diffusion rate for } O_2} = \frac{\sqrt{\text{GMW } O_2}}{\sqrt{\text{GMW } CO_2}} = \frac{\sqrt{32}}{\sqrt{44}}$$
$$= \frac{5.6}{6.6}$$

By combining Graham's and Henry's laws, it can be said that the rates of diffusion of two gases are directly proportional to the ratio of their solubility coefficients, and inversely proportional to the ratio of their gram-molecular weights. For example, when the two laws are used to determine the relative rates of diffusion of carbon dioxide and oxygen, it can be seen that carbon dioxide diffuses about 20 times faster than oxygen.

$$\frac{\text{Diffusion rate for } CO_2}{\text{Diffusion rate for } O_2} = \frac{5.6 \times 0.592}{6.6 \times 0.0244} = \frac{20}{1}$$

To summarize, the diffusion constant (D) for a particular gas is directly proportional to the solubility coefficients (S) of the gas, and inversely proportional to the square root of the GMW of the gas:

$$D = \frac{S}{\sqrt{GMW}}$$

Mathematically, by substituting the diffusion constant,

$$D = \frac{S}{\sqrt{GMW}}$$

into Fick's law:

$$\dot{V} \text{ gas} \approx \frac{A \cdot D \cdot (P_1 - P_2)}{T}$$

then Fick's law can be rewritten as:

$$\dot{V} \text{ gas} \approx \frac{A \cdot S \cdot (P_1 - P_2)}{\sqrt{GMW} \times T}$$

Clinical Application of Fick's Law

Clinically, Fick's law is confirmed by the following general statements:

- The area (A) component of the law is verified in that a decreased alveolar surface area (e.g., caused by alveolar collapse or alveolar fluid) decreases the ability of oxygen to enter the pulmonary capillary blood.
- The $P_1 - P_2$ portion of the law is confirmed in that a decreased alveolar oxygen pressure ($P_{A_{O_2}}$ or P_1) (e.g., caused by high altitudes or alveolar hypoventilation) reduces the diffusion of oxygen into the pulmonary capillary blood.
- The thickness (T) factor is confirmed in that an increased alveolar tissue thickness (e.g., caused by alveolar fibrosis or alveolar edema) reduces the movement of oxygen across the alveolar-capillary membrane.

Fick's law also suggests how certain adverse pulmonary conditions may be improved. For example, when a patient's oxygen diffusion rate is decreased because of alveolar thickening, the administration of oxygen therapy will be beneficial. As the patient's fractional concentration of inspired oxygen ($F_{I_{O_2}}$) increases, the patient's alveolar oxygen pressure (i.e., $P_{A_{O_2}}$ or the P_1) also increases, causing the movement of oxygen across the alveolar-capillary membrane to increase.

PERFUSION-LIMITED GAS FLOW

Perfusion limited means that the transfer of gas across the alveolar wall is a function of the amount of blood that flows past the alveoli. Nitrous oxide (N_2O) is an excellent gas to illustrate this concept. When N_2O moves across the alveolar wall and into the blood, it does not chemically combine with hemoglobin. Because of this, the partial pressure of N_2O in the blood plasma rises very quickly. It is estimated that the partial pressure of N_2O will equal that of the alveolar gas when the blood is only about one-tenth of the way through the alveolar-capillary system (Figure 3–8). Once the partial pressures of the N_2O in the blood and in the alveolar gas are equal, the diffusion of N_2O stops. In order for the diffusion of N_2O to resume, additional blood must enter the alveolar-capillary system. The rate of perfusion, therefore, determines the amount of diffusion of N_2O.

Figure 3–8

Nitrous oxide (N_2O) quickly equilibrates with pulmonary blood. When equilibrium occurs, the diffusion of N_2O stops. In order for the diffusion of N_2O to resume, fresh blood (pulmonary artery blood) must enter the alveolar-capillary system. This phenomenon is called *perfusion limited.* P_{N_2O} = partial pressure of N_2O in the blood.

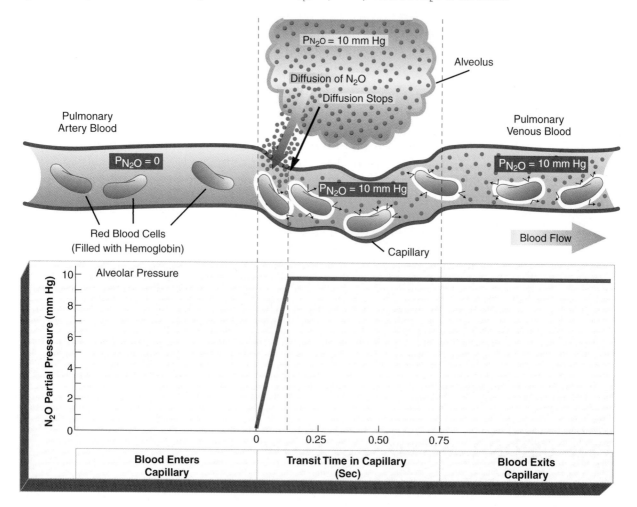

DIFFUSION-LIMITED GAS FLOW

Diffusion limited means that the movement of gas across the alveolar wall is a function of the integrity of the alveolar-capillary membrane itself. Carbon monoxide (CO) is an excellent gas to illustrate this concept. When CO moves across the alveolar wall and into the blood, it rapidly enters the red blood cells (RBCs) and tightly bonds to hemoglobin (CO has an affinity for hemoglobin that is about 210 times greater than that of oxygen).

Note that when gases are in chemical combination with hemoglobin, they no longer exert a partial pressure. Thus, because CO has a strong chemical attraction to hemoglobin, most of the CO enters the RBCs, combines with hemoglobin, and no longer exerts a partial pressure in the blood plasma. Because there is no appreciable partial pressure of CO in the blood plasma at any time (i.e., $P_1 - P_2$ stays constant), only the diffusion characteristics of the alveolar-capillary membrane, not the amount of blood flowing through the capillary, limit the diffusion of CO (Figure 3–9).

This property makes CO an excellent gas for evaluating the lung's ability to diffuse gases and is used in what is called the *diffusion capacity of carbon monoxide* (DL_{CO}) test. The DL_{CO} test measures the amount of CO that moves across the alveolar-capillary membrane into the blood in a

Figure 3–9
Carbon monoxide (CO) rapidly bonds to hemoglobin and, thus, does not generate an appreciable partial pressure (P_{CO}) in the plasma. As a result of this chemical relationship, blood flow (perfusion) does not limit the rate of CO diffusion. When the alveolar-capillary membrane is abnormal (e.g., in alveolar fibrosis), however, the rate of CO diffusion decreases. This phenomenon is called *diffusion limited*. In essence, diffusion limited means that the structure of the alveolar-capillary membrane alone limits the rate of gas diffusion.

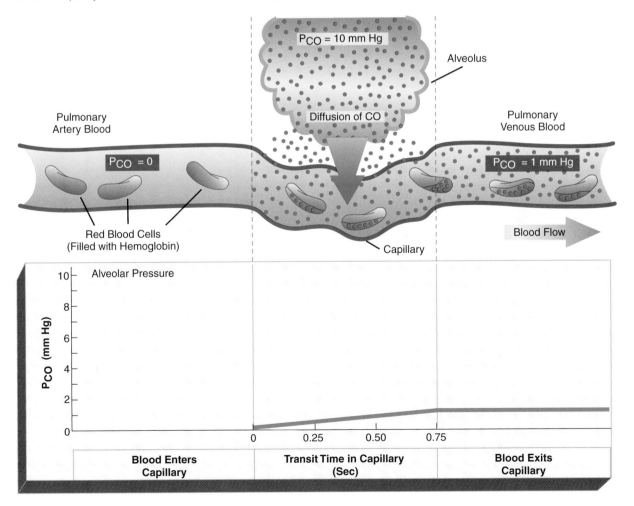

given time. In essence, this test measures the physiologic effectiveness of the alveolar-capillary membrane. The normal diffusion capacity of CO is 25 mL/min/mm Hg. Figure 3–10 shows clinical conditions that may cause problems in diffusion. See Figure 3–6 for an illustration of the diffusion of oxygen during a diffusion-limited state. Table 3–4 presents factors that affect measured DL_{CO}.

Figure 3–10

Clinical conditions that decrease the rate of gas diffusion. These conditions are known as *diffusion-limited problems.*

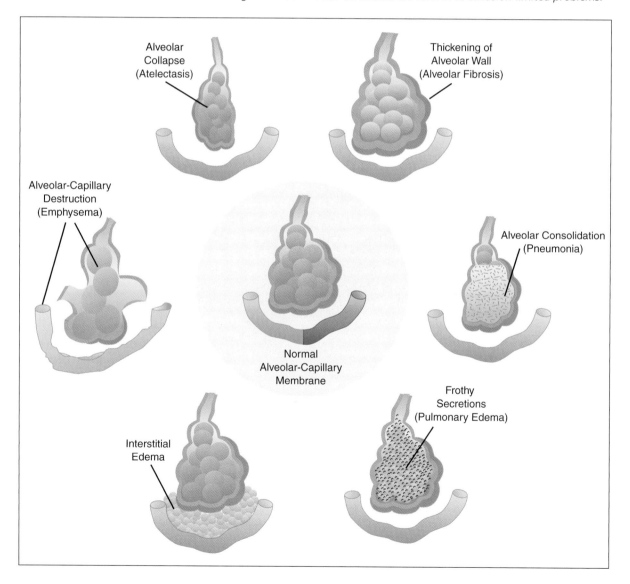

TABLE 3–4
Factors That Affect Measured $D_{L_{CO}}$

Age	The $D_{L_{CO}}$ progressively increases between birth and 20 years of age. After age 20, the $D_{L_{CO}}$ decreases as a result of the normal anatomic alterations of the lungs that reduce the overall alveolar-capillary surface area.
Lung volume	The $D_{L_{CO}}$ is directly related to an individual's lung size. Thus, the greater the subject's lung volume, the greater the $D_{L_{CO}}$.
Body size	As a general rule, the $D_{L_{CO}}$ increases with body size. The size of the lungs is directly related to the subject's ideal body size. Thus, the larger the subject, the greater the lung size and the higher the $D_{L_{CO}}$.
Body position	The $D_{L_{CO}}$ is about 15% to 20% greater when the individual is in the supine position, compared with the upright position.
Exercise	The $D_{L_{CO}}$ increases with exercise. This is most likely because of the increased cardiac output, and capillary recruitment and distention, associated with exercise.*
Alveolar P_{O_2} ($P_{A_{O_2}}$)	The $D_{L_{CO}}$ decreases in response to a high $P_{A_{O_2}}$. This is because O_2 and CO both compete for the same hemoglobin sites.[†]
Hemoglobin concentration	*Anemia:* Patients with low hemoglobin content have a low CO-carrying capacity and, therefore, a low $D_{L_{CO}}$ value. *Polycythemia:* Patients with high hemoglobin content have a high CO-carrying capacity and, therefore, a high $D_{L_{CO}}$ value.
Carboxyhemoglobin	Individuals who already have CO bound to their hemoglobin (e.g., smokers or fire fighters overcome by smoke inhalation), generate a "back pressure" to alveolar P_{CO}. This condition decreases the pressure gradient between the alveolar CO and the blood CO, which in turn reduces the $D_{L_{CO}}$ (see discussion of Fick's law).

* See Chapter 5.
[†] See Chapter 6.

HOW OXYGEN CAN BE EITHER PERFUSION OR DIFFUSION LIMITED

When oxygen diffuses across the alveolar wall and into the blood, it enters the RBCs and combines with hemoglobin—but not with the same avidity as does carbon monoxide. Hemoglobin quickly becomes saturated with oxygen and, once this occurs, oxygen molecules in the plasma can no longer enter the RBCs. This, in turn, causes the partial pressure of oxygen in the plasma to increase.

Under normal resting conditions, the partial pressure of oxygen in the capillary blood equals the partial pressure of oxygen in the alveolar gas when the blood is about one-third of the way through the capillary. Beyond this point, the transfer of oxygen is perfusion limited (Figure 3–11). When the patient has either a decreased cardiac output or a decreased

Figure 3–11

Under normal resting conditions, the diffusion of oxygen across the alveolar-capillary membrane stops when blood is about one-third of the way through the capillary. This occurs because the partial pressure of oxygen in the capillary blood (P_{O_2}) equals the partial pressure of oxygen in the alveolus ($P_{A_{O_2}}$). Once oxygen equilibrium occurs between the alveolus and capillary blood, the diffusion of oxygen is *perfusion limited.*

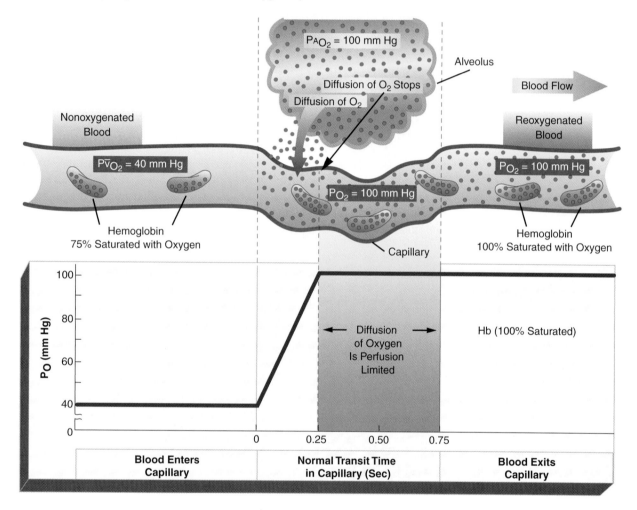

hemoglobin level (anemia), the effects of perfusion limitation may become significant.

When the diffusion properties of the lungs are impaired (see Figure 3–10), however, the partial pressure of oxygen in the capillary blood may never equal the partial pressure of the oxygen in the alveolar gas during the normal alveolar-capillary transit time. Thus, under normal circumstances the diffusion of oxygen is perfusion limited, but under certain abnormal pulmonary conditions the transfer of oxygen may become diffusion limited.

CHAPTER SUMMARY

Diffusion is the movement of gas molecules from an area of relatively high concentration of gas to one of low concentration. When several different gases are mixed together, each gas in the mixture diffuses according to its own individual partial pressure gradient. Diffusion continues until all gases in the two areas are in equilibrium. Fundamental to the understanding of the diffusion of gases are the gas laws, including the ideal gas law, Boyle's law, Charles' law, Gay-Lussac's law, and Dalton's law. The gas laws provide the basic foundation to understand (1) the gases that compose the barometric pressure, (2) the partial pressure of these gases in the air, alveoli, and blood, and (3) the ideal alveolar gas equation. Finally, essential to the knowledge base regarding the diffusion of gases across the alveolar-capillary membrane is the understanding of (1) the diffusion of oxygen and carbon dioxide across the alveolar-capillary membrane, (2) Fick's law, including how Henry's law and Graham's law are used in Fick's law, (3) perfusion-limited gas flow, (4) diffusion-limited gas flow, and (5) how oxygen can be either perfusion or diffusion limited.

1 CLINICAL APPLICATION CASE

This 68-year-old man entered the hospital in severe left ventricular heart failure and pulmonary edema (Figure 3–12).* He appeared very anxious and his lips and skin were blue. He had a frequent and strong cough, productive of moderate amounts of frothy, white and pink secretions. The patient's vital signs were blood pressure—140/88 mm Hg, heart rate—93 beats/min and weak, and respiratory rate—28 breaths/min and shallow. On auscultation, crackles and rhonchi (fluid sounds) could be heard over both lung fields. His arterial oxygen pressure (Pa_{O_2}) was 53 mm Hg (normal range is 80–100 mm Hg).

The emergency department physician administered several different heart medications and a diuretic. The respiratory therapist placed a continuous positive airway pressure (CPAP) mask over the patient's nose and mouth, and set the

Pulmonary edema refers to fluid accumulation in the alveoli and airways. Pulmonary edema is commonly associated with congestive heart failure (CHF).

pressure at +10 cm H_2O and the fractional concentration of inspired oxygen (FI_{O_2}) at 0.4. One hour later the patient was breathing comfortably. His lips and skin no longer appeared blue, and his cough was less frequent. No frothy or pink sputum was noted at this time. His vital signs were blood pressure—126/78 mm Hg, heart rate—77 beats/min, and respiratory rate—16 breaths/min. On auscultation, his breath sounds were improved. His arterial oxygen pressure (Pa_{O_2}) was 86 mm Hg.

DISCUSSION

This case illustrates both the adverse and therapeutic effects of factors presented in Fick's law (see Figure 3–7). The patient presented in the emergency department in severe left ventricular heart failure and pulmonary edema (see Figure 3–12). This means that the patient's left ventricle was failing to pump blood adequately and

(continues)

Figure 3–12
Cross sectional view of alveoli with pulmonary edema. Pathology includes (1) interstitial edema, (2) fluid engorgement throughout the alveolar wall interstitium, and (3) frothy white secretions in the alveoli.

caused blood to back up into the patient's lungs. This pathologic process, in turn, caused the patient's pulmonary blood pressure to increase. As the pulmonary blood pressure increased, fluid moved out of the pulmonary capillaries and into the extracapillary spaces, as well as into the alveoli and into the tracheobronchial tree. As a result of this process, the thickness of the alveolar-capillary membrane also increased (see Figure 3–2).

Because gas diffusion ($\dot{V}$) is *indirectly* related to thickness (T), the diffusion of oxygen across the alveolar-capillary membrane decreased (Fick's law). This fact was illustrated by the low Pa_{O_2} of 53 mm Hg when the patient first entered the hospital. The physician treated the original cause of this condition—the failing heart and fluid overload—with medications. As the cardiac function and fluid overload improved,

(continues)

the thickness of the alveolar-capillary membrane returned to normal. As the thickness of the alveolar-capillary membrane decreased, the diffusion of oxygen increased.

While the physician was treating the patient's failing heart, the respiratory therapist worked to offset the patient's poor oxygenation by increasing the patient's PA_{O_2} (P_1 of Fick's law). As Fick's law shows, the diffusion of gas is *directly* related to $P_1 - P_2$. The therapist increased the patient's PA_{O_2} by (1) increasing the pressure at the level of the patient's alveoli with the CPAP mask, and (2) increasing the inspired FI_{O_2} to 0.4.

Thus, the reduction in alveolar-capillary membrane thickness (decreased via medications), the increased pressure at the level of the alveoli (produced via CPAP), and the increased FI_{O_2} (increased P_1) all worked to enhance the diffusion of oxygen, as shown by the Pa_{O_2} of 86 mm Hg achieved 1 hour later. The patient's cardiac condition progressively improved and he was discharged from the hospital 2 days later.

2 CLINICAL APPLICATION CASE

A 78-year-old woman with a long history of chronic interstitial lung disease (alveolar thickening and fibrosis) was admitted to the hospital because of respiratory distress. She was well known to the hospital staff. She had been admitted to the hospital on several occasions, and for the 2 years prior to this admission, she had been on continuous oxygen at home (2 L/min by nasal cannula). The home care respiratory therapist made regular visits to the patient's home to check on her equipment and to assess her respiratory status. In fact, it was the respiratory therapist who alerted the physician about the patient's poor respiratory status that prompted this hospitalization.

On admission, the patient appeared anxious and agitated. Her skin was pale and blue and felt cool and clammy. Her vital signs were blood pressure—166/91 mm Hg, heart rate—105 beats/min, and respiratory rate—24 breaths/min. Her breath sounds were clear and loud. Although chest x-ray regularly showed signs of increased alveolar density (white appearance) because of her lung fibrosis, this day's chest x-ray was markedly worse.

The physician on duty felt that the chest x-ray showed an acute inflammatory condition from an undetermined cause. The physician started the patient on corticosteroids. The respiratory therapist noted that even though the patient's alveolar oxygen pressure (PA_{O_2}) was calculated to be 165 mm Hg, the patient's arterial oxygen pressure (Pa_{O_2}) was only 57 mm Hg (normal, 80–100 mm Hg). In response to the low Pa_{O_2}, the therapist increased the patient's inspired oxygen concentration (FI_{O_2}) from 2 L/min via nasal cannula (an FI_{O_2} of about 0.28) to 0.5 via an oxygen Venturi mask.

Over the next 24 hours the patient's condition progressively improved. She stated that she was breathing much better. Her skin color returned to normal and no longer felt cold or wet. Her vital signs were blood pressure—128/86 mm Hg, heart rate—76 beats/min, and respiratory rate—14 breaths/min. A second chest x-ray showed improvement, compared with the previous day's chest x-ray, and her Pa_{O_2} was 89 mm Hg, within normal limits.

DISCUSSION

This case illustrates both the acute and chronic effects of an increased alveolar-capillary membrane. As Fick's law states, the diffusion of gas is *indirectly* related to

(continues)

the thickness of the alveolar-capillary membrane, and *directly* related to $P_1 - P_2$ (see Figure 3–7). Because the patient had chronic alveolar fibrosis and thickening, her oxygen diffusion was low. This is why continuous oxygen (2 L/min) administered via nasal cannula at home was needed to offset this condition. Increasing the alveolar oxygen level (i.e., increasing the P_{AO_2} or P_1) enhanced oxygen diffusion. When the patient's usual chronic status was stable, the 2 L/min oxygen via cannula at home was usually adequate to oxygenate her alveolar-capillary blood.

Because the patient had an acute alveolar inflammatory condition overlying her chronic problem, her alveolar-capillary membrane became even thicker. As a result, her usual home oxygen administration was not enough to meet the new challenge. Over the course of her hospitalization, however, the steroid therapy reduced her alveolar inflammation. As the acute alveolar inflammation improved, the thickness of her alveolar-capillary membrane decreased. While this process was taking place, the increased oxygen concentration (P_1) worked to offset the patient's poor oxygenation status and thus worked to make her comfortable. The patient continued to improve and was discharged on day 5 of her hospital stay. She continued to use oxygen via nasal cannula at home.

REVIEW QUESTIONS

1. If a container having a volume of 375 mL and a pressure of 15 cm H_2O in it is suddenly reduced to a volume of 150 mL, what would be the pressure in the container?
   A. 17.5 cm H_2O
   B. 28 cm H_2O
   C. 37.5 cm H_2O
   D. 43 cm H_2O

2. If the gas temperature in a closed container that has a pressure of 50 cm H_2O in it is increased from 125 absolute to 235 absolute, what would be the pressure in the container?
   A. 86 cm H_2O
   B. 94 cm H_2O
   C. 102 cm H_2O
   D. 117 cm H_2O

3. Which of the following gas laws states that in a mixture of gases the total pressure is equal to the sum of the partial pressure of each gas?
   A. Dalton's law
   B. Gay-Lussac's law
   C. Charles' law
   D. Boyle's law

4. At sea level, the normal percentage of carbon dioxide (CO_2) in the atmosphere is
   A. 5%
   B. 40%
   C. 78%
   D. 0.03%

5. At sea level, the alveolar water vapor pressure is normally about
   A.   0.2 mm Hg
   B.   47 mm Hg
   C.   0.0 mm Hg
   D.   40 mm Hg

6. If a patient is receiving an $F_{I_{O_2}}$ of 0.60 on a day when the barometric pressure is 725 mm Hg, and if the Pa_{CO_2} is 50 mm Hg, what is the patient's alveolar oxygen tension ($P_{A_{O_2}}$)?
   A.   177 mm Hg
   B.   233 mm Hg
   C.   344 mm Hg
   D.   415 mm Hg

7. The normal transit time for blood through the alveolar-capillary system is about
   A.   0.25 second
   B.   0.50 second
   C.   0.75 second
   D.   1.0 second

8. Under normal resting conditions, the diffusion of oxygen and carbon dioxide is usually completed in about
   I.   0.25 second
   II.   0.50 second
   III.   0.75 second
   IV.   1.0 second
   V.   one-third of the time available
       A. II only
       B. III only
       C. IV and V only
       D. I and V only

9. Which of the following states that the rate of gas diffusion is inversely proportional to the weight of the gas?
   A.   Graham's law
   B.   Charles' law
   C.   Henry's law
   D.   Gay-Lussac's law

10. According to Fick's law, gas diffusion is
    I.   directly proportional to the thickness of the tissue
    II.   indirectly proportional to the diffusion constants
    III.   directly proportional to the difference in partial pressure of the gas between the two sides
    IV.   indirectly proportional to the tissue area
        A. I only
        B. III only
        C. IV only
        D. II and III only

CLINICAL APPLICATION QUESTIONS

CASE 1

1. As a result of the severe left heart failure and increased pulmonary blood pressure in the case, fluid moved out of the pulmonary capillaries and into the extracapillary spaces. The pathologic process caused the thickness of the alveolar-capillary membrane to _____.

2. Because gas diffusion is indirectly related to the thickness, the diffusion of oxygen across the alveolar-capillary membrane in this case _____.

3. While the physician was treating the patient's failing heart, the respiratory therapist worked to offset the patient's poor oxygenation by increasing the patient's _____, which is _____ of Fick's law.

4. The therapist achieved the goal in question 3 by (1) increasing the patient's overall _____, and (2) increasing the inspired _____.

CASE 2

1. Which factor in Fick's law confirmed why the patient's oxygenation status was chronically low in this case?

   Answer: _____

2. Which factor in Fick's law was used therapeutically to improve the patient's oxygenation status?

   Answer: _____

3. Which factor in Fick's law caused the patient's oxygenation status to acutely worsen in this case?

   Answer: _____

4. In addition to the corticosteroid therapy, what factor in Fick's law was used therapeutically to improve the patient's oxygenation status?

   Answer: _____

CHAPTER 4

Pulmonary Function Measurements

O B J E C T I V E S

By the end of this chapter, the student should be able to:

1. Define the following *lung volumes:*
   —Tidal volume
   —Inspiratory reserve volume
   —Expiratory reserve volume
   —Residual volume

2. Define the following *lung capacities:*
   —Vital capacity
   —Inspiratory capacity
   —Functional residual capacity
   —Total lung capacity
   —Residual volume/total lung capacity ratio

3. Identify the approximate lung volumes and capacities in milliliters in the average healthy man and woman between 20 and 30 years of age.

4. Compare and contrast how the following methods indirectly measure the residual volume and the capacities containing the residual volume:
   —Closed circuit helium dilution
   —Open circuit nitrogen washout
   —Body plethysmography

5. Compare and contrast the following *expiratory flow rate measurements:*
   —Forced vital capacity
   —Forced expiratory volume timed
   —Forced expiratory volume$_{1 \, sec}$/forced vital capacity ratio
   —Forced expiratory flow$_{25\%-75\%}$
   —Forced expiratory flow$_{200-1200}$

   —Peak expiratory flow rate
   —Maximum voluntary ventilation
   —Flow-volume curves

6. Identify the following average dynamic flow rate measurements for the healthy man and woman between 20 and 30 years of age:
   —Forced expiratory volume timed for periods of 0.5, 1.0, 2.0, and 3.0 seconds
   —Forced expiratory flow$_{200-1200}$
   —Forced expiratory flow$_{25\%-75\%}$
   —Peak expiratory flow rate
   —Maximum voluntary ventilation

7. Describe the *effort-dependent portion* of a forced expiratory maneuver.

8. Describe the *effort-independent portion* of a forced expiratory maneuver.

9. Explain how the *dynamic compression mechanism* limits the flow rate during the last 70 percent of a forced vital capacity, and define the *equal pressure point.*

10. Describe the diffusion capacity of carbon monoxide study.

11. Describe how the following are used to evaluate the patient's ability to maintain spontaneous, unassisted ventilation:
    —Maximum inspiratory pressure (MIP)
    —Maximum expiratory pressure (MEP)

12. Complete the review questions at the end of this chapter.

LUNG VOLUMES AND CAPACITIES

The total amount of air that the lungs can accommodate is divided into four separate volumes. Four specific combinations of these lung volumes are used to designate lung capacities (Figure 4–1).

Lung Volumes

Tidal Volume (V_T): The volume of air that normally moves into and out of the lungs in one quiet breath.

Inspiratory Reserve Volume (IRV): The maximum volume of air that can be inhaled after a normal tidal volume inhalation.

Expiratory Reserve Volume (ERV): The maximum volume of air that can be exhaled after a normal tidal volume exhalation.

Residual Volume (RV): The amount of air remaining in the lungs after a maximal exhalation.

Lung Capacities

Vital Capacity (VC): The maximum volume of air that can be exhaled after a maximal inspiration (IRV + V_T + ERV). There are two major VC measurements: the **slow vital capacity (SVC)**, in which exhalation is performed slowly; and the **forced vital capacity (FVC)**, in which maximal effort is made to exhale as rapidly as possible. A restrictive lung

Figure 4–1

Normal lung volumes and capacities. IRV = inspiratory reserve volume; V_T = tidal volume; ERV = expiratory reserve volume; RV = residual volume; VC = vital capacity; TLC = total lung capacity; IC = inspiratory capacity; FRC = functional residual capacity.

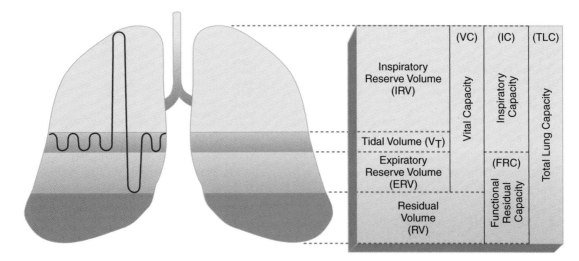

disorder causes the SVC to decrease. The FVC will be discussed in more detail later in this chapter.

Inspiratory Capacity (IC): The volume of air that can be inhaled after a normal exhalation (V_T + IRV).

Functional Residual Capacity (FRC): The volume of air remaining in the lungs after a normal exhalation (ERV + RV).

Total Lung Capacity (TLC): The maximum amount of air that the lungs can accommodate (IC + FRC).

Residual Volume/Total Lung Capacity Ratio (RV/TLC × 100): The percentage of the TLC occupied by the RV.

The amount of air that the lungs can accommodate varies primarily with the age, height, and sex of the individual. Table 4–1 lists the normal lung volumes and capacities of the average man and woman ages 20 to 30 years.

Changes in lung volumes and capacities are seen in trauma and disease. Such changes are usually classified as either an obstructive lung disorder or a restrictive lung disorder.

In an obstructive lung disorder, the RV, V_T, FRC, and RV/TLC ratio are increased; and the VC, IC, IRV, and ERV are decreased (Figure 4–2). In a restrictive lung disorder, the VC, IC, RV, FRC, V_T, and TLC are all decreased (Figure 4–3).

TABLE 4–1

Approximate Lung Volumes and Capacities in Healthy Men and Women 20 to 30 Years of Age

Measurement	Men mL	Men Approx. % of TLC	Women mL	Women Approx. % of TLC
Tidal volume (V_T)	500	8–10	400–500	8–10
Inspiratory reserve volume (IRV)	3100	50	1900	30
Expiratory reserve volume (ERV)	1200	20	800	20
Residual volume (RV)	1200	20	1000	25
Vital capacity (VC)	4800	80	3200	75
Inspiratory capacity (IC)	3600	60	2400	60
Functional residual capacity (FRC)	2400	40	1800	40
Total lung capacity (TLC)	6000	—	4200	—
Residual volume/total lung capacity ratio (RV/TLC × 100)	$\frac{1200}{6000}$	20	$\frac{1000}{4200}$	25

Figure 4–2

How obstructive lung disorders alter lung volumes and capacities. IRV = inspiratory reserve volume; V_T = tidal volume; ERV = expiratory reserve volume; RV = residual volume; VC = tidal capacity; IC = inspiratory capacity; FRC = functional residual capacity; TLC = total lung capacity.

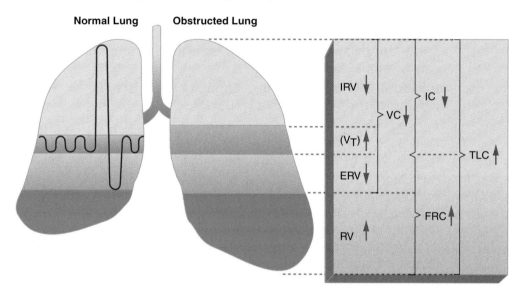

Figure 4–3

How restrictive lung disorders alter lung volumes and capacities. IRV = inspiratory reserve volume; V_T = tidal volume; ERV = expiratory reserve volume; RV = residual volume; VC = vital capacity; IC = inspiratory capacity; FRC = functional residual capacity; TLC = total lung capacity.

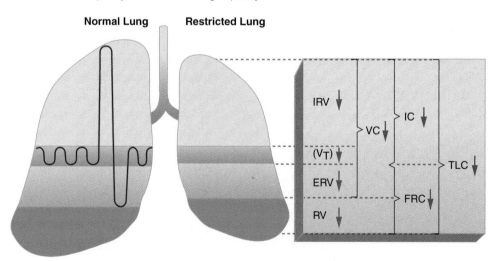

Indirect Measurements of the Residual Volume and Capacities Containing the Residual Volume

Because the *residual volume* (RV) cannot be exhaled, the RV, and lung capacities that contain the RV, are measured indirectly by one of the following methods: *closed circuit helium dilution, open circuit nitrogen washout,* or *body plethysmography.* A brief description of each of these methods follows.

The **closed circuit helium dilution** test requires the patient to rebreathe from a spirometer that contains a known volume of gas (V_1) and a known concentration (C_1) of helium (He), usually 10 percent. The patient is "switched-in" to the closed circuit system at the end of a normal tidal volume breath (i.e., the level at which only the FRC is left in the lungs). A helium analyzer continuously monitors the He concentration. Exhaled carbon dioxide is chemically removed from the system. The gas in the patient's FRC, which initially contains no He, mixes with the gas in the spirometer. This dilutes the He throughout the entire system (i.e., patient's lungs, spirometer, and circuit). The test lasts for about 7 minutes. When the He changes by less than 0.2 percent over a period of 1 second, the test is terminated. The He concentration at this point is C_2. The final volume of the entire system—the He circuit and lungs (V_2)—can be calculated by using the following formula:

$$V_1C_1 = V_2C_2$$

which is rearranged to solve for V_2 as follows

$$V_2 = \frac{V_1C_1}{C_2}$$

The FRC can then be calculated by subtracting the initial spirometer volume (V_1) from the equilibrium volume (V_2). (FRC = $V_2 - V_1$). The RV is determined by FRC − ERV. The TLC can be calculated by RV + VC.

In the **open circuit nitrogen washout** test, the patient breathes 100 percent oxygen through a one-way valve for up to 7 minutes. The patient is "switched-in" to the system at the end of a normal tidal volume (i.e., the level at which only the FRC is left in the lungs). At the beginning of the test, the nitrogen (N_2) concentration in the alveoli is 79 percent (C_1). During each breath, oxygen is inhaled and N_2-rich gas from the FRC is exhaled. Over several minutes, the N_2 in the patient's FRC is effectively washed out. In patients with normal lungs this occurs in 3 minutes or less. Patients with obstructive lung disease may not wash out completely even after 7 minutes.

During the washout period, the exhaled gas volume is measured and the average concentration of N_2 is determined with a nitrogen analyzer. The test is complete when the N_2 concentration drops from 79 to 1.5 percent or less. The FRC (V_1) can then be determined by taking the initial concentration of N_2 in the FRC gas (C_1), the total volume of gas exhaled during the washout period (V_2), and the average concentration of N_2 in the exhaled gas (C_2) and inserting the findings into the following equation:

$$V_1 = \frac{C_2 V_2}{C_1}$$

The FRC can then be calculated by subtracting the known volume of the breathing circuit (V_{bc}) and correcting for the volume of N_2 excreted into the lungs from the plasma and body tissues during the test (V_{tis}):

$$FRC = V_1 - V_{bc} + V_{tis}$$

Body plethysmography measures the gas volume within the lungs (thoracic gas volume [V_{TG}]) indirectly by using a modification of Boyle's law. During the test, the patient sits in an airtight chamber called a *body box.* Initially, the patient is permitted to breathe quietly through an open valve (shutter). Once the patient is relaxed, the test begins at the precise moment the patient exhales to the end tidal volume level (FRC). At this point, the shutter is closed and the patient is instructed to pant against the closed shutter. Pressure and volume changes are monitored during this period. The alveolar pressure changes caused by the compression and decompression of the lungs are estimated at the mouth. Because there is no airflow during this period, and because the temperature is kept constant, the pressure and volume changes can be used to determine the trapped volume (FRC) by applying Boyle's law. This method is generally considered to be the most accurate of the three methods for measuring RV.

PULMONARY MECHANICS

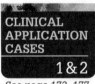

CLINICAL
APPLICATION
CASES
1 & 2
See page 173–177

In addition to measuring volumes and capacities, the rate at which gas flows in and out of the lungs can also be measured. Expiratory flow rate measurements provide data on the integrity of the airways and the severity of airway impairment, as well as indicating whether the patient has a large airway or a small airway problem. Collectively, the tests for measuring expiratory flow rates are referred to as the pulmonary mechanic measurements.

Pulmonary Mechanic Measurements
Forced Vital Capacity (FVC)

The FVC is the maximum volume of gas that can be exhaled as forcefully and rapidly as possible after a maximal inspiration (Figure 4–4). The FVC is the most commonly performed pulmonary function measurement. In the normal individual, the *total expiratory time* (TET) required to

Figure 4–4
Forced vital capacity (FVC). A = point of maximal inspiration and the starting point of an FVC.

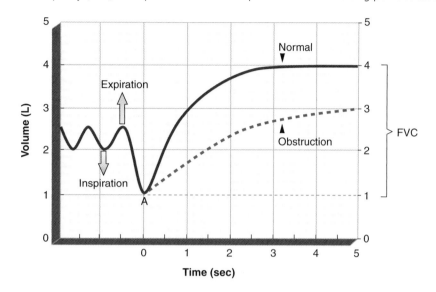

completely exhale the FVC is 4 to 6 seconds. In obstructive lung disease (e.g., chronic bronchitis), the TET increases. TETs greater than 10 seconds have been reported in these patients.

In the normal individual, the FVC and the slow vital capacity (SVC) are usually equal. In the patient with obstructive lung disease, the SVC is often normal and the FVC is usually decreased because of air trapping. The FVC is also decreased in restrictive lung disorders (e.g., pulmonary fibrosis, adult respiratory distress syndrome, pulmonary edema). This is primarily due to the low vital capacity associated with restrictive disorders. The TET needed to exhale the FVC in a restrictive disorder, however, is usually normal or even lower than normal, because the elasticity of the lung is high (low compliance) in restrictive disorders.

Forced Expiratory Volume Timed (FEV$_T$)

The FEV$_T$ is the maximum volume of gas that can be exhaled within a specific time period. This measurement is obtained from an FVC. The most frequently used time period is 1 second. Other commonly used periods are 0.5, 2, and 3 seconds (Figure 4–5). Normally, the percentage of the total FVC exhaled during these time periods is as follows: FEV$_{0.5}$, 60 percent; FEV$_1$, 83 percent; FEV$_2$, 94 percent; and FEV$_3$, 97 percent. Patients with *obstructive pulmonary disease* have a decreased FEV$_T$. Patients with *restrictive lung disease* also have a decreased FEV$_T$, primarily due to the low vital capacity associated with such disease. The FEV$_T$ decreases with age.

Figure 4–5

Forced expiratory volume timed (FEV$_T$).

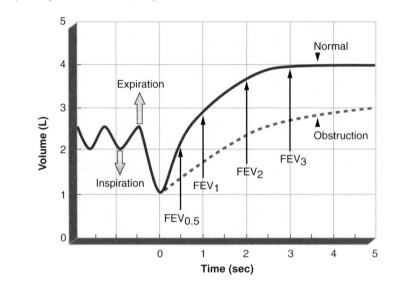

Forced Expiratory Volume$_{1\ Sec}$/Forced Vital Capacity Ratio (FEV$_1$/FVC Ratio)

The *FEV$_1$/FVC ratio* is the comparison of the amount of air exhaled in 1 second to the total amount exhaled during an FVC maneuver. Because the FEV$_1$/FVC ratio is expressed as a percentage, it is commonly referred to as a *forced expiratory volume in 1 second percentage* (FEV$_{1\%}$). As mentioned previously, the normal adult exhales 83 percent or more of the FVC in 1 second (FEV$_1$). Thus, under normal conditions the patient's FEV$_{1\%}$ should also be 83 percent or greater. Clinically, however, an FEV$_{1\%}$ of 65 percent or more is often used as an acceptable value in older patients.

Collectively, the **FVC**, **FEV$_1$**, and the **FEV$_{1\%}$** are the most commonly used pulmonary function measurements to (1) determine the severity of a patient's obstructive pulmonary disease, and (2) distinguish between an obstructive and restrictive lung disorder. The key pulmonary function differences between an obstructive and restrictive lung disorder are as follows: In obstructive lung disorders, both the FEV$_1$ and the FEV$_{1\%}$ are *decreased.* In restrictive lung disorders, the FEV$_1$ is *decreased,* but the FEV$_{1\%}$ is normal or *increased.*

Forced Expiratory Flow$_{25\%-75\%}$ (FEF$_{25\%-75\%}$)

The FEF$_{25\%-75\%}$ is the average flow rate that occurs during the middle 50 percent of an FVC measurement (Figure 4–6). This average measurement reflects the condition of *medium- to small-sized airways.* The average

Figure 4–6
Forced expiratory flow$_{25\%-75\%}$ (FEF$_{25\%-75\%}$).

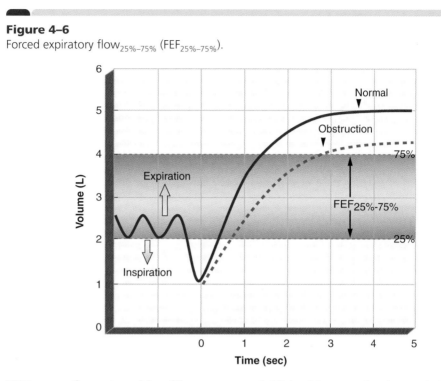

FEF$_{25\%-75\%}$ for normal healthy men aged 20 to 30 years is about 4.5 L/sec (270 L/min), and for women of the same age, about 3.5 L/sec (210 L/min). The FEF$_{25\%-75\%}$ decreases with age and in obstructive lung disease. In obstructive lung disease, flow rates as low as 0.3 L/sec (18 L/min) have been reported.

The FEF$_{25\%-75\%}$ is also decreased in patients with restrictive lung disorders, primarily because of the low vital capacity associated with restrictive lung disorders. Although the FEF$_{25\%-75\%}$ has no value in distinguishing between obstructive and restrictive disease, it is helpful in further confirming—or ruling out—an obstructive pulmonary disease in patients with borderline low FEV$_{1\%}$. Conceptually, the FEF$_{25\%-75\%}$ is similar to measuring, and then averaging, the flow rate from a water faucet when 25 and 75 percent of a specific volume of water have accumulated in a measuring container (Figure 4–7).

Forced Expiratory Flow$_{200-1200}$ (FEF$_{200-1200}$)

The FEF$_{200-1200}$ is the average flow rate that occurs between 200 and 1200 mL of the FVC (Figure 4–8). The first 200 mL of the FVC is usually exhaled more slowly than the average flow rate because of (1) the inertia involved in the respiratory maneuver, and (2) the unreliability of response time of the equipment. Because the FEF$_{200-1200}$ measures expiratory flows at high lung volumes, it is a good index of the integrity of *large airway function* (above the bronchioles). Flow rates that originate from the large airways

Figure 4–7

The $FEF_{25\%-75\%}$ is similar to measuring and then averaging the flow rate from a faucet when 1 and 3 liters of water have accumulated in a 4-liter container. Picture the flow rate from the faucet being measured when 1 liter (25%) of water has entered a 4-liter container **(A)**. Again, picture the flow rate from the faucet being measured when 3 liters (75%) of water have entered the 4-liter container **(B)**. Taking the average of the two flow rates would be similar to the $FEF_{25\%-75\%}$, which measures and then averages the flow rate when an individual exhales 25% and 75% of the FVC.

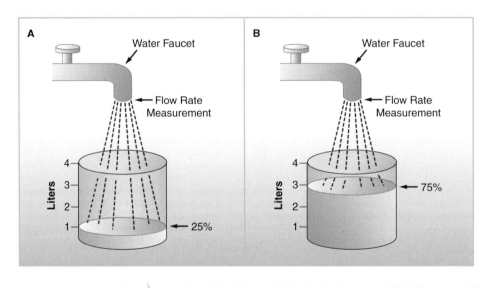

Figure 4–8

Forced expiratory flow$_{200-1200}$ ($FEF_{200-1200}$).

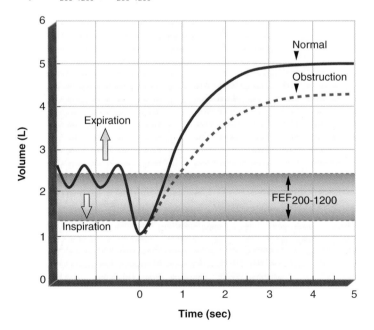

Figure 4–9
The FEF$_{200-1200}$ is similar to measuring and then averaging the flow rate of water from a faucet at the precise moment when 200 and 1200 mL of water have accumulated in a container. Picture the flow rate from the faucet being measured when 200 mL of water have entered the container **(A)**. Then picture the flow rate from the faucet being measured when 1200 mL of water have entered container **(B)**. Taking the average of the two flow rates would be similar to the FEF$_{200-1200}$, which measures and then averages the flow rate at the precise point when 200 and 1200 mL of gas have been exhaled during an FVC maneuver.

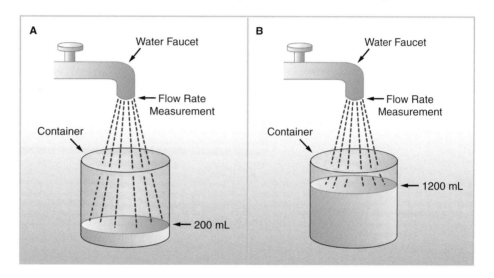

are referred to as the effort-dependent portion of the FVC.* Thus, the greater the patient effort, the higher the FEF$_{200-1200}$ value. The average FEF$_{200-1200}$ for healthy men ages 20 to 30 years is about 8 L/sec (480 L/min), and for women of the same age, about 5.5 L/sec (330 L/min).

The FEF$_{200-1200}$ decreases with age and in obstructive lung disease. Flow rates as low as 1 L/sec (60 L/min) have been reported in some patients with obstructive lung disease. The FEF$_{200-1200}$ is also decreased in patients with restrictive lung disorders. This is primarily because of the low vital capacity associated with restrictive lung disorders. Conceptually, the FEF$_{200-1200}$ is similar to measuring, and then averaging, the flow rate from a water faucet when 200 and 1200 mL have accumulated in a measuring container (Figure 4–9).

Peak Expiratory Flow Rate (PEFR)

The PEFR (also known as *peak flow rate*) is the maximum flow rate that can be achieved during an FVC maneuver (Figure 4–10). The PEFR is most commonly measured at the bedside using a small, handheld flow-sensing

See "The Effort-Dependent Portion of a Forced Expiratory Maneuver" later in this chapter.

Figure 4–10
Peak expiratory flow rate (PEFR).

device called a **peak flow meter**. Similar to the $FEF_{200-1200}$ measurement, the PEFR reflects initial flows originating from the large airways during the first part of an FVC maneuver (the effort-dependent portion of the FVC*). Thus, the greater the patient effort, the higher the PEFR value.

The average PEFR for normal healthy men ages 20 to 30 years is about 10 L/sec (600 L/min), and for women of the same age, about 7.5 L/sec (450 L/min). The PEFR decreases with age and in obstructive lung disease. The PEFR is an inexpensive and effective bedside measurement that is used both in the hospital and home care setting to evaluate gross changes in airway function and to assess the patient's response to bronchodilator therapy.

Maximum Voluntary Ventilation (MVV)

The MVV is the largest volume of gas that can be breathed voluntarily in and out of the lungs in 1 minute (the patient actually performs the test for only 12 or 15 seconds); it is also known as *maximum breathing capacity* (MBC) (Figure 4–11). The MVV is a general test that evaluates the performance of the respiratory muscles' strength, the compliance of the lung and thorax, airway resistance, and neural control mechanisms. The MVV is a broad test and only large reductions are significant. The average MVV for healthy men ages 20 to 30 years is about 170 L/min, and for women of the same age it is about 110 L/min. The MVV decreases with age and chronic obstructive pulmonary disease. The MVV

*See "The Effort-Dependent Portion of a Forced Expiratory Maneuver" later in this chapter.

Figure 4–11
Maximum voluntary ventilation (MVV).

is relatively normal in restrictive pulmonary disease. The MVV decreases with age.

Flow-Volume Loop

The flow-volume loop is a graphic presentation of a forced vital capacity (FVC) maneuver followed by a forced inspiratory volume (FIV) maneuver. When the FVC and FIV are plotted together, the illustration produced by the two curves is called a **flow-volume loop** (Figure 4–12). The flow-volume loop compares both the *flow rates* and *volume changes* produced at different points of an FVC and FIV maneuver. Although the flow-volume loop does not measure the $FEF_{200-1200}$ and $FEF_{25\%-75\%}$, it does show the *maximum flows* ($\dot{V}_{max}$) at any point of the FVC. The most commonly reported maximum flows are $FEF_{25\%}$, $FEF_{50\%}$, and $FEF_{75\%}$. In healthy individuals, the $FEF_{50\%}$ (also called the $\dot{V}_{max_{50}}$) is a straight line because the expiratory flow decreases linearly with volume throughout most of the FVC range. In subjects with obstructive lung disease, however, the flow rate decreases at low lung volumes, causing the $FEF_{50\%}$ to decrease. This causes a cuplike or scooped out effect on the flow-volume loop.

To summarize, depending on the sophistication of the equipment, several important measurements can be obtained from the flow-volume loop, including the following:

Figure 4–12

Normal flow-volume loop. PEFR = peak expiration flow rate; PIFR = peak inspiratory flow rate; FVC = forced vital capacity; $FEF_{25\%-75\%}$ = forced expiratory flow$_{25\%-75\%}$; $FEF_{50\%}$ = forced expiratory flow$_{50\%}$ (also called $\dot{V}_{max_{50}}$).

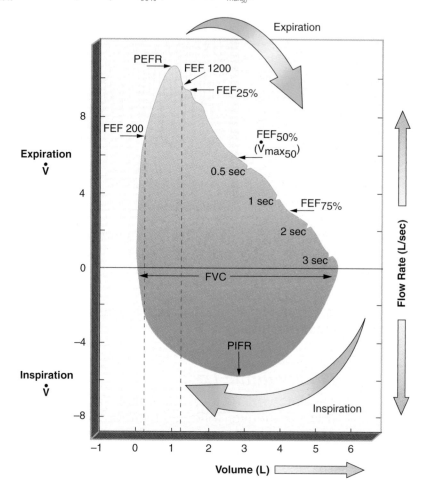

- PEFR
- PIFR
- FVC
- FEV_T

- FEV_1/FVC ratio
- $FEF_{25\%}$
- $FEF_{50\%}$ ($\dot{V}_{max_{50}}$)
- $FEF_{75\%}$.

Flow-volume loop measurements graphically illustrate both obstructive (Figure 4–13) and restrictive lung problems (Figure 4–14). Table 4–2 summarizes the average dynamic flow rate values found in healthy men and women ages 20 to 30 years.

Figure 4–13
Flow-volume loop, obstructive pattern. FVC = forced vital capacity.

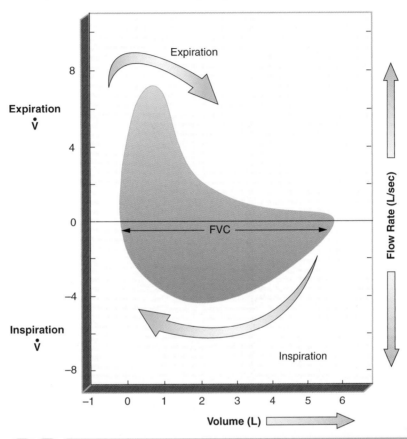

TABLE 4–2
Average Dynamic Flow Rate Measurements in Healthy Men and Women 20 to 30 Years of Age

Measurement*	Men	Women
FEV_T		
$\quad FEV_{0.5}$	60%	60%
$\quad FEV_{1.0}$	83%	83%
$\quad FEV_{2.0}$	94%	94%
$\quad FEV_{3.0}$	97%	97%
$FEF_{200-1200}$	8 L/sec (480 L/min)	5.5 L/sec (330 L/min)
$FEF_{25\%-75\%}$	4.5 L/sec (270 L/min)	3.5 L/sec (210 L/min)
PEFR	10 L/sec (600 L/min)	7.5 L/sec (450 L/min)
MVV	170 L/min	110 L/min

* See text for explanation of abbreviations.

Figure 4–14
Flow-volume loop, restrictive pattern. FVC = forced vital capacity.

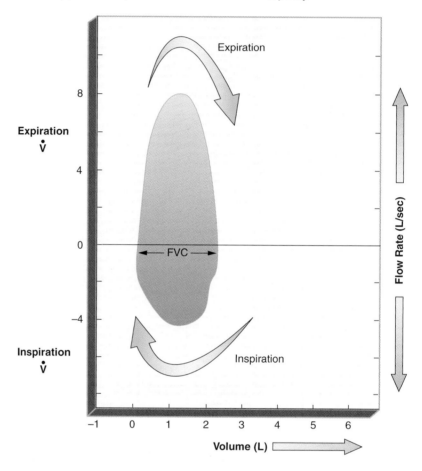

HOW THE EFFECTS OF DYNAMIC COMPRESSION DECREASE EXPIRATORY FLOW RATES

CLINICAL
APPLICATION
CASE

1

See page 173

The Effort-Dependent Portion of a Forced Expiratory Maneuver

During approximately the first 30 percent of an FVC maneuver, the maximum peak flow rate is dependent on the amount of muscular effort exerted by the individual. This portion of the FVC maneuver originates from the large airways and is referred to as **effort-dependent**. As discussed earlier, the $FEF_{200-1200}$ and PEFR measurements reflect flow rates from the large airways. Thus, the greater the patient effort, the higher the $FEF_{200-1200}$ and PEFR values.

The Effort-Independent Portion of a Forced Expiratory Maneuver

The flow rate during approximately the last 70 percent of an FVC maneuver is **effort independent**. That is, once a maximum flow rate has been attained, the flow rate cannot be increased by further muscular effort.

The lung volume at which the patient initiates a forced expiratory maneuver also influences the maximum flow rate. As lung volumes decline, flow also declines. The reduced flow, however, is the maximum flow for that particular volume.

Figure 4–15 illustrates where the effort-dependent and effort-independent portions of a forced expiratory maneuver appear on a flow-volume loop.

Figure 4–15

The effort-dependent and effort-independent portions of a forced expiratory maneuver in a flow-volume loop measurement. FVC = forced vital capacity.

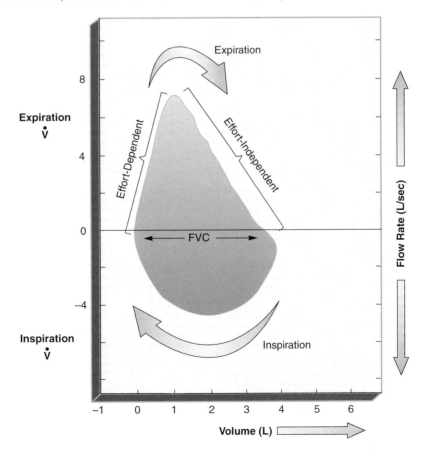

Dynamic Compression of the Bronchial Airways

The limitation of the flow rate that occurs during the last 70 percent of an FVC maneuver is due to the **dynamic compression** of the walls of the airways. As gas flows through the airways from the alveoli to the atmosphere during passive expiration, the pressure within the airways diminishes to zero (Figure 4–16A).

Figure 4–16
The dynamic compression mechanism. **(A)** During passive expiration, static elastic recoil pressure of the lungs (P_{stL}) is 10, pleural pressure (P_{pl}) at the beginning of expiration is −5, and alveolar pressure (P_{alv}) is +5. In order for gas to move from the alveolus to the atmosphere during expiration, the pressure must decrease progressively in the airways from +5 to 0. As A shows, P_{pl} is always less than the airway pressure. **(B)** During forced expiration, P_{pl} becomes positive (+10 in this illustration). When this P_{pl} is added to the P_{stL} of +10, P_{alv} becomes +20. As the pressure progressively decreases during forced expiration, there must be a point at which the pressures inside and outside the airway wall are equal. This point is the equal pressure point. Airway compression occurs downstream (toward the mouth) from this point because the lateral pressure is less than the surrounding wall pressure.

During a forced expiratory maneuver, however, as the airway pressure decreases from the alveoli to the atmosphere, there is a point at which the pressure within the lumen of the airways equals the pleural pressure surrounding the airways. This point is called the **equal pressure point**.

Downstream (i.e., toward the mouth) from the equal pressure point, the lateral pressure within the airway becomes less than the surrounding pleural pressure. Consequently, the airways are compressed. As muscular effort and pleural pressure increase during a forced expiratory maneuver, the equal pressure point moves upstream (i.e., toward the alveolus). Ultimately, the equal pressure point becomes fixed where the individual's flow rate has achieved maximum (Figure 4–16B). In essence, once dynamic compression occurs during a forced expiratory maneuver, increased muscular effort merely augments airway compression, which in turn increases airway resistance.

As the structural changes associated with certain respiratory diseases (e.g., COPD) intensify, the patient commonly responds by increasing intrapleural pressure during expiration to overcome the increased airway resistance produced by the disease. By increasing intrapleural pressure during expiration, however, the patient activates the dynamic compression mechanism, which in turn further reduces the diameter of the bronchial airways. This results in an even greater increase in airway resistance.

Flow normally is not limited to effort during inspiration. This is because the airways widen as greater inspiratory efforts are generated, thus enhancing gas flow (see Figure 2–23).

Maximum Inspiratory and Expiratory Pressure

An individual's **maximum inspiratory pressure** (MIP) and **maximum expiratory pressure** (MEP) are directly related to muscle strength. Table 4–3 shows the average MIP and MEP for the normal healthy adult. Clinically, the MIP and MEP are used to evaluate the patient's ability to maintain spontaneous, unassisted mechanical ventilation. Both the MIP and MEP are commonly measured while the patient inhales and exhales through an endotracheal tube that is attached to a pressure gauge. For the best results, the MIP should be measured at the patient's *residual volume,* and the MEP should be measured at the patient's *total lung capacity.* In general, the patient is ready for a trial of spontaneous or

TABLE 4–3
Maximum Inspiratory and Expiratory Pressures

	MIP	MEP
Male	−125 cm H_2O	230 cm H_2O
Female	−90 cm H_2O	150 cm H_2O

unassisted ventilation when the MIP is greater than -25 cm H_2O and the MEP is greater than 50 cm H_2O.

Diffusion Capacity of Carbon Monoxide (DL_{CO})

The DL_{CO} study measures the amount of carbon monoxide (CO), a diffusion-limited gas,* that moves across the alveolar-capillary membrane. CO has an affinity for hemoglobin that is about 210 times greater than that of oxygen. Thus, in individuals who have normal amounts of hemoglobin and normal ventilatory function, the only limiting factor to the diffusion of CO is the alveolar-capillary membrane. In essence, the DL_{CO} study measures the physiologic status of the various anatomic structures that compose the alveolar-capillary membrane (see Figure 3–2).

The CO single-breath technique is commonly used for this measurement. Under normal conditions, the average DL_{CO} value for the resting male is 25 mL/min/mm Hg (STPD). This value is slightly lower in females, presumably because of their smaller normal lung volumes. The DL_{CO} may increase threefold in healthy subjects during exercise. The DL_{CO} generally decreases in response to lung disorders that affect the alveolar-capillary membrane. For example, the DL_{CO} is decreased in emphysema because of the alveolar-capillary destruction associated with this lung disease. See Figure 3–10 for other common lung disorders that affect the alveolar-capillary membrane and cause the DL_{CO} to decrease.

CHAPTER SUMMARY

The total amount of air that the lungs can accommodate is divided into four separate volumes and four capacities. The lung volumes are the tidal volume (V_T), inspiratory reserve volume (IRV), expiratory reserve volume (ERV), and residual volume (RV). The capacities consist of the vital capacity (VC), inspiratory capacity (IC), functional residual capacity (FRC), and total lung capacity (TLC). In obstructive lung disorders, the RV, V_T, FRC, and RV/TLC ratio are increased; the VC, IC, IRV, and ERV are decreased. In restrictive lung disorders, the VC, IC, RV, FRC, V_T, and TLC are all decreased. Because the RV cannot be exhaled, the RV, and lung capacities that contain the RV, are measured indirectly by either the closed circuit helium dilution method, the open circuit nitrogen washout method, or by body plethymosgraphy.

In addition to measuring volumes and capacities, the rate at which gas flows into and out of the lungs can be measured. Collectively, the tests used to measure expiratory flow rates are referred to as pulmonary mechanic measurements. These tests include the forced vital capacity (FVC), forced expiratory volume time (FEV_T), forced expiratory volume 1 sec/forced vital capacity ratio (FEV_1/FVC), forced expiratory flow

*See diffusion-limited gas flow discussion, page 142.

25%–75% ($FEF_{25\%-75\%}$), forced expiratory flow$_{200-1200}$ ($FEF_{200-1200}$), peak expiratory flow rate (PEFR), and the maximum voluntary ventilation (MVV). The flow-volume loop is a graphic presentation of an FVC followed by a forced inspiratory volume (FIV) maneuver. The flow-volume loop compares both the flow rates and volume changes produced at different points of the FVC and FIV maneuver. A number of measurements can be obtained from the flow-volume loop, including the PEFR, PIFR, FVC, FEV_T, FEV_1/FVC ratio, $FEF_{25\%}$, $FEF_{50\%}$ ($\dot{V}_{max_{50}}$), and $FEF_{75\%}$. To fully understand the pulmonary mechanic measurements, the respiratory therapist must have a basic knowledge of how the effects of dynamic compression decrease expiratory flow rates, including the influences of (1) the effort-dependent portion of a forced expiratory maneuver, (2) the effort-independent portion of a forced expiratory maneuver, and (3) the dynamic compression of the bronchial airways. Finally, the maximum inspiratory pressure (MIP) and maximum expiratory pressure (MEP) are used to directly measure muscle strength, and the diffusion capacity of carbon monoxide (DL_{CO}) is routinely used to evaluate the physiologic status of the various anatomic structures of the alveolar-capillary membrane.

1 CLINICAL APPLICATION CASE

A 16-year-old girl with a long history of asthma became short of breath while playing volleyball during her high school gym class. The head coach took her out of the game and had an assistant coach watch her closely. Even though the patient inhaled a total of four puffs of the bronchodilator albuterol from a metered-dose inhaler over the next 30 minutes, her condition progressively worsened. Concerned, the coach called the patient's mother. Because the patient had had to be given mechanical ventilation on two different occasions, the patient's mother asked the coach to take her daughter directly to the emergency department of the local hospital.

In the emergency department, the patient was observed to be in severe respiratory distress. Her skin was blue and she was using her accessory muscles of inspiration. The patient stated, "My asthma is really getting bad." Her vital signs were blood pressure—180/110 mm Hg, heart rate—130 beats/min, respiratory rate—36 breaths/min, and oral temperature 37°C. While on 4 L/min oxygen via nasal cannula, her hemoglobin oxygen saturation (Sp_{O_2}), measured by pulse oximetry over the skin of her index finger, was 83 percent.

A portable chest x-ray showed that her lungs were hyperinflated and that her diaphragm was depressed (Figure 4–17). Measurement of the patient's forced vital capacity provided the following data:

Bedside Spirometry		
Parameter*	**Predicted**	**Actual**
FVC	2800 mL	1220 mL
FEV_1	>83%	44%
PEFR	400 L/min	160 L/min

*FVC = forced vital capacity; FEV_1 = forced expiratory volume in 1 second (see text); PEFR = peak expiratory flow rate.

(continues)

Figure 4–17
X-ray showing presence of asthma.

Because the respiratory therapist felt that the patient did not produce a good effort on her first FVC test, a second test was done. Even though the patient appeared to exhale much more forcefully during the second FVC test, the spirometry results were identical to the previous ones. The patient's mother stated that her daughter's "personal best" peak expiratory flow rate (PEFR) at home was 360 L/min. While the patient was in the emergency department, the nurse started an intravenous infusion. The respiratory therapist increased the patient's oxygen via nasal cannula to 6 L/min. The patient was then given a continuous bronchodilator therapy via a handheld nebulizer per the respiratory care protocol. The medical director of the respiratory care department was notified and a mechanical ventilator was placed on standby.

One hour later, the patient stated that she was breathing easier. Her skin appeared pink and she was no longer using her accessory muscles of inspiration. Her vital signs were blood pressure—122/76 mm Hg, heart rate—82 beats/min, and respiratory rate—14 breaths/min. On 2 L/min oxygen via

(continues)

nasal cannula her Sp_{O_2} was 97 percent. Her bedside spirometry results at this time were as follows:

Bedside Spirometry		
Parameter*	Predicted	Actual
FVC	2800 mL	2375 mL
FEV_1	>83%	84%
PEFR	400 L/min	345 L/min

*FVC = forced vital capacity; FEV_1 = forced expiratory volume in 1 second; PEFR = peak expiratory flow rate.

The patient continued to improve and her oxygen therapy, bronchodilator therapy, and IV were all discontinued the next morning. Her bedside spirometry results were FVC, 2810 mL; FEV_1, 87 percent; and PEFR, 355 L/min. She was discharged on the afternoon of the second day. During her exit interview, she was instructed to use her metered-dose inhaler about 15 minutes before each gym class.

DISCUSSION

This case illustrates (1) how the measurement of a patient's pulmonary mechanics can serve as an important clinical monitor; and (2) the effects and interrelationships of the following on the bronchial airways during a forced expiratory maneuver: the *effort-independent* portion of a forced expiratory maneuver, *dynamic compression*, and the *equal pressure point*.

When the patient was in the emergency department, the fact that her mother knew her daughter's "personal best" PEFR served as an important clinical indicator of the severity of the patient's asthma attack. Today, asthma patients commonly monitor their own PEFR at home to evaluate the severity of an asthmatic episode. Some physicians instruct their patients to call them or to go directly to the hospital when their PEFR decreases to a specific level.

The fact that the respiratory therapist obtained the same bedside spirometry results on the second test demonstrated the effects of *effort-independent flow rate, dynamic compression*, and the *equal pressure point* on the bronchial airways during an FVC maneuver. Remember, approximately the last 70 percent of an FVC maneuver is effort independent because of the dynamic compression of the bronchial airways. When the patient made a stronger muscular effort on the second FVC test, she only moved the equal pressure point (and dynamic compression) of her airways closer to the alveoli—which in turn further increased airway resistance and offset any increase in her FVC (see Figure 4–16).

2 CLINICAL APPLICATION CASE

A 29-year-old man with no previous history of pulmonary disease presented at his family physician's office complaining of a frequent cough and shortness of breath. He stated that his cough had started about 2 weeks prior to this visit as a result of breathing paint fumes while working in a small and confined area. Even though the patient stated that he had stopped painting in the enclosed area immediately, his cough and his ability to breathe progressively worsened. At the time of this office visit, he had been too ill to work for 2 days. The physician admitted the patient to the

(continues)

hospital and requested a pulmonary consultation.

In the hospital, the patient appeared healthy but in severe respiratory distress. His skin was blue and his hospital gown was damp from perspiration. He had a frequent and weak cough. During each coughing episode, he produced a moderate amount of thick, white and yellow sputum. His vital signs were blood pressure—155/96 mm Hg, heart rate—90 beats/min, respiratory rate— 26 breaths/min, and oral temperature of 37°C. Dull percussion notes were elicited over the lower lobe of the patient's left lung. Rhonchi were heard over both lungs during exhalation, and loud bronchial rales were heard over the left lower lobe.

On administration of 4 L/min oxygen via nasal cannula, the patient's arterial oxygen pressure (Pa_{O_2}) was 63 mm Hg (normal, 80–100 mm Hg). A chest x-ray showed several areas of alveolar collapse (*atelectasis*) throughout the left lower lobe. A pulmonary function study revealed the following results:

Pulmonary Function Study No. 1		
Parameter*	Predicted	Actual
FVC	4600 mL	2990 mL
FEV_1	>83%	67%
$FEF_{200-1200}$	470 L/min	306 L/min
PEFR	>400 L/min	345 L/min
VC	4600 mL	2900 mL
RV	1175 mL	764 mL
FRC	2350 mL	1528 mL

*FVC = forced vital capacity; FEV_1 = forced expiratory volume in first second of an FVC maneuver; $FEF_{200-1200}$ = forced expiratory flow$_{200-1200}$; see text; PEFR = peak expiratory flow rate; VC = vital capacity; RV = residual volume; FRC = functional residual capacity.

In the patient's chart, the physician noted that the excessive bronchial secretions were a result of an acute tracheobronchial tree inflammation (acute bronchitis) caused by the inhalation of noxious paint fumes. The physician also noted that the patches of atelectasis (see Figure 3–10) identified in the patient's left lower lung lobe were most likely caused by excessive airway secretions and mucous plugging.

The respiratory therapist working with the patient obtained a sputum sample and sent it to the laboratory for culture. To help mobilize and clear the excessive bronchial secretions and to offset the mucous plugging, the patient was started on aggressive bronchial hygiene therapy, which consisted of coughing and deep breathing, chest physical therapy, and postural drainage. To treat the atelectasis in the left lower lobe, the patient received lung expansion therapy (hyperinflation therapy), which consisted of incentive spirometry, coughing and deep breathing, and continuous positive airway pressure (CPAP) via a face mask.

Three days later, the patient's general appearance had improved significantly and he no longer appeared to be in respiratory distress. His skin was pink. He no longer had a cough. When the patient was asked to cough, the cough was strong and nonproductive. At this time, he was receiving antibiotic therapy for a streptococcal infection that had been identified from a sputum culture. His vital signs were blood pressure—116/66 mm Hg, heart rate—64 beats/min, respiratory rate— 12 breaths/min, and oral temperature of 37°C. Normal percussion notes were elicited over both lungs. Normal bronchial vesicular breath sounds were heard over both lungs.

On room air, the patient's Pa_{O_2} was 96 mm Hg. A chest x-ray showed no problems. A second pulmonary function study revealed

(continues)

the results shown in the table below. The patient was discharged the following day.

Pulmonary Function Study No. 2		
Parameter*	Predicted	Actual
FVC	4600 mL	4585 mL
FEV_1	>83%	83%
$FEF_{200-1200}$	470 L/min	458 L/min
PEFR	>400 L/min	455 L/min
VC	4600 mL	4585 mL
RV	1175 mL	1165 mL
FRC	2350 mL	2329 mL

*FVC = forced vital capacity; FEV_1 = forced expiratory volume in first second of an FVC maneuver; $FEF_{200-1200}$ = forced expiratory flow$_{200-1200}$; see text; PEFR = peak expiratory flow rate; VC = vital capacity; RV = residual volume; FRC = functional residual capacity.

DISCUSSION

This case illustrates both an obstructive and restrictive lung disorder. Because of the excessive bronchial secretions produced by the inhalation of paint fumes and the subsequent streptococcal infection, the patient's FVC, FEV_1, $FEF_{200-1200}$, and PEFR were all decreased at the time of admission.

In addition, the excessive bronchial secretions (and the patient's weak cough effort) caused mucous pooling, and mucous plugging, of the bronchial airways in the left lower lobe. As a result of the mucous plugging, the alveoli distal to the bronchial obstructions could not be ventilated and eventually collapsed. This condition was verified by the chest x-ray and by the decreased VC, RV, and FRC.

Fortunately, his respiratory problems were reversible with aggressive bronchial hygiene therapy and lung expansion therapy. Once the bronchial secretions were cleared, the obstructive problem was no longer present. This was verified by the increased values shown of the FVC, FEV_1, $FEF_{200-1200}$, and PEFR. When the mucous plugs were cleared and the lungs were re-expanded, the restrictive problem was no longer present. This was verified by the increased values of the VC, FRC, and RV.

REVIEW QUESTIONS

1. The volume of air that can be exhaled after a normal tidal volume exhalation is the
   A. IRV
   B. FRC
   C. FVC
   D. ERV

2. In an obstructive lung disorder, the
   I. FRC is decreased
   II. RV is increased
   III. VC is decreased
   IV. IRV is increased
      A. I and III only
      B. II and III only
      C. II and IV only
      D. II, III, and IV only

3. The PEFR in normal healthy men ages 20 to 30 years may exceed
   A.   300 L/min
   B.   400 L/min
   C.   500 L/min
   D.   600 L/min

4. Which of the following can be obtained from a flow-volume loop study?
   I.   FVC
   II.   PEFR
   III. FEV_T
   IV. $FEF_{25\%-75\%}$
   A. I and II only
   B. II and III only
   C. I, III, and IV only
   D. All of these

5. The MVV in normal healthy men ages 20 to 30 years is
   A.   60 L/min
   B.   100 L/min
   C.   170 L/min
   D.   240 L/min

6. Approximately how much of a forced expiratory maneuver is effort dependent?
   A.   20%
   B.   30%
   C.   40%
   D.   50%

7. Which of the following forced expiratory measurements reflects the status of medium-sized to small-sized airways?
   A. $FEF_{200-1200}$
   B.   PEFR
   C.   MVV
   D. $FEF_{25\%-75\%}$

8. Normally, the percentage of the total volume exhaled during an FEV_1 by a 20-year-old individual is
   A.   60%
   B.   83%
   C.   94%
   D.   97%

9. Which of the following forced expiratory measurements is a good index of the integrity of large airway function?
   A. FEV_T
   B. $FEF_{200-1200}$
   C. $FEF_{25\%-75\%}$
   D.   MVV

10. The residual volume/total lung capacity ratio in healthy men ages 20 to 30 years is
    A. 15%
    B. 20%
    C. 25%
    D. 30%

11. A 73-year-old man with a long history of smoking demonstrates the following clinical data on a pulmonary function test (PFT):

Pulmonary Function Test			
PFT	Below Normal	Normal	Above Normal
VC	X		
RV			X
FRC			X
ERV	X		
FEV_T	X		
$FEV_{1\%}$	X		
$FEF_{25\%-75\%}$	X		
PEFR	X		
MVV	X		

Based on the information shown, the patient appears to have
    A. an obstructive lung disorder
    B. a restrictive lung disorder
    C. both obstructive and restrictive lung disorders
    D. neither an obstructive or restrictive lung disorder

CLINICAL APPLICATION QUESTIONS

CASE 1

1. When the patient was in the emergency department, what pulmonary function measurement served as an important clinical indicator of the severity of the patient's asthma attack?

    Answer: _____

2. The fact that the respiratory therapist obtained the same bedside spirometry results on the second test demonstrated the presence of what three physiologic effects?

    _____

    _____

    _____

3. When the patient made a stronger muscular effort on the second FVC test, she only moved the equal pressure point of her airways

_____

_____

CASE 2

1. This patient demonstrated both obstructive and restrictive lung disorders. During the first part of the case, which pulmonary function studies verified that the patient had an obstructive pulmonary disorder?

   Answer: _____

   _____

   _____

2. Which pulmonary function studies verified that the patient had a restrictive pulmonary disorder?

   Answer: _____

   _____

   _____

3. After aggressive bronchial hygiene therapy and lung expansion therapy, the patient's FEV_1 (increased _____ ; decreased _____ ; remained the same _____), and the RV (increased _____ ; decreased _____ ; remained the same _____).

CHAPTER 5

The Anatomy and Physiology of the Circulatory System

O B J E C T I V E S

By the end of this chapter, the student should be able to:

1. Describe the function of the following specialized cells in the plasma:
   —Erythrocytes
   —Leukocytes
   —Thrombocytes
2. List the chemical components of plasma.
3. Describe the structure and function of the following components of the heart:
   —Inferior vena cava and superior vena cava
   —Right and left atria
   —Right and left ventricles
   —Pulmonary trunk
   —Pulmonary arteries
   —Pulmonary semilunar valve
   —Pulmonary veins
   —Tricuspid valve
   —Bicuspid valve (or mitral valve)
   —Aortic valve
   —Chordae tendineae
   —Papillary muscles
4. Describe the function of the major components of the pericardium.
5. Describe the major components of the heart wall, including:
   —Epicardium
   —Myocardium
   —Endocardium
6. Describe the blood supply of the heart, including:
   —Left coronary artery
   • Circumflex branch
   • Anterior interventricular branch
   —Right coronary artery
   • Marginal branch
   • Posterior interventricular branch
   —Venous drainage
   • Great cardiac veins
   • Middle cardiac vein
   • Coronary sinus
   • Thebesian vein
7. Describe how blood flows through the heart.
8. Describe the following components of the pulmonary and systemic vascular systems:
   —Arteries
   —Arterioles
   —Capillaries
   —Venules
   —Veins
9. Explain the neural control of the vascular system.
10. Describe the function of the baroreceptors.
11. Define the following types of *pressures:*
    —Intravascular pressure
    —Transmural pressure
    —Driving pressure

(continues)

12. Describe how the following relate to the *cardiac cycle* and *blood pressure:*
    —Ventricular systole
    —Ventricular diastole
13. List the *intraluminal blood pressures* throughout the pulmonary and systemic vascular systems.
14. Describe how blood volume affects blood pressure, and include the following:
    —Stroke volume
    —Heart rate
    —Cardiac output
15. Identify the percentage of blood found throughout the various parts of the pulmonary and systemic systems.
16. Describe the influence of *gravity* on blood flow, and include how it relates to
    —Zone 1
    —Zone 2
    —Zone 3

17. Define the following *determinants of cardiac output:*
    —Ventricular preload
    —Ventricular afterload
    —Myocardial contractility
18. Define *vascular resistance.*
19. Describe how the following affect the pulmonary vascular resistance:
    —Active mechanisms
      • Abnormal blood gas values
      • Pharmacologic stimulation
      • Pathologic conditions
    —Passive mechanisms
      • Increased pulmonary arterial pressure
      • Increased left atrial pressure
      • Lung volume and transpulmonary pressure changes
      • Blood volume changes
      • Blood viscosity changes
20. Complete the review questions at the end of this chapter.

The delivery of oxygen to the cells of the body is a function of blood flow. Thus, when the flow of blood is inadequate, good alveolar ventilation is of little value.

The circulatory system consists of the **blood**, the **heart** (pump), and the **vascular system**.

THE BLOOD

Blood consists of numerous specialized cells that are suspended in a liquid substance called **plasma**. The cells in the plasma include the **erythrocytes** (red blood cells), **leukocytes** (white blood cells), and **thrombocytes** (or platelets, which are actually cell fragments) (Table 5–1).

Erythrocytes

Erythrocytes constitute the major portion of the blood cells. In the healthy adult man there are about 5 million red blood cells (RBCs) in each cubic millimeter of blood (mm^3). The healthy adult woman has about

TABLE 5–1
Formed Elements of the Blood

Cell Type	Illustration	Description	Number of Cells/mm³ of Blood	Duration of Development (D) and Life Span (LS)	Function
Erythrocytes (red blood cells, RBCs)		Biconcave, anucleate disc; salmon-colored; diameter 7–8 μm	4–6 million	D: 5–7 days LS: 100–120 days	Transport oxygen and carbon dioxide
Leukocytes (white blood cells, WBCs)		Spherical, nucleated cells	4,000–11,000		
Neutrophils		Nucleus multilobed; inconspicuous cytoplasmic granules; diameter 10–14 μm	3000–7000	D: 6–9 days LS: 6 hours to a few days	Phagocytize bacteria
Eosinophils		Nucleus bilobed; red cytoplasmic granules; diameter 10–14 μm	100–400	D: 6–9 days LS: 8–12 days	Kill parasitic worms; destroy antigen-antibody complexes; inactivate some inflammatory chemicals of allergy
Basophils		Nucleus lobed; large blue-purple cytoplasmic granules; diameter 10–12 μm	20–50	D: 3–7 days LS: a few hours to a few days	Release histamine and other mediators of inflammation; contain heparin, an anticoagulant
Agranulocytes Lymphocytes		Nucleus spherical or indented; pale blue cytoplasm; diameter 5–17 μm	1500–3000	D: days to weeks LS: hours to years	Mount immune response by direct cell attack or via antibodies
Monocytes		Nucleus, U or kidney-shaped; gray-blue cytoplasm; diameter 14–24 μm	100–700	D: 2–3 days LS: months	Phagocytosis; develop into macrophages in tissues
Platelets		Discoid cytoplasmic fragments containing granules; stain deep purple; diameter 2–4 μm	250,000–500,000	D: 4–5 days LS: 5–10 days	Seal small tears in blood vessels; instrumental in blood clotting

Figure 5–1
When a blood-filled capillary tube is centrifuged, the red blood cells (RBCs) become packed at the bottom of the test tube, leaving the fluid plasma at the top of the tube. White cells and platelets form a thin, light-colored "buffy coat" at the interface between the packed RBCs and the plasma.

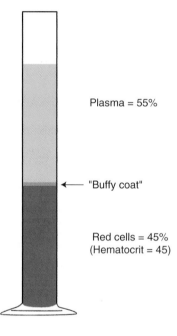

Plasma = 55%

← "Buffy coat"

Red cells = 45%
(Hematocrit = 45)

4 million RBCs/mm^3. The percentage of RBCs in relation to the total blood volume is known as the **hematocrit**. The normal hematocrit is approximately 45 percent in the adult man (Figure 5–1) and 42 percent in the adult woman. In the normal newborn, the hematocrit ranges between 45 and 60 percent.

Microscopically, the RBCs appear as biconcave discs, averaging about 7.5 μm in diameter and 2.5 μm in thickness. They are produced in the red bone marrow in the spongy bone of the cranium, bodies of vertebrae, ribs, sternum, and proximal epiphyses of the humerus and femur. It is estimated that the RBCs are produced at the rate of 2 million cells per second. An equal number of worn-out RBCs are destroyed each second by the spleen and liver. The life span of a RBC is about 120 days. The major constituent of the RBCs is **hemoglobin**, which is the primary substance responsible for the transport of oxygen.

Leukocytes

The primary function of the **leukocytes**, or **white blood cells** (WBCs), is to protect the body against bacteria, viruses, parasites, toxins, and tumors. The leukocytes are far less numerous than RBCs, averaging between 4000 and 11,000 cells/mm^3. Unlike RBCs, which are confined to the bloodstream, WBCs are able to leave the capillary blood vessels (a process called **diapedesis**) when needed for inflammatory or immune responses. Diapedesis is activated by chemical signals released by the damaged cells (**positive chemotaxis**). Once out of the bloodstream, the leukocytes form cytoplasmic extensions that move them along through the tissue spaces toward the damaged cells (**amoeboid motion**). Whenever the WBCs are mobilized for action, the body increases their production and twice the normal number may appear in the blood within a few hours. A WBC count greater than 11,000 cells/mm^3 is called **leukocytosis**. This condition is seen in patients with bacterial or viral infections.

Leukocytes are grouped into two major categories on the basis of structural and chemical characteristics: *Granulocytes* (neutrophils, eosinophils, and basophils) contain specialized membrane-bound cytoplasmic granules; *agranulocytes* (lymphocytes and monocytes) lack granules. Because the general function of the leukocytes is to combat inflammation and infection, the clinical diagnosis of an injury or infection is often assisted by a *differential count*, which is the determination of the percentage of each type of white cell (in 100 WBCs). Table 5–2 shows a normal differential count.

Granulocytes

Granulocytes, which include the neutrophils, basophils, and eosinophils, are spherical in shape and much larger than erythrocytes. They characteristically have rounded nuclear masses connected by thinner strands of nuclear material. Their membrane-bound cytoplasmic granules stain quite specifically with Wright's stain. Functionally, all granulocytes are relatively short-lived phagocytes.

Neutrophils are the most numerous of the WBCs. They typically account for half or more of the WBC population (40 to 70 percent). Neutrophils are active phagocytes that are twice the size of erythrocytes. They stain a lilac color. Neutrophils contain small granules that produce potent antibiotic-like proteins called **defensins**. They are especially found at inflammation sites caused by bacteria and some fungi, which they ingest

TABLE 5–2
Normal Differential Count

Polymorphonuclear Granulocytes		Mononuclear Cells	
Neutrophils	60–70%	Lymphocytes	20–25%
Eosinophils	2–4%	Monocytes	3–8%
Basophils	0.5–1%		

and destroy. Neutrophils kill bacteria by means of a process called a **respiratory bust**, whereby oxygen is actively metabolized to produce potent bacterial-killing oxidizing substances such as bleach and hydrogen peroxide. Defensin-mediated lysis also occurs. The number of neutrophils increases dramatically during bacterial infections.

Eosinophils account for 1 to 4 percent of all leukocytes. They are approximately the same size as neutrophils. They have large, coarse granules that stain brick red to crimson. Eosinophils lessen the severity of allergies by phagocytizing immune (antigen-antibody) complexes involved in allergic attacks. This action in turn inactivates certain inflammatory chemicals that are typically released during an allergic reaction. An elevated eosinophil count is commonly seen in asthmatic patients.

Basophils are the smallest group of WBCs, accounting for 1 percent or less of the leukocyte population. Basophils are about the same size or slightly smaller than neutrophils. Basophils also combat allergic reactions. Their cytoplasm contains large coarse histamine-containing granules that stain purplish-black. **Histamine** is an inflammatory substance that causes vasodilation and attracts other WBCs to the inflamed site.

Agranulocytes

Agranulocytes, which include the lymphocytes and monocytes, lack cytoplasmic granules. Their nuclei are typically spherical or kidney shaped. Although they are similar in structure to the granulocytes, they function differently.

Lymphocytes are the second most numerous leukocytes in the blood. Lymphocytes stain dark-purple and their nuclei are usually spherical in shape and surrounded by a thin rim of pale-blue cytoplasm. Although large numbers of lymphocytes exist in the body, only a small amount are found in the bloodstream. Most of the lymphocytes are found in the lymphoid tissues (lymph nodes), where they play an important role in immunity. **T lymphocytes** (T cells) function in the immune response by acting directly against virus-infected cells and tumors. **B lymphocytes** (B cells) give rise to *plasma cells,* which produce **antibodies** (immunoglobulins) that work to inactivate invading antigens.

Monocytes account for 4 to 8 percent of the WBCs. They have pale-blue cytoplasm and a darkly stained U-shaped or kidney-shaped nucleus. In the tissue, monocytes differentiate into highly mobile **macrophages** with large appetites. In chronic infections, such as tuberculosis, the macrophages increase in number and are actively phagocytic. Monocytes are also effective against viruses and certain intracellular bacterial parasites.

Thrombocytes

Thrombocytes, or *blood platelets,* are the smallest of the formed elements in the plasma (see Table 5–1). The normal platelet count ranges from 250,000 to 500,000/mm^3 of blood. The function of the platelets is to prevent blood loss from a traumatized area of the body involving the smallest blood vessels. They do this by virtue of an activator substance called **platelet factor**, which is a sticky substance that causes blood clotting at the traumatized site. The platelets also contain *serotonin* which, when released, causes smooth-muscle constriction and reduced blood flow.

Plasma

When all the cells are removed from the blood, a straw-colored liquid called plasma remains. Plasma constitutes about 55 percent of the total blood volume (see Figure 5–1). Approximately 90 percent of plasma consists of water. The remaining 10 percent is composed of proteins, electrolytes, food substances, respiratory gases, hormones, vitamins, and waste products. Table 5–3 outlines the chemical composition of plasma. Blood serum is plasma without its fibrinogen and several other proteins involved in clotting.

TABLE 5–3
Chemical Composition of Plasma

Water		Food Subtances	
	93% of plasma weight	Amino acids	40 mg/100 mL
		Glucose/carbohydrates	100 mg/100 mL
Proteins		Lipids	500 mg/100 mL
Albumins	4.5 g/100 mL	Individual vitamins	0.0001–2.5 mg/100 mL
Globulins	2.5 g/100 mL		
Fibrinogen	0.3 g/100 mL	**Respiratory Gases**	
		O_2	0.3 mL/100 mL
Electrolytes		CO_2	2 mL/100 mL
Cations		N_2	0.9 mL/100 mL
Na^+	143 mEq/L		
K^+	4 mEq/L	**Individual Hormones**	
Ca^{2+}	2.5 mEq/L		0.000001–0.05 mg/100 mL
Mg^{2+}	1.5 mEq/L		
Anions		**Waste Products**	
Cl^-	103 mEq/L	Urea	34 mg/100 mL
PO_4^{3-}	1 mEq/L	Creatinine	1 mg/100 mL
SO_4^{2-}	0.5 mEq/L	Uric acid	5 mg/100 mL
HCO_3^-	27 mEq/L	Bilirubin	0.2–1.2 mg/100 mL

THE HEART

The **heart** is a hollow, four-chambered, muscular organ that consists of the upper right and left **atria** and the lower right and left **ventricles** (Figure 5–2). The atria are separated by a thin muscular wall called the **interatrial septum**; the ventricles are separated by a thick muscular wall called the **interventricular septum**. The heart actually functions as two separate pumps. The right atrium and ventricle act as one pump to propel unoxygenated blood to the lungs. At the same time, the left atrium and ventricle act as another pump to propel oxygenated blood throughout the systemic circulation. Compared with the ventricles, the atria are small, thin-walled chambers. As a rule, they contribute little to the propulsive pumping activity of the heart.

Externally, the heart appears as a cone-shaped structure, weighing between 250 and 350 g. It is enclosed in the **mediastinum** and extends obliquely between the second rib and the fifth intercostal space (Figure 5–3A). The heart rests on the superior surface of the diaphragm, anterior to the vertebral column and posterior to the sternum (Figure 5–3B). Both the left and right lateral portions of the heart are flanked by the lungs, which partially obscure it (Figure 5–3C). Approximately two-thirds of the heart lies to the left of the midsternal line; the balance extends to the right.

The **base** of the heart is broad and flat, about 9 cm, and points toward the right shoulder. The **apex** points inferiorly toward the left hip. When fingers are pressed between the fifth and sixth ribs just below the left nipple, the heart beat can be felt where the apex is in contact with the internal chest wall. This site is called the **point of maximal intensity** (**PMI**).

The Pericardium

The heart is enclosed in a double-walled sac called the **pericardium** (Figure 5–4). The outer wall, the **fibrous pericardium**, is a tough, dense, connective tissue layer. Its primary function is to (1) protect the heart; (2) anchor the heart to surrounding structures, such as the diaphragm and the great vessels; and (3) prevent the heart from overfilling. The inner wall, the **serous pericardium**, is a thin, slippery, serous membrane. The serous pericardium is composed of two layers: the **parietal layer**, which lines the internal surface of the fibrous pericardium, and the **visceral layer** (also called the **epicardium**). The epicardium is an integral part of the heart often described as the outermost layer of the heart. Between the two layers of the serous pericardium there is a film of serous fluid, which allows the parietal and visceral membranes to glide smoothly against one another, which in turn permits the heart to work in a relatively friction-free environment.

Figure 5–2
(A) Anterior view of the heart; **(B)** posterior view of the heart.

Left common carotid artery
Brachiocephalic artery
Left subclavian artery
Aortic arch
Right pulmonary artery
Left pulmonary artery
Ascending aorta
Superior vena cava
Left pulmonary veins
Right pulmonary veins
Ligamentum arteriosum
Pulmonary trunk
Left atrium
Circumflex artery
Right atrium
Auricle
Right coronary artery
(in right atrioventricular groove)
Left coronary artery
(in left atrioventricular groove)
Anterior cardiac vein
Left ventricle
Right ventricle
Great cardiac vein
Marginal artery
Small cardiac vein
Anterior interventricular artery
(in anterior interventricular sulcus)
Inferior vena cava
Apex

A

Aorta
Superior vena cava
Left pulmonary artery
Left pulmonary veins
Right pulmonary artery
Auricle
Right pulmonary veins
Left atrium
Great cardiac vein
Right atrium
Inferior vena cava
Posterior vein
of left ventricle
Right coronary artery
(in right atrioventricular groove)
Coronary sinus
Left ventricle
Posterior interventricular artery
(in posterior interventricular sulcus)
Right ventricle
Apex
Middle cardiac vein

B

Figure 5–3
The relationship of the heart to the thorax: **(A)** the relationship of the heart to the sternum, ribs, and diaphragm; **(B)** cross-sectional view showing the relationship of the heart to the thorax; **(C)** relationship of the heart to the lungs and great vessels.

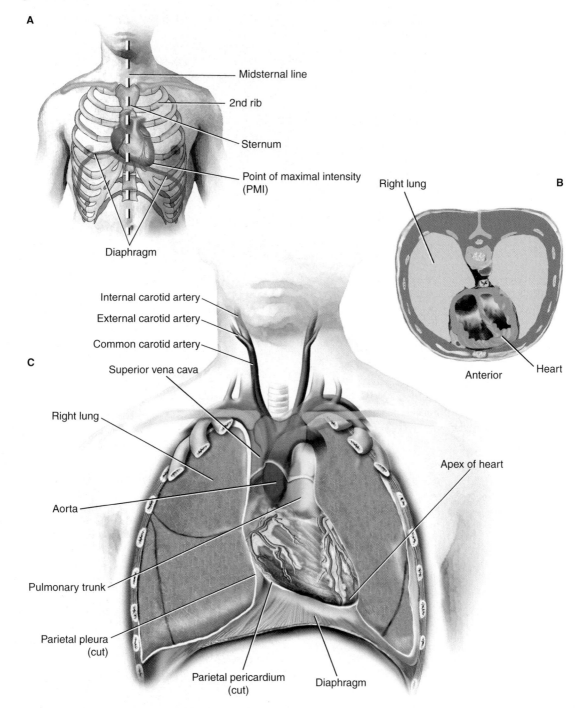

A

- Midsternal line
- 2nd rib
- Sternum
- Point of maximal intensity (PMI)
- Diaphragm

B

Right lung

Anterior

Heart

C

- Internal carotid artery
- External carotid artery
- Common carotid artery
- Superior vena cava
- Right lung
- Aorta
- Pulmonary trunk
- Parietal pleura (cut)
- Parietal pericardium (cut)
- Diaphragm
- Apex of heart

Figure 5–4
The layers of the pericardium and the heart wall.

Fibrous pericardium

Parietal layer of
serous pericardium

Pericardial cavity

Visceral layer of
serous pericardium
(epicardium)

Myocardium

Endocardium

Heart wall

Pericardium

Myocardium

Heart chamber

The Wall of the Heart

The heart wall is composed of the following three layers: epicardium (visceral pericardium), myocardium, and endocardium (see Figure 5–4).

The **epicardium**, or visceral layer of the pericardium, is composed of a single sheet of squamous epithelial cells overlying delicate connective tissue. In older patients, the epicardium layer is often infiltrated with fat.

The **myocardium** is a thick contractile middle layer of uniquely constructed and arranged muscle cells. The myocardium forms the bulk of the heart. It is the layer that actually contracts. The contractile tissue of the myocardium is composed of fibers with the characteristic cross-striations of muscular tissue. The cardiac muscle cells are interconnected to form a network spiral or circular bundles (Figure 5–5). These interlacing circular bundles effectively connect all the parts of the heart together. Collectively, the spiral bundles form a dense network called the **fibrous skeleton of the heart**, which reinforces the internal portion of the myocardium. Specifically modified tissue fibers of the myocardium constitute the conduction system of the heart (i.e., the sinoatrial [SA] node, the atrioventricular [AV] node, the AV bundle of His, and the Purkinje fibers) (discussed in more detail in Chapter 12).

Figure 5–5
View of the spiral and circular arrangement of the cardiac muscle bundles.

Cardiac muscle bundles

The **endocardium** is a glistening white sheet of squamous epithelium that rests on a thin connective tissue layer. Located in the inner myocardial surface, it lines the heart's chambers. It contains small blood vessels and a few bundles of smooth muscles. It is continuous with the endothelium of the great blood vessels—the superior and inferior vena cava.

Blood Supply of the Heart

Arterial Supply

The blood supply of the heart originates directly from the aorta by means of two arteries: the **left coronary artery** and the **right coronary artery**.

The left coronary artery divides into the **circumflex branch** and the **anterior interventricular branch** (Figure 5–6A). The circumflex branch runs posteriorly and supplies the left atrium and the posterior wall of the left ventricle. The anterior interventricular branch travels toward the apex

Figure 5–6
Coronary circulation: **(A)** arterial vessels; **(B)** venous vessels.

A   B

of the heart and supplies the anterior walls of both ventricles and the interventricular septum. The right coronary artery supplies the right atrium and then divides into the **marginal branch** and the **posterior interventricular branch**. The marginal branch supplies the lateral walls of the right atrium and right ventricle. The posterior interventricular branch supplies the posterior wall of both ventricles.

Venous Drainage

The venous system of the heart parallels the coronary arteries. Venous blood from the anterior side of the heart empties into the **great cardiac veins**; venous blood from the posterior portion of the heart is collected by the **middle cardiac vein** (see Figure 5–6B). The great and middle cardiac veins merge and empty into a large venous cavity within the posterior wall of the right atrium called the **coronary sinus**. A small amount of venous blood is collected by the **thebesian veins**, which empties directly into both the right and left atrium. The venous drainage that flows into the left atrium contributes to the normal anatomic shunt, the phenomenon whereby oxygenated blood mixes with deoxygenated blood (this concept is discussed in more detail in Chapter 6).

Blood Flow Through the Heart

As shown in Figure 5–7, the right atrium receives venous blood from the **inferior vena cava** and **superior vena cava**. A small amount of cardiac venous blood enters the right atrium by means of the thebesian veins. This blood is low in oxygen and high in carbon dioxide. A one-way valve, the **tricuspid valve**, lies between the right atrium and the right ventricle. The tricuspid valve gets it name from its three valve leaflets, or cusps. The tricuspid leaflets are held in place by tendinous cords called **chordae tendinae**, which are secured to the ventricular wall by the **papillary muscles**. When the ventricles contract, the tricuspid valve closes and blood leaves the right ventricle through the **pulmonary trunk** and enters the lungs by way of the right and left **pulmonary arteries**. The **pulmonary semilunar valve** separates the right ventricle from the pulmonary trunk.

After blood passes through the lungs, it returns to the left atrium by way of the **pulmonary veins**. These vessels are best seen in a posterior view of the heart (see Figure 5–2B). The returning blood is high in oxygen and low in carbon dioxide. The **bicuspid valve** (also called the **mitral valve**) lies between the left atrium and the left ventricle. This valve, which consists of two cusps, prevents blood from returning to the left atrium during ventricular contraction. Similar to the tricuspid valve, the bicuspid valve is also held in position by chordae tendinae and papillary muscles. The left ventricle pumps blood through the ascending **aorta**. The **aortic valve**, which lies at the base of the ascending aorta, has semilunar cusps (valves) that close when the ventricles relax. The closure

Figure 5–7
Internal chambers and valves of the heart.

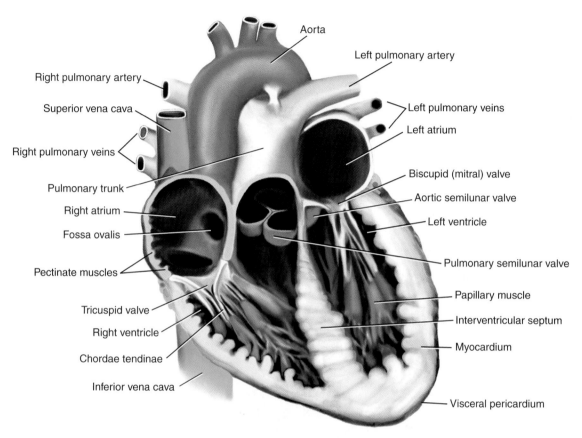

of the semilunar valves prevent the backflow of blood into the left ventricle (see Figure 5–7).

THE PULMONARY AND SYSTEMIC VASCULAR SYSTEMS

The vascular network of the circulatory system is composed of two major subdivisions: the **systemic system** and the **pulmonary system** (Figure 5–8). The pulmonary system begins with the pulmonary trunk and ends in the left atrium. The systemic system begins with the aorta and ends in the right atrium. Both systems are composed of arteries, arterioles, capillaries, venules, and veins (see Figure 1–29).

Arteries are vessels that carry blood away from the heart. The arteries are strong, elastic vessels that are well suited for carrying blood under

Figure 5–8
Pulmonary and systemic circulation. Pulmonary circulation is indicated by pink arrows; systemic circulation is indicated by blue arrows.

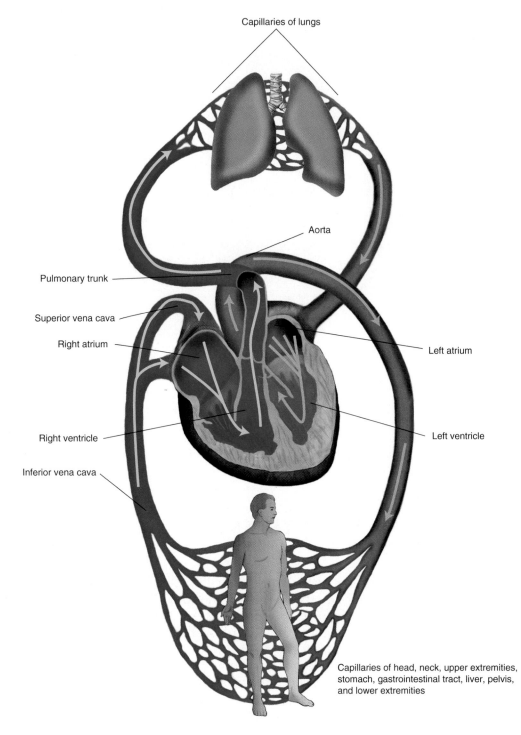

Capillaries of lungs

Aorta

Pulmonary trunk

Superior vena cava

Right atrium

Left atrium

Right ventricle

Left ventricle

Inferior vena cava

Capillaries of head, neck, upper extremities, stomach, gastrointestinal tract, liver, pelvis, and lower extremities high pressure in the systemic system. The arteries subdivide as they move away from the heart into smaller vessels and, eventually, into vessels called **arterioles**. Arterioles play a major role in the distribution and regulation of blood pressure and are referred to as the **resistance vessels**.

Gas exchange occurs in the **capillaries**. In the capillaries of the pulmonary system, gas exchange is called **external respiration** (gas exchange between blood and air). In the capillaries of the systemic system, gas exchange is called **internal respiration** (gas exchange between blood and tissues).

The **venules** are tiny veins continuous with the capillaries. The venules empty into the veins, which carry blood back to the heart. The veins differ from the arteries in that they are capable of holding a large amount of blood with very little pressure change. Because of this unique feature, the veins are called **capacitance vessels**. Approximately 60 percent of the body's total blood volume is contained within the venous system.

Neural Control of the Vascular System

The pulmonary arterioles and most of the arterioles in the systemic circulation are controlled by sympathetic impulses. Sympathetic fibers are found in the arteries, arterioles and, to a lesser degree, in the veins (Figure 5–9). The **vasomotor center**, which is located in the medulla oblongata, governs the number of sympathetic impulses sent to the vascular systems. Under normal circumstances, the vasomotor center transmits a continual stream of sympathetic impulses to the blood vessels,

Figure 5–9
Neural control of the vascular system. Sympathetic neural fibers to the arterioles are especially abundant.

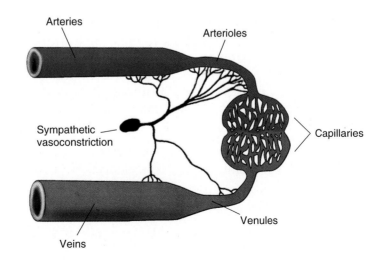

maintaining the vessels in a moderate state of constriction all the time. This state of vascular contraction is called the **vasomotor tone**.

The vasomotor center coordinates both vasoconstriction and vasodilation by controlling the number of sympathetic impulses that leave the medulla. For example, when the vasomotor center is activated to constrict a particular vascular region (i.e., more than the normal state of constriction), it does so by increasing the number of sympathetic impulses to that vascular area. In contrast, the vasomotor center initiates vasodilation by reducing the number of sympathetic impulses sent to a certain vascular region. (The major vascular beds in the systemic system that are *not* controlled by this mechanism are the arterioles of the heart, brain, and skeletal muscles. Sympathetic impulses to these vessels cause vasodilation.) In addition to the sympathetic control, blood flow through the large veins can be affected by abdominal and intrathoracic pressure changes.

Working together, the vasomotor center and the cardiac centers in the medulla oblongata regulate the arterial blood pressure in response to signals received from special pressure receptors located throughout the body. These pressure receptors are called **arterial baroreceptors**.

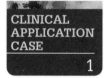

CLINICAL
APPLICATION
CASE

1

See page 220

The Baroreceptor Reflex

Specialized stretch receptors called **baroreceptors** (also called *presso-receptors*) are located in the walls of the carotid arteries and the aorta. In the **carotid arteries**, the baroreceptors are found in the carotid sinuses located high in the neck where the common carotid arteries divide into the external and internal carotid arteries (Figure 5–10). The walls of the carotid sinuses are thin and contain a large number of branching, vinelike nerve endings that are sensitive to stretch or distortion. The afferent fibers from the carotid sinuses travel with the **glossopharyngeal nerve** (ninth cranial) to the medulla. In the aorta, the baroreceptors are located in the **aortic arch** (see Figure 5–10). The afferent fibers from the aortic arch baroreceptors travel with the **vagus nerve** (tenth cranial).

The baroreceptors regulate the arterial blood pressure by initiating reflex adjustments to changes in blood pressure. For example, when the arterial pressure decreases, the neural impulses transmitted from the baroreceptors to the vasomotor and cardiac centers in the medulla also decrease. This causes the medulla to increase its sympathetic activity, which in turn causes an increase in the following:

- Heart rate
- Myocardial force of contraction
- Arterial constriction
- Venous constriction.

The net result is (1) an increased cardiac output (because of an increased heart rate and stroke volume), (2) an increase in the total

Figure 5–10
Location of
the arterial
baroreceptors.

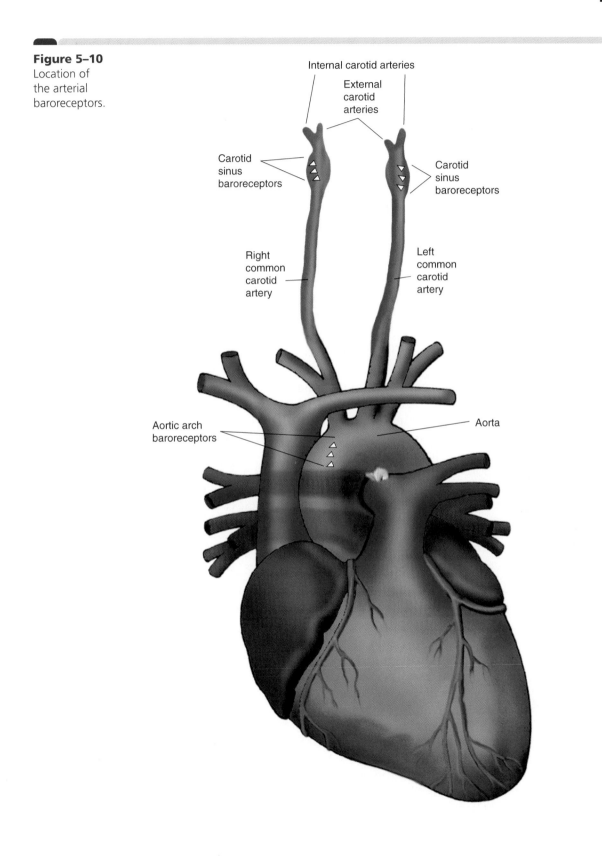

peripheral resistance (primarily induced by arterial constriction), and (3) the return of blood pressure toward normal. The vascular constriction occurs primarily in the abdominal region (including the liver, spleen, pancreas, stomach, intestine, kidneys, skin, and skeletal muscles).

In contrast, when the blood pressure increases, the neural impulses from the arterial baroreceptors increase. This causes the medulla to decrease its sympathetic activity, which in turn reduces both the cardiac output and the total peripheral resistance.

Finally, the baroreceptors function as short-term regulators of arterial blood pressure. That is, they respond instantly to any blood pressure change to restore the blood pressure toward normal (to the degree possible in the situation). If, however, the factors responsible for moving the arterial pressure away from normal persist for more than a few days, the arterial baroreceptors will eventually come to "accept" the new pressure as normal. For example, in individuals who have chronically high blood pressure (*hypertension*), the baroreceptors still operate, but at a higher level—in short, their operating point is reset at a higher level.

Other Baroreceptors

Baroreceptors are also found in the large arteries, large veins, and pulmonary vessels and the cardiac walls themselves. Functionally, most of these receptors are similar to the baroreceptors in the carotid sinuses and aortic arch in that they send an increased rate of neural transmissions to the medulla in response to increased pressure. By means of these additional receptors, the medulla gains a further degree of sensitivity to venous, atrial, and ventricular pressures. For example, a slight decrease in atrial pressure initiates sympathetic activity even before there is a decrease in cardiac output and, therefore, a decrease in the arterial blood pressure great enough to be detected by the aortic and carotid baroreceptors.

PRESSURES IN THE PULMONARY AND SYSTEMIC VASCULAR SYSTEMS

CLINICAL APPLICATION CASES

1 & 2

See pages 220–222

Three different types of pressures are used to study the blood flow: intravascular, transmural, and driving.

Intravascular pressure is the actual blood pressure in the lumen of any vessel at any point, relative to the barometric pressure. This pressure is also known as the intraluminal pressure.

Transmural pressure is the difference between the intravascular pressure of a vessel and the pressure surrounding the vessel. The transmural pressure is *positive* when the pressure inside the vessel exceeds the pressure outside the vessel, and *negative* when the pressure inside the vessel is less than the pressure surrounding the vessel.

Figure 5–11

Schematic illustration of a blood vessel and an alveolus, showing the types of blood pressures used to study blood flow. Within the blood vessel, the intravascular pressure at point A is 15 mm Hg, and the intravascular pressure at point B is 5 mm Hg. The pressure within the alveolus (which represents the pressure surrounding the blood vessel) is zero. In view of these numbers, the following can be stated: (1) The transmural pressure at point A is +15 mm Hg, (2) the transmural pressure at point B is +5 mm Hg, and (3) the driving pressure between point A and point B is 10 mm Hg.

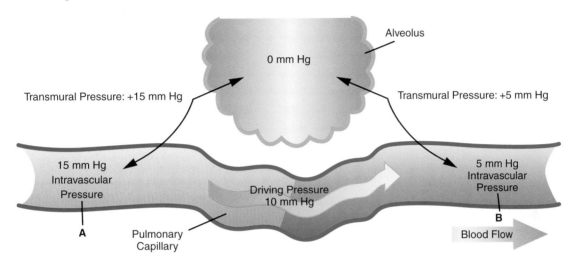

Driving pressure is the difference between the pressure at one point in a vessel and the pressure at any other point downstream in the vessel.

Figure 5–11 illustrates the different types of pressures used to study the flow of blood.

THE CARDIAC CYCLE AND ITS EFFECT ON BLOOD PRESSURE

The arterial blood pressure rises and falls in a pattern that corresponds to the phases of the cardiac cycle. When the ventricles contract (ventricular systole), blood is forced into the pulmonary artery and the aorta, and the pressure in these arteries rises sharply. The maximum pressure generated during ventricular contraction is the **systolic pressure**. When the ventricles relax (ventricular diastole), the arterial pressure drops. The lowest pressure that remains in the arteries prior to the next ventricular contraction is the **diastolic pressure** (Figure 5–12). In the systemic system, normal systolic pressure is about 120 mm Hg and normal diastolic pressure is about 80 mm Hg. In the pulmonary system, the normal systolic pressure is about 25 mm Hg and the normal diastolic pressure is about 8 mm Hg (Figure 5–13).

Figure 5–12
Sequence of cardiac contraction:
(A) ventricular diastole and atrial systole;
(B) ventricular systole and atrial diastole.

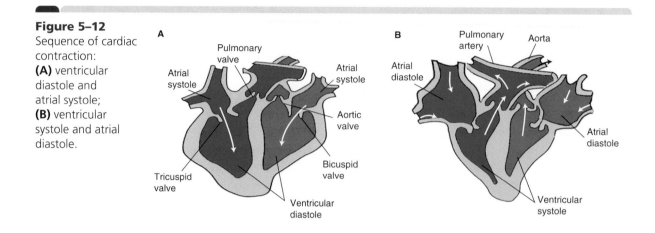

Figure 5–13
Summary of diastolic and systolic pressures in various segments of the circulatory system. Red vessels: oxygenated blood. Blue vessels: deoxygenated blood.

The mean arterial blood pressure (MAP) can be estimated by measuring the systolic blood pressure (SBP) and the diastolic blood pressure (DBP) and using the following formula:

$$MAP = \frac{SBP + (2 \times DBP)}{3}$$

For example, the mean arterial blood pressure of the systemic system, which has a systolic pressure of 120 mm Hg and a diastolic pressure of 80 mm Hg, would be calculated as follows:

$$MAP = \frac{SBP + (2 \times DBP)}{3}$$

$$= \frac{120 + (2 \times 80)}{3}$$

$$= \frac{280}{3}$$

$$= 93 \text{ mm Hg}$$

In the normal adult, the MAP ranges between 80 to 100 mm Hg. When the MAP falls below 60 mm Hg, the blood flow through the brain and kidneys is significantly reduced. Organ deterioration and failure may occur in minutes.

The pulmonary circulation is a low-pressure system. The mean pressure in the pulmonary artery is about 15 mm Hg and the mean pressure in the left atrium is about 5 mm Hg. Thus, the driving pressure needed to move blood through the lungs is 10 mm Hg. In contrast, the mean intraluminal pressure in the aorta is about 100 mm Hg and the mean right atrial pressure is about 2 mm Hg, making the driving pressure through the systemic system about 98 mm Hg. Compared with the pulmonary circulation, the pressure in the systemic system is about 10 times greater. Figure 5–14 shows the mean intraluminal blood pressures throughout both the pulmonary and systemic vascular systems.

The surge of blood rushing into the arterial system during each ventricular contraction causes the elastic walls of the arteries to expand. When the ventricular contraction stops, the pressure drops almost immediately and the arterial walls recoil. This alternating expansion and recoil of the arterial wall can be felt as a pulse in systemic arteries that run close to the skin's surface. Figure 5–15 shows the major sites where a pulse can be detected by palpation.

The Blood Volume and Its Effect on Blood Pressure

The volume of blood ejected from the ventricle during each contraction is called the **stroke volume**. Normally, the stroke volume ranges between 40 and 80 mL. The total volume of blood discharged from the ventricles

Figure 5–14
Mean intraluminal blood pressure at various points in the pulmonary and systemic vascular systems.

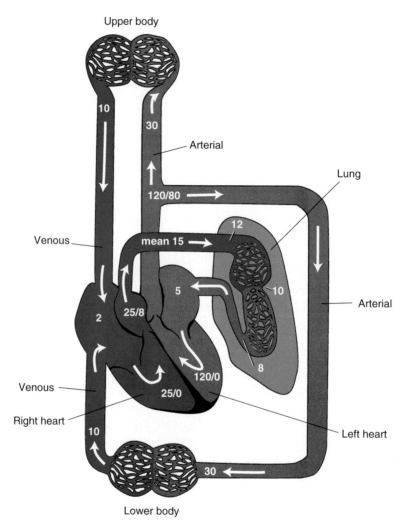

per minute is called **cardiac output**. The cardiac output (CO) is calculated by multiplying the stroke volume (SV) by the heart rate (HR) per minute (CO = SV × HR). Thus, if the stroke volume is 70 mL, and the heart rate is 72 beats per minute (bpm), the cardiac output is 5040 mL/min.

Under normal circumstances, the cardiac output directly influences blood pressure. In other words, *when either the stroke volume or heart rate increases, the blood pressure increases.* Conversely, when the stroke volume or heart rate decreases, the blood pressure decreases.

Although the total blood volume varies with age, body size, and sex, the normal adult volume is about 5 L. Of this volume, about 75 percent is

Figure 5–15
Major sites where an arterial pulse can be detected.

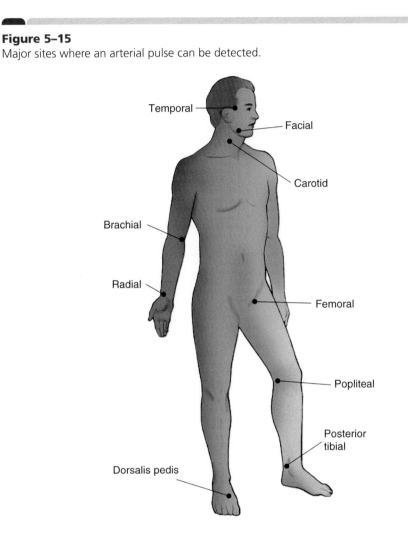

in the systemic circulation, 15 percent in the heart, and 10 percent in the pulmonary circulation. Overall, about 60 percent of the total blood volume is in the veins, and about 10 percent is in the arteries. Normally, the pulmonary capillary bed contains about 75 mL of blood, although it has the capacity of about 200 mL.

THE DISTRIBUTION OF PULMONARY BLOOD FLOW

In the upright lung, blood flow progressively decreases from the base to the apex (Figure 5–16). This linear distribution of blood is a function of (1) **gravity**, (2) **cardiac output**, and (3) **pulmonary vascular resistance**.

Figure 5–16

Distribution of pulmonary blood flow. In the upright lung, blood flow steadily increases from the apex to the base.

Apex

Base

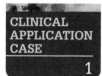

CLINICAL
APPLICATION
CASE

1

See page 220

Gravity

Because blood is a relatively heavy substance, it is **gravity dependent**; that is, it naturally moves to the portion of the body, or portion of the organ, that is closest to the ground. In the average lung, there is a distance of about 30 cm between the base and the apex. The blood that fills the lung from the bottom to the top is analogous to a column of water 30 cm long and, therefore, exerts a pressure of about 30 cm H_2O (22 mm Hg) between the base and apex. Because the pulmonary artery enters each lung about midway between the top and bottom of the lung, the pulmonary artery pressure must be greater than 15 cm H_2O (11 mm Hg) to overcome the gravitational force and, thereby, supply blood to the lung apex. For this reason, most of the blood flows through (or falls into) the lower half of the lung—the gravity-dependent portion of the lung.

As a result of the gravitational effect on blood flow, the intraluminal pressures of the vessels in the gravity-dependent area (lower lung region) are greater than the intraluminal pressures in the least gravity-dependent area (upper lung region). The high intraluminal pressure of the vessels in the gravity-dependent area causes the vessels to distend. As the vessels widen, the vascular resistance decreases and, thus, permits blood flow to increase. The fact that blood flow is enhanced as the vascular system widens is according to Poiseuille's law for flow ($\dot{V} \cong Pr^4$).

The position of the body can significantly change the gravity-dependent portion of the lungs. For example, when an individual is in the supine position (lying on the back), the gravity-dependent area is the posterior

Figure 5–17
Blood flow normally moves into the gravity-dependent areas of the lungs. Thus, body position affects the distribution of the pulmonary blood flow as illustrated in the **(A)** erect, **(B)** supine, **(C)** lateral, and **(D)** upside-down positions.

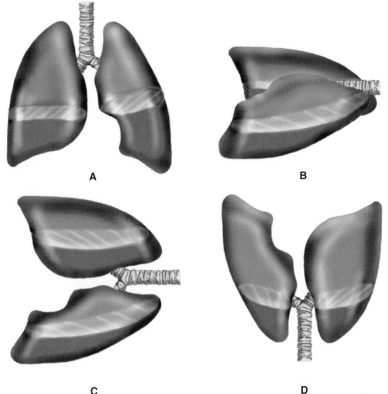

A   B

C   D

portion of the lungs; when an individual is in the prone position (lying on the stomach), the gravity-dependent region is the anterior portion of the lungs; when the person is lying on the side, the lower, lateral half of the lung nearest the ground is gravity dependent; when an individual is suspended upside down, the apices of the lungs become gravity dependent (Figure 5–17).

Figure 5–18 uses a three-zone model to illustrate the effects of gravity and alveolar pressure on the distribution of pulmonary blood flow.

In **Zone 1** (the least gravity-dependent area), the alveolar pressure is sometimes greater than both the arterial and the venous intraluminal pressures. As a result, the pulmonary capillaries can be compressed and blood is prevented from flowing through this region. Under normal circumstances, this situation does not occur, because the pulmonary arterial pressure (generated by the cardiac output) is usually sufficient to raise the blood to the top of the lungs and to overcome the alveolar pressure. There are, however, a variety of conditions—such as severe hemorrhage, dehydration, and positive pressure ventilation—that can result in the

Figure 5–18

Relationship between gravity, alveolar pressure (P_A), pulmonary arterial pressure (P_a), and pulmonary venous pressure (P_v) in different lung zones. Note: The +2 cm H_2O pressure in the alveoli (e.g., during expiration) was arbitrarily selected for this illustration.

alveolar pressure being higher than the arterial and venous pressures. When the alveoli are ventilated but not perfused, no gas exchange can occur and **alveolar dead space** is said to exist (see Figure 2–33).

In **Zone 2**, the arterial pressure is greater than the alveolar pressure and, therefore, the pulmonary capillaries are perfused. Because the alveolar pressure is greater than the venous pressure, the effective driving pressure for blood flow is determined by the pulmonary arterial pressure minus the alveolar pressure—not the normal arterial-venous pressure difference. Thus, because the alveolar pressure is essentially the same throughout all the lung regions, and because the arterial pressure progressively increases toward the gravity-dependent areas of the lung, the effective driving pressure (arterial pressure minus alveolar pressure) steadily increases down the vertical axis of Zone 2. As a result, from the beginning of the upper portion of Zone 2 (the point at which the arterial pressure equals the alveolar pressure) to the lower portion of Zone 2 (the point at which the venous pressure equals the alveolar pressure) the flow of blood progressively increases.

In **Zone 3** (gravity-dependent area), both the arterial and the venous pressures are greater than the alveolar pressure and, therefore, blood flow through this region is constant. Because the arterial pressure and venous pressure both increase equally downward in Zone 3, the arterial-venous pressure difference and, therefore, blood flow is essentially the same throughout all of Zone 3.

Determinants of Cardiac Output

As described earlier, the cardiac output is equal to the stroke volume times the heart rate (CO = SV × HR). The stroke volume is determined by (1) ventricular preload, (2) ventricular afterload, and (3) myocardial contractility.

Ventricular Preload

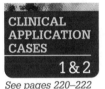

CLINICAL
APPLICATION
CASES
1 & 2
See pages 220–222

Ventricular preload refers to the degree that the myocardial fiber is stretched prior to contraction (*end-diastole*). Within limits, the more the myocardial fiber is stretched during diastole (*preload*), the more strongly it will contract during systole and, therefore, the greater the myocardial contractility will be. This mechanism enables the heart to convert an increased venous return into an increased stroke volume. Beyond a certain point, however, the cardiac output does not increase as the preload increases.

Because the degree of myocardial fiber stretch (preload) is a function of the pressure generated by the volume of blood returning to the ventricle during diastole, ventricular preload is reflected in the **ventricular end-diastolic pressure** (**VEDP**)—which, in essence, reflects the **ventricular end-diastolic volume** (**VEDV**). In other words, as the VEDV increases or decreases, the VEDP (and, therefore, the cardiac output) increases or decreases, respectively. It should be noted, however, that similar to lung compliance (C_L), VEDP and VEDV are also influenced by ventricular compliance. For example, when the ventricular compliance is decreased as a result of disease, the VEDP increases significantly more than the VEDV.

The relationship between the VEDP (degree of myocardial stretch) and cardiac output (stroke volume) is known as the **Frank-Starling curve** (Figure 5–19).

Ventricular Afterload

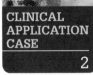

CLINICAL
APPLICATION
CASE
2
See page 221

Ventricular afterload is defined as the force against which the ventricles must work to pump blood. It is determined by several factors, including (1) the volume and viscosity of the blood ejected, (2) the peripheral vascular resistance, and (3) the total cross-sectional area of the vascular space into which blood is ejected. The arterial systolic blood pressure best reflects the ventricular afterload. For example, as the arterial systolic pressure

Figure 5–19

Frank-Starling curve. The Frank-Starling curve shows that the more the myocardial fiber is stretched as a result of the blood pressure that develops as blood returns to the chambers of the heart during diastole, the more the heart muscle will contract during systole. In addition, the heart muscle will contract with greater force. The stretch produced within the myocardium at end-diastole is called preload. Clinically, it would be best to determine the preload of the left ventricle by measuring the end-diastolic pressure of the left ventricle or left atrium. However, because this practice would be impractical at the patient's bedside, the best preload approximation of the left heart is the pulmonary capillary wedge pressure (PCWP). As shown here, the relationship of the PCWP (preload) to the left ventricular stroke work index (LVSWI) (force of contraction) may appear in four quadrants: (1) hypovolemia, (2) optimal function, (3) hypervolemia, and (4) cardiac failure.

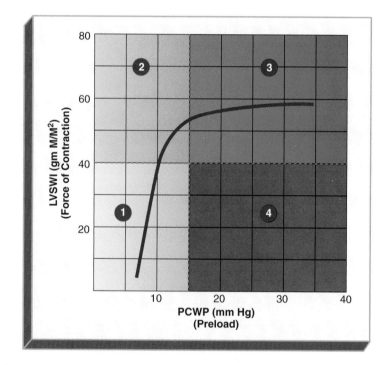

increases, the resistance (against which the heart must work to eject blood) also increases. Clinically, this condition is particularly serious in the patient with congestive heart failure and low stroke volume. By reducing the peripheral resistance (*afterload reduction*) in such patients, the stroke volume increases with little or no change in the blood pressure. This is because blood pressure (BP) is a function of the cardiac output (CO) times the systemic vascular resistance (SVR): BP = CO × SVR.

Myocardial Contractility

Myocardial contractility may be regarded as the force generated by the myocardium when the ventricular muscle fibers shorten. In general, when the contractility of the heart increases or decreases, the cardiac output increases or decreases, respectively.

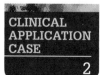

CLINICAL
APPLICATION
CASE

2

See page 221

There is no single measurement that defines contractility in the clinical setting. Changes in contractility, however, can be inferred through clinical assessment (e.g., pulse, blood pressure, skin temperature) and serial hemodynamic measurements (discussed in Chapter 15). An increase in myocardial contractility is referred to as **positive inotropism**. A decrease in myocardial contractility is referred to as **negative inotropism**.

Vascular Resistance

Circulatory resistance is approximated by dividing the mean arterial pressure (MAP) by the cardiac output (CO):

$$Resistance = \frac{MAP}{CO}$$

In general, when the vascular resistance increases, the blood pressure increases (which in turn increases the ventricular afterload). Because of this relationship, blood pressure monitoring can be used to reflect pulmonary or systemic resistance. That is, when resistance increases or decreases, the blood pressure will increase or decrease.

In the pulmonary system, there are several known mechanisms that change the vascular resistance. Such mechanisms are classified as either *active* or *passive mechanisms.*

Active Mechanisms Affecting Vascular Resistance

Active mechanisms that affect vascular resistance include abnormal blood gases, pharmacologic stimulation, and pathologic conditions that have a direct effect on the vascular system.

Abnormal Blood Gases.

- Decreased P_{O_2} (hypoxia)
- Increased P_{CO_2} (hypercapnia)
- Decreased pH (acidemia).

The pulmonary vascular system constricts in response to a decreased alveolar oxygen pressure (**hypoxia**). The exact mechanism of this phenomenon is unknown. Some investigators suggest that alveolar hypoxia causes the lung parenchyma to release a substance that produces vasoconstriction. It is known, however, that the partial pressure of oxygen in the *alveoli* ($P_{A_{O_2}}$)—not the partial pressure of oxygen of the *capillary blood* (Pc_{O_2})—controls this response. The effect of hypoxic vasoconstriction is to direct blood away from the hypoxic lung regions to lung areas that have a higher partial pressure of oxygen.

Clinically, when the number of hypoxic regions becomes significant (e.g., in the advanced stages of emphysema or chronic bronchitis), generalized pulmonary vasoconstriction can develop. This can cause a substantial increase in the pulmonary vascular resistance and in the work of the right heart. This in turn leads to right ventricular hypertrophy, or *cor pulmonale.*

Pulmonary vascular resistance increases in response to an acute increase in the P_{CO_2} level (**hypercapnia**). It is believed, however, that the vasoconstriction that occurs is most likely due to the increased hydrogen ion (H^+) concentration (*respiratory acidosis*) that develops from a sudden increase in the P_{CO_2} level, rather than to the P_{CO_2} itself. This is supported by the fact that pulmonary vasoconstriction does not occur when hypercapnia is accompanied by a normal pH (*compensated respiratory acidosis*).

Pulmonary vasoconstriction develops in response to decreased pH (increased H^+ concentration), or **acidemia**, of either metabolic or respiratory origin.

Pharmacologic Stimulation. The pulmonary vessels constrict in response to various pharmacologic agents, including:

- Epinephrine
- Norepinephrine
- Dobutamine
- Dopamine
- Phenylephrine.

Constricted pulmonary vessels relax in response to the following agents:

- Oxygen
- Isoproterenol
- Aminophylline
- Calcium-channel blocking agents.

Pathologic Conditions. Pulmonary vascular resistance increases in response to a number of pathologic conditions. Some of the more common ones are:

- Vessel blockage or obstruction (e.g., caused by a thrombus or an embolus, such as a blood clot, fat cell, air bubble, or tumor mass)
- Vessel wall diseases (e.g., sclerosis, polyarteritis, or scleroderma)
- Vessel destruction or obliteration (e.g., emphysema or pulmonary interstitial fibrosis)
- Vessel compression (e.g., pneumothorax, hemothorax, or tumor mass).

Pathologic disturbances in the pulmonary vasculary system can develop in the arteries, arterioles, capillaries, venules, or veins. When increased vascular resistance originates in the venules or veins, the transmural pressure increases and, in severe cases, causes the capillary fluid to spill into the alveoli. This is called **pulmonary edema**. Left ventricular failure will cause the same pathologic disturbances. When the resistance originates in the arteries or arterioles, the pulmonary artery pressure will increase but the pulmonary capillary pressure will be normal or low. Regardless of the origin of the pathologic disturbance, a severe and persistent pulmonary vascular resistance is ultimately followed by an elevated right ventricular pressure, right ventricular strain, right ventricular hypertrophy, and right heart failure.

Passive Mechanisms Affecting Vascular Resistance

The term *passive mechanism* refers to a secondary change in pulmonary vascular resistance that occurs in response to another mechanical change. In other words, when a mechanical factor in the respiratory system changes, a passive increase or decrease in the caliber of the pulmonary blood vessels also occurs. Some of the more common passive mechanisms are listed below.

Pulmonary Arterial Pressure Changes. As pulmonary arterial pressure increases, the pulmonary vascular resistance decreases (Figure 5–20). This is assuming that lung volume and left atrial pressure remain constant. The pulmonary vascular resistance decreases because of the

Figure 5–20
Increased mean pulmonary arterial pressure decreases pulmonary vascular resistance.

Figure 5–21

Schematic drawing of the mechanisms that may be activated to decrease pulmonary vascular resistance when the mean pulmonary artery pressure increases. **(A)** A group of pulmonary capillaries, one-half of which are not perfused; **(B)** the previously unperfused capillaries shown in A are recruited (i.e., opened) in response to the increased pulmonary artery pressure; **(C)** the increased blood pressure has distended the capillaries that are already open.

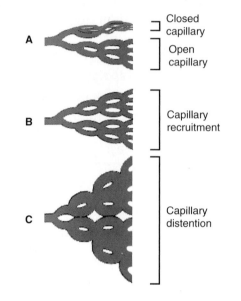

increase in intraluminal distending pressure, which increases the total cross-sectional areas of the pulmonary vascular system through the mechanisms of **recruitment** and **distention**.

As shown in Figure 5–21, *recruitment* means the opening of vessels that were closed or not being utilized for blood flow before the vascular pressure increased. *Distention,* on the other hand, means the stretching or widening of vessels that were open, but not to their full capacity. Both of these mechanisms increase the total cross-sectional area of the vascular system, which in turn reduces the vascular resistance. These mechanisms, however, have their limits.

Left Atrial Pressure Changes. As the left atrial pressure increases, while the lung volume and pulmonary arterial pressure are held constant, pulmonary vascular resistance decreases.

Lung Volume Changes. The effect of changes in lung volume on pulmonary vascular resistance varies according to the location of the vessel. Two major groups of vessels must be considered: (1) **alveolar vessels**—those vessels that surround the alveoli (*pulmonary capillaries*)—and (2) **extra-alveolar vessels**—the larger arteries and veins.

Figure 5–22

Schematic illustration of pulmonary vessels during inspiration. The alveolar vessels (pulmonary capillaries) are exposed to the intrapleural pressure change and are stretched and flattened. The extra-alveolar vessels expand as the intrapleural pressure becomes increasingly negative during inspiration.

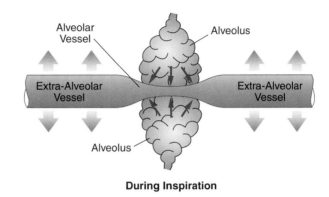

During Inspiration

Alveolar Vessels. Because the pulmonary capillary vessels are so thin, intrapleural pressure changes directly affect the anatomy of the capillaries. During normal inspiration, the alveolar vessels progressively stretch and flatten. During expiration, the alveolar vessels shorten and widen. Thus, as the lungs are inflated, the resistance offered by the alveolar vessels progressively increases (Figure 5–22). During the inspiratory phase of mechanical ventilation (*positive pressure phase*), moreover, the resistance generated by the alveolar vessels may become excessively high and, as a result, restrict the flow of pulmonary blood. The pressure difference between the alveoli and the lumen of the pulmonary capillaries is called the *transmural pressure* (see Figure 5–11).

Extra-Alveolar Vessels. The extra-alveolar vessels (the large arterioles and veins) are also exposed to the intrapleural pressure. They behave differently, however, from the pulmonary capillaries (alveolar vessels) when subjected to volume and pressure changes. That is, as the lung volume increases in response to a more negative intrapleural pressure during inspiration, the transmural pressure increases (i.e., the pressure within the vessels becomes more positive) and the extra-alveolar vessels distend (see Figure 5–22). A second factor that dilates the extra-alveolar vessels at higher lung volumes is the radial traction generated by the connective tissue and by the alveolar septa that hold the larger vessels in place throughout the lung.

Another type of extra-alveolar vessel is the so-called corner vessel, located at the junction of the alveolar septa. As the lung volume increases, the corner vessels are also pulled open (dilated) by the radial traction force created by the expansion of the alveoli (Figure 5–23).

Figure 5–23

Schematic drawing of the extra-alveolar "corner vessels" found at the junction of the alveolar septa. Expansion of the alveoli generates radial traction on the corner vessels, causing them to dilate. The alveolar vessels are compressed and flattened at high lung volumes.

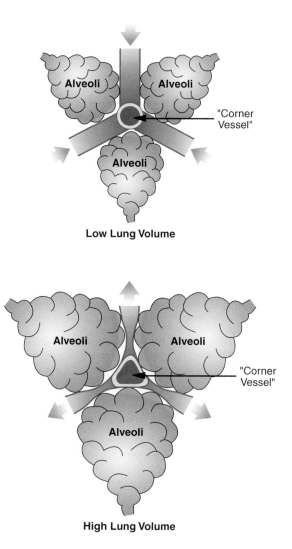

PULMONARY VASCULAR RESISTANCE

To summarize, at low lung volumes (low distending pressures), the extra-alveolar vessels narrow and cause the vascular resistance to increase. The alveolar vessels, however, widen and cause the vascular resistance to decrease. In contrast, at high lung volumes (high distending pressures), the extra-alveolar vessels dilate and cause the vascular

Figure 5–24

At low lung volumes, the extra-alveolar vessels generate a greater resistance to pulmonary blood flow; at high lung volumes, the alveolar vessels generate a greater resistance to pulmonary blood flow. When added together, the resistances of the extra-alveolar and alveolar vessels demonstrate a U-shaped curve. Pulmonary vascular resistance (PVR) is lowest near the functional residual capacity (FRC) and increases at both high and low lung volumes. RV = residual volume; TLC = total lung capacity.

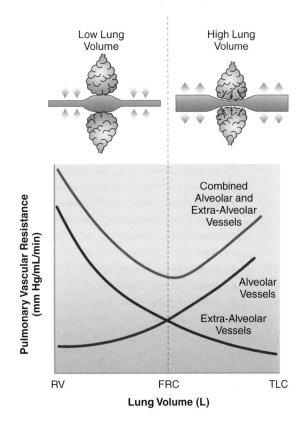

resistance to decrease. The alveolar vessels, however, flatten and cause the vascular resistance to increase.

Finally, because the alveolar and extra-alveolar vessels are all part of the same vascular system, the resistance generated by the two groups of vessels is additive at any lung volume. The effect of changes in lung volume on the total pulmonary vascular resistance is a U-shaped curve (Figure 5–24). Thus, the pulmonary vascular resistance (PVR) is lowest near the functional residual capacity (FRC) and increases in response to both high and low lung volumes.

Blood Volume Changes. As blood volume increases, the recruitment and distention of pulmonary vessels will ensue, and pulmonary vascular resistance will tend to decrease (see Figure 5–21).

Blood Viscosity Changes. The viscosity of blood is derived from the hematocrit, the integrity of red blood cells, and the composition of plasma. As blood viscosity increases, the pulmonary vascular resistance increases. Table 5–4 summarizes the active and passive mechanisms of vascular resistance.

TABLE 5–4

Summary of the Effects of Active and Passive Mechanisms on Vascular Resistance

	↑ Resistance (vascular constriction)	↓ Resistance (vascular dilation)
ACTIVE MECHANISMS		
Abnormal Blood Gases		
$\downarrow P_{O_2}$	X	
$\uparrow P_{CO_2}$	X	
$\downarrow$pH	X	
Pharmacologic Stimulation		
Epinephrine	X	
Norepinephrine	X	
Dobutamine	X	
Dopamine	X	
Phenylephrine	X	
Oxygen		X
Isoproterenol		X
Aminophylline		X
Calcium-channel blocking agents		X
Pathologic Conditions		
Vessel blockage/obstruction	X	
Vessel wall disease	X	
Vessel destruction	X	
Vessel compression	X	
PASSIVE MECHANISMS		
↑Pulmonary arterial pressure		X
↑Left atrial pressure		X
↑Lung volume (extreme)	X	
↓Lung volume (extreme)	X	
↑Blood volume		X
↑Blood viscosity	X	

↑ = increased; ↓ = decreased.

CHAPTER SUMMARY

The transport of oxygen to the cells of the body is a function of the circulatory system. The essential components of the circulatory system consist of the blood, the heart, and the pulmonary and systemic vascular systems. *Blood* consists of a variety of specialized cells that are suspended in a fluid called plasma. The cells in the plasma include the erythrocytes, leukocytes, and thrombocytes.

Essential components of the *heart* include the right and left atria, right and left ventricles, the interventricular septum, the pericardium, the walls of the heart (i.e., epicardium, myocardium, endocardium), the arterial supply of the heart (the left and right coronary artery), the venous drainage (i.e., the great cardiac veins, middle cardiac vein, coronary sinus, and thebesian veins), and the blood flow through the heart.

The *pulmonary* and *systemic vascular systems* are composed of the arteries, arterioles, capillaries, venules, and veins. The pulmonary arterioles and most of the arterioles in the systemic circulation are controlled by sympathetic impulses. Specialized stretch receptors called baroreceptors regulate the arterial blood pressure by initiating reflex adjustments to deviations in blood pressure. The following three types of pressures are used to study the blood flow in the pulmonary and systemic vascular systems: intravascular, transmural, and driving. During each cardiac cycle, the ventricular systole and diastole have a direct relationship to the blood pressure. During ventricular systole, the arterial blood pressure sharply increases; during ventricular diastole, the arterial blood pressure decreases. The high and low blood pressures generated by ventricular systole and diastole result in mean intraluminal blood pressures throughout the pulmonary and systemic circulation. The mean systemic vascular pressure is about 10 times that of the pulmonary vascular system.

The distribution of pulmonary blood flow is a function of (1) gravity, (2) cardiac output, and (3) pulmonary vascular resistance. The influence of gravity in the upper right lung is described in terms of zones 1, 2, and 3; zone 3 is the most gravity-dependent area. Determinants of cardiac output are a function of ventricular preload, ventricular afterload, and myocardial contractility. Finally, the pulmonary vascular resistance may increase or decrease as a result of active and passive mechanisms. Active mechanisms include abnormal blood gases, pharmacologic stimulation, and pathologic conditions. Passive mechanisms include increased pulmonary arterial pressure, increased left atrial pressure, lung volume changes, and blood volume and blood viscosity changes.

1 CLINICAL APPLICATION CASE

A 16-year-old girl was involved in an automobile accident on the way home from school during a freezing rain. As she drove over a bridge, her car hit a patch of ice, spun out of control, and hit a cement embankment. It took the emergency rescue team almost an hour to cut her out of her car with the "Jaws of Life." She was stabilized at the accident scene and then transported to the trauma center.

In the emergency department, the patient was unconscious and hypotensive. It was obvious that she had lost a lot of blood; her shirt and pants were soaked with blood. She had several large lacerations on her forehead, face, neck, left arm, and left leg. The patient's head was lowered and her legs were elevated. The emergency department nurse started an intravenous infusion of Ringer's lactated solution. The respiratory therapist placed a nonrebreathing oxygen mask on the patient's face and drew an arterial blood sample. The radiologic technician took several portable x-rays.

The patient had several large bruises and abrasions over her left anterior chest that were most likely caused by the steering wheel when her car hit the cement embankment. Her four upper front teeth were broken off at the gum line. Her skin was pale and blue. Her vital signs were blood pressure—78/42 mm Hg, heart rate—145 beats/min and weak, and respirations—22 breaths/min and shallow. Her breath sounds were diminished bilaterally. Her arterial oxygen pressure (Pa_{O_2}) was 72 mm Hg.

Although chest x-ray showed no broken ribs, patches of pulmonary infiltrates (increased alveolar density) could be seen over the left anterior lung. Additional x-rays showed that she had a broken left humerus and left tibia. She was taken to surgery to repair her lacerations and broken bones. Five hours later, she was transferred to the surgical intensive care unit with her left arm and left leg in a cast.

To offset the increased alveolar density noted on the chest x-ray, the respiratory therapist administered continuous positive airway pressure (CPAP) via a face mask for 20 minutes every hour. Between the CPAP treatments, the patient continued to receive oxygen via a nonrebreathing mask. Two hours later, the patient was conscious and talking to her parents. Her skin appeared normal and her vital signs were blood pressure—115/82 mm Hg, heart rate—75 beats/min and strong, and respirations—14 breaths/min. Normal vesicular breath sounds were heard throughout both lungs. Her fractional concentration of inspired oxygen (FI_{O_2}) was decreased to 0.4, and her Pa_{O_2} on this setting was 94 mm Hg.

The patient's cardiopulmonary status progressively improved and she was discharged on the sixth day of hospitalization. Although her broken bones healed adequately, she had trouble walking normally for some time after the accident. Because of this problem, she continued to receive physical therapy twice a week for 6 months on an outpatient basis. At the time of her high school graduation, she had completely recovered.

DISCUSSION

This case study illustrates (1) the activation of the baroreceptor reflex, (2) hypovolemia and how it relates to preload, (3) negative transmural pressure, and (4) the effects of gravity on blood flow.

(continues)

As shown in this chapter, the specialized stretch receptors called *baroreceptors* (see Figure 5–10) regulate the arterial blood pressure by initiating reflex adjustments to changes in blood pressure. In this case, as the patient's blood pressure decreased from the loss of blood, neural impulses transmitted from the baroreceptors to the vasomotor and cardiac centers in the medulla decreased. This action, in turn, likely caused the patient's medulla to increase its sympathetic activity, which increased the heart rate (her pulse was 145 beats/min in the emergency department).

Because *ventricular preload* is a function of the blood pressure generated by the volume of blood returning to the left or right ventricle during diastole, it can easily be seen why the patient's ventricular preload decreased as she became hypovolemic from the loss of blood. In the emergency department, the fact that the patient's ventricular preload was low was reflected by her low blood pressure (78/42 mm Hg). It should be noted that as preload decreases, cardiac output decreases.

Finally, as the patient's preload decreased (from blood loss), the *transmural pressure* in her least gravity-dependent lung areas became increasingly negative. *Transmural pressure* is the difference between the intraluminal pressure of a vessel and the pressure surrounding the vessel (see Figure 5–11). The transmural pressure is negative when the pressure surrounding the vessel is greater than the pressure inside the vessel. In this case, this pathophysiologic process was offset by (1) lowering the patient's head and elevating her legs, which used the effects of gravity to move blood to the patient's lungs, and (2) replacing the volume of blood lost by administering Ringer's lactated solution. These two procedures worked to change the negative transmural pressures to positive transmural pressures in the lung regions.

2 CLINICAL APPLICATION CASE

A 72-year-old woman presented in the intensive care unit with left ventricular heart failure and pulmonary edema (also called congestive heart failure). She had no history of respiratory disease. The patient's husband stated that she had gone to bed with no remarkable problems, but awoke with severe dyspnea after several hours of sleep. Concerned, her husband called 911.

On observation, the patient's skin was cyanotic and she was in obvious respiratory distress. Her neck veins were distended and her ankles were swollen. Her vital signs were blood pressure—214/106 mm Hg, heart rate—90 beats/min, and respirations— 28 breaths/min. On auscultation, rales and rhonchi were heard over both lung fields. She had a frequent, productive cough with frothy white secretions. Her arterial oxygen pressure (Pa_{O_2}) on 3 L/min oxygen via nasal cannula was 48 mm Hg. A portable chest x-ray showed dense, fluffy opacities (white areas) that spread outward from the hilar areas to the peripheral borders of the lungs. The chest x-ray also showed that the left ventricle was enlarged (ventricular hypertrophy).

The physician prescribed (1) *positive inotropic agents* (see Table 15–3) to improve the strength of the left ventricular contraction

(continues)

and cardiac output, and (2) a systemic *vasodilator* (see Table 15–6) to decrease the patient's elevated blood pressure. Diuretic agents were also administered to promote fluid excretion. The respiratory therapist increased the patient's oxygen levels using a partial rebreathing mask.

Two hours later, the patient's cardiopulmonary status had significantly improved. Her skin appeared normal and her neck veins were no longer distended. Her peripheral edema was no longer present. Her vital signs were blood pressure—130/87 mm Hg, heart rate—81 beats/min, and respirations—14 breaths/min. Her Pa_{O_2}, on 2 L/min oxygen via nasal cannula, was 103 mm Hg. A second chest x-ray showed that her lungs were clear and the left ventricle had returned to normal size.

DISCUSSION

This case illustrates the effects of high blood pressure on (1) ventricular afterload, (2) ventricular contractility, (3) ventricular preload, and (4) transmural pressure.

Ventricular afterload is defined as the force against which the ventricles must work to pump blood. In this case, the patient's left ventricular afterload was very high because of increased peripheral vascular resistance. Clinically, this was reflected by the patient's high blood pressure of 214/106 mm Hg. Because of the high blood pressure and high left ventricular afterload, the patient's left ventricle eventually weakened and began to fail. As the ability of the left ventricle to pump blood decreased, the blood volume (and

pressure) in the left ventricle increased. Even though the preload was increased, the left ventricle was unable to meet the increased demands created by the increased blood volume.

As this condition worsened, blood backed up into the patient's lungs, causing the *transmural pressure* in the pulmonary capillary to increase significantly. As a result of the excessively high transmural pressure, fluid leaked out of the pulmonary capillaries and into the alveoli and airways. Clinically, this was verified by the rales and rhonchi heard during auscultation, and by the white, frothy secretions produced when the patient coughed. As fluid accumulated in the patient's alveoli, the diffusion of oxygen into the pulmonary capillaries decreased. This was verified by the decreased Pa_{O_2} of 48 mm Hg.

Finally, as the blood volume and the transmural pressure in the pulmonary capillaries increased, the right ventricular afterload increased, which in turn decreased the ability of the right ventricle to pump blood despite the fact that the preload increased. This condition was reflected by the patient's distended neck veins and peripheral edema.

Fortunately, in this case the patient responded well to the positive inotropic vasodilator, and diuretic agents. The vasodilator and diuretics worked to reduce the right and left ventricular afterloads, and the inotropic agents increased the ability of the ventricles to pump blood. The patient rapidly improved and was discharged on the fourth day of her hospital stay. Presently, she is seen by her family physician every 2 months.

REVIEW QUESTIONS

1. Which of the following are granulocytes?
  I. Neutrophils
  II. Monocytes
  III. Eosinophils
  IV. Lymphocytes
  V. Basophils
   A. II only
   B. V only
   C. II and IV only
   D. I, III, and V only

2. In healthy men, the hematocrit is about
   A.   25 percent
   B.   35 percent
   C.   45 percent
   D.   65 percent

3. Which of the following agents cause pulmonary vascular constriction?
  I. Isoproterenol
  II. Epinephrine
  III. Oxygen
  IV. Dopamine
   A. III only
   B. II and IV only
   C. I, II, and IV only
   D. All of these

4. If the pressure in the pulmonary artery is 34 mm Hg and the pressure in the left atrium is 9 mm Hg, what is the driving pressure?
   A.   9 mm Hg
   B.   17 mm Hg
   C.   25 mm Hg
   D.   34 mm Hg

5. The tricuspid valve lies between the
   A.   right atrium and the right ventricle
   B.   left ventricle and the aorta
   C.   right ventricle and the pulmonary artery
   D.   left atrium and the left ventricle

6. Which of the following is usually elevated in patients with asthma?
   A.   Lymphocytes
   B.   Neutrophils
   C.   Basophils
   D.   Eosinophils

7. The mean intraluminal pressure in the pulmonary capillaries is
   A.   5 mm Hg
   B.   10 mm Hg
   C.   15 mm Hg
   D.   20 mm Hg

8. An increase in the number of which of the following suggests a bacterial infection?
   A.   Lymphocytes
   B.   Neutrophils
   C.   Monocytes
   D.   Eosinophils

9. The force the ventricles must work against to pump blood is called
   A.   myocardial contractility
   B.   ventricular afterload
   C.   negative inotropism
   D.   ventricular preload

10. Compared with the systemic circulation, the pressure in the pulmonary circulation is about
    A.   1/10 the pressure
    B.   1/4 the pressure
    C.   1/3 the pressure
    D.   1/2 the pressure

11. The difference between the pressure in the lumen of a vessel and that of the pressure surrounding the vessel is called the
    A.   driving pressure
    B.   transmural pressure
    C.   diastolic pressure
    D.   intravascular pressure

12. Which of the following cause(s) pulmonary vasoconstriction?
    I.   Hypercapnia
    II.   Hypoxia
    III.   Acidemia
    IV.   Increased H^+ concentration
    A. III only
    B. II and IV only
    C. II, III, and IV only
    D. All of these

13. The cardioinhibitor center of the medulla slows the heart by sending neural impulses by way of the
    I.   tenth cranial nerve
    II. parasympathetic nervous system
    III. sympathetic nervous system
    IV. vagus nerve
       A. IV only
       B. III only
       C. I and IV only
       D. I, II, and IV only

14. Which of the following cause(s) passive changes in the pulmonary vascular resistance?
    I.   pH changes
    II. Transpulmonary pressure changes
    III. P_{CO_2} changes
    IV. Blood viscosity changes
       A. II only
       B. III only
       C. I and III only
       D. II and IV only

15. Which of the following cause blood clotting at a traumatized site?
    A.   Thrombocytes
    B.   Basophils
    C.   Monocytes
    D.   Eosinophils

CLINICAL APPLICATION QUESTIONS

CASE 1

1. As the patient's blood pressure decreased from the loss of blood, neural impulses transmitted from the _____ to the vasomotor and cardiac centers in the medulla (decreased _____; increased _____).

2. In the emergency department, the patient's low preload was reflected by her low _____.

3. As the preload decreases, the cardiac output _____.

4. The negative transmural pressure in this case was offset by (1) _____

   _____

   and (2) _____

   _____.

CASE 2

1. In this case, the patient's left ventricular afterload was very high. This condition was reflected by the patient's _____.

2. As a result of the excessively high transmural pressure, fluid leaked out of the pulmonary capillaries and into the alveoli and airways. Clinically, this was verified by the _____ and _____ heard on auscultation.

3. As fluid accumulated in the patient's alveoli, the diffusion of oxygen into the pulmonary capillaries decreased. This was verified by the _____.

4. The increased right ventricular afterload was reflected by the patient's _____

5. The vasodilator and diuretic agents worked to reduce the right and left ventricular _____.

CHAPTER 6

Oxygen Transport

O B J E C T I V E S

By the end of this chapter, the student should be able to:

1. Calculate the quantity of oxygen that *dissolves in the plasma* of the blood.
2. Describe the major features of *hemoglobin,* including:
   —Heme portion
      • Iron
   —Globin portion
      • Four amino acid chains
         ○ Two alpha chains
         ○ Two beta chains
   —Ferrous state versus ferric state
   —Normal hemoglobin concentrations in the adult male and female and in the infant
3. Calculate the quantity of oxygen that *combines with hemoglobin.*
4. Calculate the *total amount* of oxygen in the blood.
5. Identify the abbreviations for the following:
   —Oxygen content of arterial blood
   —Oxygen content of mixed venous blood
   —Oxygen content of pulmonary capillary blood
6. Describe how the following relate to the *oxygen dissociation curve:*
   —Percentage of hemoglobin bound to oxygen
   —Oxygen pressure
   —Oxygen content
7. Describe the clinical significance of the
   —flat portion of the oxygen dissociation curve
   —steep portion of the oxygen dissociation curve
   —P_{50}
8. Identify the factors that shift the oxygen dissociation curve to the right.
9. Identify the factors that shift the oxygen dissociation curve to the left.
10. Explain the clinical significance of a right or left shift of the oxygen dissociation curve with regard to the
    —loading of oxygen in the lungs
    —unloading of oxygen at the tissues
11. Perform the following oxygen transport calculations:
    —Total oxygen delivery
    —Arterial-venous oxygen content difference
    —Oxygen consumption
    —Oxygen extraction ratio
    —Mixed venous oxygen saturation
12. Identify the factors that increase and decrease the *oxygen transport* calculations.
13. Differentiate between the following forms of *pulmonary shunting:*
    —Absolute shunts
       • Anatomic shunt
       • Capillary shunt
    —Relative shunt (shunt-like effect)
14. Explain the meaning of *venous admixture.*
15. Calculate the *shunt equation.*

(continues)

16. Describe the clinical significance of pulmonary shunting.
17. Describe the differences between *hypoxemia* and *hypoxia*.
18. Define the four main types of tissue hypoxia:
    —Hypoxic hypoxia
    —Anemic hypoxia
    —Circulatory hypoxia
    —Histotoxic hypoxia
19. Explain the meaning of
    —cyanosis
    —polycythemia
20. Complete the review questions at the end of this chapter.

An understanding of oxygen transport is essential to the study of pulmonary physiology and to the clinical interpretation of arterial and venous blood gases. Table 6–1 lists the normal blood gas values.* To fully understand this subject, the student must understand (1) how oxygen is transported from the lungs to the tissues, (2) the oxygen dissociation curve and its clinical significance, (3) how various oxygen transport calculations are used to identify the patient's cardiac and ventilatory status, and (4) the major forms of tissue hypoxia.

OXYGEN TRANSPORT

The transport of oxygen between the lungs and the cells of the body is a function of the blood and the heart. Oxygen is carried in the blood in two forms: (1) as dissolved oxygen in the blood plasma, and (2) chemically bound to the hemoglobin (Hb) that is encased in the erythrocytes, or red blood cells (RBCs).

TABLE 6–1
Normal Blood Gas Value Ranges

Blood Gas Value*	Arterial	Venous
pH	7.35–7.45	7.30–7.40
P_{CO_2}	35–45 mm Hg (Pa_{CO_2})	42–48 mm Hg ($P\bar{v}_{CO_2}$)
HCO_3^-	22–28 mEq/L	24–30 mEq/L
P_{O_2}	80–100 mm Hg (Pa_{O_2})	35–45 mm Hg ($P\bar{v}_{O_2}$)

* Technically, only the oxygen (P_O) and carbon dioxide (P_{CO}) pressure readings are "true" blood gas values. The pH indicates the balance between the bases and acids in the blood. The bicarbonate (HCO_3^-) reading is an indirect measurement that is calculated from the pH and P_{CO_2} levels.

See Appendix V for a representative example of a cardiopulmonary profile sheet used to monitor the blood gas values of the critically ill patient.

CLINICAL
APPLICATION
CASE

1

See page 263

Oxygen Dissolved in the Blood Plasma

As oxygen diffuses from the alveoli into the pulmonary capillary blood, it dissolves in the plasma of the blood. The term **dissolve** means that when a gas like oxygen enters the plasma, it maintains its precise molecular structure (in this case, O_2) and moves freely throughout the plasma in its normal gaseous state. Clinically, it is this portion of the oxygen that is measured to assess the patient's partial pressure of oxygen (P_{O_2}) (see Table 6–1).

The quantity of oxygen that dissolves in the plasma is a function of Henry's law, which states that the amount of gas that dissolves in a liquid (in this case, plasma) at a given temperature is proportional to the partial pressure of the gas. At normal body temperature, about 0.003 mL of oxygen will dissolve in 100 mL of blood for every 1 mm Hg of P_{O_2}. Thus, in the healthy individual with an arterial oxygen partial pressure (Pa_{O_2}) of 100 mm Hg, approximately 0.3 mL of oxygen is dissolved in every 100 mL of plasma (0.003 × 100 mm Hg = 0.3 mL). This is written as 0.3 volumes percent (vol%). Vol% represents the amount of O_2 in milliliters that is in 100 mL of blood (vol% = mL O_2/100 mL blood). For example, 10 vol% of O_2 means that there are 10 mL of O_2 in 100 mL of blood. In terms of total oxygen transport, a relatively small percentage of oxygen is transported in the form of dissolved oxygen.

Oxygen Bound to Hemoglobin

Hemoglobin

CLINICAL
APPLICATION
CASE

1

See page 263

Most of the oxygen that diffuses into the pulmonary capillary blood rapidly moves into the RBCs and chemically attaches to the hemoglobin. Each RBC contains approximately 280 million hemoglobin molecules, which are highly specialized to transport oxygen and carbon dioxide.

Normal adult hemoglobin, which is designated Hb A, consists of (1) four heme groups, which are the pigmented, iron-containing non-protein portions of the hemoglobin molecule, and (2) four amino acid chains (polypeptide chains) that collectively constitute globin (a protein) (Figure 6–1).

At the center of each heme group, the iron molecule can combine with one oxygen molecule in an easily reversible reaction to form oxyhemoglobin:

$$\text{Hb} \quad + \quad O_2 \quad \rightleftharpoons \quad \text{Hb}_{O_2}$$

Reduced
hemoglobin   Oxygen   Oxyhemoglobin
(uncombined or   (combined or
deoxygenated   oxygenated
hemoglobin)   hemoglobin)

Because there are four heme/iron groups in each Hb molecule, a total of four oxygen molecules can combine with each Hb molecule. When four

Figure 6–1

Schematic illustration of a hemoglobin molecule. The globin (protein) portion consists of two identical alpha (α) chains and two beta (β) chains. The four heme (iron-containing) portions are in the center of each globin molecule.

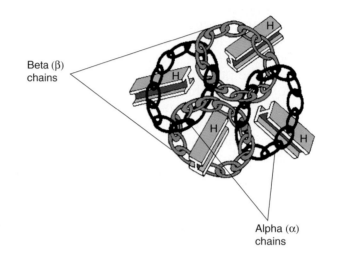

Beta (β) chains

Alpha (α) chains

oxygen molecules are bound to one Hb molecule, the Hb is said to be 100 percent saturated with oxygen; an Hb molecule with three oxygen molecules is 75 percent saturated; and so forth. Hemoglobin bound with oxygen (Hb$_{O_2}$) is called **oxyhemoglobin**. Hemoglobin not bound with oxygen (Hb) is called **reduced hemoglobin** or **deoxyhemoglobin**. The amount of oxygen bound to Hb is directly related to the partial pressure of oxygen.

The globin portion of each Hb molecule consists of two identical alpha (α) chains, each with 141 amino acids, and two identical beta (β) chains, each with 146 amino acids (α$_2$β$_2$). Normal fetal hemoglobin (Hb F) has two alpha (α) chains and two gamma (γ) chains (α$_2$γ$_2$). This increases hemoglobin's attraction to oxygen and facilitates transfer of maternal oxygen across the placenta. Fetal hemoglobin is gradually replaced with Hb A over the first year of postnatal life.

When the precise number, sequence, or spatial arrangement of the globin amino acid chains is altered, the hemoglobin will be abnormal. For example, sickle cell hemoglobin (Hb S) has a different amino acid substituted into the β chain. This causes the deoxygenated hemoglobin molecule (hemoglobin not bound to oxygen) to change the RBC shape from biconcave to a crescent or sickle form that has a tendency to form thrombi (clots). Various drugs and chemicals, such as nitrites, can change the iron molecule in the heme from the *ferrous state* to the *ferric state*, eliminating the ability of hemoglobin to transport oxygen. This type of hemoglobin is known as *methemoglobin.*

The normal hemoglobin value for the adult male is 14 to 16 g/100 mL of blood. In other words, if all the hemoglobin were to be extracted from all the RBCs in 100 mL of blood, the hemoglobin would actually weigh between 14 and 16 g. Clinically, the weight measurement of hemoglobin, in reference to 100 mL of blood, is referred to as either the *gram percent of hemoglobin* (g% Hb) or *grams per deciliter* (g/dL). The average adult female hemoglobin value is 12 to 15 g%. The average infant hemoglobin value is 14 to 20 g%. Hemoglobin constitutes about 33 percent of the RBC weight.

Quantity of Oxygen Bound to Hemoglobin

Each g% of Hb is capable of carrying approximately 1.34 mL* of oxygen. Thus, if the hemoglobin level is 15 g%, and if the hemoglobin is fully saturated, about 20.1 vol% of oxygen will be bound to the hemoglobin. The figure 20.1 is calculated using the following formula:

CLINICAL APPLICATION CASE

1

See page 263

$$O_2 \text{ bound to Hb} = 1.34 \text{ mL } O_2 \times 15 \text{ g\% Hb}$$

$$= 20.1 \text{ vol\% } O_2$$

At a normal arterial oxygen pressure (Pa_{O_2}) of 100 mm Hg, however, the hemoglobin saturation (Sa_{O_2}) is only about 97 percent because of these normal physiologic shunts:

- Thebesian venous drainage into the left atrium
- Bronchial venous drainage into the pulmonary veins
- Alveoli that are underventilated relative to pulmonary blood flow.

Thus, the amount of arterial oxygen in the preceding equation must be adjusted to 97 percent. The equation is written as follows:

$$\begin{array}{r} 20.1 \text{ vol\% } O_2 \\ \times\ 0.97 \\ \hline 19.5 \text{ vol\% } O_2 \end{array}$$

Total Oxygen Content

To determine the total amount of oxygen in 100 mL of blood, the dissolved oxygen and the oxygen bound to hemoglobin must be added together. The following case study summarizes the calculations required to compute an individual's total oxygen content.

Case Study: Anemic Patient

A 27-year-old woman with a long history of anemia (decreased hemoglobin concentration) is showing signs of respiratory distress. Her respiratory rate is 36 breaths/min, heart rate 130 beats/minute, and blood

---

The literature also reports values of 1.36, 1.38, and 1.39. The figure 1.34 is the most commonly used factor and is used in this textbook.

pressure 155/90 mm Hg. Her hemoglobin concentration is 6 g%, and her Pa_{O_2} is 80 mm Hg (Sa_{O_2} 90%).

Based on this information, the patient's total oxygen content is computed as follows:

1. Dissolved O_2:

$$\begin{array}{r} 80\ Pa_{O_2} \\ \times\ 0.003\ \text{(dissolved } O_2 \text{ factor)} \\ \hline 0.24\ \text{vol\% } O_2 \end{array}$$

2. Oxygen bound to hemoglobin:

$$\begin{array}{r} 6\ g\%\ Hb \\ \times\ 1.34\ (O_2 \text{ bound to Hb factor}) \\ \hline 8.04\ \text{vol\% } O_2\ \text{(at } Sa_{O_2} \text{ of 100\%)} \end{array}$$

$$\begin{array}{r} 8.04\ \text{vol\% } O_2 \\ \times\ 0.90\ Sa_{O_2} \\ \hline 7.236\ \text{vol\% } O_2 \end{array}$$

3. Total oxygen content:

$$\begin{array}{r} 7.236\ \text{vol\% } O_2\ \text{(bound to hemoglobin)} \\ +\ 0.24\ \ \ \text{vol\% } O_2\ \text{(dissolved } O_2) \\ \hline 7.476\ \text{vol\% } O_2\ \text{(total amount of } O_2/100\ mL\ \text{of blood)} \end{array}$$

Note that the patient's total arterial oxygen content is less than 50 percent of normal. Her hemoglobin concentration, which is the primary mechanism for transporting oxygen, is very low. Once this problem is corrected, the clinical manifestations of respiratory distress should no longer be present.

The total oxygen content of the arterial blood (Ca_{O_2}), mixed venous blood ($C\bar{v}_{O_2}$), and pulmonary capillary blood (Cc_{O_2}) is calculated as follows:

- Ca_{O_2}: Oxygen content of arterial blood
  $(Hb \times 1.34 \times Sa_{O_2}) + (Pa_{O_2} \times 0.003)$
- $C\bar{v}_{O_2}$: Oxygen content of mixed venous blood
  $(Hb \times 1.34 \times S\bar{v}_{O_2}) + (P\bar{v}_{O_2} \times 0.003)$
- Cc_{O_2}: Oxygen content of pulmonary capillary blood
  $(Hb \times 1.34)* + (P_{A_{O_2}}{}^{\dagger} \times 0.003)$

---

*It is assumed that the hemoglobin saturation with oxygen in the pulmonary capillary blood (Sc_{O_2}) is 100 percent or 1.0.
†See "Ideal Alveolar Gas Equation" section in Chapter 3.

It will be shown later in this chapter how various mathematical manipulations of the Ca_{O_2}, $C\bar{v}_{O_2}$, and Cc_{O_2} values are used in different oxygen transport calculations to reflect important factors concerning the patient's cardiac and ventilatory status.

OXYGEN DISSOCIATION CURVE

As shown in Figure 6–2, the oxygen dissociation curve is part of a nomogram that graphically illustrates the *percentage of hemoglobin* (left-hand side of the graph) that is chemically bound to oxygen at each *oxygen pressure* (bottom portion of the graph). On the right-hand side of the graph, a second scale is included that gives the precise *oxygen content* that is carried by the hemoglobin at each oxygen pressure.

The curve is S-shaped with a steep slope between 10 and 60 mm Hg and a flat portion between 70 and 100 mm Hg. The steep portion of the

Figure 6–2

Oxygen dissociation curve.

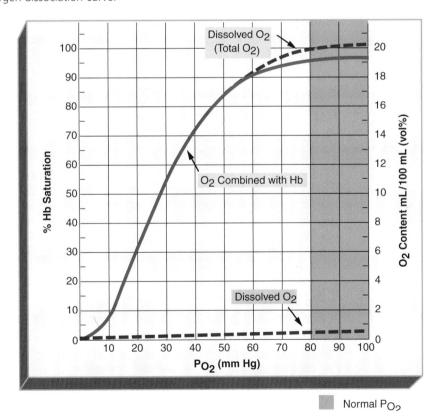

curve shows that oxygen rapidly combines with hemoglobin as the P_{O_2} increases. Beyond this point (60 mm Hg), a further increase in the P_{O_2} produces only a slight increase in oxygen-hemoglobin bonding. In fact, because the hemoglobin is already 90 percent saturated at a P_{O_2} of 60 mm Hg, an increase in the P_{O_2} from 60 to 100 mm Hg elevates the total saturaion of the hemoglobin by only 7 percent (see Figure 6–2).

Clinical Significance of the Flat Portion of the Curve

The P_{O_2} can fall from 100 to 60 mm Hg and the hemoglobin will still be 90 percent saturated with oxygen. Thus, the upper curve plateau illustrates that hemoglobin has an excellent safety zone for the loading of oxygen in the lungs.

As the hemoglobin moves through the alveolar-capillary system to pick up oxygen, a significant partial pressure difference continues to exist between the alveolar gas and the blood, even after most of the oxygen is transferred. This mechanism enhances the diffusion of oxygen during the transit time of the hemoglobin in the alveolar-capillary system.

The flat portion also means that increasing the P_{O_2} beyond 100 mm Hg adds very little additional oxygen to the blood. In fact, once the P_{O_2} increases enough to saturate 100 percent of the hemoglobin with oxygen, the hemoglobin will no longer accept any additional oxygen molecules. However, a small additional amount of oxygen continues to dissolve in the plasma as the P_{O_2} rises ($P_{O_2} \times 0.003$ = dissolved O_2).

Clinical Significance of the Steep Portion of the Curve

A reduction of P_{O_2} to below 60 mm Hg produces a rapid decrease in the amount of oxygen bound to hemoglobin. Clinically, therefore, when the P_{O_2} continues to fall below 60 mm Hg, the quantity of oxygen delivered to the tissue cells may be significantly reduced.

The steep portion of the curve also shows that as the hemoglobin moves through the capillaries of the tissue cells, a large amount of oxygen is released from the hemoglobin for only a small decrease in P_{O_2}. Thus, the diffusion of oxygen from the hemoglobin to the tissue cells is enhanced.

The P_{50}

A point of reference on the oxygen dissociation curve is the P_{50} (Figure 6–3). The P_{50} represents the partial pressure at which the hemoglobin is 50 percent saturated with oxygen—that is, when there are two oxygen molecules on each hemoglobin molecule. Normally, the P_{50} is about 27 mm Hg. Clinically, however, there are a variety of abnormal conditions that can shift the oxygen dissociation curve to either the right or left. When this

Figure 6–3

The P_{50} represents the partial pressure at which hemoglobin is 50 percent saturated with oxygen. When the oxygen dissociation curve shifts to the right, the P_{50} increases. When the oxygen dissociation curve shifts to the left, the P_{50} decreases.

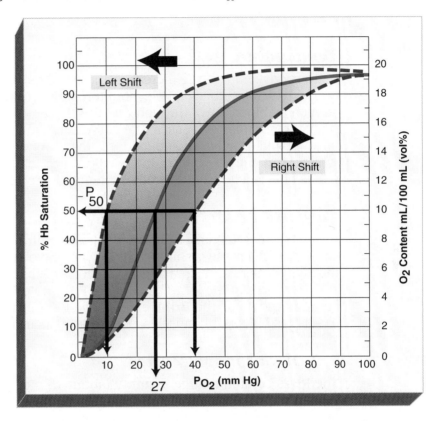

happens, the P_{50} changes. For example, when the curve shifts to the right, the affinity of hemoglobin for oxygen decreases, causing the hemoglobin to be less saturated at a given P_{O_2}. Thus, *when the curve shifts to the right, the P_{50} increases.* On the other hand, when the curve moves to the left, the affinity of hemoglobin for oxygen increases, causing the hemoglobin to be more saturated at a given P_{O_2}. Thus, *when the curve shifts to the left, the P_{50} decreases* (see Figure 6–3).

Factors That Shift the Oxygen Dissociation Curve

pH

As the blood hydrogen-ion concentration increases (decreased pH), the oxygen dissociation curve shifts to the right. This mechanism enhances the unloading of oxygen at the cellular level, because the pH decreases in this area as carbon dioxide (the acidic end-product of cellular metabolism) moves into the blood. In contrast, as the blood hydrogen-ion (H^+) concentration decreases, the curve shifts to the left. This mechanism facilitates the loading of oxygen onto hemoglobin as blood passes through the lungs, because the pH increases as carbon dioxide moves out of the blood and into the alveoli.

Temperature

As the body temperature increases, the curve moves to the right. Thus, exercise, which produces an elevated temperature, enhances the release of oxygen as blood flows through the muscle capillaries. Conversely, as the body temperature decreases, the curve shifts to the left. This mechanism partly explains why an individual's lips, ears, and fingers appear blue while swimming in very cold water. That is, their Pa_{O_2} is normal, but oxygen is not readily released from the hemoglobin at the cold tissue sites.

Carbon Dioxide

As the P_{CO_2} level increases (increased H^+ concentration), the oxyhemoglobin saturation decreases, shifting the oxyhemoglobin dissociation curve to the right, whereas decreasing P_{CO_2} levels (decreased H^+ concentrations) shift the curve to the left. The effect of P_{CO_2} and pH on the oxyhemoglobin curve is known as the **Bohr effect**. The Bohr effect is most active in the capillaries of working muscles, particularly the myocardium.

2,3-Diphosphoglycerate

The RBCs contain a large quantity (about 15 mol/g Hb) of the substance 2,3-diphosphoglycerate (2,3-DPG). 2,3-DPG is a metabolic intermediary that is formed by the RBCs during anaerobic glycolysis. Hemoglobin's affinity for oxygen decreases as the 2,3-DPG level increases. Thus, the effect of an elevated concentration of 2,3-DPG is to shift the oxygen dissociation curve to the right. Clinically, a variety of conditions affect the level of 2,3-DPG.

Hypoxia. Regardless of the cause, hypoxia increases the 2,3-DPG level.

Anemia. The 2,3-DPG level increases as the hemoglobin concentration decreases. This mechanism may explain why individuals with anemia frequently do not manifest the signs or symptoms associated with hypoxia.

pH Changes. As the pH increases, the 2,3-DPG concentration increases. Thus, the shift of the oxygen dissociation curve to the left by the increased pH is offset somewhat by the increased 2,3-DPG level, which shifts the curve to the right. Conversely, as the pH decreases, the 2,3-DPG concentration decreases. Thus, while the decreased pH shifts the curve to the right, the decreased 2,3-DPG level works to shift the curve to the left.

Stored Blood. Blood stored for as little as 1 week has been shown to have very low concentrations of 2,3-DPG. Thus, when patients receive stored blood, the oxygen unloading in their tissues may be reduced because of the decreased 2,3-DPG level.

Fetal Hemoglobin

Fetal hemoglobin (Hb F) is chemically different from adult hemoglobin. Hb F has a greater affinity for oxygen and, therefore, shifts the oxygen dissociation curve to the left (reducing the P_{50}). During fetal development, the higher affinity of Hb F enhances the transfer of oxygen from maternal blood to fetal blood. After birth, Hb F progressively disappears and is completely absent after about 1 year.

Carbon Monoxide Hemoglobin

Carbon monoxide (CO) has about 210 times the affinity of oxygen for hemoglobin. Because of this, a small amount of CO can tie up a large amount of hemoglobin (CO_{Hb}) and, as a result, prevent oxygen molecules from bonding to hemoglobin. This can seriously reduce the amount of oxygen transferred to the tissue cells. In addition, when CO_{Hb} is present, the affinity of hemoglobin for oxygen increases and shifts the oxygen dissociation curve to the left. Thus, the oxygen molecules that do manage to combine with hemoglobin are unable to unload easily in the tissues.

Figure 6–4 summarizes factors that shift the oxygen dissociation curve to the right and left and how the P_{50} is affected by these shifts.

Clinical Significance of Shifts in the O₂ Dissociation Curve

When an individual's blood Pa_{O_2} is within normal limits (80–100 mm Hg), a shift of the oxygen dissociation curve to the right or left does not significantly affect hemoglobin's ability to transport oxygen to the peripheral tissues, because shifts in this pressure range (80–100 mm Hg) occur on the flat portion of the curve. However, when an individual's blood Pa_{O_2} falls below the normal range, a shift to the right or left can have a remarkable effect on the hemoglobin's ability to pick up and release oxygen, because shifts below the normal pressure range occur on the steep portion of the curve. For example, consider the loading and unloading of oxygen during the clinical conditions discussed next.

Right Shifts—Loading of Oxygen in the Lungs

Picture the loading of oxygen onto hemoglobin as blood passes through the alveolar-capillary system at a time when the alveolar oxygen tension (PA_{O_2}) is moderately low—say, 60 mm Hg (caused, for example, by an acute asthmatic episode). Normally, when the PA_{O_2} is 60 mm Hg, the P_{O_2} of the pulmonary capillary blood (Pc_{O_2}) is also about 60 mm Hg. Thus, the

CLINICAL
APPLICATION
CASE

2

See page 265

Figure 6–4

Factors that shift the oxygen dissociation curve to the right and left. (DPG = 2,3-diphosphoglycerate; for other abbreviations, see text).

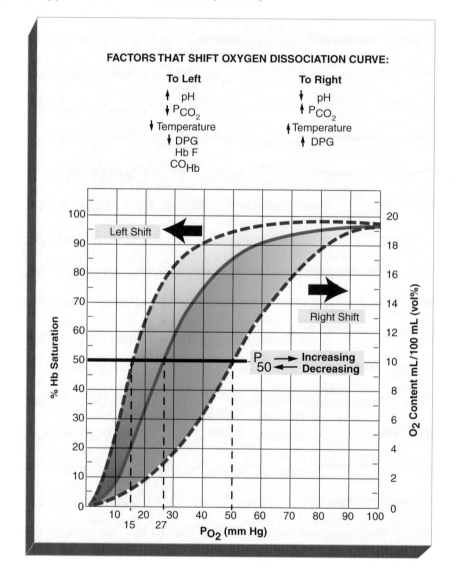

hemoglobin is about 90 percent saturated with oxygen as it leaves the alveoli (Figure 6–5). If, however, the oxygen dissociation curve shifts to the right, as indicated in Figure 6–6 (p. 240) (caused by a pH of about 7.1), the hemoglobin will be only about 75 percent saturated with oxygen as it leaves the alveoli—despite the fact that the patient's plasma P_{O_2} is still 60 mm Hg.

In view of this gas transport phenomenon, therefore, it should be stressed that *the total oxygen delivery may be much lower than indicated by*

Figure 6–5

Normally, when the $P_{A_{O_2}}$ is 60 mm Hg, the plasma P_{O_2} of the alveolar-capillary blood is also about 60 mm Hg and the hemoglobin is about 90 percent saturated with oxygen as it leaves the alveoli.

a particular Pa_{O_2} value when a disease process is present that causes the oxygen dissociation curve to shift to the right (see Figure 6–4). However, as discussed later, the unloading of oxygen at the tissue sites is actually enhanced when the oxygen dissociation curse is shifted to the right. This action helps to offset the decreased loading of oxygen between the alveoli and pulmonary capillaries when the curve is shifted to the right. Note also that when a right shift is accompanied by either a decreased cardiac output or a reduced level of hemoglobin, the patient's ability to transport oxygen will be jeopardized even more.

Figure 6–6

When the $P_{A_{O_2}}$ is 60 mm Hg at a time when the oxygen dissociation curve has shifted to the right because of a pH of 7.1, the hemoglobin will be only about 75 percent saturated with oxygen as it leaves the alveoli.

Right Shifts—Unloading of Oxygen at the Tissues

Although the total oxygen delivery may decrease in the above situation, the plasma P_{O_2} at the tissue sites does not have to fall as much to unload oxygen from the hemoglobin. For example, if the tissue cells metabolize 5 vol% oxygen at a time when the oxygen dissociation curve is in its normal position, the plasma P_{O_2} must fall from 60 mm Hg to about 35 mm Hg

Figure 6–7

Normally, when the plasma P_{O_2} is 60 mm Hg, the P_{O_2} must fall from 60 mm Hg to about 35 mm Hg to free 5 vol% oxygen from the hemoglobin for tissue metabolism.

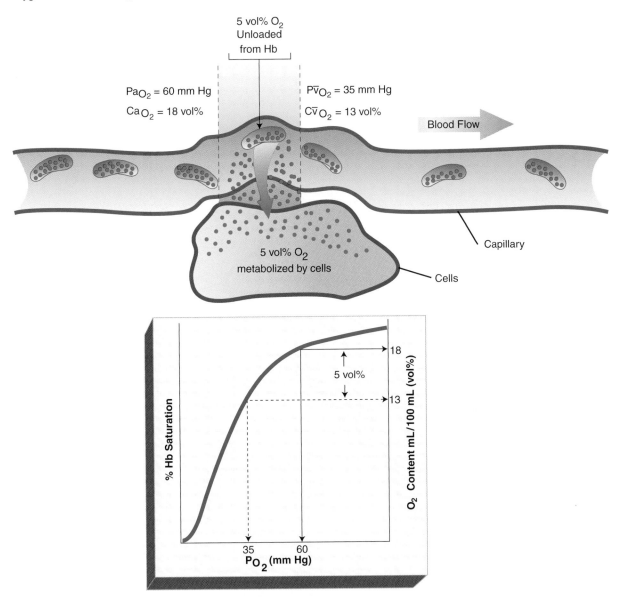

to free 5 vol% oxygen from the hemoglobin (Figure 6–7). If, however, the curve shifts to the right in response to a pH of 7.1, the plasma P_{O_2} at the tissue sites would only have to fall from 60 mm Hg to about 40 mm Hg to unload 5 vol% oxygen from the hemoglobin (Figure 6–8).

Figure 6–8

When the Pa_{O_2} is 60 mm Hg at a time when the oxygen dissociation curve has shifted to the right because of a pH of 7.1, the plasma P_{O_2} at the tissue site would have to fall from 60 mm Hg to about 40 mm Hg to unload 5 vol% oxygen from the hemoglobin.

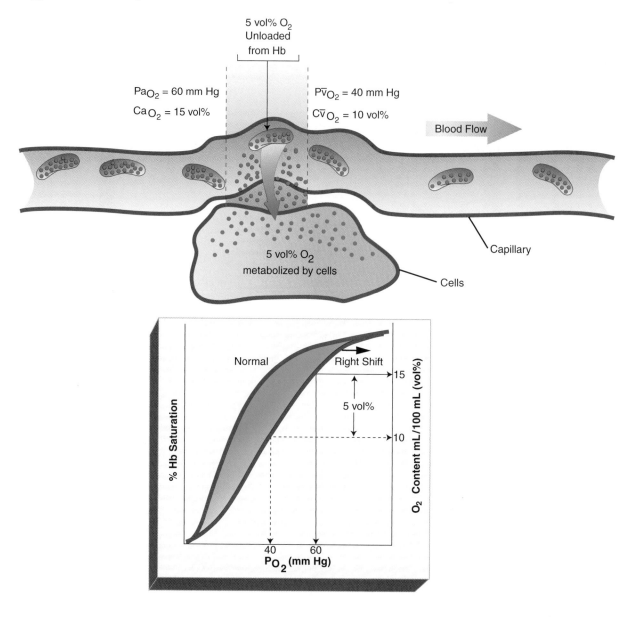

Left Shifts—Loading of Oxygen in the Lungs

If the oxygen dissociation curve shifts to the left, as indicated in Figure 6–9 (caused by a pH of about 7.6), at a time when the $P_{A_{O_2}}$ is 60 mm Hg, the hemoglobin will be about 95 percent saturated with oxygen as it leaves the alveoli, even though the patient's plasma P_{O_2} is only 60 mm Hg.

Figure 6–9

When the $P_{A_{O_2}}$ is 60 mm Hg at a time when the oxygen dissociation curve has shifted to the left because of a pH of 7.6, the hemoglobin will be about 95 percent saturated with oxygen as it leaves the alveoli.

Left Shifts—Unloading of Oxygen at the Tissues

Although the total oxygen delivery increases in the previously mentioned situation, the plasma P_{O_2} at the tissue sites must decrease more than normal in order for oxygen to dissociate from the hemoglobin. For example, if the tissue cells require 5 vol% oxygen at a time when the oxygen dissociation curve is normal, the plasma P_{O_2} will fall from 60 mm Hg to about 35 mm Hg to free 5 vol% of oxygen from the hemoglobin (see Figure 6–7). If, however, the curve shifts to the left because of a pH of 7.6, the plasma P_{O_2} at the tissue sites would have to fall from 60 mm Hg to about 30 mm Hg in order to unload 5 vol% oxygen from the hemoglobin (Figure 6–10).

Figure 6–10

When the Pa_{O_2} is 60 mm Hg at a time when the oxygen dissociation curve has shifted to the left because of a pH of 7.6, the plasma P_{O_2} at the tissue sites would have to fall from 60 mm Hg to about 30 mm Hg to unload 5 vol% oxygen from the hemoglobin.

OXYGEN TRANSPORT CALCULATIONS

CLINICAL APPLICATION CASES

1 & 2

See pages 263–267

Various mathematical manipulations of the Ca_{O_2}, $C\bar{v}_{O_2}$, and Cc_{O_2} values can serve as excellent indicators of an individual's cardiac and ventilatory status. Clinically, the most common oxygen transport studies performed are (1) total oxygen delivery, (2) arterial-venous oxygen content difference, (3) oxygen consumption, (4) oxygen extraction ratio, (5) mixed venous oxygen saturation, and (6) pulmonary shunting.*

Total Oxygen Delivery

The total amount of oxygen delivered or transported to the peripheral tissues is dependent on (1) the body's ability to oxygenate blood, (2) the hemoglobin concentration, and (3) the cardiac output ($\dot{Q}$). **Total oxygen delivery** (D_{O_2}) is calculated as follows:

$$D_{O_2} = \dot{Q}_T \times (Ca_{O_2} \times 10)$$

where $\dot{Q}_T$ is total cardiac output (L/min); Ca_{O_2} is the oxygen content of arterial blood (mL oxygen/100 mL blood); and the factor 10 is needed to convert the Ca_{O_2} to mL O_2/L blood.

For example, if an individual has a cardiac output of 5 L/min and a Ca_{O_2} of 20 vol%, the total amount of oxygen delivered to the peripheral tissues will be about 1000 mL of oxygen per minute:

$$D_{O_2} = \dot{Q}_T \times (Ca_{O_2} \times 10)$$
$$= 5\,L \times (20\,vol\% \times 10)$$
$$= 1000\,mL\,O_2/min$$

Oxygen delivery decreases when there is a decline in (1) blood oxygenation, (2) hemoglobin concentration, or (3) cardiac output. When possible, an individual's hemoglobin concentration or cardiac output will often increase in an effort to compensate for a reduced oxygen delivery.

Arterial-Venous Oxygen Content Difference

The **arterial-venous oxygen content difference**, $C(a - \bar{v})_{O_2}$, is the difference between the Ca_{O_2} and the $C\bar{v}_{O_2}$ ($Ca_{O_2} - C\bar{v}_{O_2}$). Clinically, the mixed venous blood needed to compute the $C\bar{v}_{O_2}$ is obtained from the patient's pulmonary artery (see Figure 6–1).

See Appendix V for a representative example of a cardiopulmonary profile sheet used to monitor the oxygen transport status of the critically ill patient.

Figure 6–11

Oxygen dissociation curve. The normal oxygen content difference between arterial and venous blood is about 5 vol%. Note that both the right side and the left side of the graph illustrate that approximately 25 percent of the available oxygen is used for tissue metabolism and, therefore, the hemoglobin returning to the lungs is normally about 75 percent saturated with oxygen.

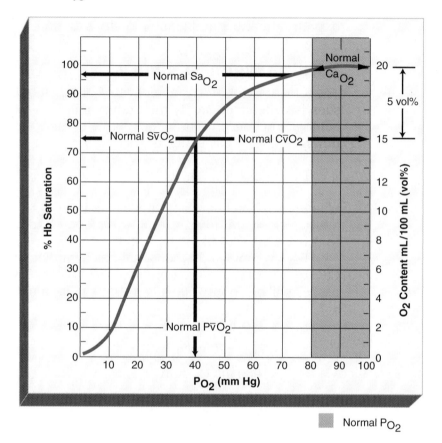

Normally, the Ca_{O_2} is about 20 vol% and the $C\bar{v}_{O_2}$ is 15 vol% (Figure 6–11). Thus, the normal $C(a - \bar{v})_{O_2}$ is about 5 vol%:

$$C(a - \bar{v})_{O_2} = Ca_{O_2} - C\bar{v}_{O_2}$$
$$= 20 \text{ vol\%} - 15 \text{ vol\%}$$
$$= 5 \text{ vol\%}$$

In other words, 5 mL of oxygen are extracted from each 100 mL of blood for tissue metabolism (50 mL O_2/L). Because the average individual has a cardiac output of about 5 L/min and a $C(a - \bar{v})_{O_2}$ of about 5 vol%,

TABLE 6–2

Factors That Increase the $C(a - \bar{v})_{O_2}$

Decreased cardiac output
Periods of increased oxygen consumption
  Exercise
  Seizures
  Shivering
  Hyperthermia

TABLE 6–3

Factors That Decrease the $C(a - \bar{v})_{O_2}$

Increased cardiac output
Skeletal muscle relaxation (e.g., induced by drugs)
Peripheral shunting (e.g., sepsis, trauma)
Certain poisons (e.g., cyanide prevents cellular metabolism)
Hypothermia

approximately 250 mL of oxygen are extracted from the blood during the course of 1 minute (50 mL O_2/L × 5 L/min).

Clinically, the $C(a - \bar{v})_{O_2}$ can provide useful information regarding the patient's cardiopulmonary status, because oxygen changes in mixed venous blood can occur earlier than oxygen changes in an arterial blood gas. Table 6–2 lists factors that can cause the $C(a - \bar{v})_{O_2}$ to increase. Factors that can cause the $C(a - \bar{v})_{O_2}$ to decrease are listed in Table 6–3.

Oxygen Consumption

The amount of oxygen extracted by the peripheral tissues during the period of 1 minute is called **oxygen consumption**, or *oxygen uptake* ($\dot{V}_{O_2}$). An individual's oxygen consumption is calculated by using this formula:

$$\dot{V}_{O_2} = \dot{Q}_T \, [C(a - \bar{v})_{O_2} \times 10]$$

where $\dot{Q}_T$ is the total cardiac output (L/min); $C(a - \bar{v})_{O_2}$ is the arterial-venous oxygen content difference ($Ca_{O_2} - C\bar{v}_{O_2}$); and the factor 10 is needed to convert the $C(a - \bar{v})_{O_2}$ to mL O_2/L.

TABLE 6–4
Factors That Increase $\dot{V}_{O_2}$
Exercise
Seizures
Shivering
Hyperthermia

TABLE 6–5
Factors That Decrease $\dot{V}_{O_2}$
Skeletal muscle relaxation (e.g., induced by drugs)
Peripheral shunting (e.g., sepsis, trauma)
Certain poisons (e.g., cyanide prevents cellular metabolism)
Hypothermia

For example, if an individual has a cardiac output of 5 L/min and a $C(a - \bar{v})_{O_2}$ of 5 vol%, the total amount of oxygen metabolized by the tissues in 1 minute will be 250 mL:

$$\dot{V}_{O_2} = \dot{Q}_T\ [C(a - \bar{v})_{O_2} \times 10]$$
$$= 5\ \text{L/min} \times 5\ \text{vol\%} \times 10$$
$$= 250\ \text{mL}\ O_2/\text{min}$$

Clinically, the oxygen consumption is usually related to the patient's body surface area (BSA) (see Appendix IV), because the amount of oxygen extracted by the peripheral cells varies with an individual's height and weight. The patient's oxygen consumption index is derived by dividing the $\dot{V}_{O_2}$ by the BSA. The average oxygen consumption index ranges between 125 to 165 mL O_2/m^2.

Factors that cause an increase in oxygen consumption are listed in Table 6–4. Table 6–5 lists factors that cause a decrease in oxygen consumption.

CLINICAL
APPLICATION
CASE

1

See page 263

Oxygen Extraction Ratio

The **oxygen extraction ratio** (O_2ER) is the amount of oxygen extracted by the peripheral tissues divided by the amount of oxygen delivered to the peripheral cells. The O_2ER is also known as the *oxygen coefficient ratio* or the *oxygen utilization ratio*.

The O_2ER is easily calculated by dividing the $C(a - \bar{v})_{O_2}$ by the Ca_{O_2}. In considering the normal Ca_{O_2} of 20 vol%, and the normal $C\bar{v}_{O_2}$ of 15 vol%

(see Figure 6–11), the O_2ER ratio of the healthy individual is about 25 percent:

$$O_2ER = \frac{Ca_{O_2} - C\bar{v}_{O_2}}{Ca_{O_2}}$$

$$= \frac{20 \text{ vol\%} - 15 \text{ vol\%}}{20 \text{ vol\%}}$$

$$= \frac{5 \text{ vol\%}}{20 \text{ vol\%}}$$

$$= 0.25$$

Under normal circumstances, therefore, an individual's hemoglobin returns to the alveoli approximately 75 percent saturated with oxygen (see Figure 6–11). In an individual with a total oxygen delivery of 1000 mL/min, an extraction ratio of 25 percent would mean that during the course of 1 minute, 250 mL of oxygen are metabolized by the tissues and 750 mL of oxygen are returned to the lungs.

Factors that cause the O_2ER to increase are listed in Table 6–6. Table 6–7 lists factors that cause the O_2ER to decrease.

TABLE 6–6
Factors That Increase the O_2ER

Decreased cardiac output
Periods of increased oxygen consumption
   Exercise
   Seizures
   Shivering
   Hyperthermia
Anemia
Decreased arterial oxygenation

TABLE 6–7
Factors That Decrease the O_2ER

Increased cardiac output
Skeletal muscle relaxation (e.g., induced by drugs)
Peripheral shunting (e.g., sepsis, trauma)
Certain poisons (e.g., cyanide prevents cellular metabolism)
Hypothermia (slows cellular metabolism)
Increased hemoglobin concentration
Increased arterial oxygenation

The O_2ER provides an important view of an individual's oxygen transport status that is not readily available from other oxygen transport measurements. For example, in an individual with normal Ca_{O_2} and normal $C\bar{v}_{O_2}$:

$$
\begin{array}{ll}
Ca_{O_2}: & 20 \text{ vol\%} \\
- C\bar{v}_{O_2}: & 15 \text{ vol\%} \\
\hline
C(a - \bar{v})_{O_2} = & 5 \text{ vol\%}
\end{array}
$$

the $C(a - \bar{v})_{O_2}$ is 5 vol% and the O_2ER is 25 percent (normal). However, in an individual with reduced Ca_{O_2} and reduced $C\bar{v}_{O_2}$:

$$
\begin{array}{ll}
Ca_{O_2}: & 10 \text{ vol\%} \\
- C\bar{v}_{O_2}: & 5 \text{ vol\%} \\
\hline
C(a - \bar{v})_{O_2} = & 5 \text{ vol\%}
\end{array}
$$

the $C(a - \bar{v})_{O_2}$ is still 5 vol% (assuming O_2 consumption remains constant), but the extraction ratio (O_2ER) is now 50 percent—clinically, a potentially dangerous situation.

Mixed Venous Oxygen Saturation

In the presence of a normal arterial oxygen saturation level (Sa_{O_2}) and hemoglobin concentration, the continuous monitoring of mixed venous oxygen saturation ($S\bar{v}_{O_2}$) is often used in the clinical setting to detect changes in the patient's $C(a - \bar{v})_{O_2}$, $\dot{V}_{O_2}$, and O_2ER. Normally, the $S\bar{v}_{O_2}$ is about 75 percent (see Figure 6–11). Clinically, an $S\bar{v}_{O_2}$ of about 65 percent is acceptable.

Factors that can cause the $S\bar{v}_{O_2}$ to decrease are listed in Table 6–8. Table 6–9 lists factors that can cause the $S\bar{v}_{O_2}$ to increase.

TABLE 6–8

Factors That Decrease the $S\bar{v}_{O_2}$*

Decreased cardiac output
Periods of increased oxygen consumption
   Exercise
   Seizures
   Shivering
   Hyperthermia

* A decreased $S\bar{v}_{O_2}$ indicates that the $C(a - \bar{v})_{O_2}$, $\dot{V}_{O_2}$, and O_2ER are increasing.

TABLE 6–9
Factors That Increase the $S\bar{v}_{O_2}$*

Increased cardiac output
Skeletal muscle relaxation (e.g., induced by drugs)
Peripheral shunting (e.g., sepsis, trauma)
Certain poisons (e.g., cyanide prevents cellular metabolism)
Hypothermia

* An increased $S\bar{v}_{O_2}$ indicates that the $C(a - \bar{v})_{O_2}$, $\dot{V}_{O_2}$, and O_2ER are decreasing.

Continuous $S\bar{v}_{O_2}$ monitoring can signal changes in the patient's $C(a - \bar{v})_{O_2}$, $\dot{V}_{O_2}$, and O_2ER earlier than routine arterial blood gas monitoring, because the Pa_{O_2} and Sa_{O_2} levels are often normal during early $C(a - \bar{v})_{O_2}$, $\dot{V}_{O_2}$, and O_2ER changes. Table 6–10 summarizes how various clinical factors may alter an individual's D_{O_2}, $\dot{V}_{O_2}$, $C(a - \bar{v})_{O_2}$, O_2ER, and $S\bar{v}_{O_2}$.

Pulmonary Shunting

Pulmonary shunting is defined as that portion of the cardiac output that moves from the right side to the left side of the heart without being exposed to alveolar oxygen (PA_{O_2}). Clinically, pulmonary shunting can be subdivided into (1) *absolute shunts* (also called *true shunt*) and (2) *relative shunts* (also called *shunt-like effects*).

Absolute Shunt

Absolute shunts (also called *true shunts*) can be grouped under two major categories: *anatomic shunts* and *capillary shunts.*

Anatomic Shunts. An **anatomic shunt** exists when blood flows from the right side of the heart to the left side without coming in contact with an alveolus for gas exchange (see Figures 6–12A and B). In the healthy lung, there is a normal anatomic shunt of about 3% of the cardiac output. This normal shunting is caused by non-oxygenated blood completely bypassing the alveoli and entering (1) the pulmonary vascular system by means of the bronchial venous drainage, and (2) the left atrium by way of the thebesian veins. The following are common abnormalities that cause anatomic shunting:

- Congenital heart disease
- Intrapulmonary fistula
- Vacular lung tumors.

TABLE 6–10
Clinical Factors Affecting Various Oxygen Transport Calculation Values

Clinical Factors	Oxygen Transport Calculations				
	D_{O_2} (1000 mL O_2/min)	$\dot{V}_{O_2}$ (250 mL O_2/min)	$C(a-\bar{v})_{O_2}$ (5 vol%)	O_2ER (25%)	$S\bar{v}_{O_2}$ (75%)

↑ O₂ Loading in the lungs
  ↑ Hb
  ↑ Pa_{O_2}
  ↓ Pa_{CO_2}
  ↑ pH
  ↑ Temperature
	↑	Same	Same	↓	↑

↓ O₂ Loading in the lungs
  ↓ Hb
  ↑ Pa_{CO_2}
  ↓ pH
  ↓ Pa_{O_2}
  Anemia
  ↑ Temperature
	↓	Same	Same	↑	↓

↑ Metabolism
  Exercise
  Seizures
  Hyperthermia
  Shivering
	Same	↑	↑	↑	↓

↓ Metabolism
  Hypothermia
  Skeletal muscle relaxation
    (e.g., drug induced)
	Same	↓	↓	↓	↑

↓ Cardiac output	↓	Same	↑	↑	↓
↑ Cardiac output	↑	Same	↓	↓	↑
Peripheral shunting (e.g., sepsis, trauma)	Same	↓	↓	↓	↑
Certain poisons (e.g., cyanide)	Same	↓	↓	↓	↑

↑ = increased; ↓ = decreased.

Congenital Heart Disease. Certain congenital defects permit blood to flow directly from the right side of the heart to the left side without going through the alveolar capillary system for gas exchange. Congenital heart defects include ventricular septum defect or newborns with persistent fetal circulation.

Figure 6–12

Pulmonary shunting: **(A)** normal alveolar-capillary unit; **(B)** anatomic shunt; **(C)** types of capillary shunts; **(D)** types of shunt-like effects.

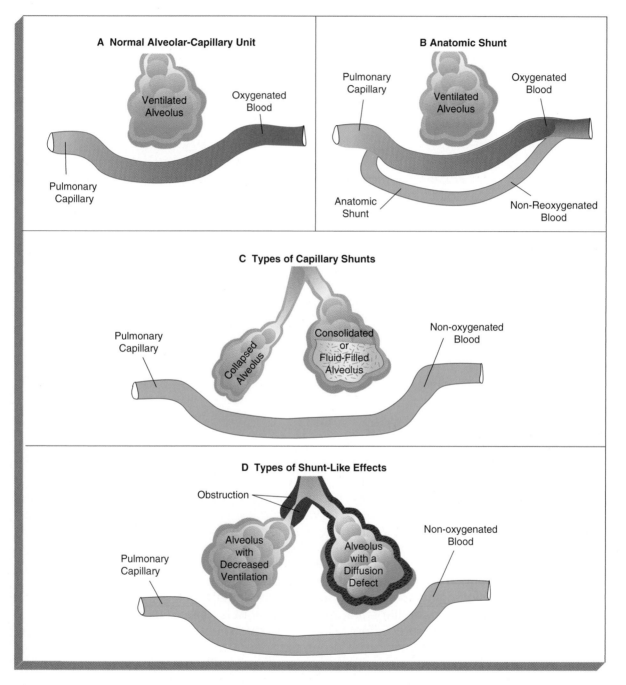

Intrapulmonary Fistula. In this type of anatomic shunting, a right-to-left flow of pulmonary blood does not pass through the alveolar-capillary system. It may be caused by chest trauma or disease. For example, a penetrating chest wound that damages both the arteries and veins of the lung can leave an arterial-venous shunt as a result of the healing process.

Vascular Lung Tumors. Some lung tumors can become very vascular. Some permit pulmonary arterial blood to move through the tumor mass and into the pulmonary veins without passing through the alveolar-capillary system.

Capillary Shunts. A **capillary shunt** is commonly caused by (1) alveolar collapse or atelectasis, (2) alveolar fluid accumulation, or (3) alveolar consolidation (Figure 6–12C).

The sum of the anatomic shunt and capillary shunt is referred to as the *absolute,* or *true, shunt.* Clinically, patients with absolute shunting respond poorly to oxygen therapy, since alveolar oxygen does not come in contact with the shunted blood. Absolute shunting is *refractory* to oxygen therapy; that is, the reduced arterial oxygen level produced by this form of pulmonary shunting cannot be treated simply by increasing the concentration of inspired oxygen, because (1) the alveoli are unable to accommodate any form of ventilation, and (2) the blood that bypasses functional alveoli cannot carry more oxygen once it has become fully saturated—except for a very small amount that dissolves in the plasma ($P_{O_2} \times 0.003 =$ dissolved O_2).

Relative Shunt

When pulmonary capillary perfusion is in excess of alveolar ventilation, a **relative shunt**, or **shunt-like effect**, is said to exist (Figure 6–12D). Common causes of this form of shunting include (1) hypoventilation, (2) ventilation/perfusion mismatches (e.g., chronic emphysema, bronchitis, asthma, and excessive airway secretions), and (3) alveolar-capillary diffusion defects (e.g., alveolar fibrosis or alveolar edema).

Even though the alveolus may be ventilated in the presence of an alveolar-capillary defect, the blood passing by the alveolus does not have enough time to equilibrate with the alveolar oxygen tension. If the diffusion defect is severe enough to completely block gas exchange across the alveolar-capillary membrane, the shunt is referred to as an *absolute* or *true shunt* (see preceding section). Relative shunting may also occur following the administration of drugs that cause an increase in cardiac output or dilation of the pulmonary vessels. Conditions that cause a shunt-like effect are readily corrected by oxygen therapy. In other words, they are not refractory to oxygen therapy.

Venous Admixture

The end result of pulmonary shunting is **venous admixture**. Venous admixture is the mixing of shunted, *non-reoxygenated blood* with *reoxygenated blood* distal to the alveoli (i.e., downstream in the pulmonary venous system) (Figure 6–13). When venous admixture occurs, the shunted, non-reoxygenated blood gains oxygen molecules while, at the same time, the reoxygenated blood loses oxygen molecules.

This process continues until (1) the P_{O_2} throughout all of the plasma of the newly mixed blood is in equilibrium, and (2) all of the hemoglobin molecules carry the same number of oxygen molecules. The end result is a blood mixture that has a higher P_{O_2} and oxygen content than the original shunted, non-reoxygenated blood, but a lower P_{O_2} and oxygen content than the original reoxygenated blood. The final outcome of venous admixture is a reduced Pa_{O_2} and Ca_{O_2} returning to the left side of the heart. Clinically, it is this oxygen mixture that is evaluated downstream (e.g., from the radial artery) to determine an individual's arterial blood gases (see Table 6–1).

Shunt Equation

Because pulmonary shunting and venous admixture are common complications in respiratory disorders, knowledge of the degree of shunting is often desirable when developing patient care plans. The amount of

Figure 6–13

Venous admixture occurs when reoxygenated blood mixes with non-reoxygenated blood distal to the alveoli.

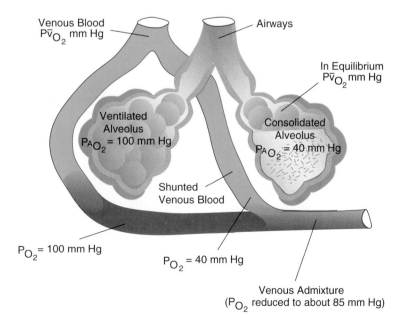

intrapulmonary shunting can be calculated by using the **classic shunt equation**, which is written as follows:

$$\frac{\dot{Q}s}{\dot{Q}\scriptsize{T}} = \frac{Cc_{O_2} - Ca_{O_2}}{Cc_{O_2} - C\bar{v}_{O_2}}$$

where $\dot{Q}s$ is cardiac output that is shunted, $\dot{Q}_T$ is total cardiac output, Cc_{O_2} is oxygen content of capillary blood, Ca_{O_2} is oxygen content of arterial blood, and $C\bar{v}_{O_2}$ is oxygen content of mixed venous blood.

To obtain the data necessary to calculate the degree of pulmonary shunting, the following clinical information must be gathered:

- P_B (barometric pressure)
- Pa_{O_2} (partial pressure of arterial oxygen)
- Pa_{CO_2} (partial pressure of arterial carbon dioxide)
- $P\bar{v}_{O_2}$ (partial pressure of mixed venous oxygen)
- Hb (hemoglobin concentration)
- PA_{O_2} (partial pressure of alveolar oxygen)*
- FI_{O_2} (fractional concentration of inspired oxygen).

Case Study: Motorcycle Crash Victim

A 38-year-old man is on a volume-cycled mechanical ventilator on a day when the barometric pressure is 750 mm Hg. The patient is receiving an FI_{O_2} of 0.70. The following clinical data are obtained:

Hb:	13 g%
Pa_{O_2}:	50 mm Hg (Sa_{O_2} = 85%)
Pa_{CO_2}:	43 mm Hg
$P\bar{v}_{O_2}$:	37 mm Hg ($S\bar{v}_{O_2}$ = 65%)

With this information, the patient's PA_{O_2}, Cc_{O_2}, Ca_{O_2}, and $C\bar{v}_{O_2}$ can now be calculated. (Remember: P_{H_2O} represents alveolar water vapor pressure and is always considered to be 47 mm Hg.)

1. $PA_{O_2} = (P_B - P_{H_2O})FI_{O_2} - Pa_{CO_2}(1.25)$

$\quad = (750 - 47)0.70 - 43(1.25)$

$\quad = (703)0.70 - 53.75$

$\quad = 492.1 - 53.75$

$\quad = 438.35 \text{ mm Hg}$

2. $Cc_{O_2} = (Hb \times 1.34)^\dagger + (PA_{O_2}{}^* \times 0.003)$

$\quad = (13 \times 1.34) + (438.35 \times 0.003)$

$\quad = 17.42 + 1.315$

$\quad = 18.735 (\text{vol}\% \; O_2)$

*See "Ideal Alveolar Gas Equation" section in Chapter 3.
†It is assumed that the hemoglobin saturation with oxygen in the pulmonary capillary blood is 100 percent or 1.0.

3. $Ca_{O_2} = (Hb \times 1.34 \times Sa_{O_2}) + (Pa_{O_2} \times 0.003)$
$= (13 \times 1.34 \times 0.85) + (50 \times 0.003)$
$= 14.807 + 0.15$
$= 14.957 (vol\% \ O_2)$

4. $C\bar{v}_{O_2} = (Hb \times 1.34 \times S\bar{v}_{O_2}) + (P\bar{v}_{O_2} \times 0.003)$
$= (13 \times 1.34 \times 0.65) + (37 \times 0.003)$
$= 11.323 + 0.111$
$= 11.434 (vol\% \ O_2)$

Based on these calculations, the patient's degree of pulmonary shunting can now be calculated:

$$\frac{\dot{Q}s}{\dot{Q}\tau} = \frac{Cc_{O_2} - Ca_{O_2}}{Cc_{O_2} - C\bar{v}_{O_2}}$$

$$= \frac{18.735 - 14.957}{18.735 - 11.434}$$

$$= \frac{3.778}{7.301}$$

$$= 0.517$$

Thus, in this case 51.7 percent of the patient's pulmonary blood flow is perfusing lung tissue that is not being ventilated.

Today, most critical care units have programmed the oxygen transport calculations into inexpensive personal computers. What was once a time-consuming, error-prone task is now quickly and accurately performed.

The Clinical Significance of Pulmonary Shunting

Pulmonary shunting below 10 percent reflects normal lung status. A shunt between 10 and 20 percent is indicative of an intrapulmonary abnormality, but is seldom of clinical significance. Pulmonary shunting between 20 and 30 percent denotes significant intrapulmonary disease and may be life threatening in patients with limited cardiovascular function.

When the pulmonary shunting is greater than 30 percent, a potentially life-threatening situation exists and aggressive cardiopulmonary supportive measures are almost always necessary.

Calculating the degree of pulmonary shunting is not reliable in patients who demonstrate (1) a questionable perfusion status, (2) a decreased myocardial output, or (3) an unstable oxygen consumption demand. This is because these conditions directly affect a patient's Ca_{O_2} and $C\bar{v}_{O_2}$ values—two major components of the shunt equation.

HYPOXIA

Hypoxemia versus Hypoxia

Hypoxemia refers to an abnormally low arterial oxygen tension (Pa_{O_2}) and is frequently associated with *hypoxia,* which is an inadequate level of tissue oxygenation (see following discussion). Although the presence of hypoxemia strongly suggests tissue hypoxia, it does not necessarily mean the absolute existence of tissue hypoxia. For example, the reduced level of oxygen in the arterial blood may be offset by an increased cardiac output. Hypoxemia is commonly classified as mild, moderate, or severe hypoxia (Table 6–11). Clinically, the presence of mild hypoxemia generally stimulates the oxygen peripheral chemoreceptors to increase the patient's breathing rate and heart rate (see Figure 9–4).

Hypoxia refers to low or inadequate oxygen for cellular metabolism. Hypoxia is characterized by tachycardia, hypertension, peripheral vasoconstriction, dizziness, and mental confusion. There are four main types of hypoxia: (1) hypoxic, (2) anemic, (3) circulatory, and (4) histotoxic (Table 6–12).

When hypoxia exists, alternate anaerobic mechanisms are activated in the tissues that produce dangerous metabolites—such as lactic acid—as a waste product. Lactic acid is a nonvolatile acid and causes the pH to decrease.

Hypoxic Hypoxia

Clinically, hypoxic hypoxia (also called hypoxemic hypoxia) refers to the condition in which there is inadequate oxygen at the tissue cells caused by low arterial oxygen tension (Pa_{O_2}). Common causes of a decreased Pa_{O_2} are (1) a low alveolar oxygen tension (PA_{O_2}), (2) diffusion

TABLE 6–11

Hypoxemia Classification*

Classification	Pa_{O_2} (mm Hg) (Rule of Thumb)
Normal	80–100
Mild hypoxemia	60–80
Moderate hypoxemia	40–60
Severe hypoxemia	<40

*The hypoxemia classifications presented in this table are generally accepted classifications. Minor variations on these values are found in the literature. In addition, a number of clinical factors often require some changes in these values (e.g., a Pa_{O_2} less than 60 mm Hg may be called severe in the patient with a very low blood volume or anemia). Nevertheless, the hypoxemia classifications and Pa_{O_2} range(s) provided in this table are useful guidelines.

TABLE 6–12
Types of Hypoxia

Hypoxia	Descriptions	Common Causes
Hypoxic hypoxia	Inadequate oxygen at the tissue cells caused by low arterial oxygen tension (Pa_{O_2})	Low PA_{O_2} caused by: • Hypoventilation • High altitude Diffusion defects Interstitial fibrosis Interstitial lung disease Pulmonary edema Pneumoconiosis Ventilation-perfusion mismatch Pulmonary shunting
Anemic hypoxia	Pa_{O_2} is normal, but the oxygen-carrying capacity of the hemoglobin is inadequate	• Decreased hemoglobin Anemia Hemorrhage • Abnormal hemoglobin Carboxyhemoglobinemia Methemoglobinemia
Circulatory hypoxia (stagnant or hypoperfusion hypoxia)	Blood flow to the tissue cells is inadequate; thus, oxygen is not adequate to meet tissue needs	• Slow or stagnant (pooling) peripheral blood flow • Arterial-venous shunts
Histotoxic hypoxia	Impaired ability of the tissue cells to metabolize oxygen	• Cyanide poisoning

defects, (3) ventilation-perfusion mismatches, and (4) pulmonary shunting. The following describe the common causes of hypoxic hypoxia in more detail:

Low Alveolar Oxygen Tension (Decreased PA_{O_2})

Because the arterial oxygen pressure (Pa_{O_2}) is determined by the alveolar oxygen pressure (PA_{O_2}), any condition that leads to a decreased PA_{O_2} will result in a reduction of the patient's Pa_{O_2}—and, subsequently, to an inadequate Ca_{O_2}. A low PA_{O_2} can develop from a variety of conditions, including (1) hypoventilation, (2) high altitudes, (3) diffusion defects, and (4) pulmonary shunting—either absolute or relative shunts.

Hypoventilation is caused by numerous conditions, such as chronic obstructive pulmonary disease, central nervous system depressants, head trauma, and neuromuscular disorders (e.g., myasthenia gravis or Guillain-Barré syndrome).

High altitudes can cause hypoxic hypoxia to develop. This is because the barometric pressure progressively decreases as altitude increases. As the barometric pressure decreases, the atmospheric oxygen tension (P_{O_2}) also decreases. In other words, the higher the altitude, the lower the oxygen pressure. Thus, the higher an individual hikes up a mountain, the lower the oxygen pressure (P_{O_2}) the person is inhaling—which, in turn, leads to a decreased Pa_{O_2} and Pa_{O_2}.

Diffusion Defects

Diffusion defects are abnormal anatomic alterations of the lungs that result in an impedance of oxygen transfer across the alveolar-capillary membrane. When a diffusion defect is present, the time available for oxygen equilibrium between the alveolus and pulmonary capillary is not adequate. Common causes of diffusion defects are chronic interstitial lung diseases, pulmonary edema, and pneumoconiosis.

Ventilation-Perfusion ($\dot{V}/\dot{Q}$ Ratio) Mismatch

When the pulmonary capillary blood is in excess of the alveolar ventilation, a decreased $\dot{V}/\dot{Q}$ ratio is said to exist. This condition causes pulmonary shunting, which in turn causes the Pa_{O_2} and Ca_{O_2} to decrease. Common causes of a decreased $\dot{V}/\dot{Q}$ ratio include chronic obstructive pulmonary disease, pneumonia, and pulmonary edema. The effects of different $\dot{V}/\dot{Q}$ relationships are discussed in greater detail in Chapter 8.

Pulmonary Shunting

The end result of pulmonary shunting and venous admixture is a decreased Pa_{O_2} and Ca_{O_2} (see earlier "Pulmonary Shunting" and "Venous Admixture" sections).

Anemic Hypoxia

In this type of hypoxia, the oxygen tension in the arterial blood is normal but the oxygen-carrying capacity of the blood is inadequate. This form of hypoxia can develop from (1) a low amount of hemoglobin in the blood or (2) a deficiency in the ability of hemoglobin to carry oxygen, as occurs in carbon monoxide poisoning or methemoglobinemia.

Anemic hypoxia develops in carbon monoxide poisoning because the affinity of carbon monoxide for hemoglobin is about 210 times greater than that of oxygen. As carbon monoxide combines with hemoglobin, the ability of hemoglobin to carry oxygen diminishes and tissue hypoxia may ensue. In methemoglobinemia, iron atoms in the hemoglobin are oxidized to the ferric state, which in turn eliminates the hemoglobin's ability to carry oxygen. Increased cardiac output is the main compensatory mechanism for anemic hypoxia.

Circulatory Hypoxia

In *circulatory hypoxia,* also called *stagnant* or *hypoperfusion hypoxia,* the arterial blood that reaches the tissue cells may have a normal oxygen tension and content, but the amount of blood—and, therefore, the amount of oxygen—is not adequate to meet tissue needs. The two main causes of circulating hypoxia are (1) slow or stagnant peripheral blood flow and (2) arterial-venous shunting.

Stagnant (hypoperfusion) hypoxia can occur when the peripheral capillary blood flow is slow or stagnant (*pooling*). This condition can be caused by (1) a decreased cardiac output, (2) vascular insufficiency, or (3) neurochemical abnormalities. When blood flow through the tissue capillaries is sluggish, the time needed for oxygen exchange increases while, at the same time, the oxygen supply decreases. Because tissue metabolism continues at a steady rate, the oxygen pressure gradient between the blood and the tissue cells can become insufficient, causing tissue hypoxia. Stagnant hypoxia is primarily associated with cardiovascular disorders and often occurs in the absence of arterial hypoxemia. It is commonly associated with a decreased $S\bar{v}_{O_2}$.

When arterial blood completely bypasses the tissue cells and moves into the venous system, an *arterial-venous shunt* is said to exist. This condition can also cause tissue hypoxia, because arterial blood is prevented from delivering oxygen to the tissue cells. Localized arterial or venous obstruction can cause a similar form of tissue hypoxia, because the flow of blood into or out of the tissue capillaries is impeded. Circulatory hypoxia can also develop when the tissues' need for oxygen exceeds the available oxygen supply.

Histotoxic Hypoxia

Histotoxic hypoxia develops in any condition that impairs the ability of tissue cells to utilize oxygen. Cyanide poisoning produces this form of hypoxia. Clinically, the Pa_{O_2} and Ca_{O_2} in the blood are normal, but the tissue cells are extremely hypoxic. The $P\bar{v}_{O_2}$, $C\bar{v}_{O_2}$, and $S\bar{v}_{O_2}$ are elevated because oxygen is not utilized.

CYANOSIS

CLINICAL APPLICATION CASES

1 & 2

See pages 263–267

When hypoxemia is severe, signs of cyanosis may develop. *Cyanosis* is the term used to describe the blue-gray or purplish discoloration seen on the mucous membranes, fingertips, and toes whenever the blood in these areas contains at least 5 g% of reduced hemoglobin per dL (100 mL). When the normal 14 to 15 g% of hemoglobin is fully saturated, the Pa_{O_2} will be about 97 to 100 mm Hg and there will be about 20 vol% of oxygen in the blood. In the patient with cyanosis with one-third (5 g%) of the hemoglobin reduced, the Pa_{O_2} will be about 30 mm Hg and there will be about 13 vol% of oxygen in the blood (Figure 6–14). In the patient with

Figure 6–14

Cyanosis may appear whenever the blood contains at least 5 g% (g/dL) of reduced hemoglobin. In the normal individual with 15 g% hemoglobin, a Pa_{O_2} of about 30 mm Hg will produce 5 g% of reduced hemoglobin. Overall, however, the hemoglobin is still about 60 percent saturated with oxygen.

polycythemia, however, cyanosis may be present at a Pa_{O_2} well above 30 mm Hg, because the amount of reduced hemoglobin is often greater than 5 g% in these patients—even when their total oxygen transport is within normal limits (about 20 vol% of O_2).

The detection and interpretation of cyanosis is difficult and there is wide individual variation between observers. The recognition of cyanosis depends on the acuity of the observer, on the lighting conditions in the examining room, and the pigmentation of the patient. Cyanosis of the nail beds is also influenced by the temperature, because vasoconstriction induced by cold may slow circulation to the point where the blood becomes bluish in the surface capillaries, even though the arterial blood in the major vessels is not oxygen poor.

POLYCYTHEMIA

When pulmonary disorders produce chronic hypoxemia, the hormone **erythropoietin** responds by stimulating the bone marrow to increase RBC production. RBC production is known as **erythropoiesis**. An increased level of RBCs is called **polycythemia**. The polycythemia that results from hypoxemia is an adaptive mechanism designed to increase the oxygen-carrying capacity of the blood.

Unfortunately, the advantage of the increased oxygen-carrying capacity in polycythemia is offset by the increased viscosity of the blood when the hematocrit reaches about 55 to 60 percent. Because of the increased viscosity of the blood, a greater driving pressure is needed to maintain a given flow. The work of the right and left ventricles must increase in order to generate the pressure needed to overcome the increased viscosity. This can ultimately lead to left ventricular hypertrophy and failure and to right ventricular hypertrophy, and cor pulmonale.

CHAPTER SUMMARY

The understanding of oxygen transport is a fundamental cornerstone to the clinical interpretation of arterial and venous blood gases. Essential components are (1) how oxygen is transported from the lungs to the tissue, including the calculation of the quantity of oxygen that is dissolved in the plasma and bound to hemoglobin; (2) the oxygen dissociation nomogram and how it relates to oxygen pressure, percentage of hemoglobin bound to oxygen, oxygen content, and right and left curve shifts; (3) how the following oxygen transport calculations are used to identify the patient's cardiac and ventilatory status: total oxygen delivery, arterial-venous oxygen content difference, oxygen consumption, oxygen extraction ratio, mixed venous oxygen saturation, and pulmonary shunting; and (4) the major forms of tissue hypoxia: hypoxic hypoxia, anemic hypoxia, circulatory hypoxia, and histotoxic hypoxia.

1 CLINICAL APPLICATION CASE

A 12-year-old girl was a victim of a "drive-by" shooting. She was standing in line outside a movie theater with some friends when a car passed by and someone inside began shooting at three boys standing nearby. Two of the boys died immediately, one was shot in the shoulder and lower jaw, and the girl was shot in the upper anterior chest. Although she was breathing spontaneously through a nonrebreathing oxygen mask when she was brought to the emergency department

25 minutes later, she was unconscious and had obviously lost a lot of blood. Her clothes were completely soaked with blood.

The patient's skin, lips, and nail beds were blue. Her skin felt cool and clammy. A small bullet hole could be seen over the left anterior chest between the second and third rib at the midclavicular line. No exit bullet hole could be seen. Her vital signs were blood pressure—55/35 mm Hg, heart rate—120 beats/min, and respiratory

(continues)

rate—22 breaths/min. Auscultation of the chest revealed normal breath sounds. A portable chest x-ray showed that the bullet had passed through the upper portion of the aorta and lodged near the spine. Her lungs were not damaged by the bullet.

Her hematocrit was 15 percent and hemoglobin was 4 g%. A unit of blood was started immediately, and a pulmonary catheter and arterial line were inserted (see Figure 15–1). Cardiac output was 6 L/min. Arterial blood gas values (on a nonrebreathing oxygen mask) were pH—7.47, Pa_{CO_2}—31 mm Hg, H_{CO_3}—23 mEq/L, and Pa_{O_2}—503 mm Hg. Her Sa_{O_2} was 98 percent. At this time, her oxygen indices were assessed (see Oxygen Transport Studies, Study No. 1).

The patient was rushed to surgery to repair her damaged aorta. Three hours later she was transferred to the surgical intensive care unit and placed on a mechanical ventilator. The surgery was considered a success, and the patient's parents were relieved to learn that a full recovery was expected. The patient was conscious and appeared comfortable and her skin felt warm and dry. Her vital signs were blood pressure—125/83 mm Hg, heart rate—76 beats/min, respiratory rate—12 breaths/min (i.e., the ventilator rate was set at 12), and

temperature 37°C. Auscultation revealed normal bronchovesicular breath sounds.

A portable chest x-ray showed no cardiopulmonary problems. Laboratory blood work showed a hematocrit of 41 percent and hemoglobin was 12 g%. Arterial blood gas values (while on the mechanical ventilation and on an inspired oxygen concentration [Fi_{O_2}] of 0.4) were pH—7.43, Pa_{CO_2}—38 mm Hg, HCO_3—24 mEq/L, and Pa_{O_2}—109 mm Hg. Sa_{O_2} was 97 percent. A second oxygen transport study showed significant improvement (see Oxygen Transport Study No. 2, above). Over the next 4 days, the patient was weaned from the ventilator and transferred from the surgical intensive care unit to the medical ward. A week later the patient was discharged from the hospital.

DISCUSSION

This case illustrates the importance of *hemoglobin* in the oxygen transport system. As a result of the gunshot wound to the chest, the patient lost a great deal of blood. Because of the excessive blood loss, the patient was unconscious, cyanotic, and hypotensive, and her skin was cool and damp to the touch. Despite the fact that the patient had an elevated Pa_{O_2} of 503 mm Hg (normal, 80–100 mm Hg) and an Sa_{O_2} of 98 percent in the emergency department, her tissue oxygenation was seriously impaired. In fact, the patient's Pa_{O_2} and Sa_{O_2} in this case were very misleading. Clinically, this was verified by the oxygen transport studies. For example, her D_{O_2} was only 316 mL (normal, about 1000 mL).*

Furthermore, note that the patient's $\dot{V}_{O_2}$ was 214 mL/min and O_2ER was 68 percent (the normal extraction ratio is 25 percent). In other words, the patient was consuming

Oxygen Transport Studies					
D_{O_2}	$\dot{V}_{O_2}$	$C(a-\bar{v})_{O_2}$	O_2ER	$S\bar{v}_{O_2}$	$\dot{Q}s \div \dot{Q}T$
Study No. 1					
316 mL	214 mL	3.58 vol%	68%	32%	3%
Study No. 2					
935 mL	245 mL	5 vol%	25%	75%	3%

D_{O_2} = total oxygen delivery; $\dot{V}_{O_2}$ = oxygen consumption, or uptake; $C(a-\bar{v})_{O_2}$ = the arterial-venous oxygen content difference; O_2ER = oxygen extraction ratio; $S\bar{v}_{O_2}$ = mixed venous oxygen saturation; $\dot{Q}s \div \dot{Q}T$ = the amount of intrapulmonary shunting.

(continues)

68 percent of the D_{O_2} (214 mL of oxygen out of a possible 316 mL of oxygen per minute). Her oxygen reserve was only about 30 percent. If this condition had not been treated immediately, she would not have survived much longer. It should be stressed that the patient's Pa_{O_2} of 503 mm Hg and Sa_{O_2} of

98 percent were very misleading—and dangerous.

$$* D_{O_2} = \dot{Q}T \times (Ca_{O_2}{}^{\dagger} \times 10)$$
$$= 6 \times (5.265 \times 10)$$
$$= 316 \; mL$$
$$^{\dagger} Ca_{O_2} = (1.34 \times 4 \, g\% \, Hb \times 0.98\%) + (503 \; mm \; Hg \times 0.003) = 5.265$$

2 CLINICAL APPLICATION CASE

An 18-year-old woman presented in the emergency department in severe respiratory distress. She was well known to the respiratory care team. She had suffered from asthma all of her life (Figure 6–15). Over the years, she had been admitted to the hospital on numerous occasions, averaging about three admissions per year. Five separate asthmatic episodes had required mechanical ventilation. Although she was usually weaned from the ventilator within 48 hours, on one occasion she was on the ventilator for 7 days. At the time of this admission, it had been over 4 years since she was last placed on mechanical ventilation.

Upon observation, the patient appeared fatigued and cyanotic, and she was using her accessory muscles of inspiration (see Figure 1–44). She was in obvious respiratory distress. Her vital signs were blood pressure—177/110 mm Hg, heart rate—160 beats/min, and respiratory rate—32 breaths/min and shallow. Her breath sounds were diminished and wheezing could be heard bilaterally. A portable chest x-ray showed that her lungs were hyperinflated and her diaphragm was depressed. Arterial blood gas values on 4 L/min oxygen via cannula were pH—7.25, Pa_{CO_2}—71, HCO_3^-—27, Pa_{O_2}—27, and Sa_{O_2}—42 percent.

Because she was in acute ventilatory failure with severe hypoxemia and was

clearly fatigued, the patient was immediately transferred to the intensive care unit, intubated, and placed on mechanical ventilation at a rate of 3 breaths/min. A pulmonary catheter and arterial line were inserted. An intravenous infusion was started and medications to treat her bronchoconstriction were administered. A hemodynamic study showed that her cardiac output ($\dot{Q}T$) was 6.5 L/min. Her hemoglobin was 13 g%. An oxygen transport study was performed at this time (see Oxygen Transport Studies, Study No. 1):

Oxygen Transport Studies					
D_{O_2}	$\dot{V}_{O_2}$	$C(a - \bar{v})_{O_2}$	O_2ER	$S\bar{v}_{O_2}$	$\dot{Q}s \div \dot{Q}T$
Study No. 1					
523 mL	314 mL	4.83 vol%	58%	24%	47%
Study No. 2					
990 mL	255 mL	5 vol%	24%	75%	3%

D_{O_2} = total oxygen delivery; $\dot{V}_{O_2}$ = oxygen consumption, or uptake; $C(a - \bar{v})_{O_2}$ = the arterial-venous oxygen content difference; O_2ER = oxygen extraction ratio; $S\bar{v}_{O_2}$ = mixed venous oxygen saturation; $\dot{Q}s \div \dot{Q}T$ = the amount of intrapulmonary shunting.

Although the patient's first day in the intensive care unit was a stormy one, her asthma progressively improved over the second day. On the morning of the third day, her skin was pink and dry and she was

(continues)

Figure 6–15

Asthma. Pathology includes (1) bronchial smooth muscle constriction, (2) inflammation and excessive production of thick, whitish bronchial secretions, and (3) alveolar hyperinflation.

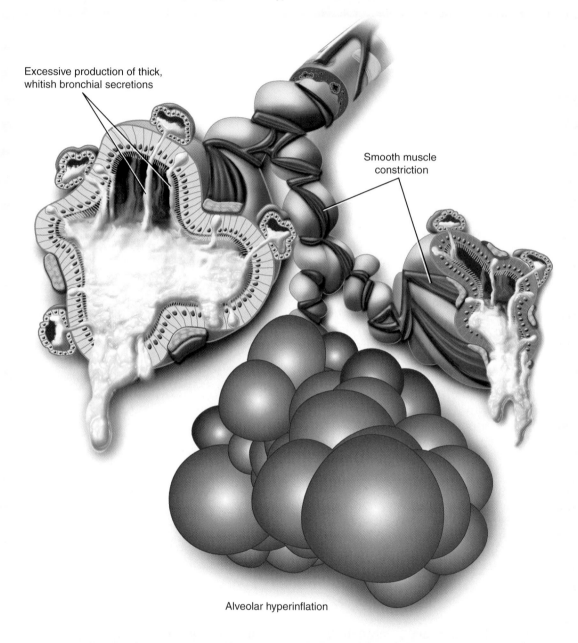

Excessive production of thick, whitish bronchial secretions

Smooth muscle constriction

Alveolar hyperinflation

resting comfortably on the mechanical ventilator. Although she was receiving 3 mechanical breaths/min, the patient was breathing primarily on her own. Her vital signs were blood pressure—125/76 mm Hg, heart rate—70 beats/min, and respiratory rate—10 breaths/min (10 spontaneous breaths between the 3 mechanical ventilations per minute). Auscultation revealed normal bronchovesicular breath sounds, and portable chest x-ray no longer showed hyperinflated lungs or a flattened diaphragm. Arterial blood gas values on an inspired oxygen concentration ($F_{I_{O_2}}$) of 0.25 were pH—7.42, Pa_{CO_2}—37, HCO_3^-—24, Pa_{O_2}—115, and Sa_{O_2}—97 percent. An oxygen transport study was performed at this time (see Oxygen Transport Study No. 2). The patient was weaned from the ventilator and was discharged from the hospital the next day.

DISCUSSION

This case illustrates the clinical significance of a *right shift* in the *oxygen dissociation curve* on (1) the loading of oxygen on hemoglobin in the lungs, and (2) the patient's total oxygen delivery (D_{O_2}). As a result of the asthmatic episode (i.e., bronchial smooth-muscle constriction, inflammation, and excessive secretions, the patient's alveolar ventilation was very poor in the emergency department. Clinically, this was verified on chest x-ray showing alveolar hyperinflation and a flattened diaphragm and by arterial blood gas analysis and the oxygen indices.

Note that alveolar "hyperinflation" does not mean the lungs are being

excessively ventilated. In fact, they are being underventilated. The lungs become hyperinflated during a severe asthmatic episode because gas is unable to leave the lungs during exhalation. As a result, "fresh" ventilation is impeded on subsequent inspirations. This condition causes the alveolar oxygen ($P_{A_{O_2}}$) to decrease and the alveolar carbon dioxide ($P_{A_{CO_2}}$) to increase (see Figure 2–40). As the $P_{A_{O_2}}$ declined, the patient's intrapulmonary shunting ($\dot{Q}s \div \dot{Q}t$) and oxygen extraction ratio (O_2ER) increased and total oxygen delivery (D_{O_2}) decreased (see Oxygen Transport Study No. 1).

In addition, as shown by the first arterial blood gas analysis, her condition was further compromised by the presence of a decreased pH (7.25) and an increased Pa_{CO_2} (72 mm Hg), which caused the oxygen dissociation curve to shift to the right. A right shift of the oxygen dissociation curve reduces the ability of oxygen to move across the alveolar-capillary membrane and bond to hemoglobin (see Figure 6–8). Because of this, the patient's hemoglobin saturation was lower than expected for a particular Pa_{O_2} level. In this case, the patient's Sa_{O_2} was only 42 percent at a time when the Pa_{O_2} was 27 mm Hg. Normally, when the Pa_{O_2} is 27 mm Hg, the hemoglobin saturation is 50 percent (see Figure 6–4). Thus, it should be emphasized that when additional factors are present that shift the oxygen dissociation curve to the right or left, the respiratory practitioner should consider these factors in the final analysis of the patient's total oxygenation status.

REVIEW QUESTIONS

1. If a patient has a Hb level of 14 g% and a Pa_{O_2} of 55 mm Hg (85 percent saturated with oxygen), approximately how much oxygen is transported to the peripheral tissues in each 100 mL of blood?
   A. 16 vol%
   B. 17 vol%
   C. 18 vol%
   D. 19 vol%

2. When the blood pH decreases, the oxygen dissociation curve shifts to the
   A. right and the P_{50} decreases
   B. left and the P_{50} increases
   C. right and the P_{50} increases
   D. left and the P_{50} decreases

3. When shunted, non-reoxygenated blood mixes with reoxygenated blood distal to the alveoli (*venous admixture*), the
   I. P_{O_2} of the non-reoxygenated blood increases
   II. Ca_{O_2} of the reoxygenated blood decreases
   III. P_{O_2} of the reoxygenated blood increases
   IV. Ca_{O_2} of the non-reoxygenated blood decreases
   A. I only
   B. IV only
   C. I and II only
   D. III and IV only

4. The normal arterial HCO_3^- range is
   A. 18–22 mEq/L
   B. 22–28 mEq/L
   C. 28–35 mEq/L
   D. 35–45 mEq/L

5. The normal calculated anatomic shunt is about
   A. 0.5–1 percent
   B. 2–5 percent
   C. 6–9 percent
   D. 10–12 percent

6. In which of the following types of hypoxia is the oxygen pressure of the arterial blood (Pa_{O_2}) usually normal?
   I. Hypoxic hypoxia
   II. Anemic hypoxia
   III. Circulatory hypoxia
   IV. Histotoxic hypoxia
   A. I only
   B. II only
   C. III and IV only
   D. II, III, and IV only

7. If a patient normally has a 12 g% Hb, cyanosis will likely appear when
   A. 10 g% Hb is saturated with oxygen
   B. 9 g% Hb is saturated with oxygen
   C. 8 g% Hb is saturated with oxygen
   D. 7 g% Hb is saturated with oxygen

8. The advantages of polycythemia begin to be offset by the increased blood viscosity when the hematocrit reaches about
   A. 30–40 percent
   B. 40–50 percent
   C. 55–60 percent
   D. 60–70 percent

9. Assuming everything else remains the same, when an individual's cardiac output decreases, the
   I. $C(a - \bar{v})_{O_2}$ increases
   II. O_2ER decreases
   III. $\dot{V}_{O_2}$ increases
   IV. $S\bar{v}_{O_2}$ decreases
     A. I only
     B. IV only
     C. II and III only
     D. I and IV only

10. Under normal conditions, the O_2ER is about
    A. 10 percent
    B. 15 percent
    C. 20 percent
    D. 25 percent

11. Case Study: Automobile Collision Victim
    A 37-year-old woman is on a volume-cycled mechanical ventilator on a day when the barometric pressure is 745 mm Hg. The patient is receiving an $F_{I_{O_2}}$ of 0.50. The following clinical data are obtained:
    Hb: 11 g%
    Pa_{O_2}: 60 mm Hg (Sa_{O_2} = 90%)
    Pv_{O_2}: 35 mm Hg ($S\bar{v}_{O_2}$ = 65%)
    Pa_{CO_2}: 38 mm Hg
    Cardiac output: 6 L/min

    Based on the above information, calculate the patient's
    A. total oxygen delivery
       Answer: _____

    B. arterial-venous oxygen content difference
       Answer: _____

    C. intrapulmonary shunting
       Answer: _____

    D. oxygen consumption
       Answer: _____

    E. oxygen extraction ratio
       Answer: _____

CLINICAL APPLICATION QUESTIONS

CASE 1

1. As a result of the gunshot wound to the chest, the patient lost a large amount of blood. Because of the excessive blood loss, the patient was:

Answer: _____

_____

2. As a result of the excessive blood loss, the patient's Pa_{O_2} of 503 mm Hg and Sa_{O_2} of 98 percent were very misleading. Which oxygen transport studies verified this fact?

Answer: _____

_____

3. In the first oxygen transport study, the patient's D_{O_2} was only 316 mL. Her $\dot{V}_{O_2}$ was 214 mL. What was her O_2ER?

Answer: _____

_____

CASE 2

1. As a result of the asthmatic episode, the patient's $P_{A_{O_2}}$ (decreased _____, increased _____), and the alveolar carbon dioxide ($P_{A_{CO_2}}$) (decreased _____, increased _____).

2. As the above condition worsened, the patient's intrapulmonary shunting ($\dot{Q}s/\dot{Q}\tau$) (decreased _____, increased _____), the oxygen extraction ratio (O_2ER) (decreased _____, increased _____), and the total oxygen delivery (D_{O_2}) (decreased _____, increased _____).

3. The patient's condition was compromised by the presence of a decreased pH (7.25) and an increased Pa_{CO_2} (72 mm Hg), which caused the oxygen dissociation curve to shift to the _____.

4. Because of the condition described in question 3, the patient's hemoglobin saturation was (higher _____, lower _____) than expected for a particular Pa_{O_2} level.

CHAPTER 7

Carbon Dioxide Transport and Acid-Base Balance

OBJECTIVES

By the end of this chapter, the student should be able to:

1. List the three ways in which carbon dioxide is transported in the *plasma*.
2. List the three ways in which carbon dioxide is transported in the *red blood cells*.
3. Describe how carbon dioxide is converted to HCO_3^- at the tissue sites and then transported in the plasma to the lungs.
4. Explain how carbon dioxide is eliminated in the lungs.
5. Describe how the *carbon dioxide dissociation curve* differs from the *oxygen dissociation curve*.
6. Explain how the *Haldane effect* relates to the carbon dioxide dissociation curve.
7. Describe how the following relate to the acid-base balance and regulation of the body:
   —Acids
   - Hydrogen ions
   - Proton donors
   - Strong and weak acids
   —Bases
   - Proton acceptors
   - Bicarbonate ions
   - Strong and weak bases
   —pH: acid-base concentration
   —The chemical buffer system's role in acid-base balance
   - Carbonic acid-bicarbonate buffer system
     ○ Henderson-Hasselbalch equation
     ○ Clinical application of the H-H equation

- Phosphate buffer system
- Protein buffer system
—The respiratory system's role in acid-base balance
—The renal system's role in acid-base balance

8. Identify the following acid-base disturbances on the $P_{CO_2}/HCO_3^-/pH$ nomogram:
   —Acute ventilatory failure (respiratory acidosis)
   —Acute ventilatory failure (with partial renal compensation)
   —Chronic ventilatory failure (with complete renal compensation)
9. Identify common causes of acute ventilatory failure.
10. Identify the following acid-base disturbances on the $P_{CO_2}/HCO_3^-/pH$ nomogram:
    —Acute alveolar hyperventilation (respiratory alkalosis)
    —Acute alveolar hyperventilation (with partial renal compensation)
    —Chronic alveolar hyperventilation (with complete renal compensation)
11. Identify common causes of acute alveolar hyperventilation.
12. Identify the following acid-base disturbances on the $P_{CO_2}/HCO_3^-/pH$ nomogram:
    —Metabolic acidosis, and include the anion gap
    —Metabolic acidosis (with partial respiratory compensation)

(continues)

—Metabolic acidosis (with complete respiratory compensation)

—Both metabolic and respiratory acidosis

13. Identify common causes of metabolic acidosis.

14. Identify the following acid-base disturbances on the P_{CO_2}/HCO_3^-/pH nomogram:

—Metabolic alkalosis

—Metabolic alkalosis (with partial respiratory compensation)

—Metabolic alkalosis (with complete respiratory compensation)

—Both metabolic and respiratory alkalosis

15. Identify common causes of metabolic alkalosis.

16. Describe base excess/deficit.

17. Complete the review questions at the end of this chapter.

An understanding of carbon dioxide (CO_2) transport is also essential to the study of pulmonary physiology and to the clinical interpretation of arterial blood gases (see Table 6–1). To fully comprehend this subject, a basic understanding of (1) how carbon dioxide is transported from the tissues to the lungs, (2) acid-base balance, (3) the P_{CO_2}/HCO_3^-/pH relationship in respiratory acid-base imbalances, and (4) the P_{CO_2}/HCO_3^-/pH relationship in metabolic acid-base imbalances is necessary.

CARBON DIOXIDE TRANSPORT

At rest, the metabolizing tissue cells consume about 250 mL of oxygen and produce about 200 mL of carbon dioxide each minute. The newly formed carbon dioxide is transported from the tissue cells to the lungs by six different mechanisms—three are in the plasma and three in the red blood cells (RBCs) (Figure 7–1).

In Plasma

- Carbamino compound (bound to protein)
- Bicarbonate
- Dissolved CO_2

Although relatively insignificant, about 1 percent of the CO_2 that dissolves in the plasma chemically combines with free amino groups of protein molecules and forms a **carbamino compound** (see Figure 7–1).

Approximately 5 percent of the CO_2 that dissolves in the plasma ionizes as **bicarbonate** (HCO_3^-). Initially, CO_2 combines with water in a process called *hydrolysis*. The hydrolysis of CO_2 and water forms carbonic acid (H_2CO_3), which in turn rapidly ionizes into HCO_3^- and H^+ ions.

$$CO_2 + H_2O \leftrightarrows H_2CO_3 \leftrightarrows HCO_3^- + H^+$$

The resulting H^+ ions are buffered by the plasma proteins. The rate of this hydrolysis reaction in the plasma is very slow and, therefore, the amount of HCO_3^- and H^+ ions that form by this mechanism is small.

Figure 7–1

How CO_2 is converted to HCO_3^- at the tissue sites. Most of the CO_2 that is produced at the tissue cells is carried to the lungs in the form of HCO_3^-.

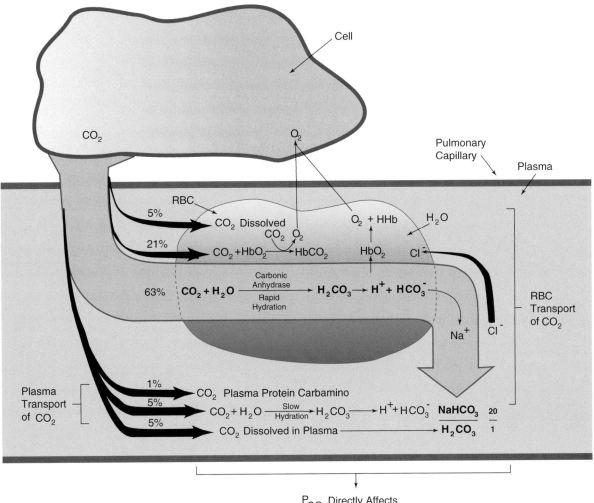

Dissolved carbon dioxide (CO_2) in the plasma accounts for about 5 percent of the total CO_2 released at the lungs. It is this portion of the CO_2 transport system in the venous blood that is measured to assess the patient's partial pressure of CO_2 (P_{CO_2}) (see Table 6–1).

Note also that the concentration of H_2CO_3 that forms in the plasma is about 1/1000 that of the physically dissolved CO_2 (P_{CO_2}) and, therefore, is proportional to the partial pressure of the CO_2. The H_2CO_3 concentration can be determined by multiplying the partial pressure of CO_2 by the factor

0.03. For example, a P_{CO_2} of 40 mm Hg generates an H_2CO_3 concentration of 1.2 mEq/L ($0.03 \times 40 = 1.2$) (see Figure 7–1).

In Red Blood Cells

- Dissolved CO_2
- Carbamino-Hb
- Bicarbonate

Dissolved carbon dioxide (CO_2) in the intracellular fluid of the red blood cells accounts for about 5 percent of the total CO_2 released at the lungs (see Figure 7–1).

About 21 percent of the CO_2 combines with hemoglobin to form a compound called **carbamino-Hb**. The O_2 that is released by this reaction is available for tissue metabolism (see Figure 7–1).

Most of the CO_2 (about 63 percent) is transported from the tissue cells to the lungs in the form of HCO_3^-. The major portion of the dissolved CO_2 that enters the RBCs is converted to HCO_3^- by the following reactions (see Figure 7–1):

1. The bulk of dissolved CO_2 that enters the RBC undergoes hydrolysis according to the following reaction (CA = carbonic anhydrase):

$$\overset{CA}{CO_2 + H_2O \leftrightarrows H_2CO_3 \leftrightarrows H^+ + HCO_3^-}$$

This reaction, which is normally a very slow process in the plasma, is greatly enhanced in the RBC by the enzyme carbonic anhydrase.

2. The resulting H^+ ions are buffered by the reduced hemoglobin.

3. The rapid hydrolysis of CO_2 causes the RBC to become saturated with HCO_3^-. To maintain a concentration equilibrium between the RBC and plasma, the excess HCO_3^- diffuses out of the RBC.

4. Once in the plasma, the HCO_3^- combines with sodium (Na^+), which is normally in the plasma in the form of sodium chloride (NaCl). The HCO_3^- is then transported to the lungs as $NaHCO_3$ in the plasma of the venous blood.

5. As HCO_3^- moves out of the RBC, the Cl^- (which has been liberated from the NaCl molecule) moves into the RBC to maintain electric neutrality. This movement is known as the **chloride shift**, or the **Hamburger phenomenon**, or as an **anionic shift to equilibrium**. During the chloride shift, some water moves into the RBC to preserve the osmotic equilibrium. This action causes the RBC to slightly swell in the venous blood.

6. In the plasma, the ratio of HCO_3^- and H_2CO_3 is normally maintained at 20:1. This ratio keeps the blood pH level within the normal range of 7.35 to 7.45. The pH of the blood becomes more alkaline as the ratio increases and less alkaline as the ratio decreases.

CARBON DIOXIDE ELIMINATION AT THE LUNGS

As shown in Figure 7–2, as the venous blood enters the alveolar capillaries, the chemical reactions occurring at the tissue level are reversed. These chemical processes continue until the CO_2 pressure is equal throughout the entire system. Table 7–1 summarizes the percentage and quantity of the total CO_2 that is transported from the tissue cells to the lungs by the six CO_2 mechanisms each minute.

Figure 7–2
How HCO_3^- is transformed back into CO_2 and eliminated in the alveoli.

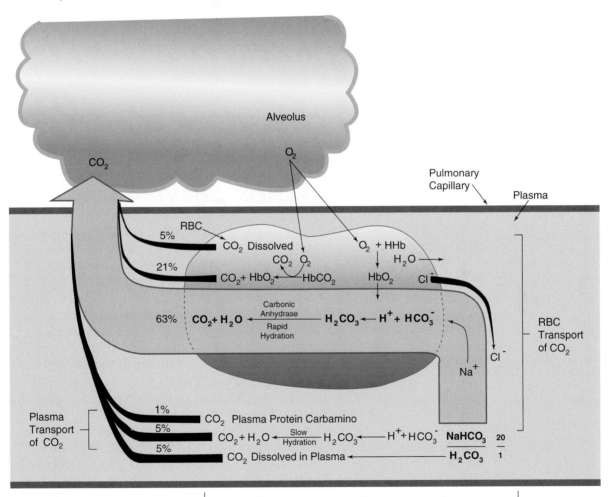

TABLE 7–1
Carbon Dioxide (CO_2) Transport Mechanisms

CO_2 Transport Mechanisms	Approx. % of Total CO_2 Transported to the Lungs	Approx. Quantity of Total CO_2 Transported to the Lungs (mL/min)
In Plasma		
Carbamino compound	1	2
Bicarbonate	5	10
Dissolved CO_2	5	10
In Red Blood Cells		
Dissolved CO_2	5	10
Carbamino-Hb	21	42
Bicarbonate	63	126
Total	**100**	**200**

CARBON DIOXIDE DISSOCIATION CURVE

Similar to the oxygen dissociation curve, the loading and unloading of CO_2 in the blood can be illustrated in graphic form (Figure 7–3). Unlike the S-shaped oxygen dissociation curve, however, the carbon dioxide curve is almost linear. This means that compared with the oxygen dissociation curve, there is a more direct relationship between the partial pressure of CO_2 (P_{CO_2}) and the amount of CO_2 (CO_2 content) in the blood. For example, when the P_{CO_2} increases from 40 to 46 mm Hg between the arterial and venous blood, the CO_2 content increases by about 5 vol% (Figure 7–4). The same partial pressure change of oxygen would increase the oxygen content only by about 2 vol% (see Figure 6–2).

The level of saturation of hemoglobin with oxygen (e.g., Sa_{O_2} or $S\overline{v}_{O_2}$) also affects the carbon dioxide dissociation curve. When the hemoglobin is 97 percent saturated with oxygen, for example, there is less CO_2 content for any given P_{CO_2} than if the hemoglobin is, say, 75 percent saturated with oxygen (Figure 7–5). The fact that deoxygenated blood enhances the loading of CO_2 is called the **Haldane effect**. Note also that the Haldane effect works the other way—that is, the oxygenation of blood enhances the unloading of CO_2.

Figure 7–6 compares both the oxygen and the carbon dioxide dissociation curves in terms of partial pressure, content, and shape.

Figure 7–3
Carbon dioxide
dissociation curve.

Figure 7–4
Carbon dioxide
dissociation curve.
An increase in the
P_{CO_2} from 40 to
46 mm Hg raises
the CO_2 content by
about 5 vol%. P_{CO_2}
changes have a
greater effect on
CO_2 content levels
than P_{O_2} changes
have on O_2 levels.

Figure 7–5

Carbon dioxide dissociation curve at two different oxygen/hemoglobin saturation levels (Sa_{O_2} of 97 and 75 percent). When the saturation of O_2 increases in the blood, the CO_2 content decreases at any given P_{CO_2}. This is known as the Haldane effect.

Figure 7–6

Comparison of the oxygen and carbon dioxide dissociation curves in terms of partial pressure, content, and shape.

ACID-BASE BALANCE AND REGULATION

Nearly all biochemical reactions in the body are influenced by the acid-base balance of their fluid environment. When the pH is either too high or too low, essentially nothing in the body functions properly. Under normal conditions, the blood pH remains within a very narrow range. The normal arterial pH range is 7.35 to 7.45. The normal venous pH range is 7.30 to 7.40. When the pH of the arterial blood is greater than 7.45, **alkalosis** or **alkalemia** is said to exist; the blood has an excess amount of bicarbonate ions (HCO_3^-). When the pH falls below 7.35, **acidosis** or **acidemia** is said to be present; the blood has an excess amount of hydrogen ions (H^+).

Most H^+ ions in the body originate from (1) the breakdown of phosphorous-containing proteins (phosphoric acid), (2) the anaerobic metabolism of glucose (lactic acid), (3) the metabolism of body fats (fatty and ketone acids), and (4) the transport of CO_2 in the blood as HCO_3^- liberates H^+ ions.

Under normal conditions, both the H^+ and HCO_3^- ion concentrations in the blood are regulated by the following three major systems: the *chemical buffer system*, the *respiratory system*, and the *renal system*.

The **chemical buffer system** responds within a fraction of a second to resist pH changes, and is called the *first line of defense*. This system is composed of (1) the *carbonic acid-bicarbonate buffer system*, (2) the *phosphate buffer system*, and (3) the *protein buffer system*. The chemical buffer system inactivates H^+ ions and liberates HCO_3^- ions in response to acidosis, or generates more H^+ ions and decreases the concentration of HCO_3^- ions in response to alkalosis.

The *respiratory system* acts within 1 to 3 minutes by increasing or decreasing the breathing depth and rate to offset acidosis or alkalosis, respectively. For example, in response to metabolic acidosis, the respiratory system causes the depth and rate of breathing to increase, causing the body's CO_2 to decrease and the pH to increase. In response to metabolic alkalosis, the respiratory system causes the depth and rate of breathing to decrease, causing the body's CO_2 to increase and the pH to decrease.

The *renal system* is the body's most effective acid-base balance monitor and regulator. The renal system requires a day or more to correct abnormal pH concentrations. When the extracellular fluids become acidic, the renal system retains HCO_3^- and excretes H^+ ions into the urine, causing the blood pH to increase. On the other hand, when the extracellular fluids become alkaline, the renal system retains H^+ and excretes basic substances (primarily HCO_3^-) into the urine, causing the blood pH to decrease.

To fully appreciate acid-base balance, and how it is normally regulated, a fundamental understanding of acids and bases, and their influences on pH, is essential.

The Basic Principles of Acid-Base Reactions and pH

Acids and Bases

Similar to salts, acids and bases are electrolytes. Thus, both acids and bases can (1) ionize and dissociate in water and (2) conduct an electrical current.

Acids

Acids are sour tasting, can react (dissolve) with many metals, and can "burn" a hole through clothing. With regard to acid-base physiology, however, an acid is a substance that releases **hydrogen ions** [H^+] in measurable amounts. Because a hydrogen ion is only a hydrogen nucleus proton, acids are defined as **proton donors**. Thus, when acids dissolve in a water solution, they release hydrogen ions (protons) and anions.

The acidity of a solution is directly related to the concentration of protons. The anions have little or no effect on the acidity. In other words, the acidity of a solution reflects only the free hydrogen ions, not those bound to anions. For example, *hydrochloric acid* (HCl), the acid found in the stomach that works to aid digestion, dissociates into a proton and a chloride ion:

$$HCl \rightarrow \underset{\text{proton}}{H^+} \quad \underset{\text{anion}}{Cl^-}$$

Other acids in the body include acetic acid ($HC_2H_3O_2$), often abbreviated as [HAc], and carbonic acid (H_2CO_3). The molecular formula for common acids is easy to identify because it begins with the hydrogen ion.

Strong and Weak Acids. First, it is important to remember that the acidity of a solution reflects only the free hydrogen ions—not the hydrogen ions still combined with anions. Thus, **strong acids**, which dissociate completely (i.e., they liberate all the H^+) and irreversibly in water, dramatically change the pH of the solution. For example, if 100 hydrochloric (HCl) acid molecules were placed in 1 mL of water, the hydrochloric acid would dissociate into 100 H^+ and 100 Cl^- ions. There would be no undissociated hydrochloric acid molecules in the solution.

Weak acids, on the other hand, do not dissociate completely in a solution and, therefore, have a much smaller effect on pH. However, even though weak acids have a relatively small effect on changing pH levels, they have a very important role in resisting sudden pH changes. Examples of weak acids are carbonic acid (H_2CO_3) and acetic acid ($HC_2H_3O_2$). If 100 acetic acid molecules were placed in 1 mL of water, the following reaction would occur:

$$100\ HC_2H_3O_2 \rightarrow 90\ HC_2H_3O_2 + \underset{\text{(hydrogen ions)}}{10\ H^+} + \underset{\text{(acetate ions)}}{10\ C_2H_3O_2^-}$$

Because undissociated acids do not alter the pH, the acidic solution will not be as acidic as the HCl solution discussed earlier. Because the dissociation of weak acids is predictable, and because the molecules of intact acids are in constant dynamic equilibrium with the dissociated ions, the dissociation of acetic acid can be written as follows:

$$HC_2H_3O_2 \leftrightarrows H^+ + C_2H_3O_2^-$$

Using this equation, it can be seen that when H^+ (released by a strong acid) is added to the acetic acid solution, the equilibrium moves to the left as some of the additional H^+ bonds with $C_2H_3O_2^-$ to form $HC_2H_3O_2$. On the other hand, when a strong base is added to the solution (adding additional OH^- and causing the pH to increase), the equilibrium shifts to the right. This occurs because the additional OH^- consumes the H^+. This causes more $HC_2H_3O_2$ molecules to dissociate and replenish the H^+. Weak acids play a very important role in the chemical buffer systems of the human body.

Bases

Bases are **proton acceptors**. Bases taste bitter and feel slippery. With regard to acid-base physiology, a base is a substance that takes up hydrogen ions [H^+] in measurable amounts. Common inorganic bases include the hydroxides, for example, magnesium hydroxide (milk of magnesia) and sodium hydroxide (lye). Similar to acids, when dissolved in water, hydroxides dissociate into **hydroxide ions** (OH^-) and cations. For example, ionization of sodium hydroxide (NaOH) results in a hydroxide ion and a sodium ion. The liberated hydroxide ion then bonds, or accepts, a proton present in the solution. This reaction produces water and, at the same time, decreases the acidity [H^+ concentration] of the solution:

$$NaOH \rightarrow \underset{\text{cation}}{Na^+} + \underset{\text{hydroxide ion}}{OH^-}$$

and then

$$OH^- + H^+ \rightarrow \underset{\text{water}}{H_2O}$$

The **bicarbonate ion (HCO_3^-)** is an important base in the body and is especially abundant in the blood. **Ammonia** (NH_3), a natural waste product of protein breakdown, is also a base. Ammonia has a pair of unshared electrons that strongly attract protons. When accepting a proton, ammonia becomes an ammonium ion:

$$NH_3 + H^+ \rightarrow \underset{\text{ammonium ion}}{NH_4^+}$$

Strong and Weak Bases. With regard to strong and weak bases, it is important to remember that bases are proton acceptors. **Strong bases** (e.g., hydroxides) dissociate easily in water and quickly tie up H^+. In contrast, **weak bases** (e.g., sodium bicarbonate or baking soda) dissociate incompletely and reversibly and are slower to accept protons. Because sodium bicarbonate accepts a relatively small amount of protons, its released bicarbonate ion is described as a weak base.

pH: Acid-Base Concentration

As the concentration of hydrogen ions in a solution increases, the more acidic the solution becomes. On the other hand, as the level of hydroxide ions increases, the more basic, or alkaline, the solution becomes. Clinically, the concentration of hydrogen ions in the body is measured in units called *pH units*. The pH scale runs from 0 to 14 and is logarithmic, which means each successive unit change in pH represents a tenfold change in hydrogen ion concentration. The **pH** of a solution, therefore, *is defined as the negative logarithm, to the base 10, of the hydrogen ion concentration [H^+] in moles per liter, or $-\log H^+$:*

$$pH = -\log_{10} [H^+]$$

When the pH is 7 ($H^+ = 10^{-7}$ mol/L), the number of hydrogen ions precisely equals the number of hydroxide ions (OH^-), and the solution is neutral—that is, neither acidic nor basic. Pure water has a neutral pH of 7, or 10^{-7} mol/L (0.0000001 mol/L) of hydrogen ions. A solution with a pH below 7, is acidic—that is, there are more hydrogen ions than hydroxide ions. For example, a solution with a pH of 6 has 10 times more hydrogen ions than a solution with a pH of 7.

A solution with a pH greater than 7 is alkaline—that is, the hydroxide ions outnumber the hydrogen ions. For example, a solution with a pH of 8 has 10 times more hydroxyl ions than a solution with a pH of 7. Thus, as the hydrogen ion concentration increases, the hydroxide ion concentration falls, and vice versa. Figure 7–7 provides the approximate pH values of several human fluids and common household substances.

The Chemical Buffer Systems and Acid-Base Balance

Chemical buffers resist pH changes and are the body's first line of defense. The ability of an acid-base mixture to resist sudden changes in pH is called its **buffer action**. The tissue cells and vital organs of the body are extremely sensitive to even the slightest change in the pH environment. In high concentrations, both acids and bases can be extremely damaging to living cells—essentially every biological process within the body is disrupted.

Figure 7–7
The pH values of representative substances. The pH scale represents the number of hydrogen ions in a substance. The concentration of hydrogen ions (H^+) and the corresponding hydroxyl concentration (OH^-) for each representative substance is also provided. Note that when the pH is 7.0, the amounts of H^+ and OH^- are equal and the solution is neutral.

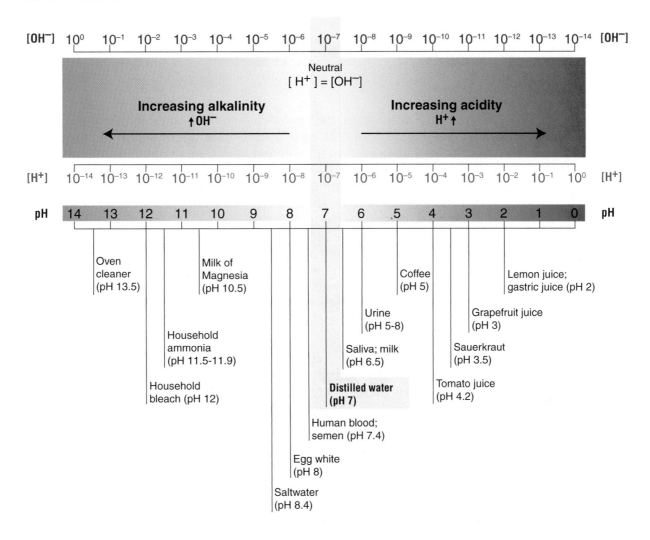

Buffers work against sudden and large changes in the pH of body fluids by (1) releasing hydrogen ions (acting as acids) when the pH increases and (2) binding hydrogen ions (acting as bases) when the pH decreases. The three major chemical buffer systems in the body are the *carbonic acid-bicarbonate buffer system, phosphate buffer system,* and the *protein buffer system.*

Carbonic Acid-Bicarbonate Buffer System and Acid-Base Balance

The **carbonic acid-bicarbonate buffer system** plays an extremely important role in maintaining pH homeostasis of the blood. Carbonic acid (H_2CO_3) dissociates reversibly and releases bicarbonate ions (HCO_3^-) and protons (H^+) as follows:

$$
\begin{array}{ccc}
 & \text{Response to an increase in pH} & \\
H_2CO_3 & \overset{\longleftarrow}{\underset{\longrightarrow}{\rule{3cm}{0pt}}} & HCO_3^- \;+\; H^+ \\
\text{H}^+\text{ donor} & \text{Response to a decrease in pH} & \text{H}^+\text{ acceptor} \quad \text{proton} \\
\text{(weak acid)} & & \text{(weak proton)}
\end{array}
$$

Under normal conditions, the ratio between HCO_3^- and H_2CO_3 in the blood is 20:1 (see Figure 7–1). The chemical equilibrium between carbonic acid (weak acid) and bicarbonate ion (weak base) works to resist sudden changes in blood pH. For example, when the blood pH increases (i.e., becomes more alkaline from the addition of a strong base), the equilibrium shifts to the right. A right shift forces more carbonic acid to dissociate, which in turn causes the pH to decrease.

In contrast, when the blood pH decreases (i.e., becomes more acidic from the addition of a strong acid), the equilibrium moves to the left. A left shift forces more bicarbonate to bind with protons. In short, the carbonic acid-bicarbonate buffer system converts (1) strong bases to a weak base (bicarbonate ion) and (2) strong acids to a weak acid (carbonic acid). As a result, blood pH changes are much less than they would be if this buffering system did not exist.

The Henderson-Hasselbalch Equation. The **Henderson-Hasselbalch (H-H) equation** mathematically illustrates how the pH of a solution is influenced by the HCO_3^- to H_2CO_3 ratio (base to acid ratio). The H-H equation is written as follows:

$$pH = pK + \log\frac{[HCO_3^-] \; (base)}{[H_2CO_3] \; (acid)}$$

The pK is derived from the dissociation constant of the acid portion of the buffer combination. The pK is 6:1 and, under normal conditions, the HCO_3^- to H_2CO_3 ratio is 20:1.

Clinically, the dissolved CO_2 ($P_{CO_2} \times 0.03$) can be used for the denominator of the H-H equation, instead of the H_2CO_3. This is possible since the dissolved carbon dioxide is in equilibrium with, and directly proportional to, the blood [H_2CO_3]. This is handy, since the patient's P_{CO_2} value can easily be obtained from an arterial blood gas. Thus, the H-H equation can be written as follows:

$$pH = pK + \log\frac{[HCO_3^-]}{[P_{CO_2} \times 0.03]}$$

H-H Equation Applied During Normal Conditions. When the HCO_3^- is 24 mEq/L, and the Pa_{CO_2} is 40 mm Hg, the base to acid ratio is 20:1 and the pH is 7.4 (normal). The H-H equation confirms the 20:1 ratio and pH of 7.4 as follows:

$$pH = pK + \log\frac{[HCO_3^-]}{[P_{CO_2} \times 0.03]}$$

$$= 6.1 + \log\frac{24 \text{ mEq/L}}{(40 \times 0.03)}$$

$$= 6.1 + \log\frac{24 \text{ mEq/L}}{(1.2 \text{ mEq/L})}$$

$$= 6.1 + \log\frac{20}{1} \quad (20\text{:}1 \text{ ratio})$$

$$= 6.1 + 1.3$$

$$= 7.4$$

H-H Equation Applied During Abnormal Conditions. When the HCO_3^- is 29 mEq/L, and the Pa_{CO_2} is 80 mm Hg, the base to acid ratio decreases to 12:1 and the pH is 7.18 (acidic). The H-H equation confirms the 12:1 ratio and the pH of 7.18 as follows:

$$pH = pK + \log\frac{[HCO_3^-]}{[P_{CO_2} \times 0.03]}$$

$$= 6.1 + \log\frac{29 \text{ mEq/L}}{(80 \times 0.03)}$$

$$= 6.1 + \log\frac{29 \text{ mEq/L}}{(2.4 \text{ mEq/L})}$$

$$= 6.1 + \log\frac{12}{1} \quad (12\text{:}1 \text{ ratio})$$

$$= 6.1 + 1.08$$

$$= 7.18$$

In contrast, when the HCO_3^- is 20 mEq/L, and the Pa_{CO_2} is 20 mm Hg, the base to acid ratio increases to 33:1 and the pH is 7.62 (alkalotic). The H-H equation confirms the 33:1 ratio and the pH of 7.62 as follows:

$$pH = pK + \log\frac{[HCO_3^-]}{[P_{CO_2} \times 0.03]}$$

$$= 6.1 + \log\frac{20 \text{ mEq/L}}{(20 \times 0.03)}$$

$$= 6.1 + \log\frac{20 \text{ mEq/L}}{(0.6 \text{ mEq/L})}$$

$$= 6.1 + \log\frac{33}{1} \quad (33\text{:}1 \text{ ratio})$$

$$= 6.1 + 1.52$$

$$= 7.62$$

Clinical Application of the H-H Equation. Clinically, the Henderson-Hasselbalch equation can be used to calculate the pH, $[HCO_3^-]$, or P_{CO_2} when any two of these three variables are known. $[HCO_3^-]$ is solved as follows:

$$[HCO_3^-] = \text{antilog}(7.40 - 6.1) \times (P_{CO_2} \times 0.03)$$

P_{CO_2} is determined as follows:

$$P_{CO_2} = \frac{[HCO_3^-]}{(\text{antilog} [pH - 6.1] \times 0.03)}$$

The H-H equation may be helpful in cross-checking the validity of the blood gas reports when the pH, P_{CO_2}, and $[HCO_3^-]$ values appear out of line. It may also be useful in estimating what changes to expect when any one of the H-H equation components is altered. For example, consider the case example that follows.

Case. A mechanically ventilated patient has a pH of 7.54, a Pa_{CO_2} of 26 mm Hg, and a HCO_3^- of 22 mEq/L. The physician asks the respiratory practitioner to adjust the patient's Pa_{CO_2} to a level that will decrease the pH to 7.45. Using the H-H equation, the Pa_{CO_2} change needed to decrease the pH to 7.45 can be estimated as follows:

$$P_{CO_2} = \frac{[HCO_3^-]}{(\text{antilog} [pH - 6.1] \times 0.03)}$$

$$= \frac{22}{\text{antilog} (7.45 - 6.1) \times 0.03}$$

$$= \frac{22}{\text{antilog} (1.35) \times 0.03}$$

$$= \frac{22}{22.38 \times 0.03}$$

$$= \frac{22}{0.67}$$

$$= 32.8 \text{ or } 33 \text{ mm Hg}$$

Thus, increasing the Pa_{CO_2} to about 33 mm Hg should move the patient's pH level close to 7.45. In this case, the respiratory practitioner would begin by either decreasing the tidal volume, or the respiratory rate, on the mechanical ventilator. After the ventilator changes are made, another arterial blood gas should be obtained in about 20 minutes. The pH and Pa_{CO_2} should be reevaluated, and followed by appropriate ventilator adjustments if necessary.

Phosphate Buffer System and Acid-Base Balance

The function of the **phosphate buffer system** is almost identical to that of the carbonic acid-bicarbonate buffer system. The primary components of the phosphate buffer system are the sodium salts of dihydrogen phosphate ($H_2PO_4^-$) and monohydrogen phosphate (HPO_4^{2-}). NaH_2PO_4 is a weak acid. Na_2HPO_4, which has one less hydrogen atom, is a weak base. When H^+ ions are released by a strong acid, the phosphate buffer system works to inactivate the acidic effects of the H^+ as follows:

$$HCl + Na_2HPO_4 \rightarrow NaH_2PO_4 + NaCl$$
$$\text{strong acid} \quad \text{weak base} \quad\quad \text{weak acid} \quad\quad \text{Salt}$$

On the other hand, strong bases are converted to weak bases as follows:

$$NaOH + NaH_2PO_4 \rightarrow Na_2HPO_4 + H_2O$$
$$\text{strong base} \quad \text{weak acid} \quad\quad \text{weak base} \quad\quad \text{water}$$

Because the phosphate buffer system is only about one-sixth as effective as that of the carbonic acid-bicarbonate buffer system in the extracellular fluid, it is not an effective buffer for blood plasma. However, it is an effective buffer system in urine and in intracellular fluid where the phosphate levels are typically greater.

Protein Buffer System and Acid-Base Balance

The body's most abundant and influential supply of buffers is the **protein buffer system**. Its buffers are found in the proteins in the plasma and cells. In fact, about 75 percent of the buffering power of body fluids is found in the intracellular proteins. Proteins are polymers of amino acids. Some of the amino acids have exposed groups of atoms known as organic acid (carboxyl) groups (—COOH), which dissociate and liberate H^+ in response to a rising pH:

$$R^*\text{—COOH} \rightarrow R\text{—COO}^- + H^+$$

R represents the entire organic molecule, which is composed of many atoms.

In contrast, other amino acids consist of exposed groups that can function as bases and accept H^+. For example, an exposed—NH_2 group can bond with hydrogen ions to form—NH_3^+:

$$R—NH_2 + H^+ \rightarrow R—NH_3^+$$

Because this reaction ties up free hydrogen ions, it prevents the solution from becoming too acidic. In addition, a single protein molecule can function as either an acid or a base relative to its pH environment. Protein molecules that have a reversible ability are called **amphoteric molecules**.

   The hemoglobin in red blood cells is a good example of a protein that works as an intracellular buffer. As discussed earlier, CO_2 released at the tissue cells quickly forms H_2CO_3, and then dissociates into H^+ and HCO_3^- ions (see Figure 7–1). At the same time, the hemoglobin is unloading oxygen at the tissue sites and becoming *reduced hemoglobin*. Because reduced hemoglobin carries a negative charge, the free H^+ ions quickly bond to the hemoglobin anions. This action reduces the acidic effects of the H^+ on the pH. In essence, the H_2CO_3, which is a weak acid, is buffered by an even weaker acid—the hemoglobin protein.

The Respiratory System and Acid-Base Balance

Although the respiratory system does not respond as fast as the chemical buffer systems, it has up to two times the buffering power of all of the chemical buffer systems combined. As discussed earlier, the respiratory system eliminates CO_2 from the body while at the same time replenishing it with O_2. The CO_2 produced at the tissue cells enters the red blood cells and is converted to HCO_3^- ions as follows:

$$CO_2 + H_2O \leftrightarrows H_2CO_3 \leftrightarrows H^+ + HCO_3^-$$

The first set of double arrows illustrates a reversible equilibrium between the dissolved carbon dioxide and the water on the left and carbonic acid on the right. The second set of arrows shows a reversible equilibrium between carbonic acid on the left and hydrogen and bicarbonate ions on the right. Because of this relationship, an increase in any of these chemicals causes a shift in the opposite direction. Note also that the right side of this equation is the same as that for the carbonic acid-bicarbonate buffer system.

   Under normal conditions, the volume of CO_2 eliminated at the lung is equal to the amount of CO_2 produced at the tissues. When the CO_2 is unloaded at the lungs, the preceding equation flows to the left, and causes the H^+ generated from the carbonic acid to transform back to water (see Figure 7–2). Because of the protein buffer system (discussed earlier), the H^+ generated by the CO_2 transport system is not permitted to increase and, therefore, has little or no effect on blood pH.

However, under abnormal conditions, the respiratory system quickly responds by either increasing or decreasing the rate and depth of breathing to compensate for acidosis or alkalosis, respectively. For example, when the pH declines (e.g., metabolic acidosis caused by lactic acids), the respiratory system responds by increasing the breathing depth and rate. This action causes more CO_2 to be eliminated from the lungs and, therefore, pushes the preceding reaction to the left and reduces the H^+ concentration. This process works to return the acidic pH back to normal. On the other hand, when the pH rises (e.g., metabolic alkalosis caused by hypokalemia), the respiratory system responds by decreasing the breathing depth and rate. This action causes less CO_2 to be eliminated from the lungs and, thus, moves the preceding reaction to the right and increases the H^+ concentration. This works to pull the alkalotic pH back to normal.

Finally, note that when the respiratory system is impaired for any reason, a serious acid-base imbalance can develop. For example, severe head trauma can cause a dramatic increase in the depth and rate of breathing that is completely unrelated to the CO_2 concentration. When this happens, the volume of CO_2 expelled from the lungs will be greater than the amount of CO_2 produced at the tissue cells. In other words, **hyperventilation** is present. This condition causes the pH to increase and **respiratory alkalosis** is said to exist. In contrast, the ingestion of barbiturates can cause a dramatic decrease in the depth and rate of breathing. When this occurs, the volume of CO_2 eliminated from the lungs is less than the amount of CO_2 produced at the tissue cells. In this case, **hypoventilation** is present. This condition causes the pH to fall and **respiratory acidosis** is said to exist. The control of ventilation is presented in Chapter 9.

The Renal System and Acid-Base Balance

Even though the chemical buffer systems can inactivate excess acids and bases momentarily, they are unable to eliminate them from the body. Similarly, although the respiratory system can expel the volatile carbonic acid by eliminating CO_2, it cannot expel other acids generated by cellular metabolism. Only the *renal system* can rid the body of acids such as phosphoric acids, uric acids, lactic acids, and ketone acids (also called fixed acids).

In addition, only the renal system can regulate alkaline substances in the blood and restore chemical buffers that are used up in managing the H^+ levels in the extracellular fluids. (For example, some HCO_3^-, which helps to adjust H^+ concentrations, is lost from the body when CO_2 is expelled from the lungs.) Basically, when the extracellular fluids become acidic, the renal system retains HCO_3^- and excretes H^+ ions into the urine, causing the blood pH to increase. On the other hand, when the extracellular fluids become alkaline, the renal system retains H^+ and excretes basic substances (primarily HCO_3^-) into the urine, causing the blood pH to decrease.

THE ROLE OF THE $P_{CO_2}/HCO_3^-/pH$ RELATIONSHIP IN ACID-BASE BALANCE

CLINICAL
APPLICATION
CASES

1 & 2

See pages 312–315

Acid-Base Balance Disturbances

As shown earlier in this chapter, the normal bicarbonate (HCO_3^-) to carbonic acid (H_2CO_3) ratio in the blood plasma is 20:1. In other words, for every H_2CO_3 ion produced in blood plasma, 20 HCO_3^- ions must be formed to maintain a 20:1 ratio (normal pH). Or, for every H_2CO_3 ion loss in the blood plasma, 20 HCO_3^- ions must be eliminated to maintain a normal pH. In other words, the H_2CO_3 ion is 20 times more powerful than the HCO_3^- ion in changing the blood pH.

Under normal conditions, the 20:1 acid-base balance in the body is automatically regulated by the chemical buffer systems, the respiratory system, and the renal system. However, these normal acid-base regulating systems have their limits. The bottom line is this: The body's normal acid-base watchdog systems cannot adequately respond to sudden, large changes in H^+ and HCO_3^- concentrations—regardless of the cause.

For example, hypoventilation causes the partial pressure of the alveolar carbon dioxide ($P_{A_{CO_2}}$) to increase, which in turn causes the plasma P_{CO_2}, HCO_3^-, and H_2CO_3 to all increase. This chemical chain of events causes the HCO_3^- to H_2CO_3 ratio to decrease, and the pH to fall (Figure 7–8). Or, when the $P_{A_{CO_2}}$ decreases, as a result of alveolar hyperventilation, the plasma P_{CO_2}, HCO_3^-, and H_2CO_3 all decrease—which, in turn, causes the HCO_3^- to H_2CO_3 ratio to increase, and the pH to rise (Figure 7–9).

Figure 7–8
Alveolar hypoventilation causes the $P_{A_{CO_2}}$ and the plasma P_{CO_2}, H_2CO_3, and HCO_3^- to increase. This action decreases the HCO_3^-/H_2CO_3 ratio, which in turn decreases the blood pH.

Figure 7–9

Alveolar hyperventilation causes the $P_{A_{CO_2}}$ and the plasma P_{CO_2}, H_2CO_3, and HCO_3^- to decrease. This action increases the HCO_3^-/H_2CO_3 ratio, which in turn increases the blood pH.

The relationship between acute P_{CO_2} changes, and the resultant pH and HCO_3^- changes that occur, is graphically illustrated in the $P_{CO_2}/HCO_3^-/pH$ nomogram (Figure 7–10). The $P_{CO_2}/HCO_3^-/pH$ nomogram is an excellent clinical tool that can be used to identify a specific acid-base disturbance.* Table 7–2 (page 293) provides an overview of the common acid-base balance disturbances that can be identified on the $P_{CO_2}/HCO_3^-/pH$ nomogram. The following sections describe (1) the common acid-base disturbances and (2) how to identify them on the $P_{CO_2}/HCO_3^-/pH$ nomogram.

Respiratory Acid-Base Disturbances

Acute Ventilatory Failure (Respiratory Acidosis)

During **acute ventilatory failure** (e.g., acute hypoventilation caused by an overdose of narcotics or barbiturates), the $P_{A_{CO_2}}$ progressively increases. This action simultaneously causes an increase in the blood P_{CO_2}, H_2CO_3, and HCO_3^- levels. Because acute changes in H_2CO_3 levels are more significant than acute changes in HCO_3^- levels, a decreased HCO_3^- to H_2CO_3 ratio develops (a ratio less than 20:1), which in turn causes the blood pH to decrease, or become acidic (see Figure 7–8). The resultant pH and HCO_3^- changes, caused by a sudden increase in the P_{CO_2} level, can be

*See Appendix VI for a pocket size $P_{CO_2}/HCO_3^-/pH$ nomogram card that can be cut out, laminated, and used as a handy arterial blood gas reference tool in the clinical setting.

Figure 7–10
Nomogram of P_{CO_2}/HCO_3^-/pH relationship.

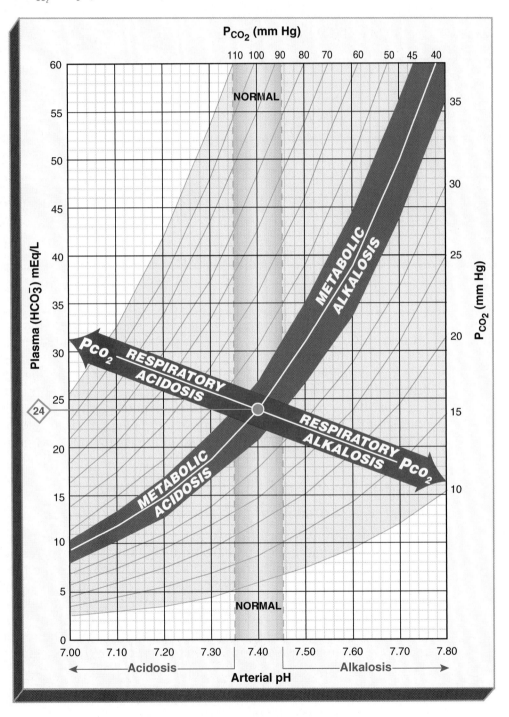

TABLE 7–2
Common Acid-Base Disturbance Classifications

- Respiratory Acid-Base Disturbances
  - Acute ventilatory failure (respiratory acidosis)
  - Acute ventilatory failure with partial renal compensation
  - Chronic ventilatory failure with complete renal compensation

  - Acute alveolar hyperventilation (respiratory alkalosis)
  - Acute alveolar hyperventilation with partial renal compensation
  - Chronic alveolar hyperventilation with complete renal compensation

- Metabolic Acid-Base Disturbances
  - Metabolic acidosis
  - Metabolic acidosis with partial respiratory compensation
  - Metabolic acidosis with complete respiratory compensation
  - Both metabolic and respiratory acidosis

  - Metabolic alkalosis
  - Metabolic alkalosis with partial respiratory compensation
  - Metabolic alkalosis with complete respiratory compensation
  - Both metabolic and respiratory alkalosis

---

easily identified by using the left side of the red-colored normal P_{CO_2} blood buffer bar located on the $P_{CO_2}/HCO_3^-/pH$ nomogram—titled RESPIRATORY ACIDOSIS in Figure 7–11.

Acute ventilatory failure is confirmed when the reported P_{CO_2}, pH, and HCO_3^- values all intersect within the red-colored RESPIRATORY ACIDOSIS bar. For example, when the reported P_{CO_2} is 80 mm Hg, at a time when the pH is 7.18 and the HCO_3^- is 28 mEq/L, acute ventilatory failure is confirmed (see Figure 7–11). This is because (1) all reported values (i.e., P_{CO_2}, HCO_3^-, and pH) intersect within the red-colored normal P_{CO_2} blood buffer bar, and (2) the pH and HCO_3^- readings are precisely what is expected for an acute increase in the P_{CO_2} to 80 mm Hg (see Figure 7–11). Table 7–3 (page 295) lists common causes of acute ventilatory failure.

Renal Compensation

In the patient who hypoventilates for a long period of time (e.g., because of chronic obstructive pulmonary disease), the kidneys will work to correct the decreased pH by retaining HCO_3^- in the blood. The presence of renal compensation is verified when the reported P_{CO_2}, HCO_3^-, and pH values all intersect in the purple-colored area shown in the upper left-hand corner of the $P_{CO_2}/HCO_3^-/pH$ nomogram of Figure 7–12 (page 296).

Acute ventilatory failure with partial renal compensation (also called partially compensated respiratory acidosis) is present when the

Figure 7–11

Acute ventilatory failure is confirmed when the reported P_{CO_2}, pH, and HCO_3^- values all intersect within the red-colored RESPIRATORY ACIDOSIS bar. For example, when the reported P_{CO_2} is 80 mm Hg, at a time when the pH is 7.18 and the HCO_3^- is 28 mEq/L, acute ventilatory failure is confirmed.

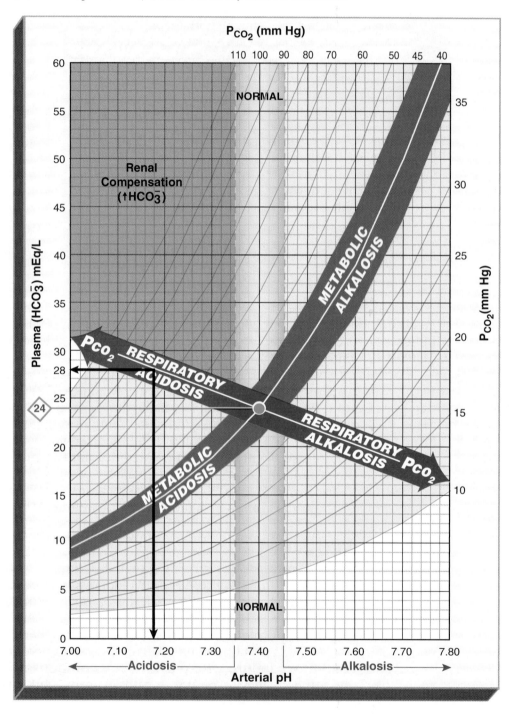

TABLE 7-3
Common Causes of Acute Ventilatory Failure

Chronic obstructive pulmonary disorders	Pulmonary disorders such as chronic emphysema and chronic bronchitis can lead to acute ventilatory failure
Drug overdose	Drugs such as narcotics or barbiturates can depress ventilation.
General anesthesia	General anesthetics can cause ventilatory failure.
Head trauma	Severe trauma to the brain can cause acute ventilatory failure.
Neurologic disorders	Neurologic disorders such as Guillain-Barré syndrome and myasthenia gravis can lead to acute ventilatory failure.

---

reported pH and HCO_3^- are both above the normal red-colored P_{CO_2} blood buffer bar (in the purple-colored area), but the pH is still less than normal. For example, when the P_{CO_2} is 80 mm Hg, at a time when the pH is 7.30 and the HCO_3 is 37 mEq/L, ventilatory failure with partial renal compensation is confirmed (see Figure 7–12).

Chronic ventilatory failure with complete renal compensation (also called compensated respiratory acidosis) is present when the HCO_3^- increases enough to cause the acidic pH to move back into the normal range, which, in this case, would be above 42 mEq/L (see Figure 7–12).

Acute Alveolar Hyperventilation (Respiratory Alkalosis)

During **acute alveolar hyperventilation** (e.g., hyperventilation due to pain and/or anxiety), the $P_{A_{CO_2}}$ will decrease and allow more CO_2 molecules to leave the pulmonary blood. This action simultaneously causes a decrease in the blood P_{CO_2}, H_2CO_3, and HCO_3^- levels. Because acute changes in H_2CO_3 levels are more significant than acute changes in HCO_3^- levels, an increased HCO_3^- to H_2CO_3 ratio develops (a ratio greater than 20:1), which, in turn, causes the blood pH to increase, or become more alkaline (see Figure 7–9). The resultant pH and HCO_3^- changes caused by an acute decrease in the P_{CO_2} level can be easily identified by using the right side of the red-colored normal P_{CO_2} blood buffer bar located on the $P_{CO_2}/HCO_3^-/pH$ nomogram titled RESPIRATORY ALKALOSIS (Figure 7–13).

Acute alveolar hyperventilation is confirmed when the reported P_{CO_2}, pH, and HCO_3^- values all intersect within the red-colored RESPIRATORY ALKALOSIS bar. For example, when the reported P_{CO_2} is 25 mm Hg, at a

Figure 7–12

Acute ventilatory failure with partial renal compensation (also called partially compensated respiratory acidosis) is present when the reported pH and HCO_3^- are both above the normal red-colored P_{CO_2} blood buffer bar (in the purple-colored area), but the pH is still less than normal. For example, when the P_{CO_2} is 80 mm Hg, at a time when the pH is 7.30 and the HCO_3 is 37 mEq/L, ventilatory failure with partial renal compensation is confirmed.

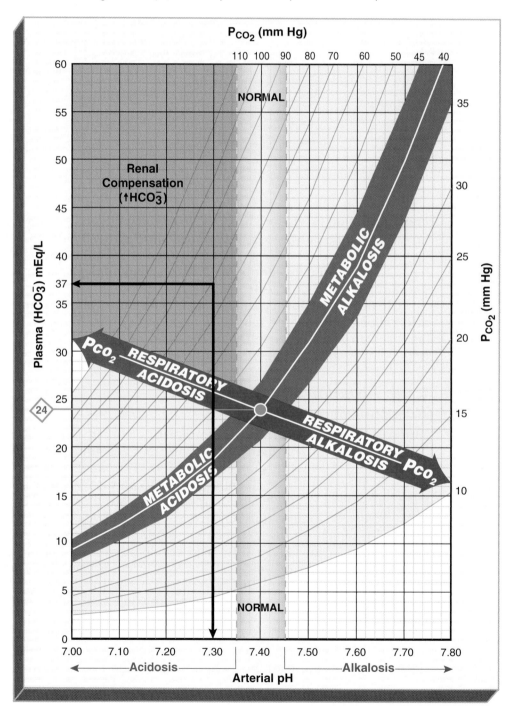

Figure 7–13

Acute alveolar hyperventilation is confirmed when the reported P_{CO_2}, pH, and HCO_3^- values all intersect within the red-colored RESPIRATORY ACIDOSIS bar. For example, when the reported P_{CO_2} is 25 mm Hg, at a time when the pH is 7.55 and the HCO_3 is 21 mEq/L, acute alveolar hyperventilation is confirmed.

> **TABLE 7–4**
> Common Causes of Acute Alveolar Hyperventilation
>
> | | |
> |---|---|
> | Hypoxia | Any cause of hypoxia (e.g., lung disorders, high altitudes, and heart disease) can cause acute alveolar hyperventilation. |
> | Pain, anxiety, and fever | Relative to the degree of pain, anxiety, and fever, hyperventilation may be seen. |
> | Brain inflammation | Relative to the degree of cerebral inflammation, hyperventilation may be seen. |
> | Stimulant drugs | Agents such as amphetamines can cause alveolar hyperventilation. |

time when the pH is 7.55 and the HCO_3 is 21 mEq/L, acute alveolar hyperventilation is confirmed (see Figure 7–13). This is because (1) all the reported values (i.e., P_{CO_2}, HCO_3^-, and pH) intersect within the red-colored normal P_{CO_2} blood buffer bar, and (2) the pH and HCO_3^- readings are precisely what is expected for an acute increase in the P_{CO_2} to 80 mm Hg (see Figure 7–13). Table 7–4 lists common causes of acute alveolar hyperventilation.

Renal Compensation

In the patient who hyperventilates for a long period of time (e.g., a patient who has been overly mechanically hyperventilated for more than 24 to 48 hours), the kidneys will work to correct the increased pH by excreting excess HCO_3^- in the urine. The presence of renal compensation is verified when the reported P_{CO_2}, HCO_3^-, and pH values all intersect in the green-colored area shown in the lower right-hand corner of the P_{CO_2}/HCO_3^-/pH nomogram of Figure 7–14.

Alveolar hyperventilation with partial renal compensation (also called partially compensated respiratory alkalosis) is present when the reported pH and HCO_3^- are both below the normal red-colored P_{CO_2} blood buffer bar (in the green-colored area), but the pH is still greater than normal. For example, when the P_{CO_2} is 20 mm Hg, at a time when the pH is 7.50 and the HCO_3^- is 15 mEq/L, alveolar hyperventilation with partial renal compensation is confirmed (see Figure 7–14).

Chronic alveolar hyperventilation with complete renal compensation (also called compensated respiratory alkalosis) is present when the HCO_3^- level decreases enough to return the alkalotic pH to normal, which, in this, case would be below 14 mEq/L (see Figure 7–14).

General Comments

As a general rule, the kidneys do not overcompensate for an abnormal pH. That is, if the patient's blood pH becomes acidic for a long period of

Figure 7–14

Alveolar hyperventilation with partial renal compensation (also called partially compensated respiratory alkalosis) is present when the reported pH and HCO_3^- are both below the normal red-colored P_{CO_2} blood buffer bar (in the green-colored area), but the pH is still greater than normal. For example, when the P_{CO_2} is 20 mm Hg, at a time when the pH is 7.50 and the HCO_3^- is 15 mEq/L, alveolar hyperventilation with partial renal compensation is confirmed.

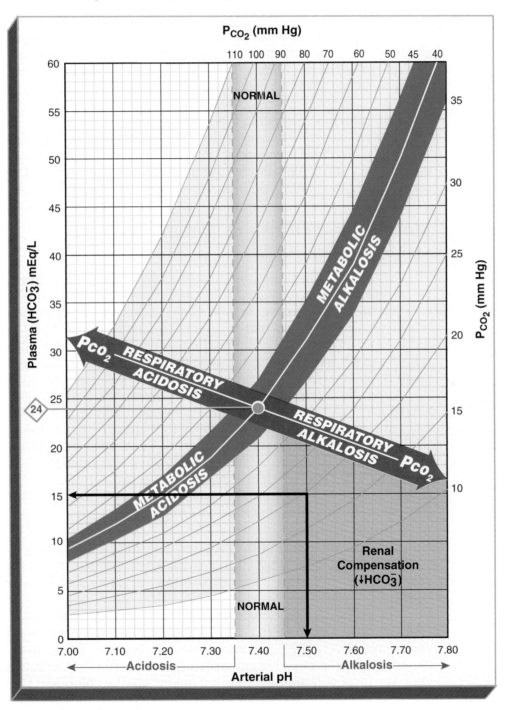

time due to hypoventilation, the kidneys will not retain enough HCO_3^- for the pH to climb higher than 7.40. The opposite is also true: Should the blood pH become alkalotic for a long period of time due to hyperventilation, the kidneys will not excrete enough HCO_3^- for the pH to fall below 7.40.

However, there is one important exception to this rule. In persons who chronically hypoventilate for a long period of time (e.g., patients with chronic emphysema or chronic bronchitis), it is not uncommon to find a pH greater than 7.40 (e.g., 7.43 or 7.44). This is due to water and chloride ion shifts that occur between the intercellular and extracellular spaces when the renal system works to compensate for a decreased blood pH. This action causes an overall loss of blood chloride (hypochloremia). Hypochloremia increases the blood pH.

To summarize, the lungs play an important role in maintaining the P_{CO_2}, HCO_3^-, and pH levels on a moment-to-moment basis. The kidneys, on the other hand, play an important role in balancing the HCO_3^- and pH levels during long periods of hyperventilation or hypoventilation.

Metabolic Acid-Base Imbalances

Metabolic Acidosis

The presence of other acids, not related to an increased P_{CO_2} level, can also be identified on the P_{CO_2}/HCO_3^-/pH nomogram. Clinically, this condition is called **metabolic acidosis**. Metabolic acidosis is present when the P_{CO_2} reading is within the normal range (35 to 45 mm Hg), but not within the red-colored normal blood buffer line when compared to the reported HCO_3^- and pH levels. This is because the pH and HCO_3^- readings are both lower than expected for a normal P_{CO_2} level.

When the reported pH and HCO_3^- levels are both lower than expected for a normal P_{CO_2} level, the P_{CO_2} reading will drop into the purple-colored bar titled METABOLIC ACIDOSIS (Figure 7–15). In short, the pH, HCO_3^-, and P_{CO_2} readings will all intersect within the purple-colored METABOLIC ACIDOSIS bar. For example, when the reported P_{CO_2} is 40 mm Hg (normal), at a time when the pH is 7.25 and the HCO_3^- is 17 mEq/L, metabolic acidosis is confirmed (see Figure 7–15). Table 7–5 (page 302) lists common causes of metabolic acidosis.

Anion Gap. The **anion gap** is used to determine if a patient's metabolic acidosis is caused by either (1) the accumulation of fixed acids (e.g., lactic acids, keto acids, or salicylate intoxication), or (2) by an excessive loss of HCO_3^-.

According to the **law of electroneutrality**, the total number of plasma positively charged ions (cations) must equal the total number of plasma negatively charged ions (anions) in the body fluids. To determine the anion gap, the most commonly measured cations are sodium (Na^+) ions. The most commonly measured anions are the chloride (Cl^-) ions and

Figure 7–15

When the reported pH and HCO_3^- levels are both lower than expected for a normal P_{CO_2} level, the P_{CO_2} reading will drop into the purple-colored bar titled METABOLIC ACIDOSIS. For example, when the reported P_{CO_2} is 40 mm Hg (normal), at a time when the pH is 7.25 and the HCO_3^- is 17 mEq/L, metabolic acidosis is confirmed.

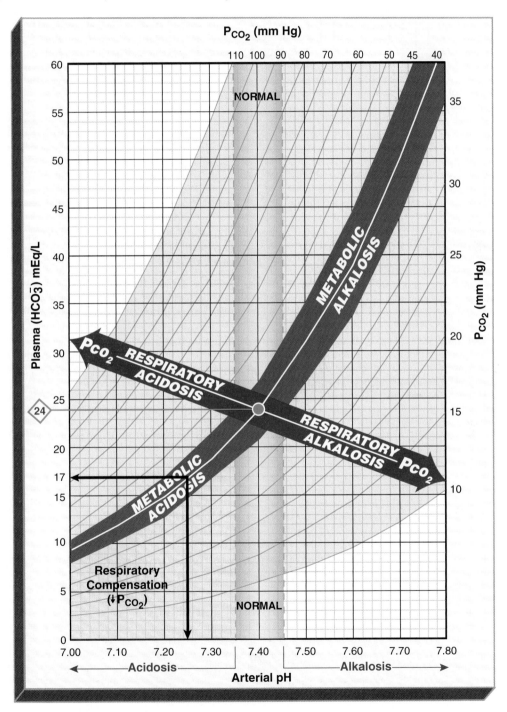

TABLE 7–5
Common Causes of Metabolic Acidosis

Lactic acidosis (fixed acids)	When the oxygen level is inadequate to meet tissue needs, alternate biochemical reactions are activated that do not utilize oxygen. This is known as **anaerobic metabolism** (non–oxygen-utilizing). Lactic acid is the end-product of this process. When these ions move into the blood, the pH decreases. Whenever an acute hypoxemia is present, the presence of lactic acids should be suspected. Lactic acids cause the anion gap to increase.
Ketoacidosis (fixed acids)	When blood insulin is low in the patient with diabetes, serum glucose cannot easily enter the tissue cells for metabolism. This condition activates alternate metabolic processes that produce **ketones** as metabolites. Ketone accumulation in the blood causes ketoacidosis. The absence of glucose because of starvation can also cause ketoacidosis. Ketoacidosis may also be seen in patients with excessive alcohol intake. The presence of ketone acids causes the anion gap to increase.
Salicylate intoxication (aspirin overdose) (fixed acids)	The excessive ingestion of aspirin leads to an increased level of salicylic acids in the blood and metabolic acidosis. Metabolic acidosis caused by salicylate intoxication causes the anion gap to increase.
Renal failure	Renal failure causes the HCO_3^- concentration to decrease and the H^+ concentration to increase. This action leads to metabolic acidosis. Metabolic acidosis caused by renal failure is associated with a normal anion gap.
Uncontrolled diarrhea	Uncontrolled diarrhea causes a loss of HCO_3 and an increased concentration of H^+. This action leads to metabolic acidosis. Metabolic acidosis caused by severe diarrhea is associated with a normal anion gap.

bicarbonate (HCO_3^-) ions. The normal plasma concentrations of these cations and anions are as follows:

Na^+ : 140 mEq/L

Cl^- : 105 mEq/L

HCO_3^- : 24 mEq/L

Mathematically, the anion gap is the calculated difference between the Na^+ ions and the sum of the HCO_3^- and Cl^- ions:

$$\text{Anion gap} = [Na^+] - ([Cl^-] + [HCO_3^-])$$
$$= 140 - (105 + 24)$$
$$= 140 - 129$$
$$= 11 \text{ mEq/L}$$

The normal anion gap range (or the range of the unmeasured ions) is 9 to 14 mEq/L. An anion gap greater than 14 mEq/L represents metabolic acidosis.

An elevated anion gap is most commonly caused by the accumulation of fixed acids (e.g., lactic acids, ketoacids, or salicylate intoxication) in the blood. This is because the H^+ ions that are generated by the fixed acids chemically react with—and are buffered by—the plasma HCO_3^-. This action causes (1) the HCO_3^- concentration to decrease and (2) the anion gap to increase.

Clinically, when the patient presents with both metabolic acidosis and an increased anion gap, the respiratory care practitioner must investigate further to determine the source of the fixed acids. This needs to be done in order to appropriately treat the patient. For example, a metabolic acidosis caused (1) by lactic acids justifies the need for oxygen therapy—to reverse the accumulation of the lactic acids—or (2) by ketone acids justifies the need for insulin—to reverse the accumulation of the ketone acids.

Interestingly, metabolic acidosis caused by an excessive loss of HCO_3^- (e.g., renal disease or severe diarrhea) does not cause the anion gap to increase. This is because, as the HCO_3^- concentration decreases, the Cl^- concentration routinely increases to maintain electroneutrality. In other words, for each HCO_3^- that is lost, a Cl^- anion takes its place (i.e., law of electroneutrality). This action maintains a normal anion gap. Metabolic acidosis caused by a decreased HCO_3^- is often called **hyperchloremic metabolic acidosis**.

To summarize, when metabolic acidosis is accompanied by an increased anion gap, the most likely cause of the acidosis is fixed acids (e.g., lactic acids, ketoacids, or salicylate intoxication). Or, when a metabolic acidosis is seen with a normal anion gap, the most likely cause of the acidosis is an excessive lose of HCO_3^- (e.g., caused by renal disease or severe diarrhea).

Metabolic Acidosis with Respiratory Compensation

Under normal conditions, the immediate compensatory response to metabolic acidosis is an increased ventilatory rate (respiratory compensation). This action causes the Pa_{CO_2} to decline. As the P_{CO_2} decreases, the H^+ concentration decreases and, therefore, works to offset the metabolic acidosis (see Figure 7–9).

As shown in Figure 7–16, when the pH, HCO_3^-, and P_{CO_2} all intersect in the yellow-colored area of the $P_{CO_2}/HCO_3^-/pH$ nomogram, **metabolic acidosis with partial respiratory compensation** is present. In other words, the Pa_{CO_2} has decreased below the normal range, but the pH is still below normal. For example, when the P_{CO_2} is 25 mm Hg, at a time when the pH is 7.30 and the HCO_3^- is 12 mEq/L, metabolic acidosis with partial respiratory compensation is confirmed (see Figure 7–16).

Figure 7–16

When the pH, HCO_3^-, and P_{CO_2} all intersect in the yellow-colored area of the $P_{CO_2}/HCO_3^-/pH$ nomogram, metabolic acidosis with partial respiratory compensation is present. For example, when the P_{CO_2} is 25 mm Hg, at a time when the pH is 7.30 and the HCO_3^- is 12 mEq/L, metabolic acidosis with partial respiratory compensation is confirmed.

Metabolic acidosis with complete respiratory compensation is present when the Pa_{CO_2} decreases enough to move the acidic pH back to the normal range, which, in this case, would be below 20 mm Hg (see Figure 7–16).

Both Metabolic and Respiratory Acidosis

When the pH, HCO_3^-, and P_{CO_2} readings all intersect in the orange-colored area of the P_{CO_2}/HCO_3^-/pH nomogram, **both metabolic and respiratory acidosis** are present (Figure 7–17). For example, if the reported P_{CO_2} is 70 mm Hg, at a time when the pH is 7.10 and the HCO_3^- is 21 mEq/L, both metabolic and respiratory acidosis are present (see Figure 7–17). Both metabolic and respiratory acidosis are commonly seen in patients with acute ventilatory failure, which causes the blood P_{CO_2} to increase (respiratory acidosis) and the Po_2 to decrease (metabolic acidosis—caused by lactic acids).

Metabolic Alkalosis

The presence of other bases, not related to a decreased P_{CO_2} level or renal activity, can also be identified on the P_{CO_2}/HCO_3^-/pH nomogram. Clinically, this condition is called **metabolic alkalosis**. Metabolic alkalosis is present when the P_{CO_2} reading is within the normal range (35 to 45 mm Hg), but not within the red normal blood buffer line when compared to the reported pH and HCO_3^- levels. This is because the pH and HCO_3^- readings are both higher than expected for a normal P_{CO_2} level.

When the reported pH and HCO_3^- levels are both higher than expected for a normal P_{CO_2} level, the P_{CO_2} reading will move up into the purple-colored bar titled METABOLIC ALKALOSIS in Figure 7–18. In other words, the pH, HCO_3^-, and P_{CO_2} readings will all intersect within the purple-colored METABOLIC ALKALOSIS bar. For example, when the reported P_{CO_2} is 40 mm Hg (normal), at a time when the pH is 7.50 and the HCO_3^- is 31 mEq/L, metabolic alkalosis is confirmed (see Figure 7–18). Table 7–6 (page 308) provides common causes of metabolic alkalosis.

Metabolic Alkalosis with Respiratory Compensation

Under normal conditions, the immediate compensatory response to metabolic alkalosis is a decreased ventilatory rate (respiratory compensation). This action causes the Pa_{CO_2} to rise. As the P_{CO_2} increases, the H^+ concentration increases and, therefore, works to offset the metabolic alkalosis (see Figure 7–8).

As shown in Figure 7–19 (page 309), when the pH, HCO_3^-, and P_{CO_2} all intersect in the pink-colored area of the P_{CO_2}/HCO_3^-/pH nomogram, metabolic alkalosis with partial respiratory compensation is present.

Figure 7–17

When the pH, HCO_3^-, and P_{CO_2} readings all intersect in the orange-colored area of the P_{CO_2}/HCO_3^-/pH nomogram, both metabolic and respiratory acidosis are present. For example, if the reported P_{CO_2} is 70 mm Hg, at a time when the pH is 7.10 and the HCO_3^- is 21 mEq/L, both metabolic and respiratory acidosis are present.

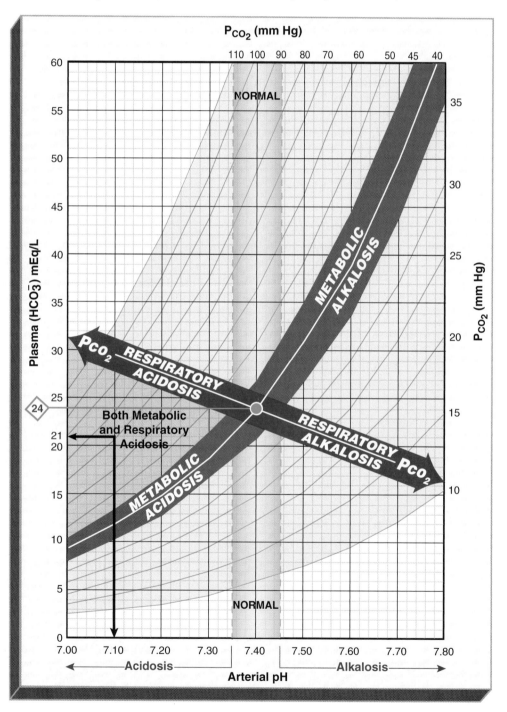

Figure 7–18

When the reported pH and HCO_3^- levels are both higher than expected for a normal P_{CO_2} level, the P_{CO_2} reading will move up into the purple-colored bar titled METABOLIC ALKALOSIS. For example, when the reported P_{CO_2} is 40 mm Hg (normal), at a time when the pH is 7.50 and the HCO_3^- is 31 mEq/L, metabolic alkalosis is confirmed.

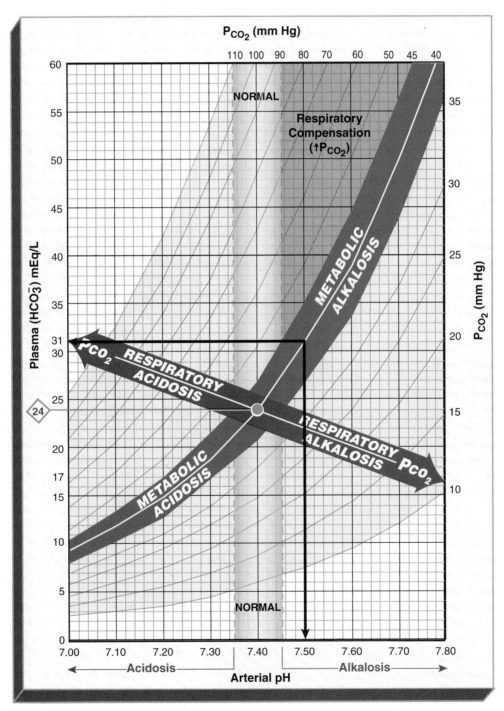

TABLE 7–6
Common Causes of Metabolic Alkalosis

Hypokalemia	The depletion of total body potassium can occur from (1) several days of intravenous therapy without adequate replacement of potassium, (2) diuretic therapy, and (3) diarrhea. Whenever the potassium level is low, the kidneys attempt to conserve potassium by excreting hydrogen ions. This mechanism causes the blood base to increase. In addition, as the potassium level in the blood decreases, intracellular potassium moves into the extracellular space in an effort to offset the reduced potassium level in the blood serum. As the potassium (K^+) cation leaves the cell, however, a hydrogen cation (H^+) enters the cell. This mechanism causes the blood serum to become more alkalotic. Patients with hypokalemia frequently demonstrate the clinical triad of (1) metabolic alkalosis, (2) muscular weakness, and (3) cardiac dysrhythmia.
Hypochloremia	When the chloride ion (Cl^-) concentration decreases, bicarbonate ions increase in an attempt to maintain a normal cation balance in the blood serum. As the bicarbonate ion increases, the patient's blood serum becomes alkalotic. The kidneys, moreover, usually excrete potassium ions when chloride ions are unavailable, which, as described above, will also contribute to the patient's metabolic alkalosis.
Gastric suction or vomiting	Excessive gastric suction or vomiting causes a loss of hydrochloric acid (HCl) and results in an increase in blood base, that is, metabolic alkalosis.
Excessive administration of corticosteroids	Large doses of sodium-retaining corticosteroids can cause the kidneys to accelerate the excretion of hydrogen ions and potassium. Excessive excretion of either one or both of these ions will cause metabolic alkalosis.
Excessive administration of sodium bicarbonate	If an excessive amount of sodium bicarbonate is administered, metabolic alkalosis will occur. This used to occur frequently during cardiopulmonary resuscitation.
Diuretic therapy	Diuretic therapy can cause increased Cl^- and H^+ excretion and HCO_3^- retention. This condition can lead to metabolic alkalosis.
Hypovolemia	A low blood volume can lead to increased H^+ excretion and metabolic alkalosis.

In other words, the Pa_{CO_2} has increased above the normal range, but the pH is still above normal. For example, when the P_{CO_2} is 60 mm Hg, at a time when the pH is 7.50 and the HCO_3^- is 46 mEq/L, metabolic alkalosis with partial respiratory compensation is present (see Figure 7–19).

Metabolic alkalosis with complete respiratory compensation is present when the Pa_{CO_2} increases enough to move the alkalotic pH back to the normal range, which, in this case, would be above 65 to 68 mm Hg (see Figure 7–19).

Figure 7–19

When the pH, HCO_3^-, and P_{CO_2} all intersect in the pink-colored area of the P_{CO_2}/HCO_3^-/pH nomogram, metabolic alkalosis with partial respiratory compensation is present. For example, when the P_{CO_2} is 60 mm Hg, at a time when the pH is 7.50 and the HCO_3^- is 46 mEq/L, metabolic alkalosis with partial respiratory compensation is present.

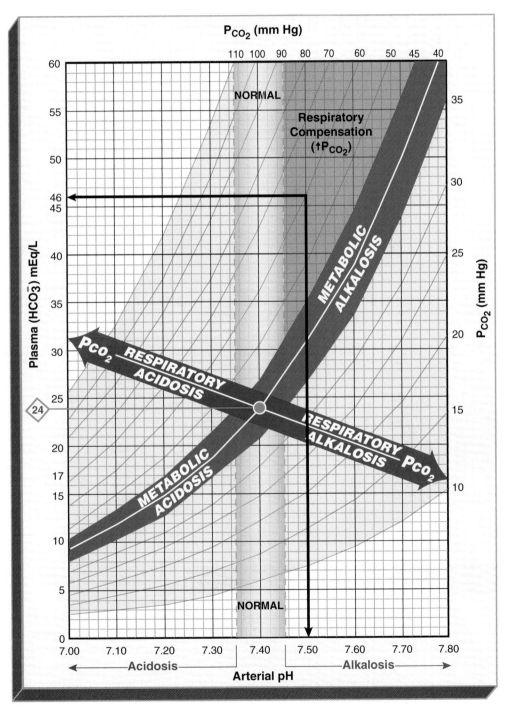

Both Metabolic and Respiratory Alkalosis

When the pH, HCO_3^-, and P_{CO_2} readings all intersect in the blue-colored area of the $P_{CO_2}/HCO_3^-/pH$ nomogram, **both metabolic and respiratory alkalosis** are present (Figure 7–20). For example, if the reported P_{CO_2} is 25 mm Hg, at a time when pH is 7.62 and the HCO_3^- is 25 mEq/L, both metabolic and respiratory alkalosis are present (see Figure 7–20).

Base Excess/Deficit

The $P_{CO_2}/HCO_3^-/pH$ nomogram also serves as an excellent tool to calculate the patient's total **base excess/deficit**. By knowing the base excess/deficit, nonrespiratory acid-base imbalances can be quantified. The base excess/deficit is reported in milliequivalents per liter (mEq/L) of base above or below the normal buffer base line of the $P_{CO_2}/HCO_3^-/pH$ nomogram.

For example, if the pH is 7.25, and the HCO_3^- is 17 mEq/L, at a time when the Pa_{CO_2} is 40 mm Hg, the $P_{CO_2}/HCO_3^-/pH$ nomogram will confirm the presence of (1) metabolic acidosis and (2) a base excess of -7 mEq/L (more properly called a base deficit of 7 mEq/L) (see Figure 7–15). Metabolic acidosis may be treated by the careful intravenous infusion of sodium bicarbonate ($NaHCO_3$).

In contrast, if the pH is 7.50, and the HCO_3^- is 31 mEq/L, at a time when the Pa_{CO_2} is 40 mm Hg, the $P_{CO_2}/HCO_3^-/pH$ nomogram will verify the presence of (1) metabolic alkalosis and (2) a base excess of 7 mEq/L (see Figure 7–18). Metabolic alkalosis is treated by (1) correcting the underlying electrolyte problem (e.g., hypokalemia or hypochloremia) or (2) administering ammonium chloride (NH_4Cl).

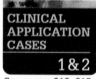

CLINICAL
APPLICATION
CASES
1 & 2

See pages 312–315

Example of Clinical Use of $P_{CO_2}/HCO_3^-/pH$ Nomogram

It has been shown that the $P_{CO_2}/HCO_3^-/pH$ nomogram is an excellent clinical tool to confirm the presence of (1) respiratory acid-base imbalances, (2) metabolic acid-base imbalances, or (3) a combination of a respiratory and metabolic acid-base imbalances. The clinical application cases at the end of this chapter further demonstrate the clinical usefulness of the $P_{CO_2}/HCO_3^-/pH$ nomogram.

CHAPTER SUMMARY

An understanding of carbon dioxide transport is also a fundamental cornerstone to the study of pulmonary physiology and the clinical interpretation of arterial blood gases. Essential components are (1) the transport of carbon dioxide from the tissues to the lungs, including the three ways in which carbon dioxide is transported in the plasma and three ways in the

Figure 7–20
When the pH, HCO_3^-, and P_{CO_2} readings all intersect in the blue-colored area of the $P_{CO_2}/HCO_3^-/pH$ nomogram, both metabolic and respiratory alkalosis are present. For example, if the reported P_{CO_2} is 25 mm Hg, at a time when pH is 7.62 and the HCO_3^- is 25 mEq/L, both metabolic and respiratory alkalosis are present.

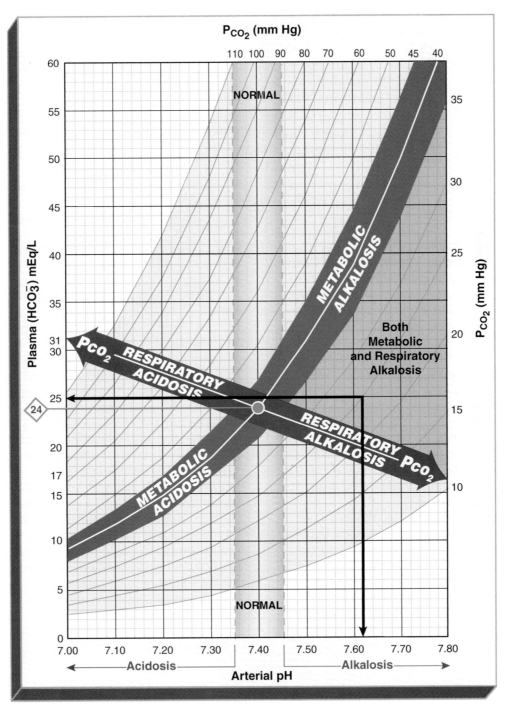

red blood cells, and how the carbon dioxide dissociation curves differ from the oxygen dissociation curve; (2) acid-base balance and regulation, including the three major buffer systems; (3) the $P_{CO_2}/HCO_3^-/pH$ relationship in respiratory acid-base imbalances, including acute ventilatory failure, chronic ventilatory failure and renal compensation, and the common causes of acute ventilatory failure; acute alveolar hyperventilation, chronic alveolar hyperventilation and renal compensation, and common causes of acute alveolar hyperventilation; (4) the $P_{CO_2}/HCO_3^-/pH$ relationship in metabolic acid-base imbalances, including metabolic acidosis, common causes of metabolic acidosis, metabolic acidosis with respiratory compensation, and both metabolic and respiratory acidosis; metabolic alkalosis, common causes of metabolic alkalosis, metabolic alkalosis with respiratory compensation, and both metabolic and respiratory alkalosis, and (5) an understanding of base excess/deficit.

1 CLINICAL APPLICATION CASE

A 36-year-old man, who had been working on his car in the garage while the motor was running, suddenly experienced confusion, disorientation, and nausea. A few minutes later he started to vomit. He called out to his wife, who was nearby. Moments later he collapsed and lost consciousness. His wife called 911. Eleven minutes later, the emergency medical team (EMT) arrived, quickly assessed the patient's condition, placed a nonrebreathing oxygen mask on the patient's face, and then transported him to the ambulance. En route to the hospital, the EMT reported that the patient continued to vomit intermittently. Because of this, the patient was frequently suctioned orally to prevent aspiration.

In the emergency department, the patient's skin was cherry red. Although he was still unconscious, he was breathing on his own through a nonrebreathing oxygen mask. A medical student assigned to the emergency department stated that it appeared that the patient was being overoxygenated—because his skin appeared cherry red—and that perhaps the oxygen

mask should be removed. The respiratory therapist working with the patient strongly disagreed.

The patient's vital signs were blood pressure—165/105 mm Hg, heart rate—122 beats/min, and respirations—36 breaths/min. His arterial blood gas values on the nonrebreathing oxygen mask were pH—7.55, Pa_{CO_2}—25 mm Hg, HCO_3^-—21 mEq/L, and Pa_{O_2}—539 mm Hg. His carboxyhemoglobin level (CO_{Hb}) was 47 percent.

The patient was transferred to the intensive care unit, where he continued to be monitored closely. Although the patient never required mechanical ventilation, he continued to receive high concentrations of oxygen for the first 48 hours. By the end of the third day he was breathing room air and was conscious and able to talk with his family and the medical staff. His vital signs were blood pressure—117/77 mm Hg, heart rate—68 beats/min, and respirations—12 breaths/min. His arterial blood gas values were pH—7.4, Pa_{CO_2}—40 mm Hg, HCO_3^-—24 mEq/L, and Pa_{O_2}—97 mm Hg. His carboxyhemoglobin level (CO_{Hb}) was

(continues)

3 percent. The patient was discharged on the fourth day.

DISCUSSION

This case illustrates (1) how clinical signs and symptoms can sometimes be very misleading, and (2) how the $P_{CO_2}/HCO_3^-/pH$ nomogram can be used to determine the cause of certain findings on arterial blood gas analysis. Even though the patient's Pa_{O_2} was very high (because of the nonrebreathing oxygen mask), the CO_{Hb} level of 47 percent had seriously impaired the patient's hemoglobin's ability to carry oxygen (see Figure 3–9). In addition, any oxygen that was being carried by the hemoglobin was unable to detach itself easily from the hemoglobin. This was because CO_{Hb} causes the oxygen dissociation curve to shift to the left (see Figure 6–4).

Thus, despite the fact that the patient's Pa_{O_2} was very high (539 mm Hg) in the emergency department, the patient's oxygen delivery system—and tissue oxygenation—was in fact very low and seriously compromised. The "cherry red" skin color noted by the medical student was a classic sign of carbon monoxide poisoning and not a sign of good skin color and oxygenation. The increased blood pressure, heart rate, and respiratory rate seen in the emergency department were compensatory mechanisms activated to counteract the decreased arterial oxygenation, that is, these mechanisms increased the total oxygen delivery (see D_{O_2} in Table 6–10).

Because it was reported that the patient had vomited excessively prior to the arterial blood gas sample being obtained in the emergency department, it was not readily apparent whether the high pH was a result of (1) the low Pa_{CO_2} caused by the acute alveolar hyperventilation (which was caused by the low oxygen delivery), or (2) a combination of both the acute alveolar hyperventilation and low Pa_{CO_2} and the loss of stomach acids (caused by the vomiting). The answer to this question can be obtained by using the $P_{CO_2}/HCO_3^-/pH$ nomogram. In this case, when the pH, Pa_{CO_2}, and HCO_3^- values are applied to the $P_{CO_2}/HCO_3^-/pH$ nomogram, it can be seen that the elevated pH was due solely to the decreased Pa_{CO_2} level, because all three variables cross through the normal buffer line (see Figure 7–13).*

See Appendix VI for a credit-card size $P_{CO_2}/HCO_3^-/pH$ nomogram that can be copied and laminated for use as a handy clinical reference tool.

---

2 CLINICAL APPLICATION CASE

During a routine physical examination, a 67-year-old man had a cardiac arrest while performing a stress test in the pulmonary rehabilitation department. The patient had a long history of chronic bronchitis and emphysema. Although the patient had been in reasonably good health for the past 3 years, he had recently complained to his family physician of shortness of breath and heart palpitations. His physician ordered a full diagnostic evaluation of the patient, which included a complete pulmonary function study and stress test.

During the interview, the patient reported that he had not performed any form of exercise in years. In fact, he jokingly stated that whenever he would start to feel as if he should start to exercise, he would

(continues)

quickly sit down and the feeling would go away. The patient was about 35 pounds overweight and, during the stress test, appeared moderately ashen and diaphoretic. When the patient collapsed, a "Code Blue" was called and cardiopulmonary resuscitation was started immediately. When the Code Blue Team arrived, the patient had an oral airway in place and was being manually ventilated, with room air only, using a face mask and bag.

An intravenous infusion was started and the patient's heart activity was monitored with an electrocardiogram (ECG). An arterial blood gas sample was obtained and showed a pH of 7.10, Pa_{CO_2}—70 mm Hg, HCO_3^-—21 mEq/L, Pa_{O_2}—38 mm Hg, and Sa_{O_2}—50 percent. Upon seeing these results, the physician evaluated the patient's chest and breath sounds. It was quickly established that the patient's head was not hyperextended appropriately (which, as a result, impeded air flow through the oral and laryngeal airways). The patient's breath sounds were very diminished, and it was also noted that the patient's chest did not rise appropriately during each manual resuscitation. The patient was immediately intubated and manually ventilated with a bag and mask with an inspired oxygen concentration (FI_{O_2}) of 1.0. Despite the fact that the patient's pH was only 7.10 at this time, no sodium bicarbonate was administered.

Immediately after the patient was intubated, breath sounds could be heard bilaterally. Additionally, the patient's chest could be seen to move upward during each manual ventilation, and his skin started to turn pink. Another arterial blood sample was then drawn. While waiting for the arterial blood gas analysis results, epinephrine and norepinephrine were administered. Moments later, normal ventricular activity was seen. The arterial blood gas values from the second sample

were pH—7.44, Pa_{CO_2}—35 mm Hg, HCO_3^-—24 mEq/L, Pa_{O_2}—360 mm Hg, and Sa_{O_2}—98 percent. Thirty minutes later, the patient was breathing spontaneously on an (FI_{O_2}) of 0.4, and he was conscious and alert. Two hours later, it was determined that the patient would not require mechanical ventilation and he was extubated. The patient was discharged from the hospital on the fourth day.

DISCUSSION

This case illustrates how the $P_{CO_2}/HCO_3^-/pH$ nomogram can be used to (1) confirm both a respiratory and metabolic acidosis and (2) prevent the unnecessary administration of sodium bicarbonate during an emergency situation. As a result of the cardiopulmonary arrest, the patient's Pa_{CO_2} rapidly increased while, at the same time, his pH and Pa_{O_2} decreased. Because the patient's head was not positioned correctly, the lungs were not ventilated adequately. As a result, the Pa_{CO_2}, pH, and Pa_{O_2} continued to deteriorate. Fortunately, this was discovered when the first arterial blood gas values were seen.

The fact that the initial pH (7.10) and HCO_3^- (21 mEq/L) were both lower than expected for an acute increase in the Pa_{CO_2} (70 mm Hg) suggested that there were additional acids present in the patient's blood (i.e., acids other than those produced by the increased Pa_{CO_2}). According to the $P_{CO_2}/HCO_3^-/pH$ nomogram, an acute increase in the patient's Pa_{CO_2} to 70 mm Hg should have caused the pH to fall to about 7.22 and the HCO_3^- level should have increased to about 28 mEq/L (see Figure 7–11). In this case, both the pH and HCO_3^- were lower than expected. According to the $P_{CO_2}/HCO_3^-/pH$ nomogram, the patient had both a respiratory and metabolic acidosis (see Figure 7–17). In this case, the most likely cause of the metabolic acidosis was the low

(continues)

Pa_{O_2} (38 mm Hg), which produces lactic acids (see Table 7–5).

The fact that the $P_{CO_2}/HCO_3^-/pH$ nomogram confirmed that the cause of the patient's lower than expected pH and HCO_3^- levels were solely due to the poor ventilation eliminated the need to administer sodium bicarbonate. In other words, because the patient's head was not positioned correctly, the patient's lungs were not being ventilated. This condition, in turn, caused the patient's Pa_{CO_2} to increase (which caused the pH to fall) and the Pa_{O_2} to decrease (which produced lactic acids and caused the pH to fall even further). In this case, therefore, the treatment of choice was to correct the cause of the respiratory and metabolic acidosis. Because the cause of the respiratory and metabolic acidosis was inadequate ventilation, the treatment of choice was aggressive ventilation.

Finally, as shown by the second arterial blood gas analysis, the arterial blood gases were rapidly corrected after intubation. In fact, the patient's Pa_{O_2} was overcorrected (360 mm Hg). The patient's inspired oxygen concentration ($F_{I_{O_2}}$) was subsequently reduced. If sodium bicarbonate had been administered to correct the patient's pH of 7.10 before the patient was appropriately ventilated, the pH and HCO_3^- readings would have been higher than normal after his Pa_{CO_2} was ventilated down from 70 mm Hg to his normal level of about 40 mm Hg.

REVIEW QUESTIONS

1. During acute alveolar hypoventilation, the blood
   - I. H_2CO_3 increases
   - II. pH increases
   - III. HCO_3^- increases
   - IV. P_{CO_2} increases
     - A. II only
     - B. IV only
     - C. II and III only
     - D. I, III, and IV only

2. The bulk of the CO_2 produced in the cells is transported to the lungs as
   - A. H_2CO_3
   - B. HCO_3^-
   - C. CO_2 and H_2O
   - D. Carbonic anhydrase

3. During acute alveolar hyperventilation, the blood
   - I. P_{CO_2} increases
   - II. H_2CO_3 decreases
   - III. HCO_3^- increases
   - IV. pH decreases
     - A. II only
     - B. IV only
     - C. I and III only
     - D. II and IV only

4. In chronic hypoventilation, renal compensation has likely occurred when the
   I. HCO_3^- is higher than expected for a particular P_{CO_2}
   II. pH is lower than expected for a particular P_{CO_2}
   III. HCO_3^- is lower than expected for a particular P_{CO_2}
   IV. pH is higher than expected for a particular P_{CO_2}
      A. I only
      B. II only
      C. I and IV only
      D. III and IV only

5. When metabolic acidosis is present, the patient's blood
   I. HCO_3^- is higher than expected for a particular P_{CO_2}
   II. pH is lower than expected for a particular P_{CO_2}
   III. HCO_3^- is lower than expected for a particular P_{CO_2}
   IV. pH is higher than expected for a particular P_{CO_2}
      A. I only
      B. II only
      C. III and IV only
      D. II and III only

6. Ketoacidosis can develop from
   I. an inadequate oxygen level
   II. renal failure
   III. an inadequate serum insulin level
   IV. anaerobic metabolism
   V. an inadequate serum glucose level
      A. I only
      B. II and III only
      C. IV and V only
      D. III and V only

7. Metabolic alkalosis can develop from
   I. hyperchloremia
   II. hypokalemia
   III. hypochloremia
   IV. hyperkalemia
      A. I only
      B. IV only
      C. I and III only
      D. II and III only

8. Which of the following HCO_3^- to H_2CO_3 ratios represent(s) an acidic pH?
   I. 18:1
   II. 28:1
   III. 12:1
   IV. 22:1
      A. I only
      B. II only
      C. III only
      D. I and III only

9. If a patient has a P_{CO_2} level of 70 mm Hg, what is the H_2CO_3 concentration?
    A. 1.3 mEq/L
    B. 1.5 mEq/L
    C. 1.7 mEq/L
    D. 2.1 mEq/L

10. The value of the pK in the Henderson-Hasselbalch equation is
    A. 1.0
    B. 6.1
    C. 7.4
    D. 20.1

11. Metabolic acidosis caused by a decreased HCO_3^- is often called
    A. hyperchloremic metabolic acidosis
    B. ketoacidosis
    C. hypokalemia
    D. lactic acidosis

12. Metabolic acidosis caused by fixed acids is present when the anion gap is greater than
    A. 9 mEq/L
    B. 14 mEq/L
    C. 20 mEq/L
    D. 25 mEq/L

13. What is the anion gap in the patient with the following clinical data?

    Na^+ 128 mEq/L

    Cl^- 97 mEq/L

    HCO_3^- 22 mEq/L

    Answer: _____

14. According to the P_{CO_2}/HCO_3^-/pH nomogram shown in Figure 7–21, if the reported P_{CO_2} is 55 mm Hg, at a time when the pH is 7.14 and the HCO_3^- is 18 mEq/L, what acid-base balance disturbance would be present?

    Answer: _____

15. According to the P_{CO_2}/HCO_3^-/pH nomogram shown in Figure 7–21, if the reported P_{CO_2} is 20 mm Hg, at a time when the pH is 7.51 and the HCO_3^- is 16 mEq/L, what acid-base balance disturbance is present?

    Answer: _____

Figure 7–21
Nomogram of P_{CO_2}/HCO_3^-/pH relationship.

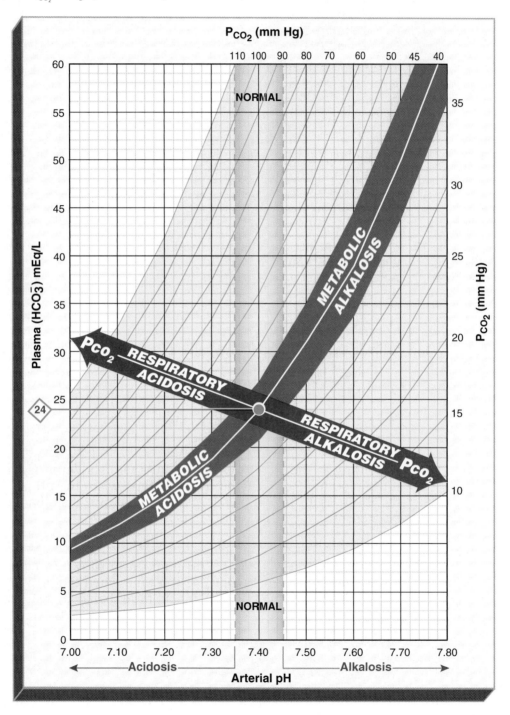

CLINICAL APPLICATION QUESTIONS

CASE 1

1. In the emergency department, even though the patient's Pa_{O_2} was very high (539 mm Hg), the CO_{Hb} level of 47 percent (enhanced _____; impaired _____) the hemoglobin's ability to carry oxygen.

2. CO_{Hb} causes the oxygen dissociation curve to shift to the _____.

3. A classic sign of carbon monoxide (CO) poisoning is a skin color that is described as _____.

4. The increased blood pressure, heart rate, and respiratory rate seen in the emergency department were compensatory mechanisms activated to counteract the decreased arterial oxygenation. These mechanisms _____

_____.

5. Initially, it was not clear why the patient's pH was so high. What were the two possible causes for the elevated pH?

   A. _____

   B. _____

6. The P_{CO_2}/HCO_3^-/pH nomogram verified that the sole cause of the elevated pH was due to the _____.

CASE 2

1. The fact that the initial pH (7.10) and HCO_3^- (21 mEq/L) were both lower than expected for an acute increase in the Pa_{CO_2} (70 mm Hg) suggested that there were additional _____ present in the patient's blood.

2. In this case, the most likely cause of the metabolic acidosis was the _____.

3. What was the treatment of choice in this case?

   Answer: _____

4. If sodium bicarbonate had initially been administered to correct the patient's low pH level, the pH and HCO_3^- readings would have been _____ than normal after the Pa_{CO_2} had been lowered to the patient's normal level.

CHAPTER 8

Ventilation-Perfusion Relationships

O B J E C T I V E S

By the end of this chapter, the student should be able to:

1. Define *ventilation-perfusion ratio.*
2. Describe the overall ventilation-perfusion ratio in the normal upright lung.
3. Explain how the ventilation-perfusion ratio progressively changes from the upper to the lower lung regions in the normal upright lung.
4. Describe how an increased and decreased ventilation-perfusion ratio affects *alveolar gases.*
5. Describe how the ventilation-perfusion ratio affects *end-capillary gases* and the *pH level.*
6. Define
   —Respiratory quotient
   —Respiratory exchange ratio
7. Identify respiratory disorders that *increase* the ventilation-perfusion ratio.
8. Identify respiratory disorders that *decrease* the ventilation-perfusion ratio.
9. Complete the review questions at the end of this chapter.

VENTILATION-PERFUSION RATIO

Ideally, each alveolus in the lungs should receive the same amount of ventilation and pulmonary capillary blood flow. In reality, however, this is not the case. Overall, alveolar ventilation is normally about 4 L/min and pulmonary capillary blood flow is about 5 L/min, making the average overall ratio of ventilation to blood flow 4:5, or 0.8. This relationship is called the **ventilation-perfusion ratio** ($\dot{V}/\dot{Q}$ ratio) (Figure 8–1).

Although the overall $\dot{V}/\dot{Q}$ ratio is about 0.8, the ratio varies markedly throughout the lung. In the normal individual in the upright position, the alveoli in the upper portions of the lungs (apices) receive a moderate amount of ventilation and little blood flow. As a result, the $\dot{V}/\dot{Q}$ ratio in the upper lung region is higher than 0.8.

In the lower regions of the lung, however, alveolar ventilation is moderately increased and blood flow is greatly increased, because blood

Figure 8–1
The normal ventilation-perfusion ratio ($\dot{V}/\dot{Q}$ ratio) is about 0.8.

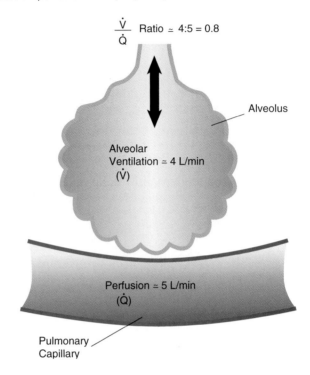

$\frac{\dot{V}}{\dot{Q}}$ Ratio ≈ 4:5 = 0.8

Alveolus

Alveolar
Ventilation ≈ 4 L/min
($\dot{V}$)

Perfusion ≈ 5 L/min
($\dot{Q}$)

Pulmonary
Capillary

flow is gravity dependent. As a result, the $\dot{V}/\dot{Q}$ ratio is lower than 0.8. Thus, the $\dot{V}/\dot{Q}$ ratio progressively decreases from top to bottom in the upright lung, and the average $\dot{V}/\dot{Q}$ ratio is about 0.8 (Figure 8–2).

How the Ventilation-Perfusion Ratio Affects the Alveolar Gases

The $\dot{V}/\dot{Q}$ ratio profoundly affects the oxygen and carbon dioxide pressures in the alveoli ($P_{A_{O_2}}$ and $P_{A_{CO_2}}$). Although the normal $P_{A_{O_2}}$ and $P_{A_{CO_2}}$ are typically about 100 and 40 mm Hg, respectively, this is not the case throughout most of the alveolar units. These figures merely represent an average.

The $P_{A_{O_2}}$ is determined by the balance between (1) the amount of oxygen entering the alveoli and (2) its removal by capillary blood flow. The $P_{A_{CO_2}}$, on the other hand, is determined by the balance between (1) the amount of carbon dioxide that diffuses into the alveoli from the capillary blood and (2) its removal from the alveoli by means of ventilation. Changing $\dot{V}/\dot{Q}$ ratios alter the $P_{A_{O_2}}$ and $P_{A_{CO_2}}$ levels for the reasons discussed in the following subsections.

Figure 8–2
In the upright lung, the $\dot{V}/\dot{Q}$ ratio progressively decreases from the apex to the base. Note, however, that although the $\dot{V}/\dot{Q}$ ratio in the lung bases is lower than $\dot{V}/\dot{Q}$ ratio in the lung apices, the absolute amounts of ventilation and perfusion are greatest in the lung bases of the upright lung.

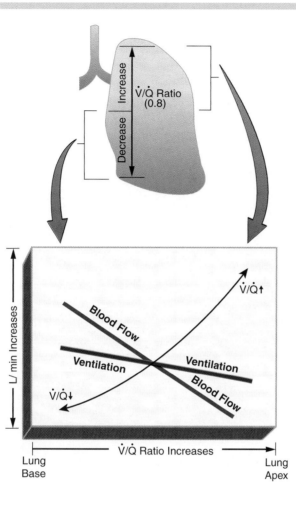

CLINICAL
APPLICATION
CASE

1

See page 331

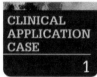

Increased $\dot{V}/\dot{Q}$ Ratio

An increased $\dot{V}/\dot{Q}$ ratio can develop from either (1) an increase in ventilation or (2) a decrease in perfusion. When the $\dot{V}/\dot{Q}$ ratio increases, the $P_{A_{O_2}}$ rises and the $P_{A_{CO_2}}$ falls. The $P_{A_{CO_2}}$ decreases because it is washed out of the alveoli faster than it is replaced by the venous blood. The $P_{A_{O_2}}$ increases because it does not diffuse into the blood* as fast as it enters (or is ventilated into) the alveolus (Figure 8–3). The $P_{A_{O_2}}$ also increases because the $P_{A_{CO_2}}$ decreases and, therefore, allows the $P_{A_{O_2}}$ to move closer to the partial pressure of atmospheric oxygen, which is about 159 mm Hg at sea level (see Table 3–2).† This $\dot{V}/\dot{Q}$ relationship is present in the upper segments of the upright lung (see Figure 8–2).

*See how oxygen can be classified as either perfusion or diffusion limited, in Chapter 3.
†See "Ideal Alveolar Gas Equation" section in Chapter 3.

Figure 8–3
When the $\dot{V}/\dot{Q}$ ratio is high, the alveolar oxygen pressure ($P_{A_{O_2}}$) increases and the alveolar carbon dioxide pressure ($P_{A_{CO_2}}$) decreases.

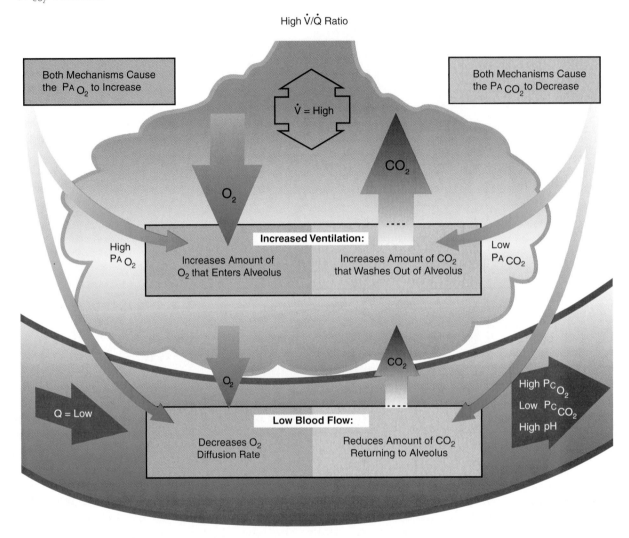

High $\dot{V}/\dot{Q}$ Ratio

Decreased $\dot{V}/\dot{Q}$ Ratio

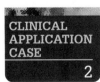

CLINICAL
APPLICATION
CASE

2

See page 332

A decreased $\dot{V}/\dot{Q}$ ratio can develop from either (1) a decrease in ventilation or (2) an increase in perfusion. When the $\dot{V}/\dot{Q}$ ratio decreases, the $P_{A_{O_2}}$ falls and the $P_{A_{CO_2}}$ rises. The $P_{A_{O_2}}$ decreases because oxygen moves out of the alveolus and into the pulmonary capillary blood faster than it is replenished by ventilation. The $P_{A_{CO_2}}$ increases because it moves out of the capillary blood and into the alveolus faster than it is washed out of the alveolus (Figure 8–4). This $\dot{V}/\dot{Q}$ is present in the lower segments of the upright lung (see Figure 8–2).

Figure 8–4

When the $\dot{V}/\dot{Q}$ ratio is low, the alveolar oxygen pressure ($P_{A_{O_2}}$) decreases and the alveolar carbon dioxide pressure ($P_{A_{CO_2}}$) increases.

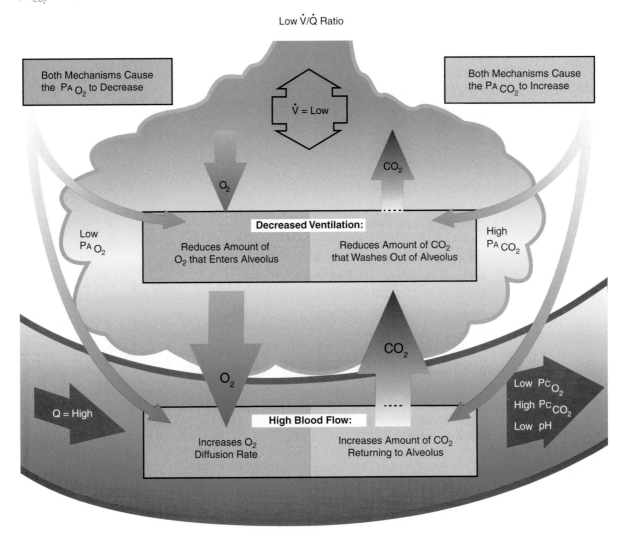

O_2–CO_2 Diagram

The effect of changing $\dot{V}/\dot{Q}$ ratios on the $P_{A_{O_2}}$ and $P_{A_{CO_2}}$ levels is summarized in the O_2–CO_2 diagram (Figure 8–5). The lines in the chart represent all the possible alveolar gas compositions as the $\dot{V}/\dot{Q}$ ratio decreases or increases. The O_2–CO_2 diagram (nomogram) shows that in the upper lung regions, the $\dot{V}/\dot{Q}$ ratio is high, the $P_{A_{O_2}}$ is increasing, and the $P_{A_{CO_2}}$ is decreasing. In contrast, the diagram shows that in the lower lung regions, the $\dot{V}/\dot{Q}$ ratio is low, the $P_{A_{O_2}}$ is decreasing, and the $P_{A_{CO_2}}$ is increasing.

Figure 8–5

The O_2–CO_2 diagram.

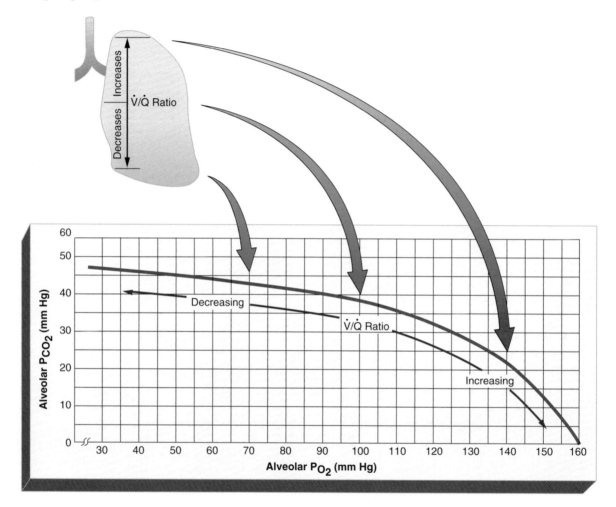

How the Ventilation-Perfusion Ratio Affects the End-Capillary Gases

The oxygen and carbon dioxide pressures in the end-capillary blood (Pc_{O_2} and Pc_{CO_2}) mirror the PA_{O_2} and PA_{CO_2} changes that occur in the lungs. Thus, as the $\dot{V}/\dot{Q}$ ratio progressively decreases from the top to the bottom of the upright lung, causing the PA_{O_2} to decrease and the PA_{CO_2} to increase, the Pc_{O_2} and Pc_{CO_2} also decrease and increase, respectively (see Figures 8–3 and 8–4).

Downstream, in the pulmonary veins, the different Pc_{O_2} and Pc_{CO_2} levels are mixed and, under normal circumstances, produce a P_{O_2} of 100 mm Hg and a Pc_{O_2} of 40 mm Hg (Figure 8–6). The result of the Pc_{O_2} and Pc_{CO_2}

Figure 8–6
The mixing of pulmonary capillary blood gases (Pc_{O_2} and Pc_{CO_2}) from the upper and lower lung regions.

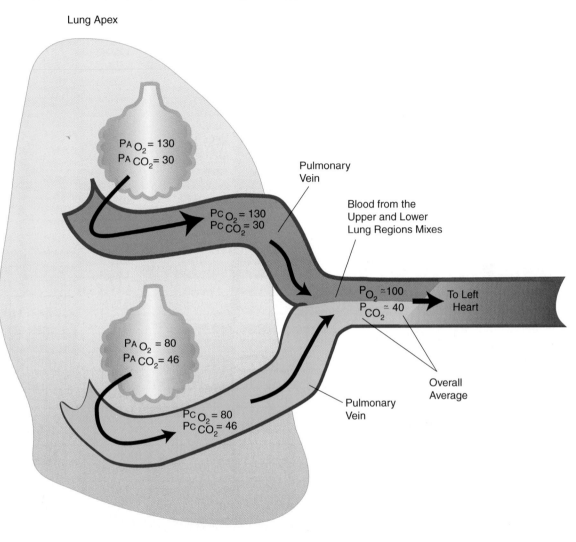

mixture that occurs in the pulmonary veins is reflected downstream in the Pa_{O_2} and Pa_{CO_2} of an arterial blood gas sample (see Table 6–1).

Note also that as the PA_{CO_2} decreases from the bottom to the top of the lungs, the progressive reduction of the CO_2 level in the end-capillary blood causes the pH to become more alkaline. The overall pH in the pulmonary veins and, subsequently, in the arterial blood is normally about 7.35 to 7.45 (see Table 6–1).

Figure 8–7 summarizes the important effects of changing $\dot{V}/\dot{Q}$ ratios.

Figure 8–7

How changes in the $\dot{V}/\dot{Q}$ ratio affect the $P_{A_{O_2}}$ and $P_{c_{O_2}}$, the $P_{A_{CO_2}}$ and $P_{c_{CO_2}}$, and the pH of pulmonary blood.

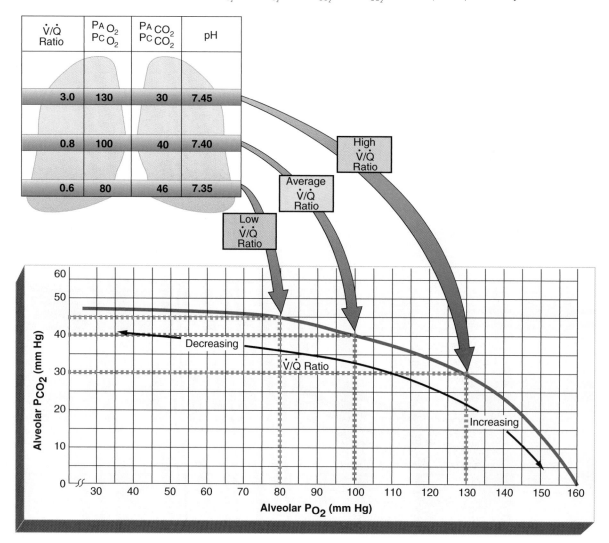

Respiratory Quotient

Gas exchange between the systemic capillaries and the cells is called **internal respiration**. Under normal circumstances, about 250 mL of oxygen are consumed by the tissues during 1 minute. In exchange, the cells produce about 200 mL of carbon dioxide. Clinically, the ratio between the volume of oxygen consumed ($\dot{V}_{O_2}$) and the volume of carbon dioxide produced ($\dot{V}_{CO_2}$) is called the **respiratory quotient** (RQ) and is expressed as follows:

$$RQ = \frac{\dot{V}_{CO_2}}{\dot{V}_{O_2}}$$

$$= \frac{200 \text{ mL } CO_2/\text{min}}{250 \text{ mL } O_2/\text{min}}$$

$$= 0.8$$

Respiratory Exchange Ratio

Gas exchange between the pulmonary capillaries and the alveoli is called **external respiration**, because this gas exchange is between the body and the external environment. The quantity of oxygen and carbon dioxide exchanged during a period of 1 minute is called the **respiratory exchange ratio** (RR). Under normal conditions, the RR equals the RQ.

How Respiratory Disorders Affect the $\dot{V}/\dot{Q}$ Ratio

In respiratory disorders, the $\dot{V}/\dot{Q}$ ratio is always altered. For example, in disorders that diminish pulmonary perfusion, the affected lung area receives little or no blood flow in relation to ventilation. This condition causes the $\dot{V}/\dot{Q}$ ratio to increase. As a result, a larger portion of the alveolar ventilation will not be physiologically effective and is said to be **wasted** or **dead space ventilation**. When the $\dot{V}/\dot{Q}$ ratio increases, the $P_{A_{O_2}}$ increases and the $P_{A_{CO_2}}$ decreases. Pulmonary disorders that increase the $\dot{V}/\dot{Q}$ ratio include:

- Pulmonary emboli
- Partial or complete obstruction in the pulmonary artery or some of the arterioles (e.g., atherosclerosis, collagen disease)
- Extrinsic pressure on the pulmonary vessels (e.g., pneumothorax, hydrothorax, presence of tumor)
- Destruction of the pulmonary vessels (e.g., emphysema)
- Decreased cardiac output.

In disorders that diminish pulmonary ventilation, the affected lung area receives little or no ventilation in relation to blood flow. This condition causes the $\dot{V}/\dot{Q}$ ratio to decrease. As a result, a larger portion of the pulmonary blood flow will not be physiologically effective in terms of gas exchange, and is said to be **shunted blood**. When the $\dot{V}/\dot{Q}$ ratio decreases, the $P_{A_{O_2}}$ decreases and the $P_{A_{CO_2}}$ increases. Pulmonary disorders that decrease the $\dot{V}/\dot{Q}$ ratio include:

- Obstructive lung disorders (e.g., emphysema, bronchitis, asthma)
- Restrictive lung disorders (e.g., pneumonia, silicosis, pulmonary fibrosis)
- Hypoventilation from any cause.

Figure 8–8 summarizes the O_2–CO_2 effects of changing $\dot{V}/\dot{Q}$ ratios in response to respiratory disorders.

Figure 8–8

Alveolar O_2 and CO_2 pressure changes that occur as a result of $\dot{V}/\dot{Q}$ ratio changes caused by respiratory disorders: **(A)** shunt unit; **(B)** normal unit; **(C)** dead space unit.

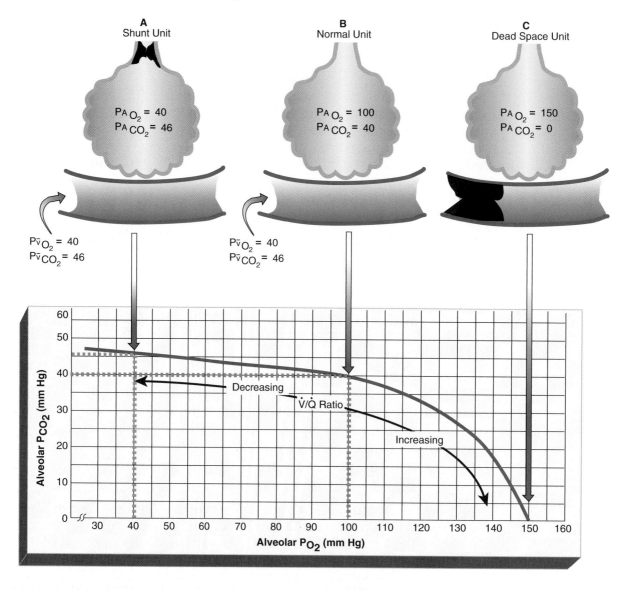

CHAPTER SUMMARY

This chapter discusses how the ventilation-perfusion $\dot{V}/\dot{Q}$ ratio can profoundly affect alveolar oxygen ($P_{A_{O_2}}$) and carbon dioxide pressures ($P_{A_{CO_2}}$). Essential components associated with this topic include (1) how the $\dot{V}/\dot{Q}$ ratio changes from the upper to lower lung regions in the normal upright lung, and (2) how an increased and decreased $\dot{V}/\dot{Q}$ ratio affects the alveolar gases and end-capillary gases and pH level. Related topics include the respiratory quotient and respiratory exchange ratio, and respiratory disorders that increase the $\dot{V}/\dot{Q}$ ratio (e.g., pulmonary emboli, decreased cardiac output) and decrease the $\dot{V}/\dot{Q}$ ratio (e.g., emphysema, bronchitis, pneumonia).

1 CLINICAL APPLICATION CASE

A 34-year-old male construction worker fell from a second-story platform and was impaled by a steel enforcement rod that was protruding vertically about 3 feet from a cement structure. The steel rod entered the side of his lower right abdomen and exited from the left side of the abdomen, about 2 cm below the twelfth rib (see x-ray below). Although the steel rod pierced the side of the descending aorta, no other major organs were seriously damaged.

The man was still conscious when workers cut through the steel rod to free him from the cement structure. While he was being cut free, an emergency medical team (EMT) inserted an intravenous infusion line, placed a nonrebreathing mask over his face, and worked to stop the bleeding as

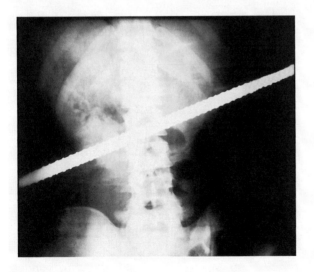

best they could. When the man was finally cut free, he was immediately transported to the trauma center. It was later estimated that he had lost about half of his blood volume at the accident site.

A full trauma team was assembled in the emergency department when the patient arrived. The patient was unconscious and very cyanotic. Even though he still had spontaneous breaths, he had an oral airway in place and was being manually ventilated with an inspired oxygen concentration ($F_{I_{O_2}}$) of 1.0. His blood pressure was 65/40 mm Hg and heart rate was 120 beats/min. The respiratory therapist intubated the patient and continued manual ventilation with an $F_{I_{O_2}}$ of 1.0.

Almost simultaneously a portable x-ray film was taken STAT to aid the trauma surgeons in the removal of the steel rod. A blood specimen was obtained for the following laboratory assays: glucose, BUN (blood urea nitrogen), creatinine, electrolytes, CBC (complete blood cell) count, and a type and screen and blood gas analysis. The emergency department physician called the laboratory to alert lab staff that 10 units of uncrossmatched O negative blood would be needed STAT, and to stay 5 units ahead at all times. The patient was rushed to surgery. The surgical team learned during the operation that the patient's hematocrit was 15.3 percent and his hemoglobin level was 5.1 g%.

(continues)

FOUR HOURS LATER

The patient was in stable condition in the surgical intensive care unit. The steel rod had been successfully removed and his aorta was repaired. Although he was still listed in critical condition, his prognosis was described as good to excellent. At this time, however, the patient was still unconscious because of the drugs administered during surgery. He was on mechanical ventilation with the following settings: tidal volume 900 mL, respirations 12 breaths/min, FI_{O_2} 0.4, continuous positive airway pressure (CPAP) 5 cm H_2O, and a positive end-expiratory pressure (PEEP) of 5 cm H_2O.

His blood pressure was 126/79 mm Hg and heart rate was 78 beats/minute. Arterial blood gas values were pH—7.44, Pa_{CO_2}—36 mm Hg, HCO_3^-—24 mEq/L, and Pa_{O_2}—136 mm Hg. Oxygen saturation measured by pulse oximeter (Sp_{O_2}) was 98 percent. His hematocrit was 44 percent and hemoglobin level was 14.6 g%. The patient's recovery progressed very well. Two days later he was conscious and no longer on the ventilator. He was discharged 6 days later.

DISCUSSION

This case illustrates an increased ventilation-perfusion ratio caused by an excessive amount of blood lost as a result of trauma (the penetrating steel rod). As the patient continued to lose blood, the blood flow through both of his lungs progressively decreased. As a result, alveolar ventilation progressively became greater than pulmonary blood flow. Thus, the patient's alveolar ventilation was becoming more and more "ineffective" physiologically. In other words, more and more of the patient's alveolar ventilation was becoming *wasted* or *dead space ventilation* (see Figure 2–33). The paradox of this condition is that even though the patient's PA_{O_2} and Pa_{O_2} increased in response to an increased ventilation-perfusion ratio, the actual amount of oxygen being transported decreased because of the reduced blood flow (see Table 6–10). Fortunately, this pathologic process was reversed in surgery.

---

2 CLINICAL APPLICATION CASE

A 4-year-old boy presented in the emergency department in severe respiratory distress. An hour earlier, the patient's mother had brought home some groceries in a large box. After removing the groceries, she noticed a silver quarter in the bottom of the box. She removed the quarter and placed it on the kitchen counter. She then gave the box to her 4-year-old son to play with. Thinking he was occupied for awhile, she went downstairs to the basement with her 10-year-old son to put a load of laundry in the washing machine. Moments later, they heard the youngest child cry.

Thinking that it was not anything serious, the mother asked the older boy to go get his brother. Seconds later, the older boy called to his mother that his brother looked blue and that he had vomited. The mother quickly went upstairs to the kitchen. She found her 4-year-old choking and expectorating frothy white sputum. She immediately knew what had happened. The quarter was gone. Her 4-year-old had put

(continues)

the quarter in his mouth and had aspirated it.

Having been trained in cardiopulmonary resuscitation (CPR), she initiated the American Heart Association's Conscious-Obstructive CPR procedure. Her son's response, however, was not favorable. In fact, his choking appeared, and sounded, worse. Frothy white secretions continued to flow out of his mouth, and a loud, brassy-like sound could be heard each time he inhaled. His inspiratory efforts were clearly labored. Alarmed, the mother immediately drove her son to the emergency department a few miles away. The 10-year-old tried to comfort his brother as they drove to the hospital.

In the emergency department, the boy was conscious, crying, and in obvious respiratory distress. His skin was cyanotic and pale. He appeared very fatigued. Inspiratory stridor could be heard without the aid of a stethoscope. He was sitting up on the side of the gurney, with his legs hanging over the edge, using his accessory muscles of inspiration. His vital signs were blood pressure—89/50 mm Hg, heart rate—105 beats/min, and respirations—6 breaths/min and labored. His breath sounds were very diminished. A portable chest x-ray film showed the quarter lodged about 2 cm above the vocal cords (see x-ray at right). Oxygen saturation measured by pulse oximetry (Sp_{O_2}) was 87 percent. The patient was immediately transferred to surgery and placed under general anethesia. The quarter was removed moments later without difficulty.

DISCUSSION

This case illustrates a decreased $\dot{V}/\dot{Q}$ ratio caused by an upper airway obstruction. Although an arterial blood sample was not drawn in this case, one can easily predict what the values would have been by considering the following factors: As a result of the upper airway obstruction, the patient had a low $\dot{V}/\dot{Q}$ ratio in both lungs. In addition, in the emergency department the patient was becoming fatigued (his respiratory rate was 6 breaths/min), which further caused the $\dot{V}/\dot{Q}$ ratio to fall.

Thus, as the patient's $\dot{V}/\dot{Q}$ ratio progressively decreased, his Pa_{O_2} decreased while, at the same time, his Pa_{CO_2} increased. This condition, in turn, caused the end-capillary oxygen pressure (Pc_{O_2}) and carbon dioxide pressure (Pc_{CO_2}) to decrease and increase, respectively. In addition, as the Pc_{CO_2} decreased, the pulmonary capillary blood pH also decreased (see Figures 8–4 and 8–7). If these arterial blood gas trends had continued, the patient would have died. Fortunately, when the quarter was successfully removed, the patient's $\dot{V}/\dot{Q}$ ratio quickly returned (increased) to normal. Today, the mother has the quarter on a charm bracelet.

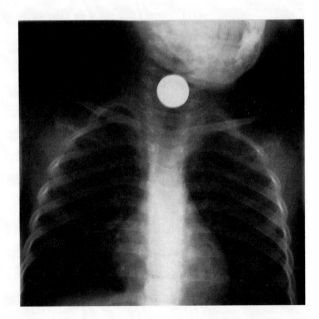

REVIEW QUESTIONS

1. Overall, the normal $\dot{V}/\dot{Q}$ ratio is about
   A. 0.2
   B. 0.4
   C. 0.6
   D. 0.8

2. In the healthy individual in the upright position, the
   I. $\dot{V}/\dot{Q}$ ratio is highest in the lower lung regions
   II. $P_{A_{O_2}}$ is lowest in the upper lung regions
   III. $\dot{V}/\dot{Q}$ ratio is lowest in the upper lung regions
   IV. $P_{A_{CO_2}}$ is highest in the lower lung regions
      A. I only
      B. II only
      C. IV only
      D. III and IV only

3. When the $\dot{V}/\dot{Q}$ ratio decreases, the
   I. $P_{A_{O_2}}$ falls
   II. $P_{c_{CO_2}}$ increases
   III. $P_{A_{CO_2}}$ rises
   IV. $P_{c_{O_2}}$ decreases
      A. I only
      B. III only
      C. II, III, and IV only
      D. All of these

4. When alveolar ventilation is 7 L/min and the pulmonary blood flow is 9.5 L/min, the $\dot{V}/\dot{Q}$ ratio is about
   A. 0.4
   B. 0.5
   C. 0.6
   D. 0.7

5. If tissue cells consume 275 mL of O_2 per minute and produce 195 mL of CO_2 per minute, what is the RQ?
   A. 0.65
   B. 0.7
   C. 0.8
   D. 0.96

CLINICAL APPLICATION QUESTIONS

CASE 1

1. As the patient continued to lose blood, his alveolar ventilation became more and more _____.

2. The patient's alveolar ventilation was _____ or _____ ventilation.

3. The paradox in this case was that even though the patient's $P_{A_{O_2}}$ and Pa_{O_2} increased in response to the increased ventilation-perfusion ratio, the actual amount of oxygen being transported (_____ decreased; _____ increased; _____ remained the same) because of the (_____ increased; _____ decreased) blood flow.

CASE 2

1. As a result of the upper airway obstruction, the patient had a (_____ low; _____ high) ventilation-perfusion in both lungs.

2. The patient's fatigue and respiratory rate of 6 breaths/min further caused the ventilation-perfusion ratio to (_____ rise; _____ fall).

3. As a result of the upper airway obstruction and subsequent ventilation-perfusion ratio, the following values:
   A. $P_{A_{O_2}}$: _____ increased; _____ decreased; _____ remained the same
   B. $P_{A_{CO_2}}$: _____ increased; _____ decreased; _____ remained the same
   C. Pc_{O_2}: _____ increased; _____ decreased; _____ remained the same
   D. Pc_{CO_2}: _____ increased; _____ decreased; _____ remained the same
   E. pH: _____ increased; _____ decreased; _____ remained the same

CHAPTER 9

Control of Ventilation

OBJECTIVES

By the end of this chapter, the student should be able to:

1. Describe the function of the following respiratory neurons of the medulla oblongata:
   —The dorsal respiratory group
   —The ventral respiratory group
2. Describe the influence of the following pontine respiratory centers on the respiratory neurons of the medulla oblongata:
   —Apneustic center
   —Pneumotaxic center
3. Describe the physiologic basis of the respiratory rhythm.
4. List conditions that can depress the respiratory neurons.
5. Describe how the following regulate the respiratory neurons:

   —Central chemoreceptors
   —Peripheral chemoreceptors
6. Describe the reflexes that influence respiration:
   —Hering-Breuer reflex
   —Deflation reflex
   —Irritant reflex
   —Juxtapulmonary-capillary receptors
   —Peripheral proprioceptor reflexes
   —Hypothalamic controls
   —Cortical controls
   —Reflexes from the aortic and carotid sinus baroreceptors
7. Complete the review questions at the end of this chapter.

The intrinsic rhythmicity of respiration is primarily controlled by specific neural areas located in the reticular substance of the medulla oblongata and pons of the brain. These neural areas possess monitoring, stimulating, and inhibiting properties that continually adjust the ventilatory patterns to meet specific metabolic needs. Also received and coordinated in these respiratory neural areas are the signals transmitted by the cerebral cortex during a variety of ventilatory maneuvers such as talking, singing, sniffing, coughing, or blowing into a woodwind instrument.

To fully understand this subject, a basic knowledge of (1) the function of the major respiratory components of the medulla, (2) the influence of the pontine respiratory centers on the medulla, (3) the major monitoring systems that influence the respiratory components of the medulla oblongata, and (4) the reflexes that influence ventilation is necessary.

THE RESPIRATORY COMPONENTS OF THE MEDULLA OBLONGATA—THE RESPIRATORY CENTERS

Although knowledge concerning this subject is incomplete, it is now believed that two groups of **respiratory neurons** in the reticular formation of the medulla oblongata are responsible for coordinating the intrinsic rhythmicity of respirations. These are (1) the dorsal respiratory groups and (2) the ventral respiratory groups (Figure 9–1). Collectively, these respiratory neurons are referred to as the *respiratory center* of the medulla.

Figure 9–1
Schematic illustration of the respiratory components of the lower brainstem (pons and medulla oblongata). PNC = pneumotaxic center; APC = apneustic center; DRG = dorsal respiratory group; VRG = ventral respiratory group; CC = central chemoreceptors.

Dorsal Respiratory Group

The **dorsal respiratory groups (DRGs)** are located dorsally in the posterior region of the medulla oblongata near the root of cranial nerve IX. The DRGs consist chiefly of **inspiratory neurons**. The DRG neurons receive inspiratory impulses from several different specialized monitoring systems throughout the body. These monitoring systems include signals from the *central chemoreceptors, peripheral chemoreceptors, stretch receptors, peripheral proprioceptors,* and *higher brain centers.* The DRG neurons continuously evaluate and prioritize the signals and, depending on the respiratory needs, send neural impulses every few seconds to the muscles of inspiration, i.e., the diaphragm and the external intercostal muscles (Figure 9–2). The DRG neurons are believed to be responsible for the basic rhythm of breathing. The DRG neurons are commonly referred to as the **pacesetting respiratory center** or the **inspiratory center**.

Under normal conditions, the DRG neurons trigger inspiratory impulses at a rate of 12 to 15 breaths/min. The neural signals of the DRGs continue for about 1 to 2 seconds and then cease abruptly, causing the muscles of inspiration to relax. During exhalation, which lasts for about 2 to 3 seconds, the natural elastic recoil forces of the lungs cause the lungs to deflate.

Ventral Respiratory Group

The **ventral respiratory groups (VRGs)** are located bilaterally in two different areas of the medulla (see Figure 9–1). The VRGs are complex networks of neurons that run between the ventral brainstem, spinal cord, and the pons and medulla systems. They contain both inspiratory and expiratory neurons. The VRG neurons are further subdivided into the nucleus ambiguus, nucleus retroambigualis, and Botzinger's complex.

The *nucleus ambiguus* contains primarily inspiratory neurons that innervate the laryngeal and pharyngeal muscles via the vagus nerve. When stimulated, the vocal cords of the larynx abduct, causing airway resistance to decrease. The *nucleus retroambigualis* is divided into the *rostral* (toward the head) and *caudal* (toward the tail) areas. The *rostral* VRG area is composed mainly of inspiratory neurons that stimulate the diaphragm and external intercostal muscles similar to the DRG neurons. The *caudal* VRG area is composed mainly of **expiratory neurons** that stimulate the internal intercostal and abdominal expiratory muscles. The *Botzinger's complex* contains only expiratory neurons that inhibit the discharge of the inspiratory neurons of the DRG and VRG.

During normal quiet breathing, the VRG is almost entirely dormant, because the lungs passively return to their original size by virtue of their own elastic recoil forces. During heavy exercise or stress, however, the expiratory neurons of the VRG actively send impulses to the muscles of exhalation (i.e., abdominal muscles) and the accessory muscles of inspiration that are innervated by the vagus nerve (see Figure 9–1).

Figure 9–2
Neural impulses from the respiratory center travel to the diaphragm by way of the right and left phrenic nerves. The cervical, thoracic, and lumbar motor nerves stimulate the external intercostal muscles (accessory muscles of inspiration).

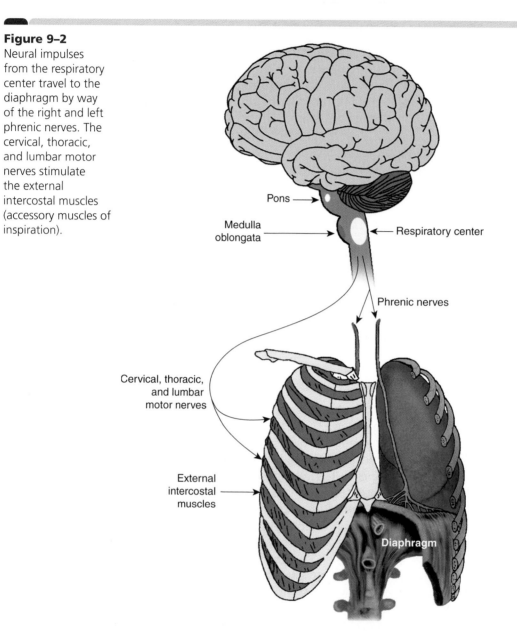

Pons

Medulla oblongata

Respiratory center

Phrenic nerves

Cervical, thoracic, and lumbar motor nerves

External intercostal muscles

Diaphragm

THE INFLUENCE OF THE PONTINE RESPIRATORY CENTERS ON THE RESPIRATORY COMPONENTS OF THE MEDULLA OBLONGATA

The pontine respiratory centers consist of the apneustic center and the pneumotaxic center. Although these centers are known to exist and can be made to operate under experimental conditions, their functional significance in humans is still not fully understood. It appears that these centers function to some degree to modify and fine-tune the rhythmicity of breathing.

Apneustic Center

The **apneustic center** is located in the lower portion of the pons (see Figure 9–1). It continually sends neural impulses that stimulate the inspiratory neurons of the DRGs and VRGs in the medulla. If unrestrained, a prolonged or gasping type of inspiration (breath hold) occurs. This inspiratory maneuver is called **apneustic breathing**. Under normal conditions, however, the apneustic center receives several different inhibitory signals that suppress its function, thus permitting expiration to occur. Research suggests that the most important inhibitory signals are elicited from the pneumotaxic center and from afferent impulses that originate from lung inflation (Hering-Breuer reflex discussed later in this chapter). Breathing becomes deep and slow when the pneumotaxic neurons are cut in animal brain-transection studies, which supports the evidence that the apneustic center is normally inhibited by the pneumotaxic center.

Pneumotaxic Center

The **pneumotaxic center** is located bilaterally in the upper one-third of the pons (see Figure 9–1), in a reticular substance called the *nucleus parabrachialis medialis* and *nucleus Kolliker-Fuse*. The pneumotaxic center receives neural impulses via the vagus from (1) the lung inflation reflex (see Hering-Breuer reflex discussed later in this chapter) and (2) the stretch receptors located in the intercostal muscle of the thorax. In response to these neural signals, the pneumotaxic center sends out inhibitory impulses to the inspiratory center of the medulla, causing the inspiratory phase to shorten. Strong signals from the pneumotaxic center decrease the inspiratory time and increase the respiratory rate. Weak signals increase the inspiratory time (increased tidal volumes) and decrease the respiratory rate.

The precise role and interaction between the apneustic and pneumotaxic center are not known. Research suggests, however, that the major function of the pneumotaxic center is to (1) limit the inspiratory phase of a ventilatory cycle, and (2) keep the apneustic center from causing an "apneustic" or gasping breathing pattern. It is believed that the pneumotaxic center works to enhance and fine-tune the rhythmicity of the breathing pattern. This is supported by animal brain-transection studies that show that when the pons is separated from the medulla, an irregular breathing pattern results. Finally, some investigators believe that the pneumotaxic center is closely related to the so-called **panting center** in animals such as dogs. For example, when a dog becomes overheated, the panting center causes it to breathe with rapid, shallow breaths that evaporate large amounts of water from the its upper airways, thus cooling the animal. In humans, the pneumotaxic center appears to have an effect similar to that of the Hering-Breuer reflex.

The Physiologic Basis of the Respiratory Rhythm

The precise physiologic basis for a rhythmic breathing pattern is not known. As discussed earlier, the DRG neurons (inspiratory center) are believed to be the pacemaker neurons, which have intrinsic automaticity and rhythmicity. Another theory suggests that it is the neural activity generated by the stretch receptors located in the lungs that controls the rhythmic respiratory pattern (see the Hering-Breuer reflex discussion later in this chapter). Another popular theory is that the rhythmic breathing pattern is established by the reciprocal inhibition of interconnected neuronal networks in the medulla. In spite of the questions surrounding the precise origin of the respiratory rhythm, it is clear that the medullary centers are intimately involved in maintaining the normal rhythm of breathing.

Conditions That Depress the Respiratory Components of the Medulla Oblongata

Several clinical conditions can depress the function of the respiratory components of the medulla, including (1) reduced blood flow through the medulla as a result of excess pressure caused by a cerebral edema or some other intracerebral abnormality, (2) acute poliomyelitis, and (3) ingestion of drugs that depress the central nervous system.

MONITORING SYSTEMS THAT INFLUENCE THE RESPIRATORY COMPONENTS OF THE MEDULLA OBLONGATA

From moment to moment, the respiratory components of the medulla (DRG and VRG) activate specific ventilatory patterns based on information received from several different monitoring systems throughout the body. The major known monitoring systems are the (1) central chemoreceptors and (2) peripheral chemoreceptors. Certain neural impulses transmitted to the respiratory neurons during exercise and certain reflexes also influence ventilation.

CLINICAL APPLICATION CASE

1

See page 352

Central Chemoreceptors

The most powerful stimulus known to influence the respiratory components (DRG and VRG) of the medulla is an excess concentration of hydrogen ions [H^+] in the cerebrospinal fluid (CSF). The **central chemoreceptors**, which are located bilaterally and ventrally in the substance of the medulla, are responsible for monitoring the H^+ ion concentration of the CSF. In fact, a portion of the central chemoreceptors is actually in direct contact with the CSF. It is believed that the central chemoreceptors transmit signals to the respiratory components of the medulla by the following mechanism:

1. As the CO_2 level increases in the arterial blood (e.g., during hypoventilation), the CO_2 molecules diffuse across a semipermeable membrane, called the **blood-brain barrier**, which separates the blood from the CSF. The blood-brain barrier is very permeable to CO_2 molecules but relatively impermeable to H^+ and HCO_3^- ions.

2. As CO_2 moves into the CSF, it forms carbonic acid by means of the following reaction:

$$CO_2 + H_2O \leftrightarrows H_2CO_3 \leftrightarrows H^+ + HCO_3^-$$

3. Because the CSF lacks hemoglobin and carbonic anhydrase and has a relatively low bicarbonate and protein level, the overall buffering system in the CSF is very slow. Because of the inefficient CSF buffering system, the H^+ generated from the preceding reaction rapidly increases and, therefore, significantly reduces the pH in the CSF.

4. The liberated H^+ ions cause the central chemoreceptors to transmit signals to the respiratory component in the medulla, which, in turn, increases the alveolar ventilation.

5. The increased ventilation reduces the Pa_{CO_2} and, subsequently, the P_{CO_2} in the CSF. As the P_{CO_2} in the CSF decreases, the H^+ ion concentration of the CSF also falls. This action decreases the stimulation of the central chemoreceptors. Thus, the neural signals to the respiratory components in the medulla also diminish; this, in turn, causes alveolar ventilation to decrease.

6. In view of the preceding sequences, it should be understood that the central chemoreceptors regulate ventilation through the indirect effects of CO_2 on the pH of the CSF (Figure 9–3).

CLINICAL APPLICATION CASES

1 & 2

See pages 352–354

Peripheral Chemoreceptors

The **peripheral chemoreceptors** are special oxygen-sensitive cells that react to the reductions of oxygen levels in the arterial blood. They are located high in the neck at the bifurcation of the internal and external carotid arteries and on the aortic arch (Figure 9–4). They are close to, but distinct from, the *baroreceptors*. The peripheral chemoreceptors are also called the *carotid* and *aortic bodies*.

The carotid and aortic bodies are composed of epithelial-like cells and neuron terminals in intimate contact with the arterial blood. When activated by a low Pa_{O_2}, *afferent* (sensory) signals are transmitted to the respiratory components in the medulla by way of the glossopharyngeal nerve (ninth cranial nerve) from the carotid bodies and by way of the vagus nerve (tenth cranial nerve) from the aortic bodies. This action, in turn, causes *efferent* (motor) signals to be transmitted to the respiratory

Figure 9–3
The relationship of the blood-brain barrier (BBB) to CO_2, HCO_3^-, and H^+. CO_2 readily crosses the BBB. H^+ and HCO_3^- do not readily cross the BBB. H^+ and HCO_3^- require the active transport system to cross the BBB. CSF = cerebrospinal fluid.

**Medulla Oblongata
(ventral surface)**

muscles, causing ventilation to increase (Figure 9–5). Compared with the aortic bodies, the carotid bodies play a much greater role in initiating an increased ventilatory rate in response to reduced arterial oxygen levels.

As shown in Figure 9–6, the peripheral chemoreceptors are not significantly activated until the oxygen content of the inspired air is low enough to reduce the Pa_{O_2} to 60 mm Hg (Sa_{O_2} about 90 percent). Beyond this point, any further reduction in the Pa_{O_2} causes a marked increase in ventilation. *Suppression* of the peripheral chemoreceptors is seen, however, when the Pa_{O_2} falls below 30 mm Hg.

In the patient with a low Pa_{O_2} and a chronically high Pa_{CO_2} level (e.g., end-stage emphysema), the peripheral chemoreceptors may be totally responsible for the control of ventilation. This is because a chronically high CO_2 concentration in the CSF inactivates the H^+ sensitivity of the central chemoreceptor—that is, HCO_3^- moves into the CSF via the active transport mechanism and combines with H^+, thus returning the pH to normal. A compensatory response to a chronically high CO_2 concentration, however, is the enhancement of the sensitivity of the peripheral chemoreceptors at higher CO_2 levels (Figure 9–7).

Finally, it is important to understand that the peripheral chemoreceptors are specifically sensitive to the P_{O_2} of the blood and relatively insensitive to the oxygen content of the blood. The precise mechanism for this exclusive P_{O_2} sensitivity is not fully understood.

Figure 9–4
Location of the carotid and aortic bodies (the peripheral chemoreceptors).

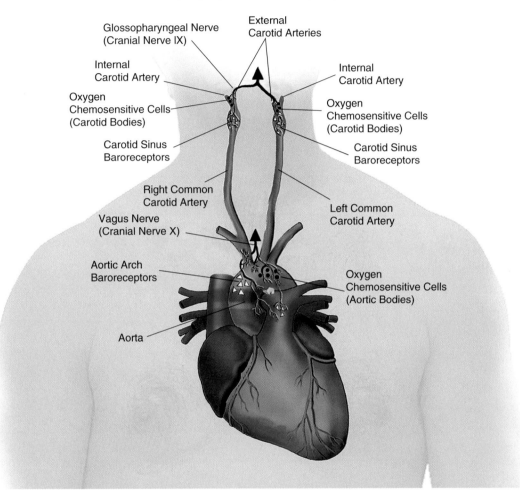

Glossopharyngeal Nerve
(Cranial Nerve IX)

External
Carotid Arteries

Internal
Carotid Artery

Internal
Carotid Artery

Oxygen
Chemosensitive Cells
(Carotid Bodies)

Oxygen
Chemosensitive Cells
(Carotid Bodies)

Carotid Sinus
Baroreceptors

Carotid Sinus
Baroreceptors

Right Common
Carotid Artery

Left Common
Carotid Artery

Vagus Nerve
(Cranial Nerve X)

Aortic Arch
Baroreceptors

Oxygen
Chemosensitive Cells
(Aortic Bodies)

Aorta

Clinically, this exclusive Pa_{O_2} sensitivity can be misleading. For example, there are certain conditions in which the Pa_{O_2} is normal (and, therefore, the peripheral chemoreceptors are not stimulated), yet the oxygen content of the blood is dangerously low. Such conditions include chronic anemia, carbon monoxide poisoning, and methemoglobinemia.

Other Factors That Stimulate the Peripheral Chemoreceptors

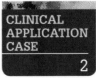

CLINICAL
APPLICATION
CASE

2

See page 353

Although the peripheral chemoreceptors are primarily stimulated by a reduced Pa_{O_2} level, they are also activated by a decreased pH (increased H^+ level). This is an important feature of the peripheral chemoreceptors,

Figure 9–5

Schematic illustration showing how a low Pa_{O_2} stimulates the respiratory components of the medulla to increase alveolar ventilation.

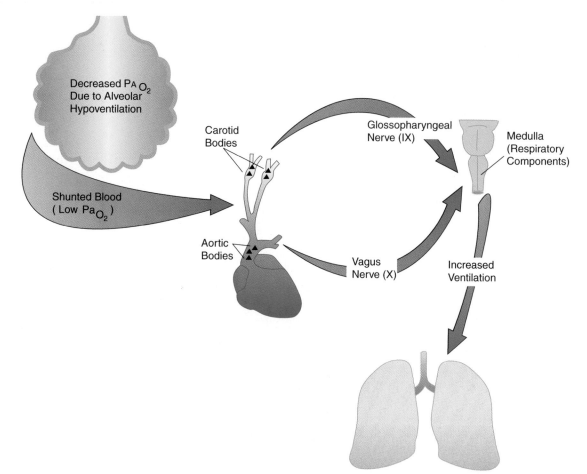

Decreased $P_A{}_{O_2}$ Due to Alveolar Hypoventilation

Shunted Blood (Low Pa_{O_2})

Carotid Bodies

Aortic Bodies

Glossopharyngeal Nerve (IX)

Vagus Nerve (X)

Medulla (Respiratory Components)

Increased Ventilation

Figure 9–6

The effect of low Pa_{O_2} levels on ventilation.

Ventilation (L/min)

Arterial P_{O_2} (mm Hg)

Figure 9–7

The effect of Pa_{O_2} on ventilation at three different Pa_{CO_2} values. Note that as the Pa_{CO_2} value increases, the sensitivity of the peripheral chemoreceptors increases.

because there are many situations in which a change in arterial H^+ ion levels can occur by means other than a primary change in the P_{CO_2}. In fact, because the H^+ ions do not readily move across the blood-brain barrier, the peripheral chemoreceptors play a major role in initiating ventilation whenever the H^+ ion concentration increases for reasons other than an increased Pa_{CO_2}. For example, the accumulation of lactic acid or ketones in the blood stimulates hyperventilation almost entirely through the peripheral chemoreceptors (Figure 9–8).

The peripheral chemoreceptors are also stimulated by (1) hypoperfusion (e.g., stagnant hypoxia), (2) increased temperature, (3) nicotine, and (4) the direct effect of Pa_{CO_2}. The response of the peripheral chemoreceptors to Pa_{CO_2} stimulation, however, is minor and not nearly so great as the response generated by the central chemoreceptors. The peripheral chemoreceptors do respond faster than the central chemoreceptors to an increased Pa_{CO_2}. This occurs because the peripheral chemoreceptors are stimulated directly by the CO_2 molecule, whereas the central chemoreceptors are stimulated by the H^+ generated by the CO_2 hydration reaction in

Figure 9–8
The accumulation of lactic acids leads to an increased alveolar ventilation primarily through the stimulation of the peripheral chemoreceptors.

↑Production of Non-CO_2 Acids (Lactic Acids)

↑Arterial (H^+)

Stimulation of Peripheral Chemoreceptors

Stimulation of Medullary Inspiration Neurons

↑ Increased Alveolar Ventilation

the CSF—a reaction that occurs slowly in the absence of carbonic anhydrase (see Figure 9–3).

Other Responses Activated by the Peripheral Chemoreceptors

In addition to the increased ventilation activated by the peripheral chemoreceptors, other responses can occur as a result of peripheral chemoreceptor stimulation, including:

- Peripheral vasoconstriction
- Increased pulmonary vascular resistance
- Systemic arterial hypertension
- Tachycardia
- Increase in left ventricular performance.

REFLEXES THAT INFLUENCE VENTILATION

A number of reflexes are known to influence the rate of ventilation.

Hering-Breuer Reflex

The Hering-Breuer reflex (also called the inflation reflex) is generated by stretch receptors, located in the visceral pleurae and in the walls of the bronchi and bronchioles, that become excited when the lungs overinflate. Signals from these receptors travel through the afferent fibers of the vagus nerve to the respiratory components in the medulla, causing inspiration to cease. In essence, the lungs themselves provide a feedback mechanism to terminate inspiration. Instead of a reflex to control ventilation, the Hering-Breuer reflex appears to be a protective mechanism that prevents pulmonary damage caused by excessive lung inflation. The significance of the Hering-Breuer reflex in the adult at normal tidal volumes is controversial; it appears to have more significance in the control of ventilation in the newborn.

Deflation Reflex

When the lungs are compressed or deflated, an increased rate of breathing results. The precise mechanism responsible for this reflex is not known. Some researchers believe that the increased rate of breathing may be due to the reduced stimulation of receptors serving the Hering-Breuer reflex rather than to the stimulation of specific deflation receptors. Others, however, think that the deflation reflex is not due to the absence of receptor stimulation of the Hering-Breuer reflex, because the reflex is still seen when the temperature of the bronchi and bronchioles is less than 8°C. The Hering-Breuer reflex is not active when the bronchi and bronchioles are below this temperature.

Irritant Reflex

When the lungs are exposed to noxious gases or accumulated mucus, the irritant receptors may also be stimulated. The irritant receptors are subepithelial mechanoreceptors located in the trachea, bronchi, and bronchioles. When the receptors are activated, a reflex vagal response causes the ventilatory rate to increase. Stimulation of the irritant receptors may also produce a reflex cough, sneeze, and bronchoconstriction.

Juxtapulmonary-Capillary Receptors

An extensive network of free nerve endings, called **C-fibers**, are located in the small conducting airways, blood vessels, and interstitial tissues between the pulmonary capillaries and alveolar walls. The C-fibers located near the alveolar capillaries are called **juxtapulmonary-capillary**

receptors, or **J-receptors**. These receptors react to certain chemicals and to mechanical stimulation. For example, they are stimulated by alveolar inflamation, pulmonary capillary congestion and edema, humoral agents (e.g., serotonin, bradykinin), lung deflation, and emboli. When the J-receptors are stimulated, a reflex response triggers a rapid, shallow breathing pattern.

Peripheral Proprioceptor Reflexes

Peripheral proprioceptors are located in the muscles, tendons, joints, and pain receptors in muscles and skin. When stimulated, the proprioceptors send neural impulses to the medulla. The medulla, in turn, sends out an increased number of inspiratory signals. This may explain, in part, why moving an individual's limbs (for example, during a drug overdose), or producing prolonged pain to the skin, stimulates ventilation. Sudden pain causes a short period of apnea, whereas prolonged pain causes the breathing rate to increase. The proprioceptors in the joints and tendons are also believed to play an important role in initiating and maintaining an increased respiratory rate during exercise. The more joints and tendons are involved, the greater the respiration rate.

Hypothalamic Controls

Strong emotions can activate sympathetic centers in the hypothalamus, which can alter respirations. For example, excitement causes the respiratory rate to increase. In addition, increased body temperature causes the respiration rate to increase, whereas decreased body temperature produces the opposite effect. For instance, a sudden cold stimulus (e.g., plunging into very cold water) can cause the cessation of breathing—or at the very least, a gasp.

Cortical Controls

Although the breathing pattern is normally controlled involuntarily by the medullary centers, one can also activate a conscious voluntary control over the rate and depth of breathing—or choose to hold the breath or take an extra deep breath.

Reflexes from the Aortic and Carotid Sinus Baroreceptors

The normal function of the aortic and carotid sinus baroreceptors, located near the aortic and carotid peripheral chemoreceptors (see Figure 5–10), is to initiate reflexes that cause (1) a decreased heart and ventilatory rate in response to an elevated systemic blood pressure and (2) an increased heart and ventilatory rate in response to a reduced systemic blood pressure.

To summarize, the *respiratory center* of the medulla oblongata coordinates both the involuntary and voluntary rhythm of breathing. The

Figure 9–9

The respiratory center receives neural and chemical stimuli on a moment to moment basis. In response to this information, the respiratory center determines the rate and depth of breathing. Excitatory stimuli (+) increase the rate and depth of breathing. Inhibitory influences (−) decrease the rate and depth of breathing. In some cases, the influences may be excitatory or inhibitory (+−), depending on which regions of the brain or receptors are activated.

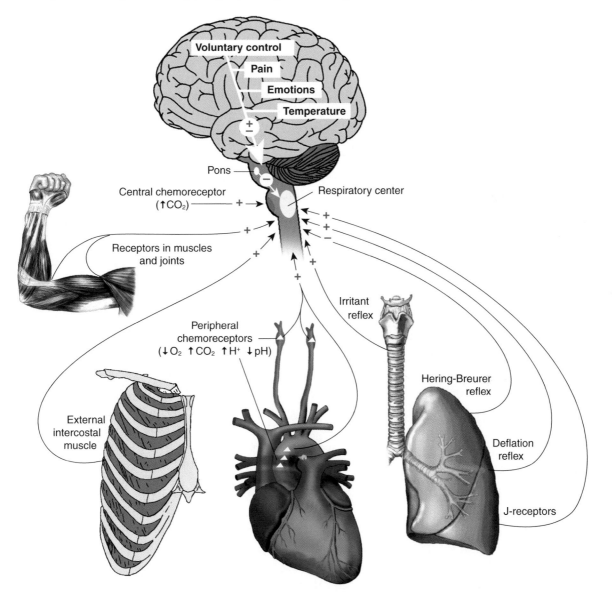

respiratory center (1) receives neural impulses from several different areas throughout the body, (2) evaluates and prioritizes these neural signals, and (3) based on the metabolic needs of the body, elicits neural impulses to the muscles of ventilation. Figure 9–9 provides an overview of the complex functions of the medulla.

CHAPTER SUMMARY

The respiratory neurons of the medulla oblongata coordinate both the involuntary and voluntary rhythm of breathing. The *respiratory center* of the medulla receives neural impulses from several different areas throughout the body, evaluates and prioritizes the signals, and elicits neural impulses to the muscles of ventilation based on the metabolic need of the body.

To fully understand this subject, the respiratory therapist must have a basic knowledge of (1) the respiratory components of the medulla, including the dorsal respiratory groups (DRGs) and ventral respiratory groups (VRGs); (2) the pontine centers on the medulla, including the apneustic center and pneumotaxic center; (3) the monitoring systems that influence the medulla, including the central chemoreceptors and peripheral chemoreceptors; and (4) the reflexes that influence ventilation, including the Hering-Breuer reflex, deflation reflex, irritant reflex, juxtapulmonary-capillary receptors, peripheral proprioceptor reflex, hypothalamic controls, cortical controls, and reflexes from the aortic and carotid sinus baroreceptors.

1 CLINICAL APPLICATION CASE

To facilitate the understanding of how the peripheral and central chemoreceptors control the ventilatory pattern, consider the following chain of events that develops when an individual who normally resides at sea level ascends to a high altitude (say, to the Colorado mountains to ski) for a period of 2 weeks.

CHANGES AT HIGH ALTITUDES

Stimulation of the Peripheral Chemoreceptors

1. As the individual ascends the mountain, the barometric pressure, and therefore the P_{O_2} of the atmosphere progressively decrease. (Remember that the oxygen percentage is still 21 percent.)

2. As the atmospheric P_{O_2} decreases, the individual's arterial oxygen pressure (Pa_{O_2}) also decreases.

3. As the individual continues to ascend the mountain, the Pa_{O_2} eventually falls low enough (to about 60 mm Hg) to activate the peripheral chemoreceptors to stimulate the medulla to increase ventilation.

4. The increased ventilation initiated by the peripheral chemoreceptors causes a secondary decrease in the Pa_{CO_2}. In other words, the individual hyperventilates in response to the reduced Pa_{O_2} level.

5. Because the peripheral chemoreceptors do not acclimate to a decreased oxygen concentration, hyperventilation will continue for the entire time the individual remains at the high altitude.

Readjustment of the Central Chemoreceptors

In response to the hyperventilation that occurs while the individual is at the high

(continues)

altitude, the central chemoreceptors readjust to the lower CO_2 level because of the following chain of events:

1. As the individual hyperventilates to offset the low atmospheric P_{O_2}, the individual's Pa_{CO_2} level decreases.

2. In response to the decreased Pa_{CO_2}, the CO_2 molecules in the CSF move into the blood until equilibrium occurs.

3. This reaction causes the pH of the CSF to increase.

4. Over the next 48 hours, however, HCO_3^- will also leave the CSF (via the active transport mechanism) to correct the pH back to normal.

In short, the individual's CSF readjusts to the low CO_2 level.

CHANGES AFTER LEAVING A HIGH ALTITUDE

Stimulation of the Central Chemoreceptors

Interestingly, even after the individual returns to a lower altitude, hyperventilation continues for a few days. The reason for this is as follows:

1. As the individual moves down the mountain, the barometric pressure steadily increases, and therefore the atmospheric P_{O_2} increases.

2. As the atmospheric P_{O_2} increases, the individual's Pa_{O_2} also increases and eventually ceases to stimulate the peripheral chemoreceptors.

3. As the stimulation of the peripheral chemoreceptors decreases, the individual's ventilatory rate decreases.

4. As the ventilatory rate declines, however, the individual's Pa_{CO_2} progressively increases.

5. As the Pa_{CO_2} increases, CO_2 molecules move across the blood-brain barrier into the CSF.

6. As CO_2 moves into the CSF, H^+ ions are formed, causing the pH of the CSF to decrease.

7. The H^+ ions liberated in the above reaction stimulate the central chemoreceptors to increase the individual's ventilatory rate.

8. Eventually, HCO_3^- ions move across the blood-brain barrier into the CSF to correct the pH back to normal. When this occurs, the individual's ventilatory pattern will be as it was before the trip to the mountains.

 2 CLINICAL APPLICATION CASE

A 44-year-old woman was found unconscious on her living room floor by her husband when he returned home from work. He immediately carried her to his car and drove her to the hospital. As he was driving, he called the hospital emergency department on his cellular telephone to alert the medical staff. He estimated that his time of arrival would be in about 15 minutes. While on the phone, he also reported that his wife had a long history of diabetes. He stated that his wife had passed out three times in the past 2 years as a result of not taking her insulin as prescribed. The husband had no idea how long his wife had been unconscious before he found her.

(continues)

Upon arrival, the patient was still unconscious and breathing very deeply and rapidly. The emergency department nurse placed an oxygen mask on the patient's face and started an intravenous infusion. A laboratory phlebotomist drew blood, and the respiratory therapist obtained an arterial blood sample from the patient's radial artery. The patient's vital signs were blood pressure—135/85 mm Hg, heart rate—97 beats/min, respirations—22 breaths/min, and temperature—37°C. The patient's respiratory pattern was charted by the respiratory therapist as Kussmaul's respiration. The patient's arterial blood gas values were pH—7.23, Pa_{CO_2}—24 mm Hg, HCO_3^-—19 mEq/L, and Pa_{O_2}—405 mm Hg. The respiratory therapist discontinued the patient's oxygen therapy. The second set of arterial blood gas values on room air were pH—7.23, Pa_{CO_2}—24 mm Hg, HCO_3^-—19 mEq/L, and Pa_{O_2}—119 mm Hg.

The laboratory report showed a blood glucose level of 837 mg/dL (normal, 70–150). The report also showed that her serum acetone level was 1:64 (normal, 0). The attending physician initiated insulin therapy. Two hours later the patient was conscious and talking with her husband. Her vital signs were blood pressure—122/68 mm Hg, heart rate—75 beats/min, respirations—12 breaths/min, and temperature—37°C. Arterial blood gas values on room air at this time were: pH—7.41, Pa_{CO_2}—39, HCO_3^-—24 mEq/L, and Pa_{O_2}—95 mm Hg. Her blood glucose level was 95 mg/dL and her acetone level was zero. The patient was discharged the next day.

DISCUSSION

This case illustrates how clinical factors other than an increased P_{CO_2} or decreased P_{O_2} can stimulate ventilation. Because the patient had not taken her insulin as prescribed, ketone acids (H^+) started to accumulate in her blood. As the ketone acid level increased, pH decreased. The excessive H^+ concentration stimulated the patient's peripheral chemoreceptors. Because the H^+ ion does not readily move across the blood-brain barrier, the peripheral chemo-receptors played a major role in causing the patient's ventilation to increase (see Figure 9–8).

In addition, note that as the patient's ventilation increased, her Pa_{CO_2} decreased (to 24 mm Hg in the emergency department). The reduction in the Pa_{CO_2} was a compensatory mechanism—i.e., the decreased Pa_{CO_2} worked to offset the acidic pH caused by the increased ketone acids. In other words, if the Pa_{CO_2} had been closer to normal level (around 40 mm Hg) in the emergency department, the pH would have been lower than 7.23.

Note also that an increased respiratory rate does not necessarily mean that patient needs oxygen therapy. In this case, however, such therapy was appropriate (because of the patient's rapid breathing) until the cause of the rapid breathing was determined. When the results of the first arterial blood gas analysis were available (Pa_{O_2} was 405 mm Hg), discontinuation of the oxygen therapy was the appropriate response.

REVIEW QUESTIONS

1. The respiratory components of the medulla consist of which of the following?
   I. Dorsal respiratory group
   II. Apneustic center
   III. Ventral respiratory group
   IV. Pneumotaxic center
      A. I only
      B. II only
      C. I and III only
      D. II and IV only

2. Which of the following has the most powerful effect on the respiratory components of the medulla?
   A. Decreased O_2
   B. Increased H^+
   C. Decreased CO_2
   D. Increased pH

3. Which of the following may cause a temporary cessation in breathing?
   I. Sudden pain
   II. Stimulation of proprioceptor
   III. Sudden cold
   IV. Inhalation of noxious gases
      A. I only
      B. II only
      C. III and IV only
      D. I and III only

4. Which of the following will readily diffuse across the blood-brain barrier?
   I. CO_2
   II. H^+
   III. HCO_3^-
   IV. H_2CO_3
      A. I only
      B. II only
      C. III only
      D. II and IV only

5. When the systemic blood pressure increases, the aortic and carotid sinus baroreceptors initiate reflexes that cause a/an
   I. increased heart rate
   II. decreased ventilatory rate
   III. increased ventilatory rate
   IV. decreased heart rate
      A. I only
      B. II only
      C. III only
      D. II and IV only

6. The peripheral chemoreceptors are significantly activated when the P_{O_2} decreases to about
   A. 75 mm Hg
   B. 70 mm Hg
   C. 65 mm Hg
   D. 60 mm Hg

7. Stimulation of the peripheral chemoreceptors can cause which of the following?
   I. Tachycardia
   II. Decreased left ventricular performance
   III. Increased pulmonary vascular resistance
   IV. Systemic arterial hypertension
      A. I only
      B. II only
      C. IV only
      D. I, III, and IV only

8. Suppression of the peripheral chemoreceptors begins when the P_{O_2} falls below
   A. 50 mm Hg
   B. 40 mm Hg
   C. 30 mm Hg
   D. 20 mm Hg

9. In addition to a low P_{O_2}, the peripheral chemoreceptors are also sensitive to a/an
   I. decreased H^+
   II. increased P_{CO_2}
   III. decreased pH
   IV. increased temperature
      A. II only
      B. III only
      C. I, II, and III only
      D. II, III, and IV only

10. Which of the following protects the lungs from excessive inflation?
    A. Juxtapulmonary-capillary receptors
    B. Hering-Breuer inflation reflex
    C. Deflation reflex
    D. Irritant reflex

CLINICAL APPLICATION QUESTIONS

CASE 1

1. True _____ False _____ As an individual ascends a mountain, both the barometric pressure and atomospheric P_{O_2} decrease.

2. True _____ False _____ The oxygen percentage decreases as an individual ascends a mountain.

3. What stimulates the medulla to increase ventilation as an individual continues to ascend a mountain?

   Answer: _____

4. As an individual continues to hyperventilate at high altitudes, the individual's Pa_{CO_2} (_____increases; _____decreases; _____remains the same).

5. After an individual returns to a lower altitude, an increased ventilation continues for a few days. What causes the individual to maintain a higher than normal respiratory rate?

   Answer: _____

CASE 2

1. Because the patient had not taken her insulin as prescribed, what type of acid accumulated in her blood?

   Answer: _____

2. What did the excess acid in the patient's blood stimulate that caused the patient's respiratory rate to increase?

   Answer: _____

3. Do H^+ ions readily move across the blood-brain barrier?

   Yes _____ No _____

4. Explain why the patient's increased ventilation was a compensatory mechanism to offset the acidic pH.

   _____

   _____

CHAPTER 10

Fetal Development and the Cardiopulmonary System

O B J E C T I V E S

By the end of this chapter, the student should be able to:

1. Describe the developmental events that occur during the following periods of fetal life:
   —Embryonic
   —Pseudoglandular
   —Canalicular
   —Terminal sac

2. Describe how the following components relate to the placenta:
   —Umbilical arteries
   —Cotyledons
   —Fetal vessels
   —Chorionic villi
   —Intervillous space
   —Spiral arterioles
   —Umbilical vein

3. List the three major reasons why oxygen transfers from maternal to fetal blood.

4. List the factors believed to cause the wide variance between the maternal and fetal P_{O_2} and P_{CO_2}.

5. Describe how the following structures relate to the fetal circulation:
   —Umbilical vein
   —Liver
   —Ductus venosus
   —Inferior vena cava
   —Right atrium
   —Superior vena cava
   —Foramen ovale

   —Pulmonary veins
   —Left ventricle
   —Right ventricle
   —Ductus arteriosus
   —Common iliac arteries
   —External and internal iliacs
   —Umbilical arteries

6. Describe what happens to the following special structures of fetal circulation after birth:
   —Placenta
   —Umbilical arteries
   —Umbilical vein
   —Ductus venosus
   —Foramen ovale
   —Ductus arteriosus

7. Describe how the fetal lung fluid is removed from the lungs at birth.

8. List the number of alveoli present at birth and at 12 years of age.

9. Describe the pressure-volume changes of the lungs of the newborn during the first 2 weeks of life.

10. Identify the average newborn values for the following:
    —Lung compliance
    —Airway resistance

11. Describe how the following circulatory changes develop at birth:
    —Decrease in pulmonary vascular resistance

(continues)

—Closure of the foramen ovale
—Constriction of the ductus arteriosus
12. Describe the role of the following in the control of ventilation of the newborn:
—Peripheral chemoreceptors
—Central chemoreceptors
—Infant reflexes
  • Trigeminal
  • Irritant
  • Head paradoxical

13. List the normal values in the newborn for
—Lung volumes and capacities
—Respiratory rate
—Heart rate
—Blood pressure
14. Complete the review questions at the end of this chapter.

FETAL LUNG DEVELOPMENT

During fetal life, the development of the lungs is arbitrarily divided into four periods: embryonic, pseudoglandular, canalicular, and terminal sac.

Embryonic Period

The **embryonic period** encompasses the developmental events that occur during the first 5 weeks after fertilization. The lungs first appear as a small bud arising from the esophagus on the 24th day of embryonic life (Figure 10–1). On about the 28th day of gestation, this bud branches into the right and left lung buds. Between the 30th and 32nd day, primitive lobar bronchi begin to appear—two on the left lung bud and three on the right lung bud. By the end of the 5th week, cartilage can be seen in the trachea, and the main stem bronchi are surrounded by primitive cellular mesoderm, which gradually differentiates into bronchial smooth muscle, connective tissue, and cartilaginous plates.

Pseudoglandular Period

The **pseudoglandular period** includes the developmental processes that occur between the 5th and the 16th week of gestation. By the 6th week, all the segments are present and the subsegmental bronchi are also well represented. The subsegmental bronchi continue to undergo further branching, and by the 16th week all the subsegmental bronchi are present.

By the 10th week, ciliated columnar epithelial cells, a deeper basal layer of irregular cells, and a primitive basement membrane appear in the conducting airways. Goblet cells also begin to appear in the trachea and large bronchi. Between the 10th and 14th weeks, there is a sudden burst of bronchial branching. It is estimated that as many as 75 percent of the conducting airways develop at this time.

At 11 weeks of gestation, cartilage begins to appear in the lobar bronchi. Cartilaginous airways continue to form until about 24 weeks of

Figure 10–1
Schematic representation of the developmental events that occur in the human lung during the embryonic and pseudoglandular periods (see text for explanation).

Anterior View   Lateral View

40 Days

28 Days

32 Days

gestation. By the 12th week, the bronchial mucous glands start to appear. Immature smooth-muscle cells are also noted at this time in the pulmonary arteries. As the tracheobronchial tree develops, new bronchial glands form until the 25th to 26th week of gestation. At birth, the concentration of bronchial glands is about 17 glands per square millimeter (mm^2). In the adult, the concentration drops to about 1 gland/mm^2, as a result of bronchial elongation and widening. By the 16th week, there are about 20 generations of bronchial airways.

Canalicular Period

The **canalicular period** includes the developmental events between the 17th and 24th week of gestation. During this time, the terminal bronchioles continue to proliferate and primitive respiratory bronchioles begin to appear. The lung mass becomes highly vascularized and the lung lobes are clearly recognizable. At about the 20th week of gestation, the lymphatic vessels begin to appear.

CLINICAL APPLICATION CASE

1

See page 373

Terminal Sac Period

The **terminal sac period** begins at the 24th week of gestation and continues until term (between the 38th and 41st week of gestation). The structures that appeared in the canalicular period continue to proliferate and the entire acinus (respiratory bronchioles, alveolar ducts, alveolar sacs, and alveoli) develops. The type I and type II alveolar cells can be identified at this time, and pulmonary surfactant begins to appear. Although pulmonary capillaries begin to appear at the 24th week, the air–blood interface between the alveoli and the pulmonary capillaries is poorly defined. By the 28th week, the air–blood interface and the quantity of pulmonary surfactant are usually sufficient to support life. By the 34th week, the respiratory acini are well developed. The smooth-muscle fibers in the conducting airways begin to appear during the last few weeks of gestation. These muscles continue to mature after birth.

PLACENTA

CLINICAL APPLICATION CASE

2

See page 375

Following conception, the fertilized egg moves down the **uterine tube** (Fallopian tube) and implants into the wall of the uterus. The placenta develops at the point of implantation. Throughout fetal life, the placenta transfers maternal oxygen and nutrients to the fetus and transfers waste products out of the fetal circulation. When fully developed, the placenta appears as a reddish brown disk about 20 cm long and 2.5 cm thick. The placenta consists of about 15 to 20 segments called **cotyledons** (Figure 10–2). Each cotyledon is composed of **fetal vessels, chorionic villi**, and **intervillous spaces** (Figure 10–3). The cotyledons provide an interface between the maternal and fetal circulation.

Deoxygenated blood is carried from the fetus to the placenta by way of two **umbilical arteries**, which are wrapped around the **umbilical vein** (see Figure 10–3). Normally, the P$_{O_2}$ in the umbilical arteries is about 20 mm Hg and the P$_{CO_2}$ is about 55 mm Hg. Once in the placenta, the

Figure 10–2
The placenta: **(A)** maternal surface; **(B)** fetal surface.

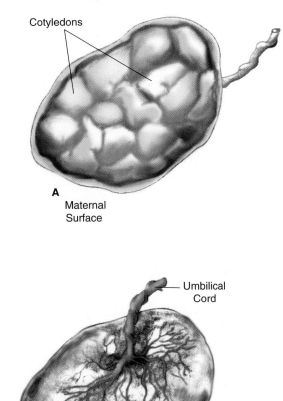

Cotyledons

A
Maternal
Surface

Umbilical
Cord

B
Fetal
Surface

umbilical arteries branch and supply each cotyledon. As the umbilical arteries enter the cotyledon, they again branch into the fetal vessels, which then loop around the internal portion of the finger-like projections of the chorionic villi. Externally, the chorionic villi are surrounded by the intervillous space (see Figure 10–3).

Maternal blood from the uterine arteries enters the intervillous space through the **spiral arterioles**. The spiral arterioles continuously spurt jets of oxygenated blood and nutrients around the chorionic villi. Although the maternal blood P_{O_2} is usually normal during the last trimester of pregnancy (80 to 100 mm Hg), the P_{CO_2} is frequently lower than expected (about 33 mm Hg). This decrease in maternal P_{CO_2} is caused by the

Figure 10–3
Anatomic structure of the placental cotyledon.

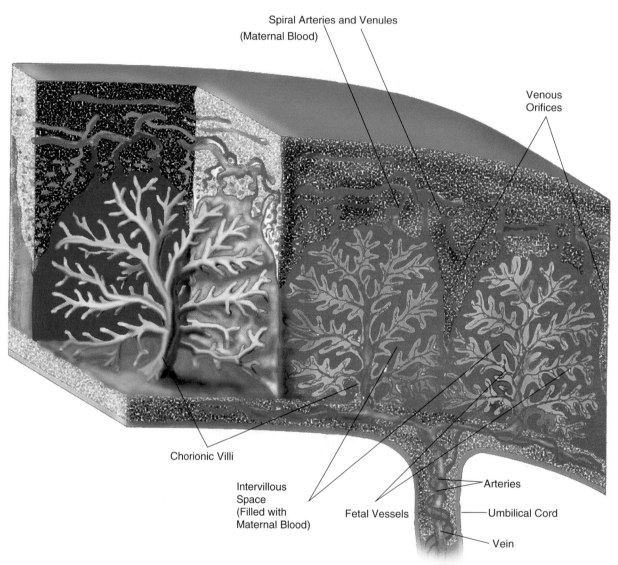

alveolar hyperventilation that develops as the growing infant restricts the mother's diaphragmatic excursion.

Once in the intervillous space, oxygen and nutrients in the maternal blood move through the tissues of the chorionic villi and enter the fetal blood. Oxygen transfers from the maternal to fetal blood because of the (1) maternal-fetal P_{O_2} gradient, (2) higher hemoglobin concentration in the fetal blood compared with that of maternal blood, and (3) greater affinity of fetal hemoglobin (Hb F) for oxygen than of adult hemoglobin (Hb A). While the maternal oxygen and nutrients are moving into the fetal blood, carbon dioxide (P_{CO_2} of about 55 mm Hg) and other waste products are moving out of the fetal blood and entering the maternal blood. The blood-to-blood barrier (chorionic villi) is about 3.5 μm thick.

Oxygenated fetal blood (actually a P_{O_2} of about 30 mm Hg and a P_{CO_2} of about 40 mm Hg) flows out of the chorionic villi via the fetal vessels and returns to the fetus by way of the umbilical vein (see Figure 10–3). The wide variance between the maternal and fetal P_{O_2} and P_{CO_2} is thought to be caused by the following factors:

- The placenta itself is an actively metabolizing organ.
- The permeability of the placenta varies from region to region with respect to respiratory gases.
- There are fetal and maternal vascular shunts.

The fetal waste products in the maternal blood move out of the intervillous space by virtue of the arteriovenous pressure gradient. The pressure in the spiral arteries is about 75 mm Hg and the pressure of the **venous orifices**, located adjacent to the spiral arteries, is about 8 mm Hg.

FETAL CIRCULATION

The umbilical vein carries oxygenated blood and nutrients from the placenta to the fetus (Figure 10–4). The umbilical vein enters the navel of the fetus and ascends anteriorly to the liver. About one-half of the blood enters the liver, and the rest flows through the **ductus venosus** and enters the **inferior vena cava**. This results in oxygenated fetal blood mixing with deoxygenated blood from the lower parts of the fetal body. The newly mixed fetal blood then travels up the inferior vena cava and enters the **right atrium**, where it again mingles with deoxygenated blood from the **superior vena cava**.

Once in the right atrium, most of the blood flows directly into the left atrium through the **foramen ovale**. While in the left atrium, the fetal blood again mingles with a small amount of deoxygenated blood from the pulmonary veins. The blood then enters the left ventricle and is pumped primarily to the heart and brain.

The rest of the blood in the right atrium moves into the right ventricle and is pumped into the pulmonary artery. Once in the pulmonary artery, most of the blood bypasses the lungs and flows directly into the aorta through the **ductus arteriosus**. A small amount of blood (about 15 percent) flows through the lungs and returns to the left atrium via the pulmonary veins. The Pa_{O_2} in the descending aorta is about 20 mm Hg. Downstream, the **common iliac arteries** branch into the **external** and **internal iliacs**. The blood in the internal iliac branch passes into the

Figure 10–4
Fetal circulation.

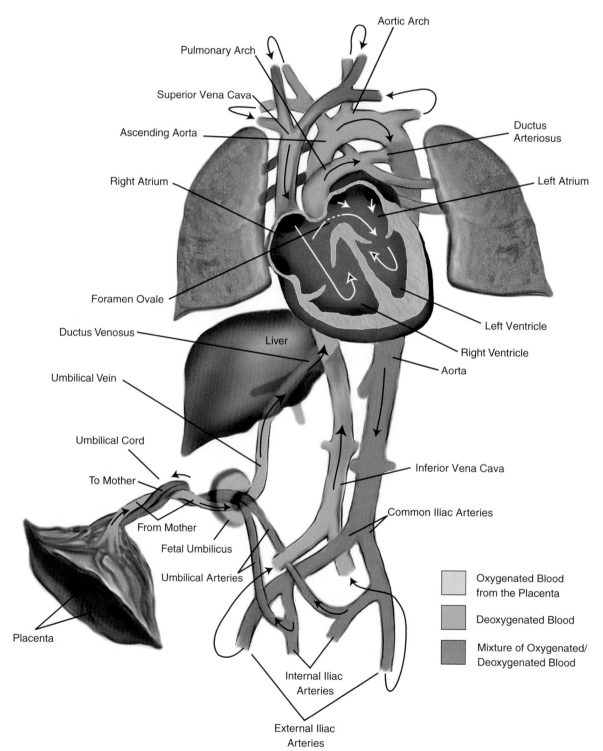

umbilical arteries and again flows back to the placenta to pick up oxygen and to drop off waste products.

After birth—and once the lungs and the renal, digestive, and liver functions are established—the special structures of the fetal circulation are no longer required. These special structures go through the following changes:

- The placenta is expelled by the mother.
- The umbilical arteries atrophy and become the lateral umbilical ligaments.
- The umbilical vein becomes the round ligament *(ligamentum teres)* of the liver.
- The ductus venosus becomes the *ligamentum venosum,* which is a fibrous cord in the liver.
- The flap on the foramen ovale usually closes (as a result of the increased left atrium blood pressure) and becomes a depression in the interatrial septum called the *fossa ovalis.*
- The ductus arteriosus atrophies and becomes the *ligamentum arteriosum.*

Fetal Lung Fluids

It is estimated that at birth, the lungs are partially inflated with liquid approximately equal to the newborn's functional residual capacity. It was once thought that this liquid originated from the aspiration of amniotic fluid, because the fetus normally demonstrates periods of rapid and irregular breathing during the last trimester of gestation. It is now known, however, that this is not the case. The fluid apparently originates from the alveolar cells during fetal development. At birth the fluid is removed from the lungs during the first 24 hours of life primarily by the following mechanisms:

- About one-third of the fluid is squeezed out of the lungs as the infant passes through the birth canal.
- About one-third of the fluid is absorbed by the pulmonary capillaries.
- About one-third of the fluid is removed by the lymphatic system.

Number of Alveoli at Birth

About 24 million primitive alveoli are present at birth. This number, however, represents only about 10 percent of the adult gas exchange units. The number of alveoli continue to increase until about 12 years of age. Thus, it is important to note that respiratory problems during childhood can have a dramatic effect on the anatomy and physiology of the mature pulmonary system.

BIRTH

Moments after birth, an intriguing and dramatic sequence of anatomic and physiologic events occurs. The function of the placenta is suddenly terminated, the lungs rapidly establish themselves as the organs of gas exchange, and all the features of adult circulation are set in place.

First Breath

At birth, the infant is bombarded by a variety of external sensory stimuli (e.g., thermal, tactile, visual). At the same time, the placenta ceases to function, causing the fetal blood P_{O_2} to decrease, the P_{CO_2} to increase, and the pH to decrease. Although the exact mechanism is unknown, the sensitivity of both the central and the peripheral chemoreceptors of the newborn increases dramatically at birth. In response to all these stimuli, the infant *inhales.*

To initiate the first breath, however, the infant must generate a remarkable negative intrapleural pressure to overcome the viscous fluid in the lungs. It is estimated that the intrapleural pressure must decrease to about −40 cm H_2O before any air enters the lungs. Intrapleural pressures as low as −100 cm H_2O have been reported. About 40 mL of air enter the lungs during the first breath. On exhalation, the infant expels about one-half of the volume obtained on the first breath, thus establishing the first portion of the residual volume. Figure 10–5 illustrates the typical pressure-volume changes of the lungs that occur in the newborn during the first 2 weeks of life. The average *lung compliance* of the newborn is about 0.005 L/cm H_2O (5 mL/cm H_2O; the *airway resistance* is about 30 cm H_2O/L/sec.

Circulatory Changes at Birth

As the infant inhales for the first time, the pulmonary vascular resistance falls dramatically. The major mechanisms that account for the decreased pulmonary vascular resistance are (1) the sudden increase in the alveolar P_{O_2}, which offsets the hypoxic vasoconstriction; (2) the removal of fluid from the lungs, reducing the external pressure on the pulmonary vessels, and (3) the mechanical increase in lung volume, which widens the caliber of the extra-alveolar vessels.

As the pulmonary vascular resistance decreases, a greater amount of blood flows through the lungs and, therefore, more blood returns to the left atrium. This causes the pressure in the left atrium to increase and the flap of the foramen ovale to close. The closure of the foramen ovale is further aided by the fall in pressure that occurs in the right atrium as the umbilical flow ceases. A few minutes later, the smooth muscles of the ductus arteriosus constrict in response to the increased P_{O_2}.

Figure 10–5
The pressure-volume changes of the newborn's lungs during the first 2 weeks of life.

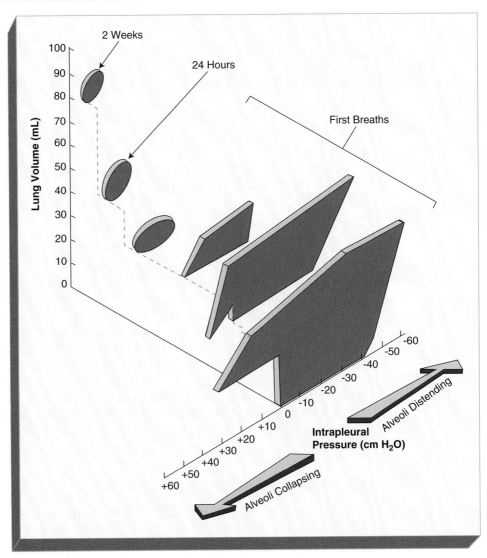

CLINICAL
APPLICATION
CASE
1
See page 373

Clinically, however, the newborn's P_{O_2} must increase to more than 45 to 50 mm Hg in order for the ductus arteriosus to close. If this P_{O_2} level is not reached, the ductus arteriosus will remain open, and the pulmonary vascular resistance will remain elevated, producing the syndrome known as **persistent pulmonary hypertension of the neonate (PPHN)** (previously known as persistent fetal circulation). Furthermore, should the fetal P_{O_2} increase sufficiently to close the ductus arteriosus but then fall within the first 24 to 48 hours after birth, the ductus arteriosus will reopen.

It is believed that other substances released at birth (such as bradykinin, serotonin, and prostaglandin inhibitors) contribute to the constriction of the ductus arteriosus.

CONTROL OF VENTILATION IN THE NEWBORN

Within moments after birth, the newborn infant initiates the first breath. Although they are inhibited during fetal life, the peripheral and central chemoreceptors play a major role in activating the first breath. It is not precisely understood why these chemoreceptors are dormant during fetal life but suddenly activated at birth.

Peripheral Chemoreceptors

The exact role of the peripheral chemoreceptors in the newborn is not clearly defined. It is known, however, that in both preterm and term infants, hypoxia elicits a transient rise in ventilation, followed by a marked fall. The magnitude of the increase is similar whether the infant is in the rapid eye-movement (REM) state, quiet sleep state, or awake state. The late fall, however, is less marked or is absent when the infant is in the quiet sleep state. One to 2 weeks after birth, the infant demonstrates the adult response of sustained hyperventilation. The response to hypoxia is greater and more sustained in the term infant than in the preterm infant. Although it is known that the peripheral chemoreceptors of the adult are responsive to CO_2, little information is available about the peripheral chemoreceptors' sensitivity to changes in CO_2 and pH during the neonatal period.

Central Chemoreceptors

The central chemoreceptors of the newborn respond to the elevated CO_2 levels in a manner similar to that of the adult. The response to an increased CO_2 level is primarily an increased tidal volume, with little change in inspiratory time or ventilatory rate. The response of the central chemoreceptors may be more marked with increasing gestational age.

Infant Reflexes

Trigeminal Reflex

Stimulation of the newborn's trigeminal nerve (i.e., the face and nasal and nasopharyngeal mucosa) causes a decrease in the infant's respiration and heart rate. It has been reported that even gentle stimulation of the malar region in both preterm and term infants may cause significant respiratory slowing. Thus, various procedures (such as nasopharyngeal suctioning) may be hazardous to the newborn. Clinically, facial cooling has been used as a means of terminating paroxysms of supraventricular tachycardia in the newborn.

Irritant Reflex

Epithelial irritant receptors, located throughout the airways, respond to direct tactile stimulation, lung deflation, and irritant gases. This response is mediated by myelinated vagal fibers. Based on gestational age, these receptors elicit different responses. In preterm infants of less than 35 weeks' gestation, tracheal stimulation (e.g., endotracheal suctioning or intubation) is commonly followed by respiratory slowing or apnea. In the term infant, however, stimulation causes marked hyperventilation. The inhibitory response seen in the preterm infant may be due to vagal nerve immaturity (i.e., the vagal nerves are not adequately myelinated). Unmyelinated neurons are unable to transmit high-frequency discharges.

Head Paradoxical Reflex

The head paradoxical reflex is a deep inspiration that is elicited by lung inflation. In other words, the infant inhales and then tops the inspiration with a deep breath before exhalation occurs. This reflex is seen in the term infant and is thought to be mediated by the irritant receptors. The head paradoxical reflex may play a role in sighing, which is frequently seen in the newborn. This reflex is thought to be valuable in maintaining lung compliance by offsetting alveolar collapse.

CLINICAL PARAMETERS IN THE NORMAL NEWBORN

Table 10–1 lists the average pulmonary function findings of the newborn. The vital signs of the normal newborn are listed in Table 10–2. Figure 10–6 illustrates graphically the average pH, Pa_{CO_2}, HCO_3^-, and Pa_{O_2} values of the normal infant over a period of 72 hours after birth.

TABLE 10–1

Approximate Lung Volumes (mL) and Capacities of the Normal Newborn

Tidal volume (V_T)	15	Vital capacity (VC)	115
Residual volume (RV)	40	Functional residual capacity (FRC)	80
Expiratory reserve volume (ERV)	40	Inspiratory capacity (IC)	75
Inspiratory reserve volume (IRV)	60	Total lung capacity (TLC)	155

TABLE 10–2
Vital Sign Ranges of the Normal Newborn

Respiratory rate (RR)	35–50/min
Heart rate (HR)	130–150/min
Blood pressure (BP)	60/40–70/45 mm Hg

Figure 10–6
The average pH, Pa_{CO_2}, HCO_3^-, and Pa_{O_2} values of the normal infant during the first 72 hours of life.

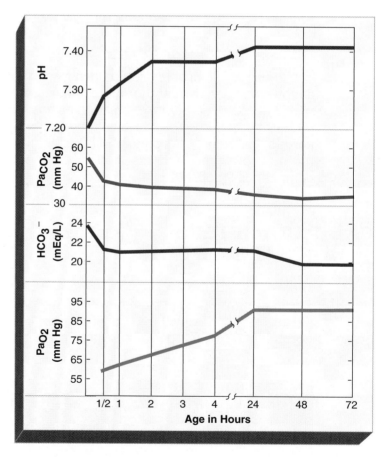

CHAPTER SUMMARY

The major cardiopulmonary physiology of the fetus and the newborn develop during four periods: embryonic, pseudoglandular, canalicular, and terminal sac. The primary components of the placenta include the cotyledons, fetal vessels, chorionic villi, intervillous spaces, umbilical arteries, umbilical vein, and spiral arterioles. The major components of fetal circulation include the umbilical vein, ductus venosus, inferior vena cava, right atrium, superior vena cava, foramen ovale, ductus ateriosus, common iliac arteries, and external and internal iliacs. Finally, the respiratory care practitioner needs a knowledge base of the anatomic and physiologic sequences occurring at birth, including the first breath, circulatory changes, and persistent pulmonary hypertension of the neonate (PPHN); control of ventilation in the newborn, including the peripheral chemoreceptors, central chemoreceptors, and infant reflexes; and the clinical parameters in the normal newborn, including approximate lung volumes and capacities and vital sign ranges.

1 CLINICAL APPLICATION CASE

A 1620 g (3 lb, 9 oz) boy was born 12 weeks early (at 28 weeks gestation). His Apgar scores at delivery were 4 and 5.* The baby's skin was cyanotic and he was in obvious respiratory distress. He demonstrated nasal flaring and intercostal retractions. A gruntlike sound could be heard without the aid of a stethoscope during each exhalation. The baby was transferred to the neonatal intensive care unit and placed on continuous positive airway pressure (CPAP) via nasal prongs at a pressure setting of 3 cm H_2O and an inspired oxygen concentration ($F_{I_{O_2}}$) of 0.4.

The Apgar score evaluates five factors: heart rate, respiratory effort, muscle tone, reflex irritability, and color. Each factor is rated either 0, 1, or 2. The scoring system provides a clinical picture of the infant's condition following delivery. An Apgar score is taken at 1 minute after delivery. A second Apgar score is taken at 5 minutes after delivery to assess the infant's ability to recover from the stress of birth and adapt to extrauterine life. The baby is usually considered to be out of danger when the score is greater than 7.

The baby's vital signs were respirations—64 breaths/min, blood pressure—48/22 mm Hg, and apical heart rate—175 beats/min. On auscultation bilateral crackles could be heard. A portable chest x-ray showed a "ground-glass" appearance and air bronchogram throughout both lung fields, consistent with infant respiratory distress syndrome (IRDS). Umbilical arterial blood gas values were pH—7.53, Pa_{CO_2}—28 mm Hg, HCO_3^-—21 mEq/L, and Pa_{O_2}—41 mm Hg. The neonatologist entered the following diagnosis in the infant's progress notes: "IRDS and PPHN" (persistent pulmonary hypertension of the neonate).

During the next 72 hours the infant's clinical progress was stormy. Three hours after the baby was born, he was intubated and placed on a time-cycled, pressure-limited synchronized intermittent mandatory ventilation (SIMV) rate of

(continues)

35 breaths/min, inspiratory time 0.5 second, peak inspiratory pressure (PIP) of 22 cm H_2O, an $F_{I_{O_2}}$ of 0.8, and positive end-expiratory pressure (PEEP) of 7 cm H_2O. The baby received Survanta® treatments (a synthetic pulmonary surfactant) through his endotracheal tube on day 2. On day 4, his clinical condition stabilized.

Although the baby was still intubated on day 5, he no longer required SIMV. The ventilator was set on the CPAP mode at a pressure setting of 3 cm H_2O with an $F_{I_{O_2}}$ of 0.4. The baby's vital signs were blood pressure—73/48 mm Hg, heart rate (apical) 122 beats/min, and respiratory rate—40 breaths/min. Normal vesicular breath sounds were heard over both lung fields. Chest x-ray showed substantial improvement throughout both lungs. The baby's umbilical arterial blood gas values were pH—7.41, Pa_{CO_2}—38 mm Hg, HCO_3^-—24 mEq/L, and Pa_{O_2}—158 mm Hg. The $F_{I_{O_2}}$ was decreased to 0.3. The neonatologist wrote the following assessment in the patient's chart: "IRDS has significantly improved and PPHN no longer appears to be present." The baby progressively improved and was discharged 3 days later.

DISCUSSION

This case illustrates the possible adverse effects of a premature birth on the infant's (1) alveolar-capillary gas exchange units and (2) pulmonary circulation. During fetal development, the alveolar-capillary system and the quantity of pulmonary surfactant usually are not sufficient to support life until the 28th week of gestation or beyond. In this case, the baby was born at the very beginning of this time period. Thus, because of the immaturity of the baby's alveolar-capillary system, the ability of the type II cells to produce pulmonary surfactant was inadequate (see Figure 1–26).

As a result of the insufficient amount of pulmonary surfactant, the pathologic processes of a common newborn respiratory disease called infant respiratory distress syndrome (IRDS) developed. The anatomic alterations of the lungs associated with IRDS include interstitial and intra-alveolar edema and hemorrhage, alveolar consolidation, intra-alveolar hyaline membrane formation, and atelectasis. All of these pathologic processes cause the alveolar-capillary membrane's thickness to increase. As this condition progressively worsened, the diffusion of oxygen between the alveoli and the pulmonary capillary blood decreased (see Figure 3–6), and the infant's lung compliance decreased (see Figure 2–11). Clinically, the decreased diffusion of oxygen was manifested by cyanosis, increased respiration rate and heart rate, and decreased Pa_{O_2}. The decreased lung compliance was manifested by nasal flaring, intercostal retractions, exhalation grunting, bilateral crackles, and a ground-glass appearance and air bronchogram on the chest x-ray.

Finally, because the baby's Pa_{O_2} was less than 45 mm Hg shortly after birth, the ductus arteriosus remained patent, producing the syndrome known as *persistent pulmonary hypertension of the neonate* (PPHN). As the infant's condition improved and his Pa_{O_2} increased, the ductus arteriosus closed and the signs and symptoms associated with PPHN disappeared. At the time of this writing, the baby was a perfectly normal 3-year-old boy who was attending half-day preschool sessions 5 days per week.

2 CLINICAL APPLICATION CASE

While in her third trimester of pregnancy, a 28-year-old woman experienced vaginal bleeding, abdominal pain, uterine tenderness, and uterine contractions. Concerned, she alerted her husband, who immediately drove her to the hospital. In the emergency department, a provisional diagnosis of *abruptio placentae* (premature partial or total separation of the placenta from the uterus) was made. Because of the excessive hemorrhage, the medical staff felt that the abruptio placentae was extensive and that both the mother and the fetus were in a life-threatening situation. The patient received medication—STAT—for shock and blood replacement. She was then transferred to surgery and prepped for a cesarean section. Shortly after the delivery of the baby (and placenta), the bleeding stopped. The presence of a near-total abruptio placentae was confirmed during the surgery.

The initial assessment of the baby showed a premature female infant born 6 weeks early (at 34 weeks gestation). She weighed only 1610 g (3 lb, 7 oz). Her first Apgar score at delivery was 4. Her heart rate was less than 100 beats/min, respiratory rate was weak and irregular, skin color was blue, she demonstrated no grimace reflex when suctioned, and her muscle tone showed only moderate flexion. The baby was manually ventilated aggressively with an inspired oxygen concentration (FI_{O_2}) of 1.0 and responded favorably within a few minutes. The second Apgar score was 8. Her heart rate was greater than 100 beats/min, she had a strong cry, her skin was pink, she demonstrated a grimace reflex when suctioned, and her muscle tone was improved.

The baby was transferred to the neonatal intensive care unit for close observation. Two hours later the baby's vital signs were respirations—44 breaths/min, blood pressure—66/42 mm Hg, and apical heart rate—135 beats/min. On auscultation, normal vesicular breath sounds were heard bilaterally. A portable chest x-ray was normal. The baby's umbilical arterial blood gas values were pH—7.33, Pa_{CO_2}—44 mm Hg, HCO_3^-—23 mEq/L, and Pa_{O_2}—52 mm Hg. Four days later, both the mother and the baby were discharged in good health.

DISCUSSION

This case illustrates the important function of the placenta as a lifeline between the mother and the baby during fetal life. Because the placenta separated from the wall of the uterus, the maternal–placentae–fetal interface was seriously compromised. In short, the ability of the fetus to absorb oxygen, nutrients, and other substances and excrete carbon dioxide and other wastes was interrupted. Complete separation brings about immediate death of the fetus. Bleeding from the site of separation may cause abdominal pain, uterine tenderness, and uterine contraction. Bleeding may be concealed within the uterus or may be evident externally, sometimes as sudden massive hemorrhage (as in this case). In severe cases, shock and death can occur in minutes. Cesarean section must be performed immediately. Fortunately, in this case the mother and the baby were treated in a timely manner.

REVIEW QUESTIONS

1. During the embryonic period, the lungs first appear at about the
    A. 10th day after fertilization
    B. 24th day after fertilization
    C. 6th week after fertilization
    D. 12th week after fertilization

2. The lungs are usually sufficiently mature to support life by the
    A. 24th week of gestation
    B. 28th week of gestation
    C. 32nd week of gestation
    D. 36th week of gestation

3. At birth, the number of alveoli represent about how much of the total adult gas exchange units?
    A. 10 percent
    B. 20 percent
    C. 30 percent
    D. 40 percent

4. The number of alveoli continues to increase until about
    A. 6 years of age
    B. 8 years of age
    C. 10 years of age
    D. 12 years of age

5. The average P_{O_2} in the umbilical arteries during fetal life is about
    A. 20 mm Hg
    B. 40 mm Hg
    C. 60 mm Hg
    D. 80 mm Hg

6. The average P_{O_2} in the umbilical vein during fetal life is about
    A. 20 mm Hg
    B. 30 mm Hg
    C. 40 mm Hg
    D. 50 mm Hg

7. The average P_{CO_2} in the umbilical arteries during fetal life is about
    A. 25 mm Hg
    B. 35 mm Hg
    C. 45 mm Hg
    D. 55 mm Hg

8. In the placenta, maternal blood is continuously pumped through the
    A. umbilical arteries
    B. chorionic villi
    C. fetal vessels
    D. intervillous space

9. In the fetal circulation, once blood enters the right atrium, most of the blood enters the left atrium by passing through the
    A.   ductus arteriosus
    B.   ductus venosus
    C.   pulmonary arteries
    D.   foramen ovale

10. Shortly after birth the ductus arteriosus constricts in response to
    I.   increased P_{O_2}
    II.   decreased P_{CO_2}
    III. increased pH
    IV.   prostaglandins
        A. I only
        B. II only
        C. III and IV only
        D. I and IV only

CLINICAL APPLICATION QUESTIONS

CASE 1

1. During fetal development, the alveolar-capillary system and the quantity of pulmonary surfactant usually are not sufficient to support life until the _____ week of gestation.

2. As a result of the insufficient amount of pulmonary surfactant, the pathologic processes of a common newborn respiratory disease called _____ developed.

3. In this case, what are the major anatomic alterations of the lungs associated with the respiratory disease that developed in the infant?

    _____

    _____

    _____

    _____

    _____

    _____

4. Describe the pathophysiology that develops as the conditions listed in question 3 worsen.

    _____

    _____

    _____

5. Describe how the following conditions are manifested in the clinical setting:

Decreased pulmonary diffusion:_____

_____

_____

Decreased lung compliance:_____

_____

_____

6. Why did PPHN develop in the infant in this case? How did this condition improve?

_____

_____

_____

CASE 2

1. Describe why the maternal–placentae–fetal interface was seriously compromised in this case. _____

_____

_____

2. Describe what condition(s) bleeding from the site of maternal–placenta separation may cause to the mother. _____

_____

3. What may develop when the maternal–placenta separation is severe? What procedure must be performed immediately? _____

_____

CHAPTER 11

Aging and the Cardiopulmonary System

OBJECTIVES

By the end of this chapter, the student should be able to:

1. Describe the effects of aging on the following components of the *respiratory system:*
   —Static mechanical properties
   • Elastic recoil of the lungs
   • Lung compliance
   • Thoracic compliance
   —Lung volumes and capacities
   —Dynamic maneuvers of ventilation
   —Pulmonary diffusing capacity
   —Alveolar dead space ventilation
   —Pulmonary gas exchange
   —Arterial blood gases
   —Arterial-venous oxygen content difference
   —Hemoglobin concentration
   —Control of ventilation
   —Defense mechanisms
   —Exercise tolerance
   —Pulmonary diseases in the elderly

2. Describe the effects of aging on the following components of the *cardiovascular system:*
   —Structure of the heart
   —Work of the heart
   —Heart rate
   —Stroke volume
   —Cardiac output
   —Peripheral vascular resistance
   —Blood pressure
   —Aerobic capacity

3. Complete the review questions at the end of this chapter.

The aging process is normal, progressive, and physiologically irreversible. Aging occurs despite optimal nutrition, genetic background, environmental surroundings, and activity patterns. The biological aging process, however, may demonstrate altered rates of progression in response to an individual's genetic background and daily living habits.

Between the years 2010 and 2030, those born from 1946 to 1964 during the post–World War II baby boom (the biggest baby boom in history) will be turning 65 years old. During this period, it is estimated that the number of people over 65 years of age will increase from the present

25 million to 50 million. By the year 2020, the 75-and-over population, who have specific activity limitations due to chronic ailments, will increase 2.5-fold (to 10.7 million). Figure 11–1 illustrates the actual and projected population of persons age 55 years and older for four different age groups from 1900 to 2040.

It is also projected that the number of annual short-stay hospital days of persons 65 years and older will increase from the 105,358 of 1980 to over 286,000 by the year 2050 (Figure 11–2). Because the mortality and

Figure 11–1

The actual and projected population of adults age 55 years and older for four different age groups (1900 to 2040).

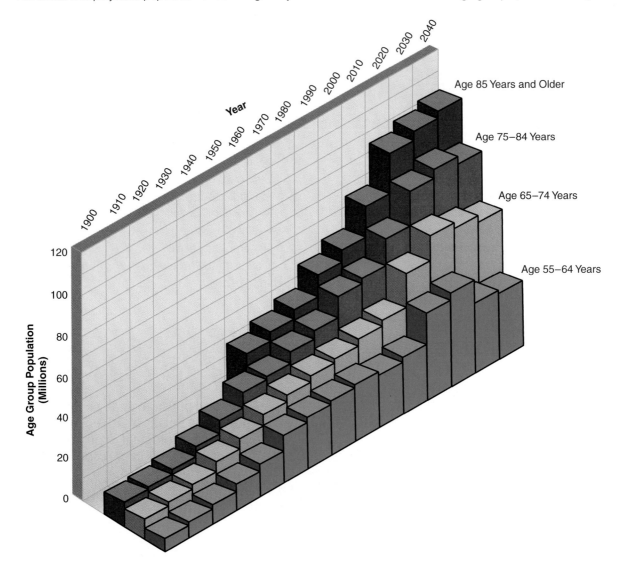

Figure 11–2

The actual and projected annual short-stay hospital days for adults age 65 years and older (1980 to 2050).

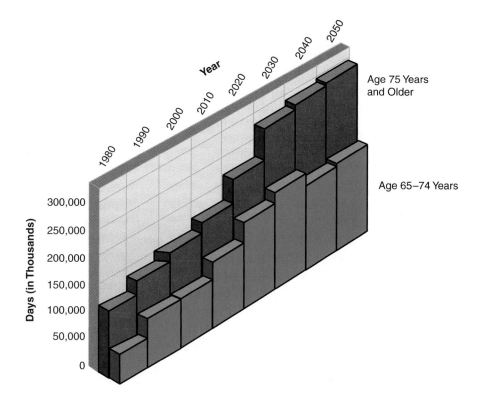

morbidity rates rise sharply after age 65, the large size of this population will undoubtedly pose a tremendous challenge to the health care industry. A basic understanding of how the aging process affects the cardiopulmonary system is critical for the respiratory care practitioner.

THE EFFECTS OF AGING ON THE RESPIRATORY SYSTEM

The growth and development of the lungs is essentially complete by about 20 years of age. Most of the pulmonary function indices reach their maximum levels between 20 and 25 years of age and then progressively decline. The precise effects of aging on the respiratory system are difficult to determine, because the changes associated with time are often indistinguishable from those caused by disease. For example, factors such as long-term exposure to environmental pollutants, recurring pulmonary infections, smoking, and some working conditions can cause alterations in the respiratory system that are not easily differentiated from changes due to aging alone. Despite these difficulties, the conclusions reached here appear to be well founded.

Static Mechanical Properties

The **functional residual capacity** is the volume remaining in the lungs when the elastic recoil of the lungs exactly balances the natural tendency of the chest wall to expand. With aging, the elastic recoil of the lungs decreases, causing lung compliance to increase. This is illustrated graphically as a shift to the left (steeper slope) of the volume-pressure curve (Figure 11–3). The decrease in lung elasticity develops because the alveoli progressively deteriorate and enlarge after age 30. Structurally, the alveolar changes resemble the air sac changes associated with emphysema.

Even though the potential for greater lung expansion exists as an individual ages, it cannot be realized because of the structural limitations that develop in the chest wall. With aging the costal cartilages progressively calcify, causing the ribs to slant downward, and this structural change causes the thorax to become less compliant. Because of these anatomic changes, the transpulmonary pressure difference, which is responsible for holding the airways open, is diminished with age.

Finally, the reduction in chest wall compliance is slightly greater than the increase in lung compliance, resulting in an overall moderate decline

Figure 11–3
Comparison of the pressure-volume curve of a 60-year-old adult with that of a 20-year-old adult.

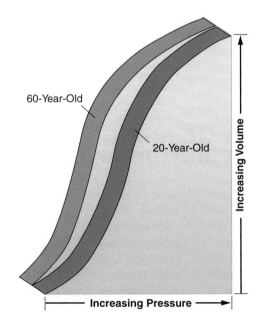

in total compliance of the respiratory system. It is estimated that the work expenditure of a 60-year-old individual to overcome static mechanical forces during normal breathing is 20 percent greater than that of a 20-year-old. The decreased compliance of the respiratory system associated with age is offset by increased respiratory frequency, rather than by increased tidal volume during exertion.

Lung Volumes and Capacities

Figure 11–4 shows the changes that occur in the lung volumes and capacities with aging. Although studies differ, it is generally agreed that the total lung capacity (TLC) essentially remains the same throughout life. Should the TLC decrease, however, it is probably due to the decreased height that typically occurs with age.

It is well documented that the residual volume (RV) increases with age. This is primarily due to age-related alveolar enlargement and to small airway closure. As the RV increases, the RV/TLC ratio also increases. The RV/TLC ratio increases from approximately 20 percent at age 20 to about 35 percent at age 60. This increase occurs predominantly after age 40.

Figure 11–4

Schematic representation of the changes that occur in lung volumes and capacities with aging.

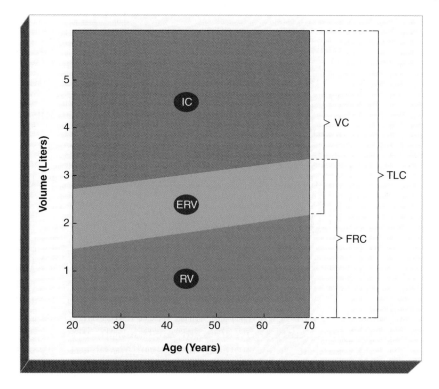

Moreover, as the RV increases, the expiratory reserve volume (ERV) decreases. Most studies show that the functional residual capacity (FRC) increases with age, but not as much as the RV and the RV/TLC. Because the FRC typically increases with age, the inspiratory capacity (IC) decreases.

Because the vital capacity (VC) is equal to the TLC minus the RV, the VC inevitably decreases as the RV increases. It is estimated that in men, the VC decreases about 25 mL/year. In women, the VC decreases about 20 mL/year. In general, the VC decreases about 40 to 50 percent by age 70.

Dynamic Maneuvers of Ventilation

Because of the loss of lung elasticity associated with aging, there inevitably is a marked effect on the dynamics of ventilation. In fact, one of the most prominent physiologic changes associated with age is the reduced efficiency in forced air expulsion. This normal deterioration is reflected by a progressive decrease in the following dynamic lung functions:

- Forced vital capacity (FVC)
- Peak expiratory flow rate (PEFR)
- Forced expiratory flow$_{25-75\%}$ (FEF$_{25-75\%}$)
- Forced expiratory volume in 1 second (FEV$_1$)
- Forced expiratory volume in 1 second/forced vital capacity ratio (FEV$_1$/FVC ratio)
- Maximum voluntary ventilation (MVV)

It is estimated that these dynamic lung functions decrease approximately 20 to 30 percent throughout the average adult's life. For example, it is reported that the FEV$_1$ decreases about 30 mL/year in men and about 20 mL/year in women after about age 20. Initially, the yearly decline in FEV$_1$ is relatively small, but accelerates with age. The FVC decreases about 15 to 30 mL/year in men and 15 to 25 mL/year in women. Precisely what causes the flow rates to decline is still being debated. However, because gas flow is dependent on (1) the applied pressure and (2) the airway resistance, changes in either or both of these factors could be responsible for the reduction of gas flow rates seen in the elderly.

Pulmonary Diffusing Capacity

The pulmonary diffusing capacity (D$_{L_{CO}}$) progressively decreases after about 20 years of age. It is estimated that the D$_{L_{CO}}$ falls about 20 percent over the course of adult life. In men, it is reported that D$_{L_{CO}}$ declines at a rate of about 2 mL/min/mm Hg; in women the decline is about 1.5 mL/min/mm Hg. This decline results from decreased alveolar surface area caused by alveolar destruction, increased alveolar wall thickness, and decreased pulmonary capillary blood flow, all of which are known to occur with aging.

Alveolar Dead Space Ventilation

Alveolar dead space ventilation increases with advancing age. This is due, in part, to (1) the decreased cardiac index associated with aging and (2) the structural alterations of the pulmonary capillaries that occur as a result of normal alveolar deterioration. In other words, the natural loss of lung elasticity results in an increase in lung compliance, which, in turn, leads to an increase in dead space ventilation. It is estimated that the alveolar dead space ventilation increases about 1 mL/year throughout adult life.

PULMONARY GAS EXCHANGE

The alveolar-arterial oxygen tension difference $P_{(A-a)O_2}$ progressively increases with age. Factors that may increase the $P_{(A-a)O_2}$ include the physiologic shunt, the mismatching of ventilation and perfusion, and a decreased diffusing capacity.

ARTERIAL BLOOD GASES

In the normal adult, the Pa_{O_2} should be greater than 90 mm Hg up to 45 years of age. After 45 years of age, the Pa_{O_2} generally declines. The minimum low Pa_{O_2}, however, should be greater than 75 mm Hg—regardless of age. Contrary to earlier beliefs, it is now documented that the Pa_{O_2} progressively decreases between the ages of 45 and 75 years, and then often increases slightly and levels off.

The Pa_{CO_2} remains constant throughout life. A possible explanation for this is the greater diffusion ability of carbon dioxide through the alveolar-capillary barrier. Because the Pa_{CO_2} remains the same in the healthy older adult, the pH and HCO_3^- levels also remain constant.

Arterial-Venous Oxygen Content Difference

The maximum arterial-venous oxygen content difference $C(a - \bar{v})_{O_2}$ tends to decrease with age. Contributory factors include (1) decline in physical fitness, (2) less efficient peripheral blood distribution, and (3) reduction in tissue enzyme activity.

Hemoglobin Concentration

Anemia is a common finding in the elderly. Several factors predispose the elderly to anemia. Red bone marrow has a tendency to be replaced by fatty marrow, especially in the long bones. Gastrointestinal atrophy, which is commonly associated with advancing age, may slow the absorption of iron or vitamin B_{12}. Gastrointestinal bleeding is also more prevalent in the elderly. Perhaps the most important reasons for anemia in the elderly are sociologic rather than medical—for example, insufficient income to purchase food or decreased interest in cooking and eating adequate meals.

Control of Ventilation

Ventilatory rate and heart rate responses to hypoxia and hypercapnia diminish with age. This is due to (1) a reduced sensitivity and responsiveness of the peripheral and central chemoreceptors and (2) the slowing of central nervous system pathways with age. In addition, age slows the neural output to respiratory muscles and lower chest wall and reduces lung mechanical efficiency. It is estimated that the ventilatory response to hypoxia is decreased more than 50 percent in the healthy male over 65 years of age; the ventilatory response to hypercapnia is decreased by more than 40 percent. These reductions increase the risk of pulmonary diseases (e.g., pneumonia, chronic obstructive pulmonary disease, and obstructive sleep apnea.)

Defense Mechanisms

The rate of the mucociliary transport system declines with age. In addition, there is a decreased cough reflex in more than 70 percent of the elderly population. The decreased cough reflex is caused, in part, by the increased prevalence of medication use (e.g., sedatives) and neurologic diseases associated with the elderly. In addition, dysphagia (impaired esophageal motility), which is commonly seen in the elderly, increases the risk for aspiration and pneumonia.

Exercise Tolerance

In healthy individuals of any age, respiratory function does not limit exercise tolerance. The oxygen transport system is more critically dependent on the cardiovascular system than on respiratory function. The maximal oxygen uptake ($\dot{V}_{O_2max}$), which is the parameter most commonly used to evaluate an individual's aerobic exercise tolerance, peaks at age 20 and progressively and linearly decreases with age. Although there is considerable variation among individuals, it is estimated that from 20 to 60 years of age, a person's maximal oxygen uptake decreases by approximately 35 percent. Evidence indicates, however, that regular physical conditioning throughout life increases oxygen uptake and, therefore, enhances the capacity for exertion during work and recreation.

Pulmonary Diseases in the Elderly

Although the occurrence of pulmonary diseases increases with age, it is difficult to determine the precise relationship aging has to pulmonary disease. This is because aging is also associated with the presence of chronic diseases (e.g., lung cancer, bronchitis, emphysema). It is known, however, that the incidence of serious infectious pulmonary diseases is significantly greater in the elderly. Although the incidence of pneumonia has decreased dramatically in recent years, pneumonia is still a major cause of death in the elderly. Evidence suggests that this is partly owing to the impaired defense mechanisms in the elderly.

THE EFFECTS OF AGING ON THE CARDIOVASCULAR SYSTEM

A variety of adverse changes develops in the cardiovascular system with age. In fact, the major causes of death in the aging population are diseases of the cardiovascular system. The major changes in the cardiovascular system that develop as a function of age are discussed next.

Structure of the Heart

Between 30 and 80 years of age, the thickness of the left ventricular wall increases by about 25 percent. Cardiac hypertrophy, however, is not considered a primary change associated with aging. In the ventricles, the muscle fiber size progressively increases. Fibrosis develops in the lining of the chambers and fatty infiltration occurs in the wall of the chambers. The amount of connective tissue increases, causing the heart to become less elastic. Thus, the compliance of the heart is reduced and the heart functions less efficiently as a pump. The heart valves thicken from calcification and fibrosis. This structural change causes the valves to become more rigid and less effective. As the valves become more rigid and distorted, the blood flow may be impeded and systolic murmurs may develop.

Work of the Heart

The work of the heart, which is defined as stroke volume times mean systolic blood pressure, decreases approximately 1 percent per year (Figure 11–5).

Heart Rate

Although the effects of age on the resting heart rate are debated, it is known that the increase in heart rate in response to stress is less in the elderly. The maximum heart rate can be estimated by the following formula:

Maximum heart rate = 220 − age

Thus, the maximum heart rate for a 60-year-old is about 160 (220 − 60 = 160) beats/min. (Recent research has shown that some older subjects

Figure 11–5
Schematic representation of the effects of aging on the work of the heart. LVSWI = left ventricular stroke work index.

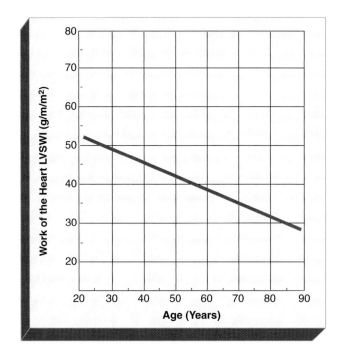

can achieve higher heart rates than those predicted by this method.) The reasons for the decreased maximum heart rate are unclear (Figure 11–6). It may be because of the diminished myocardial oxygen supply associated with advanced age. Another possibility is the decreased compliance of the heart in the elderly. The increase in heart rate in response to stress may be impaired because of increased connective tissue in the sinoatrial and atrioventricular junction and in the bundle branches. The number of catecholamine receptors on the muscle fibers may also be reduced.

With aging, moreover, it not only takes more time for the heart to accelerate, but it also takes more time to return to normal after a stressful event. Because of this, the expected increase in pulse rate in response to certain clinical situations (e.g., anxiety, pain, hemorrhage, and infectious processes) is often not as evident in the elderly.

Stroke Volume

The stroke volume diminishes with age. The precise reason for the reduction in the stroke volume is unknown. It is suggested, however, that it may be a reflection of poor myocardial perfusion, decreased cardiac compliance, and poor contractility. As the stroke volume declines, the *stroke volume index* (stroke volume divided by body surface area) also decreases.

Figure 11-6
Schematic representation of the effects of aging on the maximum heart rate.

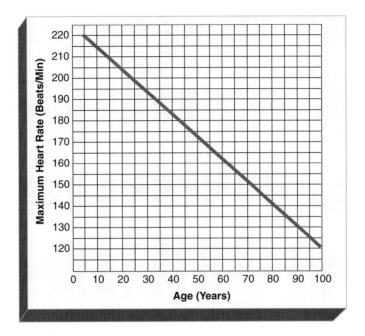

Cardiac Output

As the stroke volume diminishes, the cardiac output inevitably declines (cardiac output = stroke volume × heart rate). After age 20, the cardiac output decreases in a linear fashion about 1 percent per year (Figure 11–7). Between the ages of 30 and 80, the cardiac output decreases about 40 percent in both men and women. As the cardiac output declines, the *cardiac index* (cardiac output divided by body surface area) also decreases.

Peripheral Vascular Resistance

It is well documented that the elasticity of the major blood vessels decreases with advancing age. Both the arteries and veins undergo age-related changes. The intima thickens and the media becomes more fibrotic (see Figure 1–29). Collagen and extracellular materials accumulate in both the intima and media. As the peripheral vascular system becomes stiffer, its ability to accept the cardiac stroke volume declines. This age-related development increases the *resting pulse pressure* and the *systolic blood pressure*. It is estimated that the *total* peripheral vascular resistance increases about 1 percent per year (Figure 11–8).

As the peripheral vascular resistance increases, the perfusion of the body organs decreases. This progressive decline in organ perfusion partly explains the many organ debilities seen in elderly people. As the vascular

Figure 11-7
Schematic representation of the effects of aging on cardiac output.

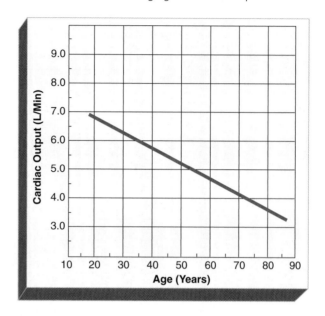

Figure 11-8
Schematic representation of the effects of aging on total peripheral vascular resistance.

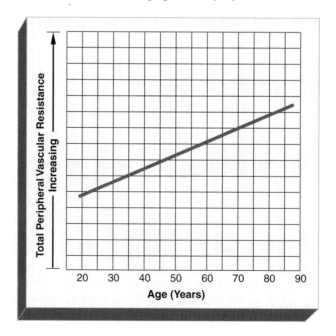

system becomes stiffer with age, its tolerance to change diminishes. For example, a sudden move from the horizontal to the vertical position may cause a marked drop in systemic blood pressure, causing dizziness, confusion, weakness, and fainting. Arterial stiffening also makes the baroreceptors, located in the carotid sinuses and aortic arch, sluggish and less able to moderate blood pressure changes.

Blood Pressure

As described previously, factors associated with aging that increase blood pressure are increasing stiffness of large arteries and increasing total peripheral resistance. Other factors, such as obesity, sodium intake, and stress, can also elevate blood pressure.

Aerobic Capacity

Aerobic capacity decreases about 50 percent between 20 and 80 years of age. This is primarily due to the reduction in muscle mass and strength associated with aging. Other possible causes include the inadequate distribution of blood flow to working muscles and the decreased ability of the tissue cells to extract oxygen.

CHAPTER SUMMARY

A fundamental knowledge base of the effects of aging on the cardiopulmonary system is an important part of respiratory care. The major components are the influence of aging on the respiratory system, including the static mechanical properties of the lungs, lung volumes and capacities, dynamic maneuvers of ventilation, pulmonary diffusing capacity, and alveolar dead space ventilation, as well as pulmonary gas exchange, arterial blood gases, arterial-venous oxygen content difference, hemoglobin concentration, control of ventilation, defense mechanisms, exercise tolerance, and presence of pulmonary diseases. The knowledge base should also include the effects of aging on the cardiovascular system, including the structure of the heart, work of the heart, heart rate, stroke volume, cardiac output, peripheral vascular resistance, blood pressure, and aerobic capacity.

REVIEW QUESTIONS

1. As an individual ages, the
    A. residual volume decreases
    B. expiratory reserve volume increases
    C. functional residual capacity decreases
    D. vital capacity decreases

2. Most of the lung function indices reach their maximum levels between
   A. 5–10 years of age
   B. 10–15 years of age
   C. 15–20 years of age
   D. 20–25 years of age

3. With advancing age, the
   I. lung compliance decreases
   II. chest wall compliance increases
   III. lung compliance increases
   IV. chest wall compliance decreases
      A. II only
      B. III only
      C. I and II only
      D. III and IV only

4. As an individual ages, the
   I. forced vital capacity increases
   II. peak expiratory flow rate decreases
   III. forced expiratory volume in 1 second increases
   IV. maximum voluntary ventilation increases
      A. I only
      B. II only
      C. II and IV only
      D. III and IV only

5. With advancing age, the
   I. Pa_{CO_2} increases
   II. Pa_{O_2} decreases
   III. $P_{(A-a)O_2}$ decreases
   IV. $C(a - \bar{v})_{O_2}$ decreases
      A. I only
      B. II only
      C. III and IV only
      D. II and IV only

6. The maximum heart rate of a 45-year-old person is
   A. 155 beats/min
   B. 165 beats/min
   C. 175 beats/min
   D. 185 beats/min

7. Over the course of life, the diffusion capacity decreases by about
   A. 5 percent
   B. 10 percent
   C. 15 percent
   D. 20 percent

8. Between 30 and 80 years of age, the cardiac output decreases by about
   A.   10 percent
   B.   20 percent
   C.   30 percent
   D.   40 percent

9. With advancing age, the
   I.   blood pressure increases
   II. stroke volume decreases
   III. cardiac output increases
   IV. heart work decreases
        A. I only
        B. II only
        C. III and IV only
        D. I, II, and IV only

10. Between 20 and 60 years of age, the RV/TLC ratio
    A.   increases from 20 to 25 percent
    B.   increases from 20 to 30 percent
    C.   increases from 20 to 35 percent
    D.   increases from 20 to 40 percent

SECTION TWO

ADVANCED CARDIOPULMONARY CONCEPTS AND RELATED AREAS—THE ESSENTIALS

CHAPTER 12

Electrophysiology of the Heart

OBJECTIVES

By the end of this chapter, the student should be able to:

1. Describe the electrophysiology of the heart, including:
   —Action potential
   • Phase 0
   • Phase 1
   • Phase 2
   • Phase 3
   • Phase 4
2. Describe the properties of the cardiac muscle, including:
   —Automaticity
   —Excitability
   —Conductivity
   —Contractility
3. Explain the following refractory periods of the heart:
   —Absolute refractory period
   —Relative refractory period
   —Nonrefractory period
4. Identify the major components of the conductive system of the heart, including:
   —Sinoatrial node
   —Atrioventricular junction
   —Bundle of His
   —Right and left bundle branches
   —Purkinje fibers
5. Describe the cardiac effects of the
   —Sympathetic nervous system
   —Parasympathetic nervous system
6. Complete the review questions at the end of this chapter.

The heart contracts by generating and propagating **action potentials**, which are electrical currents that travel across the cell membranes of the heart. The electrical events of an action potential are identical in skeletal muscles, cardiac muscle, and neurons. In neurons, however, a transmitted action potential is called a **nerve impulse**. When the heart is relaxed (i.e., not generating an action potential), the cardiac muscle fibers are in what is called their **polarized** or **resting state**. During this period, there is an electrical charge difference across the fibers of the heart cells. This electrical difference between the electrolytes inside the cell membranes and the electrolytes outside of the cell membranes is called the **resting membrane potential (RMP)**.

The primary electrolytes responsible for the electrical difference across the RMP are **potassium (K⁺)**, **sodium (Na⁺)**, and **calcium (Ca²⁺)**. Similar to all the cells in the body, the concentration of K⁺ is greatest inside the cardiac cell—about 151 mEq/L—and the concentration of K⁺ outside the cardiac cell is about 4 mEq/L. For Na⁺ and Ca²⁺, the opposite is true. The concentration of Na⁺ outside the cardiac cell is about 144 mEq/L and about 7 mEq/L inside the cell; the concentration of Ca²⁺ is about 5 mEq/L outside the cell and less than 1 mEq/L inside the cell.

When the cardiac cell is in its resting or polarized state, the inside of the cell is negatively charged with the K⁺ cation and the outside of the cell is positively charged with the Na⁺ cation. The way in which this relationship (i.e., negative inside the cell and positive outside of the cell) develops with two cations (positive ions) is as follows: In the polarized state, the Na⁺/K⁺ pump establishes (1) an increased Na⁺ concentration outside of the cell and (2) an increased K⁺ concentration inside of the cell. Both ions then diffuse along their concentration gradients, i.e., K⁺ diffuses out of the cell while, at the same time, Na⁺ diffuses into the cell. For every 50 to 75 K⁺ ions that diffuse out of the cell, only one Na⁺ diffuses into the cell. This exchange ratio results in a deficiency of positive cations inside the cell, i.e., an electrical difference (RMP) between the electrolytes inside the cell and the electrolytes outside the cell is generated (Figure 12–1).

Figure 12–1
The polarized state. For each Na⁺ ion that diffuses into the cell, about 75 K⁺ ions diffuse out of the cell. The result is a deficiency of positive cations inside the cell; this is a cell with a negative charge.

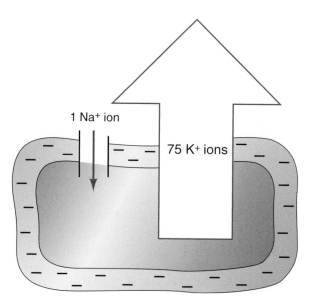

1 Na⁺ ion

75 K⁺ ions

The potential force of the RMP is measured in millivolts (mV) (1 mV = 0.001 V). The RMP of the myocardial cells is about −90 mV. A cornerstone to the understanding of the electrophysiology of the heart are the five electrophysiologic phases of the action potential. An electrocardiogram (ECG) is used to record the five phases of the action potential. A variety of heart abnormalities can disrupt any of these five electrophysiologic phases and, therefore, disrupt and alter the configuration of a normal ECG tracing.

THE FIVE PHASES OF THE ACTION POTENTIAL

Depolarization

Depolarization is the trigger for myocardial contraction.

Phase 0: Rapid depolarization (early phase). Under normal conditions, the ventricular muscle fibers are activated between 60 and 100 times/min by an electrical impulse initiated by the sinoatrial (SA) node. This action changes the RMP and allows a rapid inward flow of Na^+ into the cell through specific Na^+ channels. This process causes the inside of the cell to become positively charged. The voltage inside the cell at the end of depolarization is about +30 mV. This electrophysiologic event produces a rapid up-stroke in the action potential (see Figure 12–2).

Repolarization

Repolarization is the process by which the cells of the heart return to their resting state.

Phase 1: Initial repolarization. Immediately after phase 0, the channels for K^+ open and permit K^+ to flow out of the cell, an action which produces an early, but incomplete, repolarization (repolarization is slowed by the phase 2 influx of Ca^{2+} ions). Phase 1 is illustrated as a short downward stroke in the action potential curve just before the plateau (see Figure 12–2).

Phase 2: Plateau state. During this period, there is slow inward flow of Ca^{2+}, which, in turn, significantly slows the outward flow of K^+. The plateau phase prolongs the contraction of the myocardial cells (see Figure 12–2).

Phase 3: Final rapid repolarization. During this period, the inward flow of Ca^{2+} stops, the outward flow of K^+ is again accelerated, and the rate of repolarization accelerates (see Figure 12–2).

Phase 4: Resting or polarized state. During this period, the voltage-sensitive ion channels return to their pre-depolarization permeability. The excess Na^+ inside the cell (that occurred during depolarization) and the loss of K^+ (that occurred during

Figure 12–2
The action potential and the Na$^+$, K$^+$, and Ca^{2+} changes during phases 0, 1, 2, 3, and 4.

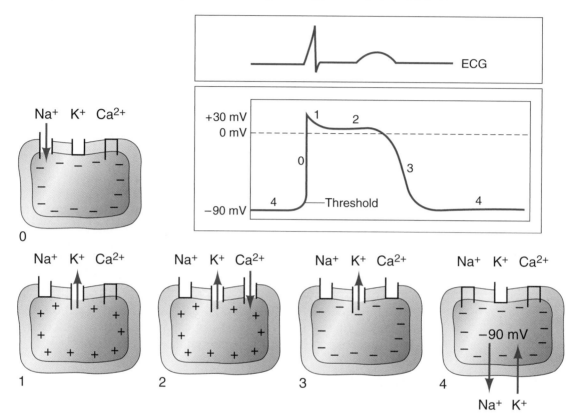

repolarization) are returned to normal by the Na$^+$ and K$^+$ ion pumps. An additional Na$^+$ and Ca^{2+} pump removes the excess of Ca^{2+} from the cell (see Figure 12–2).

PROPERTIES OF THE CARDIAC MUSCLE

The heart is composed of two types of cardiac cells: **contractile muscle fibers** and specialized "pacemaker cells" called **autorhythmic cells**. The myocardial contractile fiber cells dmake up the bulk of the musculature of the myocardium and are responsible for the pumping activity of the heart. Approximately 1 percent of the heart is composed of the autorhythmic cells, the majority of which are located in the SA node. These cells have the unique ability to initiate an action potential spontaneously, which, in turn, triggers the myocardial fibers to contract. The cardiac cells of the heart have four specific properties: automaticity, excitability, conductivity, and contractility.

Automaticity

Automaticity is the unique ability of the cells in the SA node (pacemaker cells) to generate an action potential without being stimulated. This occurs because the cell membranes of the pacemaker cells permit Na^+ to leak into the cell during phase 4. As Na^+ enters the cell, the RMP slowly increases. When the threshold potential (TP) of the pacemaker cells is reached (between -40 and -60 mV), the cells of the SA node rapidly depolarize (Figure 12–3). Under normal conditions, the unique automaticity of the pacemaker cells stimulates the action potential of the heart's conductive system (i.e., atria, atrioventricular [AV] junction, bundle branches, Purkinje fibers, ventricles) at regular and usually predictable intervals (Figure 12–4).

Excitability

Excitability (irritability) is the ability of a cell to reach its threshold potential and respond to a stimulus or irritation. The lower the stimulus needed to activate a cell, the more excitable the cell; conversely, the greater the stimulus needed, the less excitable the cell. The presence of ischemia and hypoxia cause the myocardial cell to become more excitable.

Conductivity

Conductivity is the unique ability of the heart cells to transmit electrical current from cell to cell throughout the entire conductive system.

Contractility

Contractility is the ability of cardiac muscle fibers to shorten and contract in response to an electrical stimulus.

Figure 12–3

Schematic representation comparing action potential of pacemaker and nonpacemaker (working) myocardial cells.

Figure 12–4
Conductive system of the heart.

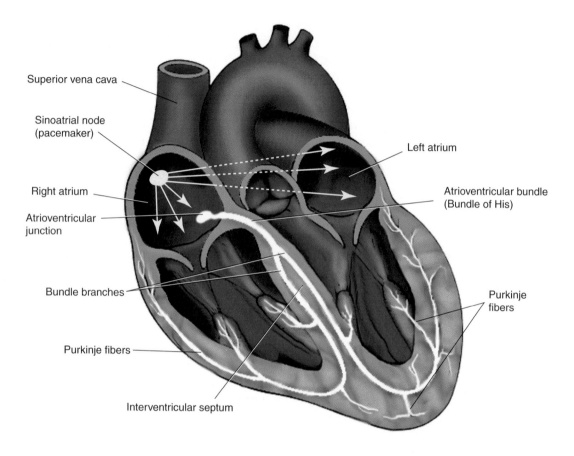

Superior vena cava

Sinoatrial node
(pacemaker)

Left atrium

Right atrium

Atrioventricular bundle
(Bundle of His)

Atrioventricular
junction

Bundle branches

Purkinje
fibers

Purkinje fibers

Interventricular septum

Refractory Periods

Additional properties of the myocardial contractile fibers and autorhythmic cells are refractory periods, which entail (1) the ionic composition of the cells during different phases of the action potential and (2) the ability of the cells to accept a stimulus.

The **absolute refractory period** is the time in which the cells cannot respond to a stimulus. The ionic composition of the cells is not in place to receive a stimulus. Phases 0, 1, 2, and about half of phase 3 represent the absolute refractory period (see Figure 12–2).

The **relative refractory period** is the time in which repolarization is almost complete and a strong stimulus may cause depolarization of some of the cells. Some cells may respond normally, some in an abnormal way, and some not at all. The second half of phase 3 represents the relative refractory period of the action potential (see Figure 12–2).

The **nonrefractory period** occurs when all the cells are in their resting or polarized state. The cells are ready to respond to a stimulus in a normal fashion. Phase 4 represents the nonrefractory period (see Figure 12–2).

The duration of each refractory period may vary in response to use of medications or recreational drugs, or presence of disease, electrolyte imbalance, myocardial ischemia, or myocardial injury.

The Conductive System

As shown in Figure 12–4, the components of the conductive system include the **sinoatrial node** (SA node), **atrioventricular junction** (AV junction), **bundle of His**, the **right** and **left bundle branches**, and the **Purkinje fibers**. The electrical cycle of the heart begins with the SA node, or pacemaker. The SA node initiates the cardiac contraction by producing an electrical impulse that travels through the right and left atria. In the right atrium, the electrical impulse is conducted through the **anterior internodal tract**, **middle internodal tract**, and **posterior internodal tract**. All three internodal pathways become one at the AV junction. The **Bachmann's bundle** conducts electrical impulses from the SA node directly to the left atrium. The electrical impulse generated by the SA node cause the right and left atria to contract simultaneously. This action in turn forces the blood in the atria to move into the ventricles.

The AV junction is located just behind the tricuspid in the lower portion of the right interatrial septum. The AV junction relays the electrical impulse from the atria to the ventricles via the bundle of His (also called the AV bundle). The bundle of His enters the intraventricular septum and divides into the left and right bundle branches. At the heart's apex, the Purkinje fibers sprend throughout the posterior portion of the ventricle and head back toward to the base of the heart. In the normal heart, the total time required for an electrical impulse to travel from the SA node to the end of the Purkinje fibers is about 0.22 second. In other words, the entire heart depolarizes in about 0.22 second.

Autonomic Nervous System

Even though the conductive system of the heart has its own intrinsic pacemaker, the autonomic nervous system plays an important role in the rate of impulse formation, conduction, and contraction strength. The regulation of the heart is controlled by neural fibers from both the sympathetic and parasympathetic nervous system.

Sympathetic neural fibers innervate the atria and ventricles of the heart. When stimulated, the sympathetic fibers cause an *increase* in the heart rate, AV conduction, cardiac contractility, and excitability. **Parasympathetic** neural fibers, via the vagus nerve, innervate the SA node, atrial muscle fibers, and the AV junction. The parasympathetic system has little or no

TABLE 12–1

Cardiac Response to Autonomic Nervous System Changes

Sympathetic Stimulation	Sympathetic Block	Parasympathetic Stimulation	Parasympathetic Block
↑ Heart rate	↓ Heart rate	↓ Heart rate	↑ Heart rate

influence on the ventricular musculature. Stimulation of the parasympathetic system causes a *decrease* in heart rate, AV conduction, contractility, and excitability.

Under normal circumstances, the heart action is maintained in a state of balanced control because of the opposing effects of the sympathetic and parasympathetic systems. However, a variety of dysrhythmias can develop when the autonomic nervous system is influenced by medications or abnormal conditions. When the sympathetic nervous system is stimulated by a drug (e.g., epinephrine), the heart rate will increase. On the other hand, when a drug (i.e., propranol) blocks the sympathetic nervous system, the parasympathetic nervous system takes control and the heart rate decreases. Table 12–1 summarizes cardiac response to autonomic nervous system changes.

CHAPTER SUMMARY

Cardiac contractions are a function of action potentials (electrical currents) that sweep across the cell membranes of the heart. Each action potential consists of five phases: phases 0, 1, 2, 3, and 4. Phase 0 represents depolarization and phases 1, 2, 3, and 4 represent different stages of repolarization. The cardiac cells of the heart have four specific properties: automaticity, excitability, conductivity, and contractility. Automaticity is the unique ability of the cells in the sinoatrial (SA) node (pacemaker cells) to generate an action potential without being stimulated. Excitability (irritability) is the ability of a cell to reach its threshold potential and respond to a stimulus or irritation. Conductivity is the ability of the heart cells to transmit electrical current from cell to cell throughout the entire conductive system. Contractility is the ability of cardiac muscle fibers to shorten and contract in response to an electrical stimulus.

An additional property of the myocardial contractile fibers and autorhythmic cells are refractory periods, which include (1) the ionic composition of the cells during different phases of the action potential and (2) the ability of the cells to accept a stimulus. The absolute refractory period is the phase in which the cells cannot respond to a stimulus. The relative refractory period is the time in which repolarization is partially complete and a strong stimulus may cause depolarization of some of the cell. The nonrefractory period is when all the cells are in their resting or polarized state and are ready to respond to a stimulus in a normal fashion. The components of the conductive system are the sinoatrial node (SA node), atrioventricular junction (AV junction), bundle of His, the right and left bundle branches, and the Purkinje fibers. Finally, although the conductive system of the heart has its own intrinsic pacemaker, the autonomic nervous system plays an important role in the rate of impulse formation, conduction, and contraction strength. The regulation of the heart is controlled by neural fibers from both the sympathetic and parasympathetic nervous systems.

REVIEW QUESTIONS

DIRECTIONS: On the line next to the item under Column A, match the item under Column B. Items under Column B may be used once, more than once, or not at all.

COLUMN A

1. _____ Resting membrane potential

2. _____ Action potential

3. _____ Phase 4

4. _____ Phase 2

5. _____ Conductivity

6. _____ Relative refractory period

7. _____ Pacemaker

8. _____ Parasympathetic nervous system

9. _____ Phase 0

10. _____ Phase 3

COLUMN B

A. A rapid up-stroke in the action potential
B. The inward flow of Ca^{2+} into the heart cells stop
C. Sinoatrial node
D. Plateau stage
E. Slow the heart rate and AV conduction
F. A strong stimulus may cause depolarization
G. Resting state
H. Ability to transmit electrical current from cell to cell
I. An electrical difference across the fibers of the heart
J. The entire sequence of electrical changes during depolarization and repolarization

CHAPTER 13

The Standard 12-ECG System

O B J E C T I V E S

By the end of this chapter, the student should be able to:

1. Describe the components of the standard limb leads, including:
   —Standard limb leads
   - Bipolar leads
     ○ Lead I
     ○ Lead II
     ○ Lead III
   - Unipolar leads
     ○ aVR
     ○ aVL
     ○ aVF
   —Axes
   —Einthoven's triangle

2. Describe how an electrical impulse of the heart is recorded when it
   —Moves toward a positive electrode
   —Moves away from a positive electrode (toward a negative electrode)
   —Moves perpendicular to a positive and negative electrode

3. Identify how the following limb leads monitor the frontal plane of the heart:
   —Left lateral leads
   —Inferior leads

4. Describe the components of the precordial (chest) leads, including:
   —V1
   —V2
   —V3
   —V4
   —V5
   —V6

5. Identify how the following precordial leads monitor the horizontal plane of the heart:
   —Anterior leads
   —Lateral leads

6. Describe the modified chest lead.

7. Describe the normal electrocardiogram (ECG) configurations and their expected measurements, including:
   —The components of the ECG paper
   —P wave
   —PR interval
   —QRS complex
   —ST segment
   —T wave
   —U wave
   —QT interval

8. Complete the review questions at the end of this chapter.

The electrocardiogram (ECG) is a graphic representation of the electrical activity of the heart's conductive system recorded over a period of time. Under normal conditions, ECG tracings have very predictable directions, durations, and amplitudes. Because of this fact, the various components of the ECG tracing can be identified, assessed, and interpreted as to normal or abnormal function. The ECG is also used to monitor the heart's response to therapeutic interventions. Because the ECG is such a useful tool in the clinical setting, the respiratory care practitioner must have a basic and appropriate understanding of ECG analysis. The essential knowledge components required for a systematic 12-ECG interpretation are discussed.

THE STANDARD 12-ECG SYSTEM

The standard 12-ECG system consists of four limb electrodes and six chest electrodes. Collectively, the electrodes (or leads) view the electrical activity of the heart from 12 different positions—6 *standard limb leads* and 6 *precordial (chest) leads* (Table 13–1). Each lead (1) views the electrical activity of the heart from a different angle, (2) has a positive and negative component, and (3) monitors specific portions of the heart from the point of view of the positive electrode in that lead.

Standard Limb Leads

As shown in Figure 13–1, the *standard limb leads* are **leads I**, **II**, **III**, **aVR**, **aVL**, and **aVF**. They are called the limb leads because they are derived from electrodes attached to the arms and legs. Leads I, II, and III are **bipolar leads**, which means they use two electrodes to monitor the heart, one positive and one negative. As illustrated in Figure 13–2, an imaginary line

TABLE 13–1
ECG Lead Systems

Standard Limb Leads		Precordial (Chest) Leads
Bipolar Leads	**Unipolar Leads**	**Unipolar Leads**
Lead I	aVR	V1
Lead II	aVL	V2
Lead III	aVF	V3
		V4
		V5
		V6

Figure 13–1

The standard limb leads—leads I, II, III, aVR, aVL, and aVF. Each of the standard limb electrodes can function as either a positive or negative electrode.

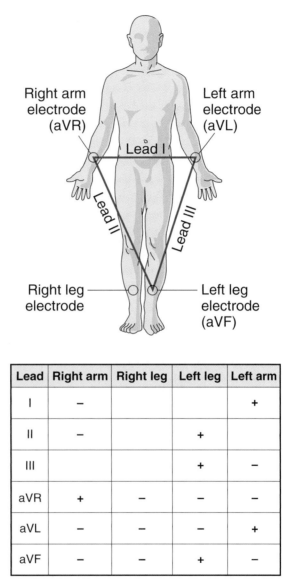

Lead	Right arm	Right leg	Left leg	Left arm
I	–			+
II	–		+	
III			+	–
aVR	+	–	–	–
aVL	–	–	–	+
aVF	–	–	+	–

can be drawn between the positive and negative electrodes for leads I, II, and III. These lines represent the **axis** of each lead. The triangle formed around the heart by the three axes is called *Einthoven's triangle.*

Electrical impulses that travel more toward the positive electrode (relative to the axis of the lead) are recorded as positive deflections in that lead (see Lead I, Figure 13–3A). When an electrical current travels

Figure 13–2
Leads I, II, and III axes form Einthoven's triangle.

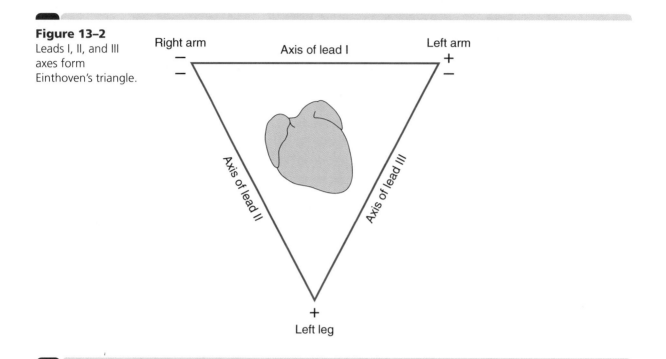

Figure 13–3
Einthoven's triangle around the heart. The arrow represents an electrical impulse moving across the surface of the heart. **(A)** In lead I, the impulse is moving toward the positive electrode and is recorded as a positive deflection. **(B)** In lead II, the impulse is moving perpendicular to the lead axis and an equiphasic or straight line is recorded. **(C)** In lead III, the impulse is moving toward the negative electrode and is recorded as a negative deflection.

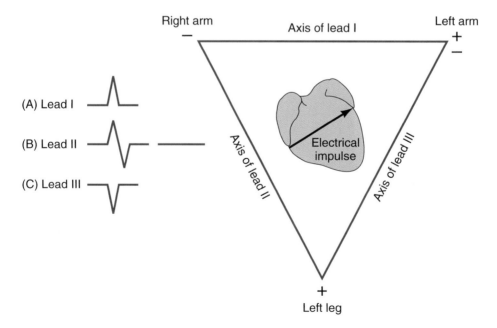

perpendicular to the lead axis, an equiphasic (half up and half down deflection) or a straight line is recorded (see Lead II, Figure 13–3B). Electrical impulses that move away from the positive electrode (or more toward the negative electrode) are recorded as negative deflections in that lead (see Lead III, Figure 13–3C). In the normal heart, the largest electrical impulse travels from the base of the heart to the apex, in a right to left direction (Figure 13–4).

The aVR, aVL, and aVF leads are **unipolar leads** (see Figure 13–1). Unipolar leads monitor the electrical activity of the heart between the positive electrode (i.e., aVR, aVL, aVF) and the zero electrical reference point at the center of the heart. In essence, the center of the heart functions as a negative electrode. Thus, the axis for these leads is drawn from the electrode and the center of the heart. When the negative electrodes are eliminated in the aVR, aVL, and aVF, the amplitude of the ECG recordings is augmented by 50 percent. This is the reason for the letter *a*, which stands for augmentation; the *V* represents voltage. The letters *R, L,* and *F* represent where the positive electrode is placed.

Collectively, the limb leads monitor the electrical activity of the heart in the **frontal plane**, which is the electrical activity that flows over the

Figure 13–4
In the normal heart, the dominant electrical current in the heart flows from the base to the apex in a right to left direction.

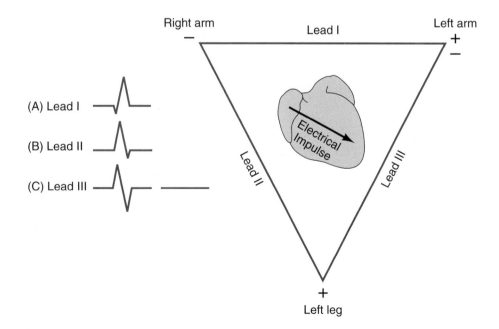

Figure 13–5
The frontal plane and the limb leads.

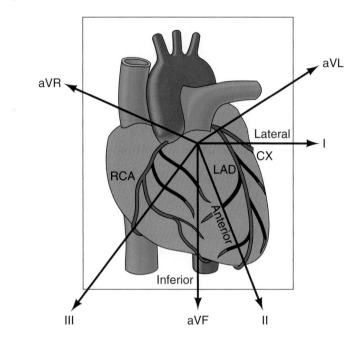

anterior surface of the heart; from the **base to the apex of the heart**, in a **right to left** direction. Leads I and aVL are called **left lateral leads**, because they monitor the left lateral side of the heart. Leads II, III, and aVF view the lower surfaces of the heart and are called **inferior leads**. The aVR lead does not contribute much information for the 12-ECG interpretation and because of this fact, it is generally ignored. Figure 13–5 summarizes the frontal plane and the limb leads.

Precordial (Chest) Leads

Figure 13–6 shows the chest position of the *precordial leads,* which are also unipolar leads (i.e., the center of the heart functions as the negative reference point, similar to the aVR, aVL, and aVF leads). Figure 13–7 shows the axes of the six precordial leads. The precordial leads monitor the heart from the **horizontal plane**, which means they record electrical activity that transverses the heart. Leads V1 and V2 monitor the right ventricle, V3 and V4 monitor the ventricle septum, and V5 and V6 view the left ventricle. Leads V1, V2, V3, and V4 are also called **anterior leads**, and leads V5 and V6 are also called **lateral leads**. Figure 13–8 summarizes the horizontal plane and its leads.

Figure 13–6
(A) The position of the electrodes on the rib thorax; **(B)** the precordial leads as they reflect the surface of the myocardium.

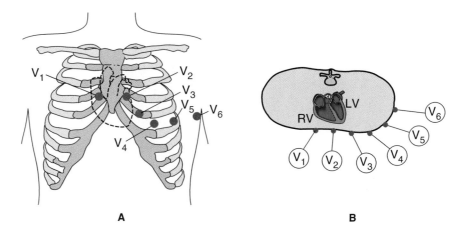

A   B

Figure 13–7
The axes of the six precordial leads.

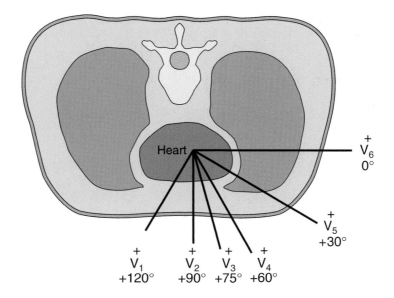

Modified Chest Lead

The *modified chest lead* (MCL$_1$) is a bipolar chest lead similar to the precordial lead V1. The positive electrode is placed on the chest (in the same position as V1) and the negative electrode is placed on the left arm or left shoulder area (Figure 13–9). The MCL$_1$ may be helpful in visualizing some waveforms.

Figure 13–8
The horizontal plane and its leads.

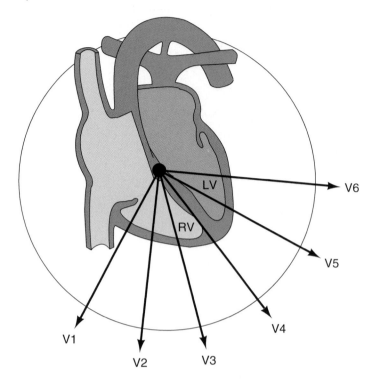

Figure 13–9
The position of the electrodes for the monitoring system MCL$_1$.

NORMAL ECG CONFIGURATIONS AND THEIR EXPECTED MEASUREMENTS (LEAD II)

The ECG Paper

All ECG systems use the same standard paper and run at the same speed of 25 mm/sec (Figure 13–10). From left to right, each **small square** has a duration of 0.04 second. Each **large square**, delineated by the darker lines, has five small squares, and a duration of 0.20 second. The paper on all ECG monitors runs at a speed of 5 large squares per second, or 300 large squares per minute (5 large squares × 60 seconds = 300 squares/min). The vertical portion of each small square also represents an **amplitude** (or voltage) of 0.1 **millivolt** (mV), and **1 millimeter** (1 mm) in distance. Prior to each test, the ECG monitor is standardized so that 1 mV is equal to 10 mm (10 small vertical squares). As shown in Figure 13–11, most ECG paper has small vertical line marks in the margins every 15 large

Figure 13–10

The ECG monitoring paper, with the blocks enlarged to illustrate the minimum units of measurement. The smallest of the blocks has three values (see solid red block): 0.04 second in duration (horizontal measurement), 0.1 mV in amplitude (vertical measurement), and 1 mm in height (also a vertical measurement). Five blocks on the horizontal would measure 0.20 second. Five blocks on the vertical would measure 5 mm and/or 0.5 mV. Note the darker lines that delineate five of the smallest blocks.

0.04 second
0.1 mV
1 mm

Figure 13–11
ECG monitoring paper showing markers indicating 3- and 6-second intervals. There are 15 blocks in 3 seconds and 30 blocks in 6 seconds.

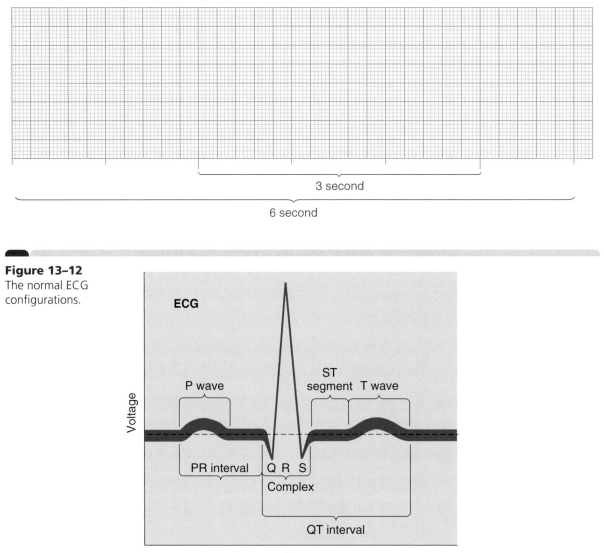

3 second

6 second

Figure 13–12
The normal ECG configurations.

squares, or every 3 seconds (0.20 × 15 = 3 seconds). Fundamental to the evaluation and interpretation of ECG recordings is the ability to measure the duration and amplitude of the waveforms.

The electrical activity of the heart is monitored and recorded on the ECG paper. As illustrated in Figure 13–12, the normal ECG configurations are composed of **waves**, **complexes**, **segments**, and **intervals** recorded as voltage (on a vertical axis) against time (on a horizontal axis). A single *waveform* begins and ends at the baseline. When the waveform continues past the baseline, it changes into another waveform. Two or more waveforms together are a *complex.* A flat, straight, or isoelectric line is called a *segment.* A waveform, or complex, connected to a segment is called an *interval.* All ECG tracings above the baseline are described as **positive** deflections. Waveforms below the baseline are **negative** deflections.

The P Wave

The normal cycle of electrical activity in the heart begins with atrial depolarization and is recorded as the *P wave.* The shape of the P wave is usually symmetrical and upright. The P wave is followed by a short pause while the electrical current passes through the AV node. This is seen on the ECG tracing as a flat, or isoelectric, line (a segment) after the P wave. The normal duration of the P wave is 0.08 to 0.11 second (2 to $2\frac{1}{2}$ small horizontal squares). The normal amplitude of the P wave is 0.2 and 0.3 mV (2 to 3 small vertical squares) (Figure 13–13).

An increased duration or amplitude of the P wave indicates the presence of atrial abnormalities, such as hypertension, valvular disease, or congenital heart defect. Repolarization of the atria is usually not recorded on an ECG tracing, because atrial repolarization normally occurs when the ventricles are depolarizing, which is a greater electrical activity. When depolarization of the atria occurs from outside the SA node, the P wave configuration appears different than an SA node-induced P wave. The rhythm of the SA

Figure 13–13
The durations of the normal ECG configurations.

wave will also be disrupted and reset. When the atria depolarize in response to a stimulus outside the SA node, the wave is called a *P prime* (P′) *wave.*

The PR Interval

The *PR interval* starts at the beginning of the P wave and ends at the beginning of the QRS complex. The normal duration of the PR interval is 0.12 to 0.20 second (3 to 5 small horizontal squares). The PR interval represents the total atrial (supraventricular) electrical activity prior to the activation of the bundle of His, ventricular branches, and Purkinje fiber system (see Figure 13–13).

The QRS Complex

The *QRS complex* represents ventricular depolarization. Because the muscle mass of the ventricles is greater than that of the atria, the amplitude of the QRS complex is higher than the P wave. The QRS complex consists of three separate waveforms: **Q wave**, **R wave**, and **S wave**. The first negative defection (below the baseline) after the P wave is the *Q wave* (Figure 13–14A). The next tall positive deflection (above the baseline) is the *R wave* (Figure 13–14B). The *S wave* is the small negative deflection (below the baseline) that follows the R wave (Figure 13–14C).

Relative to the ECG lead, the QRS complex may not have a Q wave or an S wave. Under normal conditions, the duration of the QRS complex is less than 0.10 second ($2\frac{1}{2}$ little squares) (see Figure 13–13). Abnormal ventricular-induced QRS complex waves are longer than 0.10 second. Other characteristics of an abnormal QRS complex include premature ventricular contractions (PVCs), increased amplitude, and T waves of opposite polarity.

The ST Segment

The *ST segment* represents the time between ventricular depolarization and repolarization (see Figure 13–13). The ST segment begins at the end of the QRS complex (called the J point) and ends at the beginning of the T wave. Normally, the ST segment measures 0.12 second or less. The ST segment may be elevated or depressed due to myocardial injury, ischemia, and certain cardiac medications. A flat, horizontal ST segment above or below the baseline is highly suggestive of ischemia. Figure 13–15 shows four different ST segment variations.

Figure 13–14
(A) Q waveform of the QRS complex; **(B)** R waveform of the QRS complex; **(C)** S waveform of the QRS complex.

Figure 13–15
(A) The ST segment highlighted within cardiac complex. Note the variations in ST segments in **(B)** at the baseline. **(C)** 3-mm ST segment ↑. **(D)** 3-mm ST segment ↓.

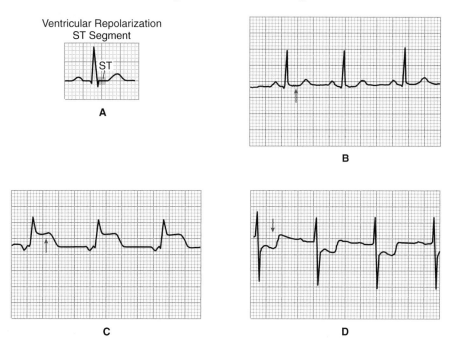

Ventricular Repolarization
ST Segment

The T Wave

The *T wave* represents ventricular repolarization, rest, and recovery (see Figure 13–13). Normally, the T wave has a positive deflection of about 0.5 mV, although it may have a negative deflection. It may, however, be of such low amplitude that it is difficult to read. The duration of the T wave normally measures 0.20 second or less.

At the beginning of the T wave, the ventricles are in their effective refractory period. At about the peak of the T wave, the ventricles are in their relative refractory period and, thus, are vulnerable to stimulation (see Figure 13–13). T waves are sensitive indicators for the presence of a number of abnormalities, including acid-base imbalances, hyperventilation, hyperkalemia, ischemia, and the use of various drugs. Figure 13–16 shows common T wave variations.

The U Wave

The *U wave* follows the T wave and has the same polarity (deflection) as the T wave (Figure 13–17). Its origin and mechanism are not known. Because of its low voltage, the U wave usually is flat and not seen; however, it often becomes prominent in the presence of certain electrolyte disturbances, certain medications, and heart disease.

Figure 13–16
(A) The T wave representing venticular depolarization; **(B)** measuring the T wave with ST segment elevation; **(C)** measuring an inverted T wave with ST segment depression.

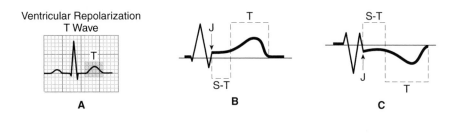

Figure 13–17
The U wave highlighted (arrow) within the cardiac complex. U waves plot only with other U waves, just as P waves plot with P waves, and QRS plots with the QRS complex.

The QT Interval

The *QT interval* is measured from the beginning of the QRS complex to the end of the T wave (see Figure 13–13). The QT interval represents total ventricular activity, i.e., ventricular depolarization (QRS) and repolarization (ST segment and the T wave). The normal QT interval measures about 0.38 second, and varies in males and females and with age. As a general rule, the QT interval should be about 40 percent of the measured RR interval.

Finally, note that the QT interval varies indirectly to the heart rate; that is, the faster the heart rate, the shorter the QT interval time. This is because when the heart rate is fast, repolarization is also faster. The QT interval time is longer with slower heart rates. The QT interval often varies with use of certain cardiac drugs that alter the heart's action potential and refractory times.

CHAPTER SUMMARY

The electrocardiogram (ECG) is a graphic representation of the electrical activity of the heart's conductive system monitored and recorded over a period of time. The essential knowledge components for the standard

TABLE 13–2
Summary of Normal ECG Configurations and Heart Activity

ECG Configuration	Heart Activity
P wave	Atrial depolarization
PR interval	Total atrial electrical activity prior to activation of the bundle of His, ventricular branches, and Purkinje fiber system
QRS complex	Ventricular depolarization
ST segment	Time between ventricular depolarization and repolarization
T wave	Ventricular repolarization
U wave	Usually is flat or not seen. Often prominent in the presence of certain electrolyte disturbances, certain medications, and heart disease
QT interval	Total ventricular activity (QRS complex, ST segment, and T wave)

12-ECG system include (1) the standard limb leads—leads I, II, III, aVR, aVL, and aVF; (2) how an electrical impulse of the ventricle is recorded; (3) the precordial (chest) leads—V_1, V_2, V_3, V_4, V_5, and V_6; and (4) the normal ECG configurations. Table 13–2 summarizes the normal ECG configurations and corresponding activity of the heart.

REVIEW QUESTIONS

1. Which of the following is (are) unipolar leads?
   I. aVL
   II. Lead II
   III. V6
   IV. Lead III
   V. aVR
      A. III only
      B. I and V only
      C. II and IV only
      D. I, III, and V only

2. The imaginary line that can be drawn between the positive and negative electrodes in leads I, II, and III is called the
   A. axis
   B. vector
   C. equiphasic line
   D. baseline

3. Which of the following monitor the electrical activity of the heart in the frontal plane?
   I. aVL
   II. Lead II
   III. aVR
   IV. Lead III
   V. aVF
      A. I and III only
      B. I, IV, and V only
      C. II, III, IV, and V only
      D. All of these

4. Which of the following monitor the left ventricle?
   I. V1
   II. V2
   III. V3
   IV. V5
   V. V6
      A. I only
      B. V only
      C. II and III only
      D. IV and V only

5. The small squares on the standard ECG paper represent
   A. 0.02 second
   B. 0.04 second
   C. 0.06 second
   D. 0.08 second

6. The normal duration of the P wave is no longer than
   A.   0.80 second
   B.   0.11 second
   C.   0.15 second
   D.   0.20 second

7. The normal duration of the PR interval is no longer than
   A.   0.12 second
   B.   0.15 second
   C.   0.20 second
   D.   0.50 second

8. The normal duration of the QRS complex is less than
   A.   0.01 second
   B.   0.05 second
   C.   0.10 second
   D.   0.15 second

9. The normal duration of the ST segment is
   A.   0.12 second or less
   B.   0.15 second or less
   C.   0.20 second or less
   D.   0.50 second or less

10. The normal duration of the T wave is
    A.   0.05 second or less
    B.   0.10 second or less
    C.   0.15 second or less
    D.   0.20 second or less

CHAPTER 14

ECG Interpretation

OBJECTIVES

By the end of this chapter, the student should be able to:

1. Describe the systematic approach to ECG interpretation, including:
   —General inspection
   —Analysis of ventricular activity
   —Analysis of atrial activity
   —Assessment of atrioventricular relationship

2. Describe the P wave, PR interval, QRS complex, QRS rate, and QRS rhythm in the normal sinus rhythm.

3. Describe the P wave, PR interval, QRS complex, QRS rate, and QRS rhythm in the following abnormal sinus mechanisms:
   —Sinus bradycardia
   —Sinus tachycardia
   —Sinus arrhythmia
   —Sinus block
   —Sinus arrest

4. Describe the P wave, PR interval, QRS complex, QRS rate, and QRS rhythm in the following abnormal atrial mechanisms:
   —Premature atrial complex
   —Atrial bigeminy
   —Atrial tachycardia
   —Atrial flutter
   —Atrial fibrillation

5. Describe the P wave, PR interval, QRS complex, QRS rate, and QRS rhythm for the following abnormal ventricular mechanisms:
   —Premature ventricular complex
   • Uniform PVCs
   • Multiform PVCs
   • Paired PVCs
   • Bigeminal PVCs
   • Trigeminal PVCs
   —Ventricular tachycardia
   —Ventricular flutter
   —Ventricular fibrillation
   —Asystole

6. Describe the P wave, PR interval, QRS complex, QRS rate, and QRS rhythm in the following atrioventricular (AV) defects:
   —Sinus rhythm with first-degree AV block
   —Sinus rhythm with second-degree AV block
   —Complete AV block

7. Complete the review questions at the end of the chapter.

HOW TO ANALYZE THE WAVEFORMS

There are many correct ways in which to approach electrocardiograph (ECG) interpretation. Fundamental to all good methods is a consistent, systematic approach. Some practitioners, for example, begin by looking at the P waves and then move on to the QRS complexes, whereas others start by looking at the QRS complexes and then the P waves. Both approaches are correct. The key is to be systematic and consistent. Table 14–1 provides an overview of the steps involved in a good systematic approach to ECG analysis. A short discussion of this approach follows.

Step 1: Does the General Appearance of the ECG Tracing Appear Normal or Abnormal?

Closely scan the ECG tracing and identify each of the wave components. Note any specific wave abnormalities. Are there any abnormalities—in terms of appearance or duration—in the P waves, QRS complexes, ST segments, or T waves? Do the complexes appear consistent from one beat to the next? Does the rate appear too slow or too fast? Does the rhythm appear regular or irregular? Are there any extra beats or pauses? It is often helpful to circle any possible abnormalities during Step 1. This initial process helps to pinpoint problem areas that can be inspected more carefully during the steps discussed next.

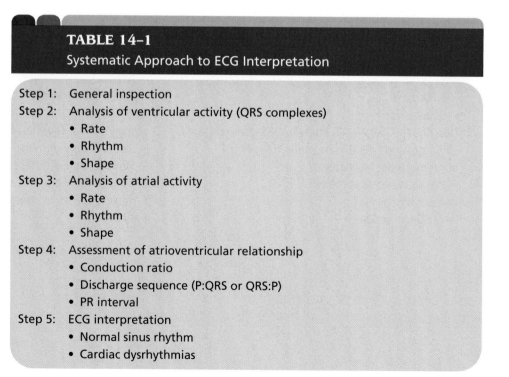

TABLE 14–1
Systematic Approach to ECG Interpretation

Step 1: General inspection
Step 2: Analysis of ventricular activity (QRS complexes)
- Rate
- Rhythm
- Shape
Step 3: Analysis of atrial activity
- Rate
- Rhythm
- Shape
Step 4: Assessment of atrioventricular relationship
- Conduction ratio
- Discharge sequence (P:QRS or QRS:P)
- PR interval
Step 5: ECG interpretation
- Normal sinus rhythm
- Cardiac dysrhythmias

Step 2: Does the Ventricular Activity (QRS Complexes) Appear Normal or Abnormal?

Rate

When the ventricular heart rate is **regular**, the rate can be determined by counting the number of large squares between two consecutive QRS complexes, and then dividing 300 by the number of large squares. For example, if there are three large squares between two QRS complexes, then the ventricular rate would be 100/min (300 ÷ 3 = 100) (Figure 14–1). Table 14–2 shows the estimated heart rate for different numbers of large

Figure 14–1

ECG recording with markers denoting the number of large squares (blocks) between the QRS complexes (RR interval). Because there are three such blocks between QRS complexes, dividing 3 into 300 provides the estimated rate of 100 per minute.

TABLE 14–2
Calculating Heart Rate by Counting the Number of Large ECG Squares

Distance Between Two QRS Complexes (number of large squares)	Estimated Heart Rate (per min)
1	300
2	150
3	100
4	75
5	60
6	50

squares between two QRS complexes. Appendix VII provides a more complete presentation of the estimated heart rate for different numbers of large squares between two QRS complexes.

When the ventricular heart rate is **irregular**, the rate can be calculated by using the vertical 3-second marks in the upper margins of the ECG paper. This is done by counting the number of QRS complexes in a 6-second interval (two 3-second marks), then multiplying this number by 10. For example, if seven QRS complexes are present in two 3-second intervals (6 seconds), then the ventricular rate is about 70 beats/min (bpm) (7 × 10 = 70). Normal *adult* heart rate is between 60 and 100 bpm. A heart rate of less than 60 bpm is classified as **bradycardia**. A heart rate greater than 100 bpm is called **tachycardia**.

Rhythm

The ventricular rhythm is determined by comparing the shortest RR intervals with the longest RR intervals. When the time variation between the shortest RR interval and the longest RR interval is greater than 0.12 second, the rhythm is *irregular*; a variation of 0.12 or less is a *regular* rhythm.

Shape

Finally, determine if the shape of the QRS complexes is identical from one complex to another. Are the QRS complexes of the expected polarity, considering the monitoring lead? The shape as well as the duration of the QRS complex help to determine the origin of the ventricular depolarization. The normal QRS duration is 0.10 second (2.5 little squares) or less. A QRS complex that is narrow and lasts 0.10 second or less represents a **supraventricular origin** (i.e., sinoatrial [SA] node or atrial source) and normal intraventricular conduction. When the QRS complex is greater than 0.10 second and the shape is distorted (e.g., increased amplitude, opposite polarity, slurred), then an abnormal electrical source (ectopic focus) is likely to be present within the ventricle.

Step 3: Does the Atrial Activity Appear Normal or Abnormal?

Similar to the assessment of the QRS complexes, the rate, rhythm, and shape of the atrial activity (P waves) are evaluated. The **rate** of the atrial activity is calculated in the same way as the QRS complexes (see Table 14–2). Normally, the P wave rate and the QRS rate are the same. The atrial **rhythm** is calculated in the same way as the QRS rhythm, except that in this case PP intervals are used. The **shape** of the P waves is then evaluated. Abnormalities may include P waves that are not of expected polarity, atrial flutter, fibrillation, or P prime (P′) waves (i.e., waves initiated outside the SA node).

Step 4: Does the Atrioventricular (AV) Relationship Appear to be Normal?

Is the AV conduction ratio 1:1? In other words, is a P wave followed by a QRS complex? When the AV conduction ratio is greater than 1:1 (e.g., 2:1, 3:1), not all the atrial impulses are being conducted to the ventricles. For example, an AV conduction ratio of 2:1 or 3:1 indicates that every second or third atrial impulse is being blocked. In some cases, the AV conduction is completely blocked and the P waves and QRS complexes are totally unrelated. The best method to determine the AV conduction ratio is to ask these two questions:

1. Is each P wave followed by a QRS complex?
2. Is each QRS complex preceded by a single P wave?

When the answers to the above questions are no, evaluate the rhythm to determine if a pattern exists. An excellent method to determine this is to measure the PR intervals to see if the intervals are fixed or variable. The PR interval is measured from the beginning of the P wave to the start of the QRS complex. The PR interval represents the time between the start of atrial depolarization to the beginning of ventricular depolarization. During a normal sinus rhythm, the PR interval is constant from one beat to the next and is no longer than 0.20 second. A PR interval greater than 0.20 second represents an abnormal delay in AV conduction.

Step 5: What Is the ECG Interpretation?

Normal Sinus Rhythm

If there are no variations from the normal sinus rhythm (NSR)—the gold standard by which most ECG dysrhythmias are measured, compared, and analyzed—then the ECG tracing is normal. When the ECG tracing varies from the normal sinus rhythm, however, the interpretation must incorporate all the information that describes the abnormal electrical activity of the heart. Thus, in view of these facts, the recognition of the normal sinus rhythm is an essential prerequisite to the interpretation of abnormal ECG tracings. The following summarizes the ECG characteristics of the normal sinus rhythm, as viewed from lead II:

- **P wave:** The P waves are positive (upright) and uniform. A QRS complex follows every P wave.
- **PR interval:** The duration of the PR interval is between 0.12 and 0.20 second and is constant from beat to beat.
- **QRS complex:** The duration of the QRS complex is 0.10 second or less. A P wave precedes every QRS complex.
- **QRS rate:** Between 60 and 100 bpm
- **QRS rhythm:** Regular

Figure 14–2 shows an ECG tracing of a normal sinus rhythm.

Figure 14–2
ECG tracing of a normal sinus rhythm.

COMMON CARDIAC DYSRHYTHMIAS

The most common cardiac dysrhythmias can be subdivided into the following four major categories: sinus mechanisms, atrial mechanisms, ventricular mechanisms, and AV conduction defects. Table 14–3 provides an overview of the major dysrhythmias found under each of these categories.

The Sinus Mechanisms

Sinus Bradycardia

Bradycardia means "slow heart." In *sinus bradycardia*, the heart rate is less than 60 bpm. The ECG characteristics of sinus bradycardia in lead II are as follows:

- **P wave:** The P waves are positive and uniform. Each P wave is followed by a QRS complex.
- **PR interval:** The PR interval has a normal duration between 0.12 and 0.20 second and is constant from beat to beat.
- **QRS complex:** The QRS complex duration is 0.10 second or less. P wave precedes every QRS complex.
- **QRS rate:** Less than 60 bpm
- **QRS rhythm:** Regular

Figure 14–3 shows an ECG tracing of sinus bradycardia. Figure 14–4 shows the presence of sinus bradycardia in two leads in a healthy adult.

Sinus bradycardia is often normal in athletes who have increased their cardiac stroke volume through physical conditioning. Common pathologic causes of sinus bradycardia include a weakened or damaged SA node, severe or chronic hypoxemia, increased intracranial pressure,

TABLE 14–3
Common Cardiac Dysrhythmias

Sinus Mechanisms	Atrial Mechanisms	Ventricular Mechanisms	AV Conduction Defects
Sinus bradycardia	Premature atrial complex (PAC)	Premature ventricular complex (PVC)	Sinus rhythm with first-degree AV block
Sinus tachycardia	Atrial bigeminy	Uniform PVCs	Sinus rhythm with second-degree AV block
Sinus arrhythmia	Atrial tachycardia	Multiform PVCs	Complete AV block
Sinus block	Atrial flutter	Paired PVCs	
Sinus arrest	Atrial fibrillation	Bigeminal PVCs	
		Trigeminal PVCs	
		Ventricular tachycardia	
		Ventricular flutter	
		Ventricular fibrillation	
		Asystole	

Figure 14–3
An ECG tracing showing one (+) P wave to the left of each QRS complex; the PR interval is consistent and the heart rate is less than 60 bpm. These computations represent a sinus bradycardia.

Figure 14–4
An ECG tracing showing sinus bradycardia in two leads from a physically fit adult.

obstructive sleep apnea, and use of certain drugs (most notably beta-blocking agents). Sinus bradycardia may lead to a decreased cardiac output and lowered blood pressure. In severe cases, sinus bradycardia may lead to a decreased perfusion and tissue hypoxia. The individual may have a weak or absent pulse, poor capillary refill, cold and clammy skin, and a depressed sensorium.

Sinus Tachycardia

Tachycardia means "fast heart." In *sinus tachycardia*, the heart rate is between 100 and 160 bpm and the rhythm is regular. The ECG characteristics of sinus tachycardia in lead II are as follows:

- **P wave:** The P waves are positive and uniform. Each P wave is followed by a QRS complex.
- **PR interval:** The PR interval has a normal duration between 0.12 and 0.20 second and is constant from beat to beat.
- **QRS complex:** The QRS complex duration is 0.10 second or less. A P wave precedes every QRS complex.
- **QRS rate:** Between 100 and 160 bpm
- **QRS rhythm:** Regular

Figure 14–5 shows an ECG tracing of sinus tachycardia.

In adults, sinus tachycardia is the normal physiologic response to exercise, emotions, fever, pain, fear, anger, and anxiety. Sinus tachycardia is also caused by physiologic stress such as hypoxemia, hypovolemia, severe anemia, hyperthermia, massive hemorrhage, hyperthyroidism, and any condition that leads to an increased sympathetic stimulation. Pathologic conditions associated with sinus tachycardia include congestive heart failure, cardiogenic shock, myocardial ischemia, heart valve disorders, pulmonary embolism, hypertension, and infarction.

Figure 14–5

An ECG tracing from an exercising adult. Note there is a single (+) P wave to the left of each QRS complex; the rate is 150 bpm.

Sinus Arrhythmia

In *sinus arrhythmia*, the heart rate varies by more than 10 percent. The P-QRS-T pattern is normal, but the interval between groups of complexes (e.g., the PP or RR intervals) vary. The ECG characteristics in sinus arrhythmia in lead II are as follows:

- **P wave:** The P waves are positive and uniform. Each P wave is followed by a QRS complex.
- **PR interval:** The PR interval has a normal duration between 0.12 and 0.20 second and is constant from beat to beat.
- **QRS complex:** The QRS complex duration is 0.10 second or less. A P wave precedes every QRS complex.
- **QRS rate:** Varies by more than 10 percent.
- **QRS rhythm:** Irregular

Figure 14–6 shows an ECG tracing of a sinus arrhythmia.

A sinus arrhythmia is normal in children and young adults. The patient's pulse will often increase during inspiration and decrease during expiration. No treatment is required unless there is a significant alteration in the patient's arterial blood pressure.

Sinus (SA) Block

In a *sinus (SA) block*, also called a *sinus exit block*, the SA node initiates an impulse but the electrical current through the atria is blocked. Thus, the atria—and the ventricles—do not depolarize or contract, resulting in no P wave or QRS complex. The next P-QRS-T complex, however, appears at the precise time it would normally appear if the sinus block had not occurred. In other words, the ECG shows that the heart has skipped a beat. The ECG characteristics for sinus block in lead II are as follows:

- **P wave:** The P waves are positive and uniform; however, an entire P-QRS-T complex is missing.

Figure 14–6
An ECG tracing of sinus arrhythmia 54 to 71 bpm.

- **PR interval:** The PR interval has a normal duration between 0.12 and 0.20 second and is constant from beat to beat, except for the pause when an entire cycle is missing. The PR interval may be slightly shorter after the pause.
- **QRS complex:** Except for the missing cycle, the QRS complex duration is 0.10 second or less, and a P wave precedes every QRS complex.
- **QRS rate:** The rate may vary according to the number and position of missing P-QRS-T cycles.
- **QRS rhythm:** The rhythm may be regular or irregular according to the number and position of missing P-QRS-T cycles.

Figure 14–7 shows an ECG tracing of a sinus block.

Sinus Arrest

Sinus arrest (SA node arrest) is the sudden failure of the SA node to initiate an impulse (i.e., no P wave). It is common to see two, three, or four P-QRS-T complexes missing following a normal P-QRS-T complex. This period of inactivity is then followed by a normal sinus rhythm. Generally, there is no pattern of frequency of occurrence; that is, the individual may demonstrate one or two periods of sinus arrests, and then demonstrate a normal sinus rhythm for minutes, or even hours, before another sinus arrest appears. When the sinus arrest is excessively long, the AV node usually takes over and initiates a new (but slower) rhythm called an escape rate. The ECG characteristics for sinus arrest in lead II are as follows:

- **P wave:** No P wave.
- **PR interval:** The PR interval has a normal duration between 0.12 and 0.20 second and is constant from beat to beat.
- **QRS complex:** The QRS complex duration is 0.10 second or less. After a sinus arrest, however, the QRS duration may be greater than 0.10 second when the escape rhythm is initiated by the AV node.

Figure 14–7
An ECG tracing showing SA block.

Figure 14–8
An ECG tracing from an 82-year-old patient showing sinus arrest. The patient required insertion of an electronic pacemaker.

- **QRS rate:** Normal sinus rhythm during nonsinus arrest periods.
- **QRS rhythm:** The QRS complexes before and after the sinus arrest are regular. The escape rate may be regular or irregular.

Figure 14–8 shows an ECG tracing of a sinus arrest.

The Atrial Mechanisms

Premature Atrial Complex

A *premature atrial complex* (PAC) results when abnormal electrical activity in the atria causes the atria to depolarize before the SA node fires. An electrical current that originates outside the SA node is called an **ectopic focus**. An ectopic focus in the atria results in a **P prime** (P′) on the ECG tracing. The P′ is usually easy to identify. It will be early or premature and it will usually vary in size and shape from the normal sinus P wave. PACs also disrupt the sinus rate and rhythm. When the sinus node regains control, the rate and rhythm will return to normal. The QRS configuration is usually normal. The ECG characteristics of a PAC in lead II are as follows:

- **P wave:** The P′ wave will appear different than a normal SA node-induced P wave. The P′ may be hidden, or partially hidden, in the preceding T wave. P′ waves hidden in the T wave often distort or increase the amplitude of the T wave. A PAC may not successfully move into the ventricles if the AV node or bundle branches are in their complete refractory period. This is called a *blocked* or *nonconducted* PAC.
- **PR interval:** The P′R interval may be normal or prolonged, depending on the timing of the PAC. Most often, however, the P′R interval is different from the normal SA node rhythm.
- **QRS complex:** Except for the abnormal cycle generated by the P′ wave, the QRS complex duration is 0.10 second or less, and a normal P wave precedes every QRS complex.

- **QRS rate:** Varies
- **QRS rhythm:** Irregular

Figure 14–9 shows an ECG tracing of a sinus rhythm with PAC. Figure 14–10 is an ECG tracing illustrating a sinus rhythm with two nonconducted PACs.

Depending on their severity and frequency, PACs may be of no clinical significance or they may result in harmful atrial arrhythmias. Causes of PACs include hypoxemia, impending heart failure, right coronary artery disease, excessive use of digitalis, pericarditis, ingestion of stimulants or caffeine, and recreational drug abuse. PACs are commonly seen in patients with chronic obstructive pulmonary disease (COPD) when the disease is

Figure 14–9

An ECG tracing showing one (+) P wave to the left of each of the first three sinus beats, a sinus rhythm at 96 bpm. The next QRS complex is similar to the sinus QRSs but is premature and has a (+) P′ superimposed on the previous T wave. The sinus P waves do not plot through the event. The PACs recur (arrow) each time, disturbing sinus rhythm. The ECG interpretation would be sinus rhythm at 96 bpm with frequent PACs.

Figure 14–10

An ECG tracing showing one (+) P wave to the left of each of the first two sinus beats, a sinus rhythm. A sudden pause occurs in the cadence of the sinus mechanism. Look back at the last T wave and note the increased amplitude. The height of the T wave is a combination of P wave and T wave amplitudes. The sinus P waves do not plot through the event, and the cadence of the sinus rhythm resumes at about 75 bpm. The ECG interpretation would be sinus rhythm at 75 bpm with frequent, nonconducted PACs.

accompanied by increased pulmonary vascular resistance. PACs are also frequently seen in females during the third trimester of pregnancy, because of the increased workload of the mother's heart, which develops primarily because (1) the mother's blood volume increases by as much as 50 percent during the third trimester and (2) the additional perfusion of the fetus and placenta causes the peripheral vascular resistance to increase.

Atrial Bigeminy

Atrial bigeminy are said to be present when every other beat is an ectopic atrial beat—a PAC. In other words, the ECG tracing shows a PAC, a normal sinus beat, a PAC, a normal sinus beat, and so on (Figure 14–11). Atrial bigeminy are often one of the first signs of congestive heart failure. Patients with atrial bigeminy should be assessed for peripheral edema, sudden weight gain, and adventitious breath sounds.

Atrial Tachycardia

Atrial tachycardia is present when an atrial ectopic focus depolarizes the atria at a rate of 130 to 250 bpm. Generally, the AV node delays many of the atrial ectopic beats and the resulting ventricular rate is usually normal. The ventricular rhythm may be regular or irregular. When atrial tachycardia appears suddenly and then disappears moments later, it is referred to as **paroxysmal atrial tachycardia**. The ECG characteristics of atrial tachycardia in lead II are as follows:

- **P′ wave:** Starts abruptly, at rates of 130 to 250 bpm. The P′ wave may or may not be seen. Visible P′ waves differ in configuration from the normal sinus P wave. At more rapid rates, the P′ is hidden in the preceding T wave and cannot be seen as a separate entity.
- **P′R interval:** The PR interval has a normal duration between 0.12 and 0.20 second and is constant from beat to beat. The P′R interval is difficult to measure at rapid rates.

Figure 14–11

An ECG tracing showing a sinus mechanism with one (+) P for each QRS. However, not all the P waves are similar. In fact, there appear to be premature QRS complexes, each with a premature P′ wave, creating a pattern; every other beat is an ectopic. When every other beat is an ectopic, this is *bigeminy.* In this case, the ectopic has its origin in the atria. Thus, the ECG interpretation would be sinus rhythm at 86 bpm with *atrial bigeminy.*

- **QRS complex:** The QRS complex duration is 0.10 second or less. A P wave usually precedes every QRS complex, although a 2:1 AV conduction ratio is often seen. The QRS complexes during atrial tachycardia may be normal or abnormal, depending on the degree of ventricular refractoriness and AV conduction time.
- **QRS rate:** Very regular
- **QRS rhythm:** Atrial tachycardia begins suddenly and is very regular.

Figure 14–12 shows an example of atrial tachycardia. Figure 14–13 shows an example of paroxysmal atrial tachycardia.

Atrial tachycardia is associated with conditions that stimulate the sympathetic nervous system, such as anxiety, excessive ingestion of caffeine or alcohol, and smoking. Unlike sinus tachycardia, which generally

Figure 14–12

An example of the onset of atrial tachycardia. In the beginning, the tracing shows a sinus rhythm at 100 bpm. A PAC (arrow) begins the sudden change in rate at 188 bpm.

Figure 14–13

An ECG tracing showing a narrow QRS complex of similar configuration throughout. Plotting out the P waves, the atrial rate is 86 bpm for the first two complexes. The rate changes suddenly. Note the PAC (arrow) at the beginning of the tachycardia. The rate here is 136 bpm, and T waves are distorted and lumpy, indicating the atrial ectopics. The rate changes again, beginning with a pause and reverting to a sinus rhythm. The visible sudden onset and end of the tachycardia is called *paroxysm*. The identification is sinus at 86 → atrial tachycardia (PAT) at 136 per minute → sinus at 86 per minute. The sinus P waves do not plot through this event.

goes unnoticed by the patient, the patient "feels" the sudden onset of atrial tachycardia. Young adults sometimes have sudden periods of paroxysmal atrial tachycardia. Atrial tachycardia is also associated with the early stages of menopause.

Atrial Flutter

A consequence of PACs is the development of *atrial flutter*. In atrial flutter, the normal P wave is absent and replaced by two or more regular sawtooth-like waves, called *flutter* or *ff waves*. The QRS complex is normal and the ventricular rate may be regular or irregular, depending on the relationship of the atrial to ventricular beats. Figure 14–14 shows an atrial flutter with a regular rhythm and with a 4:1 conduction ratio (i.e., four atrial beats for every ventricular beat). Usually, the atrial rate is constant between 200 and 300 bpm, whereas the ventricular rate is in the normal range. The ECG characteristics of atrial flutter in lead II are as follows:

- **ff waves:** Atrial depolarization is regular. Commonly has a sawtooth-like or sharktooth-like appearance.
- **P'R interval:** The P'R interval of the ff waves is typically 0.24 to 0.40 second and consistent with the QRS complex.
- **QRS complex:** The QRS complex duration is usually 0.10 second or less. Depending on the degree of ventricular refractoriness, the QRS may be greater than 0.10 second. When this is the case, the ff waves distort the QRS complexs and T waves.
- **QRS rate:** The QRS rate is a function of the degree of ventricular refractoriness and of the AV conduction time.
- **QRS rhythm:** Depending on AV conduction, the QRS rhythm may be regular or irregular.

Figure 14–15 shows three different examples of atrial flutter.

Figure 14–14
Atrial flutter with a 4:1 conduction ratio.

Figure 14–15
(A) ECG showing new-onset atrial flutter in a patient; **(B)** a continuous ECG tracing from a patient with recurrent atrial flutter. The patient was taking lanoxin 0.25 mg daily for 37 days.

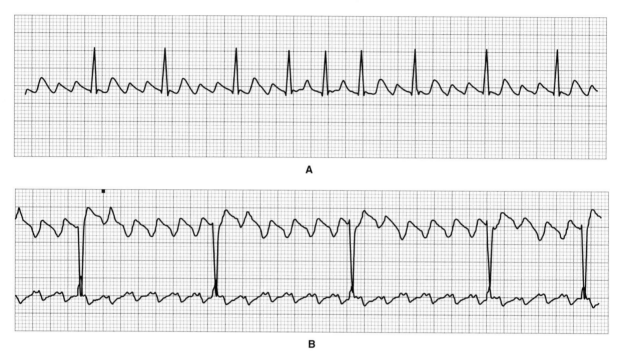

A

B

Atrial flutter is frequently seen in patients over 40 years of age with COPD (e.g., emphysema, chronic bronchitis), chronic heart disease (e.g., congestive heart failure, valvular heart disease), chronic hypertension, myocardial ischemia, myocardial infarction, hypoxemia, quinidine excess, pulmonary embolus, and hepatic disease.

Atrial Fibrillation

Another consequence of PACs is the development of *atrial fibrillation*, which is a chaotic, disorganized, and ineffective state occurring within the atria. During atrial fibrillation, the AV node is bombarded by hundreds of atrial ectopic impulses at various rates and amplitudes. Atrial fibrillation is usually easy to identify and is often referred to as *coarse fibrillation*. Unlike atrial flutter, atrial fibrillation is commonly seen in the clinical setting. The atrial rate cannot be measured because it often reaches rates between 300 and 600 bpm. The atrial P' waves are called *fib* or *ff* waves. Atrial fibrillation may reduce the cardiac output by as much as 20 percent because of the atrial quivering and loss of atrial filling

Figure 14–16
ECG tracing showing narrow QRS complex with an irregular rhythm. The chaotic pattern between the QRS complexes is the atrial fibrillation. This *coarse* pattern is easily seen.

(the so-called atrial kick). The characteristics of atrial fibrillation seen on ECG are:

- **ff waves:** Atrial depolarization is chaotic and irregular.
- **PR interval:** There are no PR intervals.
- **QRS complex:** The QRS complex duration is usually 0.10 second or less. The ff waves often distort the QRS complexes and T waves.
- **QRS rate:** The QRS rate is a function of the degree of ventricular refractoriness and conduction time.
- **QRS rhythm:** Depending on AV conduction, the QRS rhythm may be regular or irregular.

Figure 14–16 shows an example of atrial fibrillation with an irregular QRS rhythm.

Atrial fibrillation is associated with COPD, valvular heart disease, congestive heart failure, ischemic heart disease, and hypertensive heart disorders. Paroxysmal atrial fibrillation may also occur as a result of emotional stress, excessive alcohol consumption, and excessive straining and vomiting.

The Ventricular Mechanisms

Premature Ventricular Complex (PVC)

A *premature ventricular complex* (PVC) is the result of abnormal electrical activity arising within the ventricles. The QRS complex is not preceded by a P wave; rather it is wide, bizarre, and unlike the normal QRS complex. The QRS has an increased amplitude with a T wave of opposite polarity; that is, a positive QRS complex is followed by a negative T wave. The characteristics of a PVC seen on ECG are:

- **P wave:** There is no P wave before a PVC. The P waves of the dominant rhythm are normal.

- **PR interval:** There is no PR interval before a PVC. The PR interval of the dominant rhythm is normal.
- **QRS complex:** The QRS complex is wide (long duration), bizarre, and unlike the normal QRS complex. The QRS of the PVC usually has an increased amplitude with a T wave of opposite polarity. The QRS-T may also present with diminished amplitude and be narrow (short duration).
- **QRS rate:** The QRS rate is that of the underlying rhythm.
- **QRS rhythm:** The rhythm is that of the underlying rhythm, and PVCs disturb the regularity.

Figure 14–17 shows an ECG tracing with a PVC.

PVCs may occur in various forms, including **uniform PVCs**, **multiform PVCs**, **paired PVCs**, **bigeminal PVCs**, and **trigeminal PVCs**. *Uniform PVCs* (also called unifocal) orginate from one focus. All the PVCs on an ECG tracing are similar in appearance, size, and amplitude (see Figure 14–17). *Multiform PVCs* (also called multifocal) originate from more than one focus. When this occurs, the PVCs take on different shapes and amplitudes (Figure 14–18). *Paired PVCs* (also called couplets) are two closely

Figure 14–17

An ECG tracing of rhythm and two premature ventricular complexes (PVCs). Note the difference in morphology in the QRS complexes: The QRS of the premature complex is different from the dominant QRSs because it does not use the ventricular conduction pathways. The premature ventricular QRS is opposite from its T wave. The sinus P waves plot through the events because sinus cadence is undisturbed. The PVCs are similar to each other and are *uniform* in appearance. The ECG interpretation would be sinus rhythm at 86 bpm with frequent, uniform PVCs.

Figure 14–18
Note the difference between the PVCs. The ECG interpretation would be sinus rhythm about 78 bpm with frequent, *multiformed* PVCs.

Figure 14–19

An ECG tracing showing sinus rhythm with frequent, uniform PVCs and two examples of *paired* PVCs or *couplets*. Couplets indicate the beginning of reentry and are regarded as dangerous.

Figure 14–20

ECG tracing illustrating ventricular *bigeminy* (every other complex is a PVC).

coupled PVCs in a row. Paired PVCs are dangerous because the second PVC can occur when the ventricle is refractory and may cause ventricular fibrillation (Figure 14–19). Ventricular *bigeminy* is a PVC every other beat (i.e., a normal sinus beat, PVC, sinus beat, PVC, etc.) (Figure 14–20). Ventricular *bigeminy* is often seen in patients receiving digitalis. *Trigeminy* occurs when every third beat is a PVC (see Figure 14–21).

Common causes of PVCs include intrinsic myocardial disease, electrolyte disturbances (e.g., hypokalemia), hypoxemia, acidemia, hypertension, hypovolemia, stress, and congestive heart failure. PVCs may also develop as a result of use of caffeine or certain medications such as digitalis, isoproterenol, dopamine, and epinephrine. PVCs may also be a sign of theophylline, alpha-agonist, or beta-agonist toxicity.

Figure 14–21
ECG tracing illustrating *trigeminy* (every third complex is a PVC).

Ventricular Tachycardia

Three or more PVCs occurring in a row represent *ventricular tachycardia*. The QRS complex is wide and bizarre in appearance, making it difficult or impossible to identify the P waves and the T waves. The rate is regular, or slightly irregular, between 100 and 170 bpm. Ventricular tachycardia is often initiated by a PVC that is significantly premature, although it may occur suddenly after a normal sinus rhythm. When ventricular tachycardia appears suddenly and then disappears moments later, it is referred to as **paroxysmal** or **intermittent** ventricular tachycardia. When the ECG tracing shows only ventricular tachycardia, it is called *sustained ventricular tachycardia* or *V-tach*. The blood pressure level is often decreased during ventricular tachycardia. The characteristics of ventricular tachycardia seen on ECG are:

- **P wave:** The P wave usually cannot be identified during ventricular tachycardia.
- **PR interval:** The PR interval cannot be measured.
- **QRS complex:** The QRS duration is usually greater than 0.12 second and bizarre in appearance. The T wave usually cannot be identified.
- **QRS rate:** Between 100 and 170 bpm. Three or more consecutive PVCs constitute ventricular tachycardia.
- **QRS rhythm:** Regular or slightly irregular.

Figure 14–22 shows an ECG tracing of ventricular tachycardia.

Ventricular Flutter

In ventricular flutter, the ECG shows poorly defined QRS complexes. The rhythm is regular or slightly irregular, and the rate is 250 to 350 bpm. Ventricular flutter is rarely seen in the clinical setting because it usually deteriorates quickly into ventricular fibrillation. There is usually no

Figure 14–22

An ECG tracing from a 55-year-old patient with ventricular tachycardia. The patient responded to antiarrhythmic medication and was reportedly successfully reperfused.

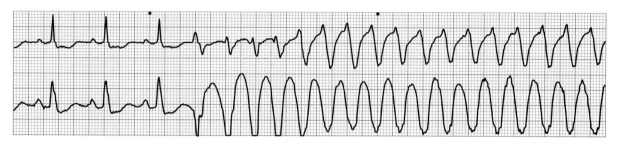

Figure 14–23

An ECG tracing showing a sinus beat followed by an R-on-T PVC, which caused ventricular flutter as confirmed on a 12-lead ECG.

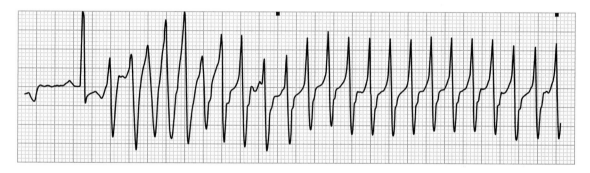

discernible peripheral pulse. The characteristics of ventricular flutter seen on ECG are:

- **P wave:** The P wave is usually not distinguishable.
- **PR interval:** The PR interval is not measurable.
- **QRS complex:** The QRS duration is usually greater than 0.12 second and bizarre in appearance. The T wave is usually not separated from the QRS complex.
- **QRS rate:** Between 250 and 350 bpm
- **QRS rhythm:** Regular or slightly irregular

Figure 14–23 shows an ECG tracing of ventricular flutter.

Ventricular Fibrillation

Ventricular fibrillation is characterized by multiple and chaotic electrical activities of the ventricles. The ventricles literally quiver out of control with no beat-producing rhythm. Ventricular fibrillation is a terminal rhythm. It may follow PVCs, ventricular tachycardia, and ventricular flutter. During ventricular fibrillation, there is no cardiac output or blood pressure and, without treatment (defibrillation), the patient will die in minutes. The characteristics of ventricular fibrillation seen on ECG are:

- **P wave:** The P waves cannot be identified.
- **PR interval:** The PR interval is not measurable.
- **QRS complex:** The QRS complex cannot be identified.
- **QRS rate:** A rate cannot be calculated.
- **QRS rhythm:** The rhythm is chaotic because of multiple, disorganized ventricular contractions.

Figure 14–24 shows three different examples of ventricular fibrillation.

Figure 14–24
ECG tracings from three patients with ventricular fibrillation.

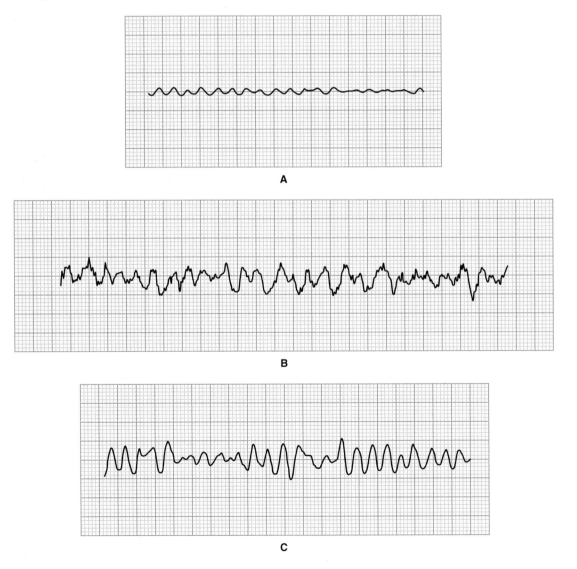

A

B

C

Figure 14–25
ECG tracings from the same patient: **(A)** An apparent asystole or fine ventricular fibrillation; **(B)** ventricular fibrillation confirmed on lead I.

Asystole (Cardiac Standstill)

Asystole is the complete absence of electrical and mechanical activity. As a result, the cardiac output stops and the blood pressure falls to about 5 to 7 mm Hg. The ECG tracing appears as a flat line and indicates severe damage to the heart's electrical conduction system (Figure 14–25). Occasionally, periods of disorganized electrical and mechanical activity may be generated during long periods of asystole; this is referred to as an *agonal rhythm* or a *dying heart*.

AV Conduction Defects
Sinus Rhythm with First-Degree AV Block

When the atrial impulse is delayed as it moves through the AV node, the PR interval increases. When the PR interval is consistently greater than 0.20 second, a *first-degree AV block* is said to exist. The ECG characteristics of first-degree AV block in lead II are:

- **P wave:** The P waves are positive and uniform. Each P wave is followed by a QRS complex.

Figure 14–26
An ECG tracing illustrating a sinus rhythm at 60 bpm with a consistently prolonged PR interval that is greater than 0.20 second. Note the PR segment is greater than 0.12 second. The ECG interpretation would be sinus rhythm at 60 bpm with first-degree AV block.

- **PR interval:** The PR interval is consistently greater than 0.20 second from beat to beat.
- **QRS complex:** The duration of the QRS complex is 0.10 second or less. Each QRS complex is preceded by a P wave.
- **QRS rate:** The rate is usually based on the normal sinus rhythm and is constant between 60 and 100 bpm.
- **QRS rhythm:** The rhythm is dependent on the sinus rhythm. When a sinus arrhythmia is present, the rhythm will vary accordingly.

Figure 14–26 shows a first-degree AV block. Note the only variation from a normal sinus rhythm is the prolonged PR interval.

Causes of first-degree AV block include right coronary artery disease, endocarditis, myocarditis, electrolyte disturbances, and aging.

Sinus Rhythm with Second-Degree AV Block: The Wenckebach Phenomenon

The **Wenckebach phenomenon** is a progressive delay in the conduction of the atrial impulse through the AV junction until, eventually, an atrial impulse is completely blocked from the ventricles. In other words, in a sinus rhythm progressive lengthening of the PR segment occurs until a P wave is not conducted. This is because the progressive prolongation of the PR interval ultimately causes the P wave to occur during the refractory period of the ventricles, resulting in a missed QRS complex. The next P wave occurs right on time. The first PR interval immediately after the missed QRS complex is the first PR interval of the next Wenckebach cycle. The Wenckebach phenomenon may repeat itself with variations in the

Figure 14–27

An ECG tracing showing progressive prolongation of the PR interval until the sinus P wave does not conduct into the ventricles. There is no ventricular depolarization, hence the missed QRS. The PR after the dropped beat is consistent with each instance. The ECG interpretation would be sinus rhythm at 86 bpm with second-degree AV block, Wenckebach, probably type I (QRS 0.08 second) inverted T waves, and ventricular rate 57 to 75 bpm.

number of conducted beats. The characteristics of the Wenckebach phenomenon seen on ECG are:

- Progressive prolongation of the PR interval
- The complex Wenckebach cycle begins and ends with a P wave
- There is one more P wave than QRS complexes in a cycle
- Irregular or decreasing RR intervals

Figure 14–27 shows an ECG tracing of the Wenckebach phenomenon.

Complete AV Block

When the pathology of the AV junction is severe, all the sinus impulses may be blocked. When a **complete AV block** is present, the *bundle of His* takes control of the ventricular rhythm at a rate of 40 to 60 bpm. This mechanism is referred to as the *escape junctional pacemaker*. The ventricular rhythm is regular. The sinus rhythm continues at its normal rate (60 to 100 bpm), completely independent of the ventricular rhythm. The sinus rhythm is regular.

When the complete AV block is caused by pathology below the bundle of His, the ventricular rhythm is controlled by what is called a ventricular escape mechanism. The rate of the ventricular escape mechanism is between 20 and 40 bpm. Similar to complete AV block above the bundle of His, the atrial and ventricular rates will be independent of each other and regular in rhythm.

To summarize, in complete AV block, the atrial rate is faster and completely independent of the ventricular rate. There is no relationship between the P and QRS complexes and there are no PR intervals. The atria remain under the control of the SA node, and the ventricles are under the control of the bundle of His or of a ventricular escape mechanism. The ECG characteristics of complete AV block in lead II are as follows:

- **P wave:** The P waves are positive and uniform. There is no relationship between the P waves and the QRS complexes. The atrial rate is faster than the ventricular escape rate.
- **PR interval:** There are no measurable PR intervals because there is no relationship between the P waves and QRS complexes.
- **QRS complex:** The duration of the QRS complex may be normal or greater than 0.12 second. When the pathology is above the bundle of His, the QRS complex is usually normal (<0.10 second). When the pathology is below the bundle of His, the duration of the QRS complexes will be greater than 0.12 second.
- **QRS rate:** The atrial rate is faster and completely independent of the ventricular rate. A junctional escape pacemaker produces a rate between 40 and 60 bpm. A ventricular escape pacemaker produces a rate between 20 and 40 bpm.
- **QRS rhythm:** Both a junctional escape pacemaker and a ventricular escape pacemaker produce a regular rhythm.

Figure 14–28 shows an ECG tracing with complete AV block.

Figure 14–28
An ECG illustrating complete AV block, probably at the level of the AV node because the QRS is 0.06 second. The atrial rate is faster than the QRS rate, and the P waves and QRS complexes are independent of each other. There are no consistent PR intervals. The ECG interpretation would be sinus rhythm at 50 bpm with complete AV block, a junctional rhythm with a ventricular rate at 40 bpm.

CHAPTER SUMMARY

A consistent, systematic approach is fundamental to all good methods of ECG interpretation. This chapter presented a five-step systematic approach to ECG interpretation: *Step 1* is the *general inspection*, which requires the examiner to closely scan the ECG tracing to determine if the general appearance of the ECG tracing looks normal or abnormal. *Step 2* is the *analysis of ventricular activity* for rate, rhythm, and shape. *Step 3* is the *analysis of atrial activity* for rate, rhythm, and shape. *Step 4* is the *assessment of the atrioventricular relationship,* which includes the conduction ratio, discharge sequence, and PR interval. *Step 5* is the *ECG interpretation* which determines if there is a normal sinus rhythm or cardiac dysrhythmias present.

The common cardiac dysrhythmias are the *sinus mechanisms*, which include sinus bradycardia, sinus tachycardia, sinus arrhythmia, sinus block, and sinus arrest; the *atrial mechanisms*, which include premature atrial complex, atrial bigeminy, atrial tachycardia, atrial flutter, and atrial fibrillation; *ventricular mechanisms*, which include premature ventricular complex (PVC), uniform PVCs, multiform PVCs, paired PVCs, bigeminal PVCs, trigeminal PVCs, ventricular tachycardia, ventricular flutter, ventricular fibrillation, and asystole; and *AV conduction defects*, which include sinus rhythm with first-degree AV block, sinus rhythm with second-degree AV block, and complete AV block.

REVIEW QUESTIONS

1.

QRS duration: _____ QT duration: _____

Ventricular rate & rhythm: _____

Atrial rate & rhythm: _____

PR interval: _____

Interpretation: _____

2.

QRS duration: _____ QT duration: _____

Ventricular rate & rhythm: _____

Atrial rate & rhythm: _____

PR interval: _____

Interpretation: _____

3.

QRS duration: _____ QT duration: _____

Ventricular rate & rhythm: _____

Atrial rate & rhythm: _____

PR interval: _____

Interpretation: _____

4.

QRS duration: _____ QT duration: _____

Ventricular rate & rhythm: _____

Atrial rate & rhythm: _____

PR interval: _____

Interpretation: _____

5.

QRS duration: _____ QT duration: _____

Ventricular rate & rhythm: _____

Atrial rate & rhythm: _____

PR interval: _____

Interpretation: _____

6.

QRS duration: _____ QT duration: _____

Ventricular rate & rhythm: _____

Atrial rate & rhythm: _____

PR interval: _____

Interpretation: _____

7.

QRS duration: _____ QT duration: _____

Ventricular rate & rhythm: _____

Atrial rate & rhythm: _____

PR interval: _____

Interpretation: _____

8.

QRS duration: _____ QT duration: _____

Ventricular rate & rhythm: _____

Atrial rate & rhythm: _____

PR interval: _____

Interpretation: _____

9.

QRS duration: _____ QT duration: _____

Ventricular rate & rhythm: _____

Atrial rate & rhythm: _____

PR interval: _____

Interpretation: _____

10.

QRS duration: _____ QT duration: _____

Ventricular rate & rhythm: _____

Atrial rate & rhythm: _____

PR interval: _____

Interpretation: _____

CHAPTER 15

Hemodynamic Measurements

OBJECTIVES

By the end of this chapter, the student should be able to:

1. List the abbreviations and normal ranges of the following hemodynamic values *directly* measured by means of the pulmonary artery catheter:
   —Central venous pressure
   —Right atrial pressure
   —Mean pulmonary artery pressure
   —Pulmonary capillary wedge pressure
   —Cardiac output

2. List the abbreviations and normal ranges of the following *computed* hemodynamic values:
   —Stroke volume
   —Stroke volume index
   —Cardiac index
   —Right ventricular stroke work index
   —Left ventricular stroke work index

   —Pulmonary vascular resistance
   —Systematic vascular resistance

3. List factors that increase and decrease the following:
   —Stroke volume
   —Stroke volume index
   —Cardiac output
   —Cardiac index
   —Right ventricular stroke work index
   —Left ventricular stroke work index

4. List the factors that increase and decrease the *pulmonary vascular resistance*.

5. List the factors that increase and decrease the *systematic vascular resistance*.

6. Complete the review questions at the end of this chapter.

HEMODYNAMIC MEASUREMENTS DIRECTLY OBTAINED BY MEANS OF THE PULMONARY ARTERY CATHETER

The term **hemodynamics** is defined as the study of the forces that influence the circulation of blood. With the advent of the pulmonary artery catheter (Figure 15–1), the hemodynamic status of the critically ill patient can be

Figure 15–1

Insertion of the pulmonary catheter. The insertion site of the pulmonary catheter may be the basilic, brachial, femoral, subclavian, or internal jugular veins. The latter two are the most common insertion sites. As the catheter advances, pressure readings and waveforms are monitored to determine the catheter's position as it moves through the right atrium (RA), right ventricle (RV), pulmonary artery (PA), and finally into a pulmonary capillary "wedge" pressure (PCWP) position. Immediately after a PCWP reading, the balloon is deflated to allow blood to flow past the tip of the catheter. When the balloon is deflated, the catheter continuously monitors the pulmonary artery pressure.

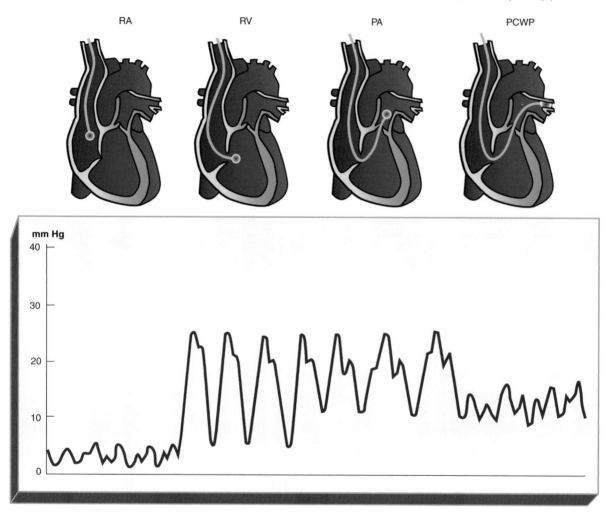

accurately determined at the bedside.* The pulmonary artery catheter has enabled the respiratory care practitioner to measure several hemodynamic parameters directly. These direct measurements, in turn, can be used to compute other important hemodynamic values. Table 15–1 lists the major hemodynamic values that can be measured directly.

*See Appendix V for a representative example of a cardiopulmonary profile sheet used to monitor the hemodynamic status of the critically ill patient.

TABLE 15–1

Hemodynamic Values Directly Obtained by Means of the Pulmonary Artery Catheter

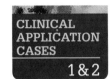

CLINICAL
APPLICATION
CASES

1 & 2

See pages 466–469

Hemodynamic Value	Abbreviation	Normal Range
Central venous pressure	CVP	0–8 mm Hg
Right atrial pressure	RAP	0–8 mm Hg
Mean pulmonary artery pressure	PA	9–18 mm Hg
Pulmonary capillary wedge pressure	PCWP	
(also pulmonary artery wedge;	PAW	4–12 mm Hg
pulmonary artery occlusion)	PAO	
Cardiac output	CO	4–8 L/min

HEMODYNAMIC VALUES COMPUTED FROM DIRECT MEASUREMENTS

Table 15–2 lists the major hemodynamic values that can be calculated from the direct measurements listed in Table 15–1. Today, such calculations are obtained either from a programmed calculator or by using the specific hemodynamic formula and a simple handheld calculator. Note, moreover, that because the hemodynamic parameters vary with the size of an individual, some hemodynamic values are "indexed" by body surface area (BSA). Clinically, the BSA is obtained from a height–weight nomogram (see Appendix IV). The normal adult BSA is 1.5 to 2 m^2.

TABLE 15–2

Computed Hemodynamic Values

Hemodynamic Value	Abbreviation	Normal Range
Stroke volume	SV	60–130 mL
Stroke volume index	SVI	30–65 mL/beat/m^2
Cardiac index	CI	2.5–4.2 L/min/m^2
Right ventricular stroke work index	RVSWI	7–12 g m/m^2
Left ventricular stroke work index	LVSWI	40–60 g m/m^2
Pulmonary vascular resistance	PVR	20–120 dynes $\times$ sec $\times$ cm^{-5}
Systemic vascular resistance	SVR	800–1500 dynes $\times$ sec $\times$ cm^{-5}

Stroke Volume

The stroke volume (SV) is the volume of blood ejected by the ventricles with each contraction. The preload, afterload, and myocardial contractility are the major determinants of stroke volume. Stroke volume is derived by dividing the cardiac output (CO) by the heart rate (HR).

$$SV = \frac{CO}{HR}$$

For example, if an individual has a cardiac output of 4.5 L/min (4500 mL/min) and a heart rate of 75 beats/min, the stroke volume would be calculated as follows:

$$SV = \frac{CO}{HR}$$

$$= \frac{4500 \text{ mL/min}}{75 \text{ beats/min}}$$

$$= 60 \text{ mL/beat}$$

Table 15–3 lists factors that increase and decrease the stroke volume.

Stroke Volume Index

CLINICAL APPLICATION CASE

2

See page 468

The stroke volume index (SVI) (also known as stroke index) is derived by dividing the stroke volume (SV) by the body surface area (BSA).

$$SVI = \frac{SV}{BSA}$$

For example, if a patient has a stroke volume of 60 mL and a body surface area of 2 m², the stroke volume index would be determined as follows:

$$SVI = \frac{SV}{BSA}$$

$$= \frac{60 \text{ mL/beat}}{2 \text{ m}^2}$$

$$= 30 \text{ mL/beat/m}^2$$

Assuming that the heart rate remains the same, as the stroke volume index increases or decreases, the cardiac index also increases or decreases. The stroke volume index reflects the (1) contractility of the heart, (2) overall blood volume status, and (3) amount of venous return. Table 15–3 lists factors that increase and decrease the stroke volume index.

TABLE 15–3

Factors Increasing and Decreasing Stroke Volume (SV), Stroke Volume Index (SVI), Cardiac Output (CO), Cardiac Index (CI), Right Ventricular Stroke Work Index (RVSWI), and Left Ventricular Stroke Work Index (LVSWI)

Increases	Decreases
Positive Inotropic Drugs (Increased Contractility)	**Negative Inotropic Drugs (Decreased Contractility)**
Dobutamine	Propranolol
Epinephrine	Timolol
Dopamine	Metoprolol
Isoproterenol	Atenolol
Digitalis	Nadolol
Amrinone	
	Abnormal Conditions
Abnormal Conditions	Septic shock (late stages)
Septic shock (early stages)	Congestive heart failure
Hyperthermia	Hypovolemia
Hypervolemia	Pulmonary emboli
Decreased vascular resistance	Increased vascular resistance
	Myocardial infarction
	Hyperinflation of Lungs
	Mechanical ventilation
	Continuous positive airway pressure (CPAP)
	Positive end-expiratory pressure (PEEP)

Cardiac Index

CLINICAL APPLICATION CASES

1 & 2

See pages 466–469

The cardiac index (CI) is calculated by dividing the cardiac output (CO) by the body's surface area (BSA).

$$CI = \frac{CO}{BSA}$$

For example, if a patient has a cardiac output of 5 L/min and a body surface area of 2 m^2, the cardiac index is computed as follows:

$$CI = \frac{CO}{BSA}$$

$$= \frac{5 \text{ L/min}}{2 \text{ m}^2}$$

$$= 2.5 \text{ L/min/m}^2$$

See Table 15–3 for a list of factors that increase and decrease the cardiac index.

Right Ventricular Stroke Work Index

The right ventricular stroke work index (RVSWI) measures the amount of work required by the right ventricle to pump blood. The RVSWI is a reflection of the contractility of the right ventricle. In the presence of normal right ventricular contractility, increases in afterload (e.g., caused by pulmonary vascular constriction) cause the RVSWI to increase, until a pleateau is reached. When the contractility of the right ventricle is diminished by the presence of disease, the RVSWI does not increase appropriately. The RVSWI is derived from the following formula:

$$RVSWI = SVI \times (PA - CVP) \times 0.0136 \text{ g/mL}$$

where SVI is stroke volume index, PA is mean pulmonary artery pressure, CVP is central venous pressure, and the density of mercury factor 0.0136 g/mL is needed to convert the equation to the proper units of measurement—i.e., gram meters/m^2 (g m/m^2).

For example, if a patient has an SVI of 35 mL, a PA of 20 mm Hg, and a CVP of 5 mm Hg, the patient's RVSWI is calculated as follows:

$$RVSWI = SVI \times (PA - CVP) \times 0.0136 \text{ g/mL}$$

$$= 35 \text{ mL/beat/m}^2 \times (20 \text{ mm Hg} - 5 \text{ mm Hg}) \times 0.0136 \text{ g/mL}$$

$$= 35 \text{ mL/beat/m}^2 \times 15 \text{ mm Hg} \times 0.0136 \text{ g/mL}$$

$$= 7.14 \text{ g m/m}^2$$

Factors that increase and decrease the RVSWI index are listed in Table 15–3.

Left Ventricular Stroke Work Index

The left ventricular stroke work index (LVSWI) measures the amount of work required by the left ventricle to pump blood. The LVSWI is a reflection of the contractility of the left ventricle. In the presence of normal left ventricular contractility, increases in afterload (e.g., caused by systemic vascular constriction) cause the LVSWI to increase until a plateau is reached. When the contractility of the left ventricle is diminished by the presence of disease, the LVSWI does not increase appropriately. The following formula is used for determining this hemodynamic variable:

$$LVSWI = SVI \times (MAP - PCWP) \times 0.0136 \text{ g/mL}$$

where SVI is stroke volume index, MAP is mean arterial pressure, PCWP is pulmonary capillary wedge pressure, and the density of mercury factor 0.0136 g/mL is needed to convert the equation to the proper units of measurement—i.e., g m/m^2.

For example, if a patient has an SVI of 30 mL, an MAP of 100 mm Hg, and a PCWP of 5 mm Hg, then:

$$LVSWI = SVI \times (MAP - PCWP) \times 0.0136 \text{ g/mL}$$

$$= 30 \text{ mL/beat/m}^2 \times (100 \text{ mm Hg} - 5 \text{ mm Hg}) \times 0.0136 \text{ g/mL}$$

$$= 30 \text{ mL/beat/m}^2 \times (95 \text{ mm Hg}) \times 0.0136 \text{ g/mL}$$

$$= 38.76 \text{ g m/m}^2$$

Table 15–3 lists factors that increase and decrease the LVSWI.

Vascular Resistance

As blood flows through the pulmonary and the systemic vascular system there is resistance to flow. The pulmonary system is a *low-resistance* system, whereas the systemic vascular system is a *high-resistance* system.

Pulmonary Vascular Resistance (PVR)

The PVR measurement reflects the afterload of the right ventricle. It is calculated by the following formula:

$$PVR = \frac{PA - PCWP}{CO} \times 80$$

where PA is the mean pulmonary artery pressure, PCWP is the pulmonary capillary wedge pressure, CO is the cardiac output, and 80 is a conversion factor for adjusting to the correct units of measurement (dyne $\times$ sec $\times$ cm^{-5}).

For example, to determine the PVR of a patient who has a PA of 15 mm Hg, a PCWP of 5 mm Hg, and a CO of 5 L/min:

$$PVR = \frac{PA - PCWP}{CO} \times 80$$

$$= \frac{15 \text{ mm Hg} - 5 \text{ mm Hg}}{5 \text{ L/min}} \times 80$$

$$= \frac{10 \text{ mm Hg}}{5 \text{ L/min}} \times 80$$

$$= 160 \text{ dynes} \times \text{sec} \times \text{cm}^{-5}$$

Table 15–4 lists factors that increase the pulmonary vascular resistance. Factors that decrease the pulmonary vascular resistance are listed in Table 15–5.

TABLE 15–4
Factors That Increase Pulmonary Vascular Resistance (PVR)

Chemical Stimuli
Decreased alveolar oxygenation
  (alveolar hypoxia)
Decreased pH (acidemia)
Increased P_{CO_2} (hypercapnia)

Pharmacologic Agents
Epinephrine
Norepinephrine
Dobutamine
Dopamine
Phenylephrine

Hyperinflation of Lungs
Mechanical ventilation
  Continuous positive airway pressure (CPAP)
  Positive end-expiratory pressure (PEEP)

Pathologic Factors
Vascular blockage
  Pulmonary emboli
  Air bubble
  Tumor mass

Vascular wall disease
  Sclerosis
  Endarteritis
  Polyarteritis
  Scleroderma

Vascular destruction
  Emphysema
  Pulmonary interstitial fibrosis

Vascular compression
  Pneumothorax
  Hemothorax
  Tumor

Humoral Substances
Histamine
Angiotensin
Fibrinopeptides
Prostaglandin $F_{2\alpha}$
Serotonin

TABLE 15–5

Factors That Decrease Pulmonary Vascular Resistance (PVR)

Pharmacologic Agents	Humoral Substances
Oxygen	Acetylcholine
Isoproterenol	Bradykinin
Aminophylline	Prostaglandin E
Calcium-channel blocking agents	Prostacyclin (prostaglandin I_2)

Systemic or Peripheral Vascular Resistance (SVR)

CLINICAL
APPLICATION
CASES

1 & 2

See pages 466–469

The SVR measurement reflects the afterload of the left ventricle. It is calculated by the following formula:

$$SVR = \frac{MAP - CVP}{CO} \times 80$$

where MAP is the mean arterial pressure, CVP is the central venous pressure, CO is the cardiac output, and 80 is a conversion factor for adjusting to the correct units of measurement (dyne $\times$ sec $\times$ cm^{-5}). (Note: The right atrial pressure [RAP] can be used in place of the CVP value.)

For example, if a patient has an MAP of 80 mm Hg, a CVP of 5 mm Hg, and a CO of 5 L/min, then:

$$SVR = \frac{MAP - CVP}{CO} \times 80$$

$$= \frac{80 \text{ mm Hg} - 5 \text{ mm Hg}}{5 \text{ L/min}} \times 80$$

$$= \frac{75 \text{ mm Hg} \times 80}{5 \text{ L/min}}$$

$$= 1200 \text{ dynes} \times \text{sec} \times \text{cm}^{-5}$$

Table 15–6 lists factors that increase and decrease the systemic vascular resistance.

TABLE 15–6

Factors That Increase and Decrease Systemic Vascular Resistance (SVR)

Increases SVR	Decreases SVR
Vasoconstricting Agents	**Vasodilating Agents**
Dopamine	Nitroglycerin
Norepinephrine	Nitroprusside
Epinephrine	Morphine
Phenylephrine	Inamrinone
	Hydralazine
Abnormal Conditions	Methyldopa
Hypovolemia	Diazoxide
Septic shock (late stages)	Phentolamine
$\downarrow P_{CO_2}$	
	Abnormal Conditions
	Septic shock (early stages)
	$\uparrow P_{CO_2}$

$\uparrow$ increased, $\downarrow$ decreased

CHAPTER SUMMARY

The hemodynamic status of the critically ill patient can be directly measured at the bedside using a pulmonary catheter. Direct hemodynamic measurements include the central venous pressure (CVP), right atrial pressure (RAP), mean pulmonary artery pressure (PA), pulmonary capillary wedge pressure (PCWP), and cardiac output (CO). The direct hemodynamic measurements, in turn, can be used to compute the following hemodynamic values: stroke volume (SV), stroke volume index (SVI), cardiac index (CI), right ventricular stroke work index (RVSI), left ventricular stroke work index (LVSWI), pulmonary vascular resistance (PVR), and systemic vascular resistance (SVR). Currently, these calculations are obtained either from a programmed calculator or by using the hemodynamic formula and a handheld calculator.

1 CLINICAL APPLICATION CASE

A 71-year-old woman reported sudden chest pain to her husband while working in her garden. Moments later she collapsed; her husband called 911 immediately. Upon arrival, the paramedics charted these vital signs: blood pressure—64/35 mm Hg, heart rate—32 beats/min, and respirations—4 breaths/min and shallow. Cardiopulmonary resuscitation

(CPR) was initiated and the patient was transferred to the hospital. En route to the hospital an intravenous line was inserted and a bolus of epinephrine was administered.

In the emergency department, the patient's vital signs were blood pressure—78/50 mm Hg, heart rate—42 beats/min, and spontaneous respirations—16 breaths/min. Dopamine was administered and the heart rate increased to 60 beats/min. Despite the improved heart rate, however, the patient's blood pressure remained low and her skin was cold and clammy. After administration of 3 L/min oxygen via nasal cannula, the patient's arterial blood gas values were: pH—7.54, Pa_{CO_2}—25 mm Hg, HCO_3^-—22 mEq/L, Pa_{O_2}—62 mm Hg.

Her electrocardiogram (ECG) showed a complete heart block.* The patient was immediately transferred to the coronary care unit (CCU). At the bedside, a transvenous cardiac pacing wire was placed under fluoroscopy and the ventricles were paced at a rate of 80 beats/min. A pulmonary catheter was then inserted (see Figure 15–1) and a hemodynamic profile was obtained (see Hemodynamic Profile No. 1).

After evaluating the first hemodynamic profile, the physician made the diagnosis of cardiogenic shock and prescribed nitroprusside for the patient. One hour later, while on an inspired oxygen concentration (FI_{O_2}) of 0.5, the patient's arterial blood gas values were pH—7.43, Pa_{CO_2}—33 mm Hg, HCO_3^-—24 mEq/L, and Pa_{O_2}—108 mm Hg. Urine output was 35 mL/hr. The patient's skin was warm and dry, and respirations were 12 breaths/min. At this time, a second hemodynamic profile was obtained (see Hemodynamic Profile No. 2).

DISCUSSION

This case illustrates the adverse "ripple" effects of an elevated *afterload* (see Chapter 5)

* *The ventricles were contracting independently from the sinus atrial node rhythm (see Figure 14–28).*

Hemodynamic Profile		
Parameter*	Profile No. 1	Profile No. 2
BP	88/54	91/55
HR	80 paced	80 paced
CVP	9	9
RAP	10	10
PA	18	16
PCWP	21	13
CI	1.1	1.8
SVR	2295	1670
Urine output (mL/hr)	0	35

*BP = blood pressure; HR = heart rate; CVP = central venous pressure; RAP = right atrial pressure; PA = mean pulmonary artery pressure; PCWP = pulmonary capillary wedge pressure; CI = cardiac index; SVR = systemic vascular resistance. Normal ranges are given in Tables 15–1 and 15–2.

on a patient's hemodynamic parameters. The very high SVR and PCWP and low CI in Hemodynamic Profile No. 1 showed that the patient's afterload was elevated. Although dopamine is a good agent to increase the patient's CI (cardiac index), in larger doses it causes the SVR (peripheral vascular resistance) to increase. Because the SVR was already high, nitroprusside (a vasodilator) was used to reduce the patient's afterload.

After the administration of the nitropruside, the patient's blood pressure essentially remained the same in the second hemodynamic profile, while her PCWP, CI, SVR, and urine output all improved significantly. In short, as the patient's SVR decreased in response to the nitroprusside, the left ventricular afterload also decreased. This action in turn allowed blood to be more readily ejected from the left ventricle. A cardiac pacemaker was permanently implanted and the patient progressively improved. The patient was discharged after 7 days.

2 CLINICAL APPLICATION CASE

A 35-year-old man was found unconscious, face down, in about 4 inches of water at a local beach. He had fallen asleep on the beach at low tide while intoxicated. His pulse was weak and he was not breathing. Someone called 911 and the lifeguard started cardiopulmonary resuscitation (CPR). When the paramedics arrived, CPR was continued with an inspired oxygen concentration (FI_{O_2}) of 1.0, and the patient was transferred to the local hospital.

In the emergency department, the patient was semiconscious. Although he demonstrated spontaneous respirations of 8 breaths/min, his breathing was labored and shallow. His pulse rate was 115 beats/min and blood pressure was 95/60 mm Hg. Chest x-ray showed a normal-size heart, but patches of alveolar infiltrates (white areas) were visible throughout both lung fields. The laboratory report showed that the patient's alcohol level was 0.53, complete blood cell (CBC) count was normal, and hemoglobin level was normal, at 15 g% (see Chapter 6). On an FI_{O_2} of 1.0, his arterial blood gas values were pH—7.27, Pa_{CO_2}—62 mm Hg, HCO_3^-—26 mEq/L, and Pa_{O_2}—38 mm Hg.

The patient was intubated and transferred to the intensive care unit. At the time of intubation, sand and seaweed were suctioned from the patient's trachea. A pulmonary artery catheter and arterial line were inserted (see Figure 15–1). The patient was placed on a mechanical ventilator with the following settings: tidal volume—750 mL, respiration rate 12—breath/min, FI_{O_2}—1.0, and positive end-expiratory pressure (PEEP)—5 cm H_2O. The patient's arterial blood gas values on these settings were pH—7.47, Pa_{CO_2}—28 mm Hg, HCO_3^-—22 mEq/L, Pa_{O_2}—57 mm Hg, and Sa_{O_2}—91 percent. At this time, a hemodynamic profile and arterial blood sample were obtained (see Hemodynamic Profile No. 1).

Hemodynamic Profile			
Parameter*	Profile No. 1 PEEP 5 cm H_2O	Profile No. 2 PEEP 10 cm H_2O	Profile No. 3 PEEP 5 cm H_2O
BP	90/60	95/68	91/62
HR	107	105	98
CI	1.9	1.5	1.9
CO	3.83	3.1	3.82
SVI	36	31	37
SVR	1490	170	1493

*BP = blood pressure; HR = heart rate; CI = cardiac index; CO = cardiac output; SVI = stroke volume index; SVR = systemic vascular resistance.

After reviewing the clinical data in the first hemodynamic profile, the physician had the respiratory therapist decrease the patient's tidal volume to 650 mL to increase the patient's Pa_{CO_2}, which had been reduced too much by the first ventilator settings (the decreased Pa_{CO_2} was the cause of elevated pH). Because the patient's Pa_{O_2} was still very low on an FI_{O_2} of 1.0, the PEEP was increased to 10 cm H_2O. A second arterial blood gas analysis showed the following values: pH—7.42, Pa_{CO_2}—36 mm Hg, HCO_3^-—23 mEq/L, Pa_{O_2}—61 mm Hg, and Sa_{O_2}—90 percent. A second hemodynamic profile was then obtained (see Hemodynamic Profile No. 2).

After reviewing the patient's second arterial blood gas analysis and second hemodynamic profile, the physician had the respiratory therapist decrease the PEEP back to 5 cm H_2O. Fifteen minutes later a third arterial blood gas analysis showed a pH of 7.42, Pa_{CO_2}—36 mm Hg, HCO_3^-—23 mEq/L, Pa_{O_2}—59 mm Hg, and Sa_{O_2}—90 percent. A third hemodynamic profile was then obtained (see Hemodynamic Profile No. 3). Despite the fact that the patient's Pa_{O_2} was less than satisfactory at this time, the physician asked the respiratory therapist to maintain the above treatment parameters.

DISCUSSION

This case illustrates that the best level of PEEP (commonly referred to as "best PEEP") was the PEEP level that produced the least depression of cardiac output and the maximum total oxygen delivery. Inspection of the three hemodynamic profiles shows that 5 cm H_2O was the most effective by these criteria.* Despite the fact that the patient's clinical course was stormy, he was eventually weaned from the ventilator 16 days after his admission. Although he did regain consciousness, he was amnesic. He was also diagnosed to have moderate to severe mental and neuro-muscular disorders. He was transferred to the rehabilitation unit where at the time of this writing progress was reported as slow.

* Chapter 6 shows how the patient's oxygen delivery for each level of PEEP can be calculated by using the total oxygen delivery (D_{O_2}) formula. It is strongly recommended that the reader calculate and compare the D_{O_2} when the patient was on 5 cm H_2O PEEP versus 10 cm H_2O PEEP. The D_{O_2} formula will show that even though the patient's Pa_{O_2} was less than desirable at 5 cm H_2O of PEEP, the cardiac output (and, therefore, the total oxygen delivery) was greater.

REVIEW QUESTIONS

Directions: On the line next to the hemodynamic parameters in Column A, match the normal range from Column B. Items in Column B may be used once, more than once, or not at all.

COLUMN A
Hemodynamic Parameters

1. _____ Mean pulmonary artery pressure
2. _____ Pulmonary vascular resistance
3. _____ Cardiac output
4. _____ Left ventricular stroke work index
5. _____ Central venous pressure
6. _____ Stroke volume index
7. _____ Pulmonary capillary wedge pressure
8. _____ Systemic vascular resistance
9. _____ Right atrial pressure
10. _____ Cardiac index

COLUMN B
Normal Range

a. 4–8 L/min
b. 800–1500 dynes $\times$ sec $\times$ cm^{-5}
c. 60–130 mL
d. 0–8 mm Hg
e. 20–120 dynes $\times$ sec $\times$ cm^{-5}
f. 9–18 mm Hg
g. 30–65 mL/beat/m^2
h. 80 mm Hg
i. 2.5–4.2 L/min/m^2
j. 4–12 mm Hg
k. 40–60 g m/m^2
l. 7–12 g m/m^2

11. Which of the following increases an individual's cardiac output?
    I. Epinephrine
    II. Hypovolemia
    III. Mechanical ventilation
    IV. Hyperthermia
       A. I only
       B. II only
       C. III only
       D. I and IV only

12. Pulmonary vascular resistance increases in response to
    I. acidemia
    II. oxygen
    III. mechanical ventilation
    IV. epinephrine
       A. II only
       B. III only
       C. I and III only
       D. I, III, and IV only

13. An individual's systemic vascular resistance increases in response to
    I. morphine
    II. hypovolemia
    III. an increased P_{CO_2}
    IV. epinephrine
       A. I only
       B. II only
       C. III only
       D. II and IV only

14. Which of the following decreases an individual's stroke volume index?
    I. Dobutamine
    II. Mechanical ventilation
    III. Propranolol
    IV. Congestive heart failure
       A. II only
       B. IV only
       C. I and III only
       D. II, III, and IV only

15. An individual's pulmonary vascular resistance decreases in response to
    I. bradykinin
    II. emphysema
    III. norepinephrine
    IV. hypercapnia
       A. I only
       B. II only
       C. III and IV only
       D. II and III only

CLINICAL APPLICATION QUESTIONS

CASE 1

1. Although dopamine is a good agent to increase the patient's CI, in larger doses it causes _____

_____

2. Why was nitroprusside administered in this case?

_____

_____

3. Why did the patient's PCWP, CI, SVR, and urine output all improve after the administration of nitroprusside?

_____

_____

CASE 2

1. Why was a PEEP of 5 cm H_2O the "best PEEP" in this case?

_____

_____

2. Using the total oxygen delivery formula (D_{O_2}) (discussed in Chapter 6), calculate and compare the D_{O_2} when the patient was receiving 5 cm H_2O PEEP compared with 10 cm H_2O PEEP.

_____

_____

CHAPTER 16

Renal Failure and Its Effects on the Cardiopulmonary System

O B J E C T I V E S

By the end of this chapter, the student should be able to:

1. Describe how the following relate to the kidney:
   —Hilum
   —Ureters
   —Cortex
   —Medulla
   —Renal pelvis
   —Major calyces
   —Minor calyces
   —Renal papillae
   —Renal pyramid
   —Nephrons

2. Describe how the following relate to the nephron:
   —Glomerulus
   —Proximal tubule
   —Loop of Henle
   —Distal tubule
   —Bowman's capsule
   —Renal corpuscle
   —Proximal convoluted tubule
   —Descending limb of the loop of Henle
   —Ascending limb of the loop of Henle
   —Distal convoluted tubule
   —Collecting duct

3. Describe how the following blood vessels relate to the nephron:
   —Renal arteries
   —Interlobar arteries
   —Arcuate arteries
   —Interlobular arteries
   —Afferent arterioles
   —Efferent arterioles
   —Peritubular capillaries
   —Interlobular veins
   —Arcuate vein
   —Interlobar vein
   —Renal vein

4. Describe the role of the following in the formation of urine:
   —Glomerular filtration
   —Tubular reabsorption
   —Tubular secretion

5. Describe the role of the following in the control of urine concentration and volume:
   —Countercurrent mechanism
   —Selective permeability

6. Describe the role of the kidneys in regulating the following:
   —Sodium
   —Potassium
   —Calcium, magnesium, and phosphate
   —Acid-base balance

7. Describe the role of the following in controlling the blood volume:
   —Capillary fluid shift system
   —The renal system

8. Identify common causes of renal disorders, including the following:
   —Congenital disorders

(continues)

—Infections
—Obstructive disorders
—Inflammation and immune responses
—Neoplasms

9. Identify causes of the following types of renal disorders:
—Prerenal conditions
—Renal conditions
—Postrenal conditions

10. Describe how mechanical ventilation alters urinary output.

11. Describe cardiopulmonary problems that can develop with renal failure, including the following:
—Hypertension and edema
—Metabolic acidosis
—Electrolyte abnormalities
  • Chloride
  • Potassium
—Anemia
—Bleeding
—Cardiovascular problems

12. Complete the review questions at the end of this chapter.

The composition of blood is largely determined by what the kidneys retain and excrete. The kidneys filter dissolved particles from the blood and selectively reabsorb the substances that are needed to maintain the normal composition of body fluids. When the renal system fails, a variety of indirect cardiopulmonary problems develop, including hypertension, congestive heart failure, pulmonary edema, anemia, and changes in acid-base balance. Because of this fact, a basic understanding of the cause, classification, and clinical manifestations of renal failure is essential in respiratory care.

THE KIDNEYS

The kidneys are two bean-shaped organs located against the posterior wall of the abdominal cavity, one on each side of the vertebral column (Figure 16–1). In the adult, each kidney is about 12 cm long, 6 cm wide, and 3 cm thick. Medially, in the central concave portion of each kidney there is a longitudinal fissure called the **hilum**. The renal artery, renal vein, and nerves enter and leave kidneys through the hilum. The **ureters**, which transport urine from the kidneys to the bladder, also exit the kidneys through the hilum.

As shown in Figure 16–2, the **cortex**, which is the outer one-third of the kidney, is a dark brownish red layer. The middle two-thirds of the kidney, the **medulla**, can be seen as a light-colored layer. Within the kidney, the ureter expands to form a funnel-shaped structure called the **renal pelvis**. The renal pelvis subdivides into two or three tubes called **major calyces** (singular, **calyx**), which in turn divide into several smaller tubes called **minor calyces**. A series of small structures called **renal**

Figure 16–1

The organs of the urinary system. Urine is formed by the kidneys and flows through the ureters to the bladder, where it is eliminated via the urethra.

papillae (or *papillary ducts*) extends from the calyx toward the cortex of the kidney to form a triangular-shaped structure called the **renal pyramid**. The peripheral portions of the papillary ducts serve as collecting ducts for the waste products selectively filtered and excreted by the **nephrons**.

Figure 16–2
Cross-section of the kidney.

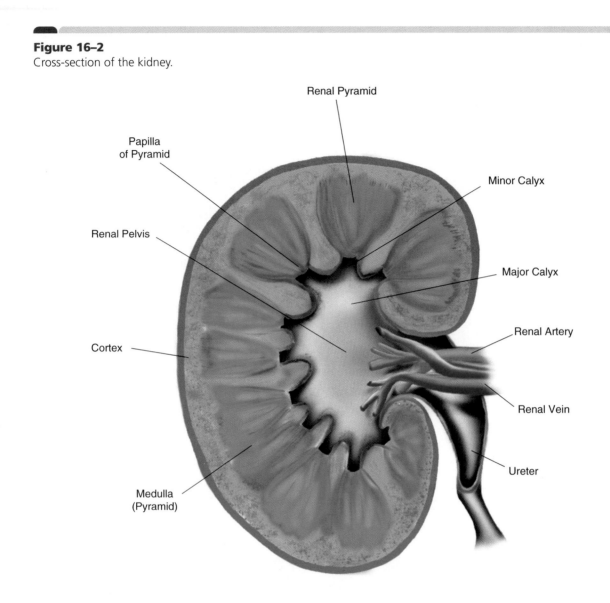

THE NEPHRONS

The nephrons are the functional units of the kidneys (Figure 16–3). Each kidney contains about one million nephrons. Each nephron consists of a **glomerulus**, **proximal tubule**, **loop of Henle**, and **distal tubule**. The distal tubules empty into the collecting ducts. Although the collecting ducts technically are not part of the renal pyramid, they are considered a functional part of the nephron because of their role in urine concentration, ion salvaging, and acid-base balance.

Figure 16–3
The nephron.

The glomerulus consists of a network of interconnected capillaries encased in a thin-walled, saclike structure called **Bowman's capsule**. The glomerulus and Bowman's capsule constitute what is known as a **renal corpuscle**. Urine formation begins with the filtration of fluid and low-molecular-weight particles from the glomerular capillaries into

Bowman's capsule. The substances that are filtered pass into the **proximal convoluted tubule**, which lies in the cortex.

The proximal tubule dips into the medulla to form the *descending* limb of the loop of Henle. The tubule then bends into a U-shaped structure to form the loop of Henle. As the tubule straightens, it ascends back toward the cortex as the *ascending* limb of the loop of Henle. The tubule again becomes convoluted as it enters the cortex. This portion of the nephron is called the **distal convoluted tubule** (see Figure 16–3). The distal convoluted tubule empties into the **collecting duct**. The collecting duct then passes through the renal pyramid to empty into the minor and major calyces, which in turn drain into the renal pelvis (see Figure 16–2). From the renal pelvis, the mixture of waste products (collectively referred to as urine) drains into the ureter, where it is carried by peristalsis to the urinary bladder. The urine is stored in the urinary bladder until it is discharged from the body through the urethra (see Figure 16–3).

BLOOD VESSELS OF THE KIDNEYS

As shown in Figure 16–4, the right and left **renal arteries** carry blood to the kidneys. Shortly after passing through the hilum of the kidney, the renal artery divides into several branches called the **interlobar arteries**. At the base of the renal pyramids, the interlobar arteries become the **arcuate arteries**. Divisions of the arcuate arteries form a series of **interlobular arteries**, which enter the cortex and branch into the **afferent arterioles**.

The afferent arterioles deliver blood to the capillary cluster that forms the glomerulus. After passing through the glomerulus, the blood leaves by way of the efferent arterioles. The efferent arterioles then branch into a complex network of capillaries called the **peritubular capillaries**, which surround the various portions of the renal tubules of the nephron (see Figure 16–3).

The peritubular capillaries reunite to form the **interlobular veins**, followed by the **arcuate vein**, the **interlobar vein**, and the **renal vein**. The renal vein eventually joins the inferior vena cava as it courses through the abdominal cavity.

URINE FORMATION

The formation of urine involves glomerular filtration, tubular reabsorption, and tubular secretion.

Glomerular Filtration

Urine formation begins in the renal corpuscle. Water and dissolved substances such as electrolytes are forced out of the glomerular capillaries by means of the blood pressure (*hydrostatic pressure*). The filtration of

Figure 16–4
Blood vessels of the kidney.

substances through the capillary membrane of the glomerulus is similar to the filtration in other capillaries throughout the body. The permeability of the glomerular capillary, however, is much greater than that of the capillaries in other tissues. As the filtrate leaves the glomerular capillaries, it is received in Bowman's capsule.

The rate of filtration is directly proportional to the hydrostatic pressure of the blood. The hydrostatic pressure in the glomerular capillary is about 55 mm Hg. This pressure, however, is partially offset by the hydrostatic pressure in Bowman's capsule of about 15 mm Hg. The osmotic pressure of the plasma is another important factor that offsets glomerular filtration. In other words, in the capillaries the hydrostatic pressure

TABLE 16–1

Forces of Glomerular Filtration

Factors	Force
Enhances Filtration	
Glomerular capillary blood pressure	+55 mm Hg
Opposes Filtration	
Fluid pressure in Bowman's capsule	−15 mm Hg
Osmotic force (caused by the protein concentration difference)	−30 mm Hg
Net Filtration Pressure	+10 mm Hg

acting to move water and dissolved particles outward is opposed by the inward osmotic pressure generated by the presence of protein in the plasma. Under normal conditions, the osmotic pressure is about 30 mm Hg. As shown in Table 16–1, the net filtration pressure, which is the algebraic sum of the three relevant forces, is about 10 mm Hg. The glomeruli filter about 125 mL of fluid per minute (about 180 L/day). Of this 125 mL, however, only about 1 mL is excreted as urine. The average urine output is about 60 mL/hour, or 1440 mL/day.

Tubular Reabsorption

As the glomerular filtrate passes through the (1) proximal convoluted tubule, (2) loop of Henle, and (3) distal convoluted tubule, water, sodium, glucose, and other substances leave the tubule and enter the blood in the peritubular capillaries. Some substances, such as glucose and amino acids, are completely reabsorbed. About 99 percent of the filtered water and sodium is reabsorbed. About 50 percent of urea is reabsorbed and the electrolyte reabsorption is generally a function of need.

Although tubular reabsorption occurs throughout the entire renal tubule system, the bulk of it occurs in the proximal convoluted portion. Certain sections of the tubule, however, reabsorb specific substances, using particular modes of transport. For example, the proximal tubule reabsorbs glucose by means of *active transport,* whereas water reabsorption occurs throughout the renal tubule by *osmosis.*

Tubular Secretion

Tubular secretion is the mechanism by which various substances are transported from the plasma of the peritubular capillaries to the fluid of the renal tubule (the *opposite* direction of tubular reabsorption). In essence, this mechanism constitutes a second pathway through which fluid can gain entrance into the renal tubule (the first being *glomerular filtration*). The most important substances transported into the tubules by means of secretion are hydrogen (H^+) and potassium (K^+) ions. In fact, most of the hydrogen and potassium ions found in the urine enter the tubules by secretion. Thus, the mechanisms that control the rates of tubular hydrogen and potassium secretion regulate the level of these substances in the blood.

URINE CONCENTRATION AND VOLUME

The composition and volume of extracellular fluids are controlled by the kidneys' ability to produce either a dilute or concentrated urine. The kidneys are able to do this by two mechanisms: the **countercurrent mechanism** and the **selective permeability of the collecting ducts**.

Countercurrent Mechanism

The countercurrent mechanism controls water reabsorption in the distal tubules and collecting ducts. It accomplishes this through the unique anatomic position of certain nephrons. About one in every five nephrons descends deep into the renal medulla. These nephrons are called **juxtamedullary nephrons**. The normal osmolality of the glomerular filtrate is approximately 300 mOsm/L.* The osmolality of the interstitial fluid increases from about 300 mOsm/L in the cortex to about 1200 mOsm/L as the juxtamedullary nephron descends into the renal medulla. This sets up a strong active transport of sodium out of the descending limb of the loop of Henle. The increased amount of sodium in the interstitial fluid, in turn, prevents water from returning to the peritubular capillaries surrounding the tubules.

Selective Permeability

As shown in Figure 16–5, the permeability of the collecting ducts is regulated by the antidiuretic hormone (ADH), which is produced in the hypothalamus and is released by the pituitary gland. The hypothalamic cells manufacture ADH in response to input from numerous vascular baroreceptors, particularly a group found in the left atrium (see Figure 16–5). When the atrial blood volume and, therefore, pressure increase, the baroreceptors are activated to transmit neural impulses to the hypothalamus, causing the production of ADH to be inhibited. This causes tubules to be impermeable to water and the urine to be greater in volume and more dilute.

*Milliosmols (mOsm/L) = 1000 milliosmols equal 1 osmol, which is the unit in which osmotic pressure is expressed. We speak of osmols or milliosmols per liter.

Figure 16–5

The pathway by which antidiuretic hormone (ADH) is controlled. When the baroreceptors in the left atrium sense an increased pressure (increased plasma volume), they send neural impulses to the hypothalamus, causing the production of ADH to decrease. In contrast, a decreased pressure (decreased plasma volume) causes the production of ADH to increase.

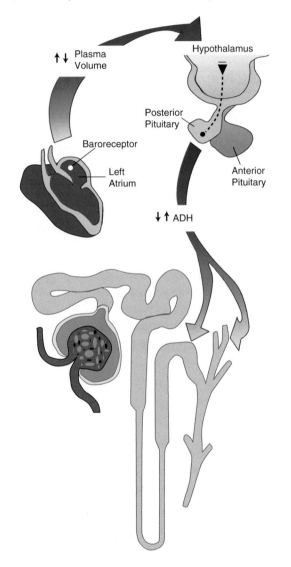

In contrast, decreased atrial pressure (*dehydration*) decreases the neural impulses originating from the baroreceptors and causes the production of ADH to increase. The result is the rapid movement of water out of these portions of the tubules of the nephron and into the interstitium of the medullary area by osmosis. This causes the urine volume to decrease and its concentration to increase.

The specific gravity (*osmolality*) of urine varies with its concentration of solutes. The urine produced by the healthy kidney has a specific gravity of about 1.003 to 1.030 under normal conditions. During periods of diminished renal function, the urine specific gravity may fall to levels of 1.008 to 1.012.

REGULATION OF ELECTROLYTE CONCENTRATION

The kidneys play a major role in maintaining a normal cellular environment by regulating the concentration of various ions. Some of the more important ions regulated by the kidneys are sodium, potassium, calcium, magnesium, and phosphate.

Sodium Ions

Sodium ions (Na^+) account for over 90 percent of the positively charged ions in the extracellular fluid. Because the sodium ions cause almost all of the osmotic pressure of the fluids, it follows that the sodium ion concentration directly affects the osmolality of the fluids. Thus, when the sodium concentration increases, there is a corresponding increase in the extracellular fluid osmolality. In contrast, the extracellular fluid osmolality decreases when there is a decreased sodium concentration.

The kidneys control the concentration of sodium primarily by regulating the amount of water in the body. When the sodium level becomes too high, the amount of water in the body increases by (1) secretion of ADH, which causes the kidney to retain water, and (2) stimulation of thirst, which causes the individual to drink liquids.

Potassium Ions

A balanced potassium (K^+) level is essential for normal nerve and muscle function. When the potassium level becomes too low, muscle weakness, diarrhea, metabolic alkalosis, and tachycardia develop. An excessively high potassium concentration causes muscle weakness, metabolic acidosis, and life-threatening arrhythmias. In response to a high K^+ level, the kidneys work to return the concentration to normal by means of two negative feedback control mechanisms: (1) the direct effect the excess potassium has on the epithelial cells of the renal tubules to cause an increased transport of potassium out of the peritubular capillaries and into the tubules of the nephrons, where it is subsequently passed in the urine; and (2) the stimulating effect the elevated potassium level has on the adrenal cortex, causing it to release increased quantities of *aldosterone*. Aldosterone stimulates the tubular epithelial cells to transport potassium ions into the nephron tubules and, hence, into the urine. The extracellular potassium concentration is normally 3.5 to 5 mEq/L.

Calcium, Magnesium, and Phosphate Ions

The precise mechanisms by which calcium, magnesium, and phosphate concentrations are regulated by the kidneys are not well understood. It is known, however, that elevated levels of any one of these ions in the extracellular fluid cause the tubules to decrease reabsorption and to pass the substances into the urine. In contrast, when any one of these substances is low in concentration, the tubules rapidly reabsorb the substance until its concentration in the extracellular fluids returns to normal.

ROLE OF THE KIDNEYS IN ACID-BASE BALANCE

In addition to the natural acid-base buffers (see Chapter 7) of the body fluids (e.g., HCO_3^-, phosphate, and protein buffers), and the respiratory system's ability to regulate the elimination of CO_2, the renal system also plays an important role in maintaining a normal acid-base balance by its ability to regulate the excretion of hydrogen ions and the reabsorption of bicarbonate ions.

All the renal tubules are capable of secreting hydrogen ions. The rate of secretion is directly proportional to the hydrogen ion concentration in the blood. Thus, when the extracellular fluids become too acidic, the kidneys excrete hydrogen ions into the urine. In contrast, when the extracellular fluids become too alkaline, the kidneys excrete basic substances (primarily sodium bicarbonate) into the urine.

This principle is illustrated in Figure 16–6, which shows that at point A, the pH of the extracellular fluid is 7.55. Because this is alkaline, the pH of the urine is also alkaline (pH 7.5), because the kidneys excrete alkaline substances from the body fluids. In contrast, the extracellular pH at point B is 7.25 and the pH of the urine is very acidic (pH 5.25), because of excretion of large quantities of acidic substances (primarily hydrogen ions) from the body fluids. In both of these examples, the excretion of either acidic or alkaline substances moves the pH toward normal.

BLOOD VOLUME

In the adult, the normal blood volume is about 5 L, and it rarely increases or decreases more than a few hundred milliliters from that value. The capillary fluid shifts and the renal system are the two major mechanisms responsible for this constancy of the blood volume.

Capillary Fluid Shift System

Under normal circumstances, the pressure in the systemic capillaries is about 17 mm Hg. When the pressure rises above this value, fluid begins to leak into the tissue spaces, causing the blood volume to decrease toward

Figure 16–6
The effect of extracellular fluid pH on urine pH.

normal. In contrast, when the blood volume falls, the capillary pressure decreases and fluid is then absorbed from the interstitial spaces, causing the blood volume to move back toward normal. This mechanism, however, has its limitations, because the tissue spaces cannot expand indefinitely when the blood volume becomes too high, nor can the tissue spaces supply an inexhaustible amount of fluid when the blood volume is too low.

The Renal System

When the blood volume increases, the glomerular pressure in the kidney rises, causing the amount of the glomerular filtrate and the volume of the urine to increase. In addition, the pressure in the peritubular capillaries decreases fluid reabsorption from the tubules, which further increases the volume of urine.

Increased blood volume increases the glomerular pressure (normally 60 mm Hg) by means of two mechanisms: (1) the increased blood volume increases the blood flow through the afferent arterioles that lead into the kidneys and thus increases the intrarenal pressure, and (2) the increased blood volume stretches the atria of the heart, which contain stretch receptors called **volume receptors**. When the volume receptors in the atria are stretched, a neural reflex is initiated which causes the renal afferent arterioles to dilate. This causes the blood flow into the kidneys to increase and thus increases the amount of urine formed. Furthermore, when the volume receptors are stretched, the secretion of ADH by the posterior pituitary gland is inhibited, which in turn increases the urine output.

RENAL FAILURE

The renal system is subject to the same types of disorders as other organs. The more common causes of renal failure are (1) congenital disorders, (2) infections, (3) obstructive disorders, (4) inflammation and immune responses, and (5) neoplasms.

Common Causes of Renal Disorders

Congenital Disorders

Approximately 10 percent of infants are born with a potentially life-threatening malformation of the renal system. Such abnormalities include unilateral renal agenesis, renal dysplasia, and polycystic disease of the kidney.

Infections

Urinary tract infections are the second most common type of bacterial infections (after respiratory tract infections). Urinary tract infections are seen more often in women than men. Approximately 20 percent of all women will develop at least one urinary tract infection during their lifetime. These infections range from bacteriuria to severe kidney infections that cause irreversible damage to the kidneys.

Obstructive Disorders

Urinary obstruction can affect all age groups and can occur in any part of the urinary tract. About 90 percent of obstructions are located below the level of the glomerulus. Some factors that predispose individuals to urinary flow obstruction are listed in Table 16–2. Persons who have a urinary obstruction are prone to infections, a heightened susceptibility to calculus formation, and permanent kidney damage.

Inflammation and Immune Responses

Kidney inflammation is caused by altered immune responses, drugs and related chemicals, and radiation. Inflammation can cause significant alterations in the glomeruli, tubules, and interstitium. The various forms of glomerulonephritis are believed to be caused by natural immune responses.

TABLE 16–2
Factors That Obstruct Urinary Flow

Calculi (bladder or kidney stones)
Normal pregnancy
Prostatic hypertrophy
Infection and inflammation causing scar tissue
Neurologic disorders (e.g., spinal cord injury, diabetic neuropathy)

Neoplasms

Cancer of the kidneys accounts for 1 to 2 percent of all cancers. Although cancer of the kidneys is relatively rare in the adult, one form of cancer—Wilms' tumor—accounts for about 70 percent of all cancers of early childhood.

Classification of Renal Disorders

Renal disorders are commonly classified according to the anatomic portion of the renal system responsible for the renal decline. The major classifications are (1) prerenal, (2) renal, and (3) postrenal.

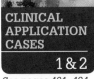

CLINICAL APPLICATION CASES

1 & 2

See pages 491–494

Prerenal Conditions

Prerenal conditions consist of abnormalities that impair blood flow to the kidneys. Prerenal problems are the most common and generally are reversible if identified and treated early. Table 16–3 lists some common prerenal causes of renal failure.

Normally, about 20 to 25 percent of the cardiac output is filtered by the kidneys. When the volume of blood falls (e.g., in cardiac failure or hemorrhage), the blood flow to the kidneys may decrease sharply. Thus, one of the early clinical manifestations of prerenal failure is a sharp reduction in urine output.

Renal Conditions

Renal abnormalities involve conditions that obstruct flow through the kidneys. Table 16–4 lists the five categories of renal abnormalities.

Postrenal Conditions

An obstruction of the urinary tract at any point between the calyces and the urinary meatus is known as a postrenal obstruction. Table 16–5 lists some abnormalities included in the postrenal category.

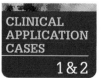

CLINICAL APPLICATION CASES

1 & 2

See pages 491–494

TABLE 16–3
Prerenal Abnormalities

Hypovolemia
    Decrease of gastrointestinal tract fluid
    Hemorrhage
    Fluid sequestration (e.g., burns)
Septicemia
Heart failure
Renal artery atherosclerosis

TABLE 16–4
Renal Abnormalities

Renal ischemia
Injury to the glomerular membrane caused by nephrotoxic agents
    Aminoglycoside agents (e.g., gentamicin, kanamycin)
    Heavy metals (e.g., lead, mercury)
    Organic solvents (e.g., ethylene glycol)
    Radiopaque contrast media
    Sulfonamides
Acute tubular necrosis
Intratubular obstruction
    Uric acid crystals
    Hemolytic reactions (e.g., blood transfusion reactions)
Acute inflammatory conditions
    Acute pyelonephritis
    Necrotizing papillitis

TABLE 16–5
Postrenal Abnormalities

Ureteral obstruction (e.g., calculi, tumors)
Bladder outlet obstruction (e.g., prostatic hypertrophy)

Mechanical Ventilation As a Cause of Renal Failure

It is well documented that mechanical ventilation can alter urinary output. *Positive pressure ventilation* decreases urinary output, whereas *negative pressure ventilation* increases urinary output. It is believed that this is due in part to the blood pressure changes that occur in response to mechanical ventilation. In positive pressure ventilation, the venous return is often impeded, causing the blood volume and, therefore, the pressure in the atria to diminish. The reduced pressure stimulates the volume receptors in the atria to send more impulses to the pituitary gland, causing more ADH to be released. As the concentration of ADH increases, the amount of urine formed by the kidneys decreases.

CARDIOPULMONARY DISORDERS CAUSED BY RENAL FAILURE

In chronic renal failure, a variety of cardiopulmonary problems can develop. In acute renal failure, the body's ability to eliminate nitrogenous wastes, water, and electrolytes is impaired. As the renal system declines further, the blood urea nitrogen (BUN), creatinine, potassium, and phosphate levels rapidly increase, and metabolic acidosis develops. Water retention gives rise to peripheral edema and pulmonary congestion. During the end-stage renal failure, virtually every portion of the body is affected. In terms of specific cardiopulmonary problems, the following problems can be expected in patients with renal failure.

Hypertension and Edema

When the renal function is impaired, the kidneys lose their ability to excrete sodium. Consequently, the ingestion of sodium leads to hypertension and edema.

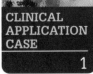

CLINICAL APPLICATION CASE

1

See page 491

Metabolic Acidosis

With the decline in renal function, the kidneys' ability to secrete hydrogen ions (H^+) and to conserve bicarbonate (HCO_3^-) progressively decreases. Furthermore, during the more advanced stages of renal failure, hyperkalemia is a frequent finding. Thus, because of the increased H^+ and K^+ ion levels and the loss of HCO_3^-, *metabolic acidosis* is an almost inevitable clinical manifestation in end stage renal failure (see Metabolic Acidosis, page 300).

Renal Acid-Base Disturbances Caused by Electrolyte Abnormalities

Chloride abnormalities can lead to acid-base disturbances through the renal system. For example, when the plasma chloride (Cl^-) level falls below normal, the amount of Cl^- available for glomerular filtration decreases. Under normal circumstances, when the positive sodium ion (Na^+) is reabsorbed by the tubules, the negative Cl^- ion must also be reabsorbed to maintain electrical neutrality. In the absence of adequate amounts of Cl^-, however, the electrical balance is maintained by the secretion of hydrogen ions (H^+). The loss of H^+ results in *hypochloremic alkalosis*. In contrast, when the plasma Cl^- level is higher than normal, the secretion of H^+ ions is reduced. This in turn causes a reduction in bicarbonate reabsorption and *hyperchloremic acidosis*.

Potassium abnormalities can also lead to acid-base disturbances through the renal system. For example, under normal conditions the potassium ion (K^+) behaves similarly to the H^+ ion in that it is secreted in the renal tubules in exchange for Na^+. In the absence of Na^+, neither K^+ nor H^+ can be secreted. When the K^+ level is higher than normal, however, the competition with H^+ for Na^+ exchange increases. When this happens, the amount of H^+ ions secreted is reduced, which in turn decreases the amount of HCO_3^- reabsorption. The end-product of this process is *hyperkalemic acidosis*. When the K^+ level is lower than normal, the competition with H^+ for Na^+ exchange decreases. Consequently, the amount of H^+ secreted is increased, which in turn increases the amount of HCO_3^- reabsorption. The end-product of this process is *hypokalemic alkalosis*.

CLINICAL APPLICATION CASE

1

See page 491

Anemia

The kidneys are a primary source of the hormone *erythropoietin*, which stimulates the bone marrow to produce red blood cells (RBCs). When the renal system fails, the production of erythropoietin is often inadequate to stimulate the bone marrow to produce a sufficient amount of RBCs. In addition, the toxic wastes that accumulate as a result of renal failure also suppress the ability of bone marrow to produce RBCs. Both of these mechanisms contribute to the anemia seen in chronic renal failure.

Bleeding

Approximately 20 percent of persons with chronic renal failure have a tendency to bleed as a result of platelet abnormalities. Clinically, this is manifested by epistaxis (nosebleed), gastrointestinal bleeding, and bruising of the skin and subcutaneous tissues.

Cardiovascular Problems

Hypertension is often an early sign of renal failure. In severe cases, the increased extracellular fluid volume, caused by sodium and water retention, gives rise to edema, congestive heart failure, and pulmonary edema. Pericarditis is also seen in about 50 percent of persons with chronic renal failure. This condition develops as a result of the pericardium being exposed to the metabolic end-products associated with renal decline.

CHAPTER SUMMARY

When the renal system fails, a number of indirect cardiopulmonary problems can develop, such as hypertension, congestive heart failure, pulmonary edema, anemia, and changes in acid-base balance. Because of this fact, a basic understanding of the cause, classification, and clinical manifestations of renal failure is essential to advanced respiratory care. The primary content areas are the kidneys, including the hilum, ureters, cortex, medulla, renal pelvis, major calyces, renal papillae, and the renal pyramid; the nephrons, including the glomerulus, proximal tubule, loop of Henle, distal tubule, Bowman's capsule, renal corpuscle, proximal convoluted tubule, distal convoluted tubule, and collecting duct; and the blood vessels of the kidneys, including the renal arteries, interlobar arteries, arcuate arteries, interlobular arteries, afferent and efferent arterioles, peritubular capillaries, interlobular veins, arcuate vein, interlobar vein, and renal vein.

In addition, the respiratory care practitioner needs a strong knowledge base of urine formation, including glomerular filtration, tubular reabsorption, and tubular secretion; urine concentration and volume, including countercurrent mechanism and selective permeability of the collecting ducts; the regulation of electrolyte concentration, including sodium, potassium, calcium, magnesium, and phosphate ions; and the role of the kidneys in acid-base balance and blood volume, including the capillary fluid shift system and the renal system. Causes of renal failure include congenital disorders, infections, obstructive disorders, inflammation and immune responses, neoplasms (tumors), and mechanical ventilation. Finally, chronic renal failure may lead to a variety of cardiopulmonary problems, including hypertension and edema, metabolic acidosis, electrolyte abnormalities, anemia, bleeding, and cardiovascular disorders.

1 CLINICAL APPLICATION CASE

A 73-year-old woman was admitted to the hospital for severe renal failure and left ventricular heart failure. An electrocardiogram (ECG) revealed a slow, irregular sinus rhythm with occasional premature ventricular contractions (PVCs). Her ankles, hands, and eyelids were swollen. Her skin was pale, damp, and cool. She had a spontaneous cough, productive of a small amount of white, frothy sputum. A chest x-ray showed white, fluffy patches that spread outward from the hilar areas to the

(continues)

peripheral borders of both lungs. Her left ventricle appeared moderately enlarged.

The patient's vital signs were blood pressure—183/97 mm Hg, heart rate—101 beats/min, respirations—18 breaths/min and deep, and temperature—37°C. The laboratory report showed that the patient's blood urea nitrogen (BUN), creatinine, potassium, and phosphate levels were all higher than normal. The patient had no urine output. On room air, her arterial blood gas values were pH—7.29, Pa_{CO_2}—32 mm Hg, HCO_3^-—17 mEq/L, and Pa_{O_2}—64 mm Hg. The respiratory therapist started the patient on 4 L/min of oxygen via a nasal cannula and drew a second arterial blood sample 25 minutes later. The results showed a pH of 7.28, Pa_{CO_2}—30, HCO_3^-—16, and Pa_{O_2}—86 mm Hg. No remarkable change was seen in the patient's vital signs.

Although the patient received aggressive medical treatment to correct her cardiac and renal problems, her pulmonary congestion did not significantly improve until she started to produce urine, 24 hours after admission. On day 4 the patient's condition was upgraded. Her skin color was normal and her skin was warm and dry to the touch. She no longer had a productive cough. When the patient was asked to produce a strong cough, no sputum was produced.

Her peripheral edema was resolved and her vital signs were blood pressure—132/84 mm Hg, heart rate—74 beats/min, and respirations—10 breaths/min. Her laboratory report showed no remarkable problems, and her ECG was normal. A second chest x-ray showed normal lungs and normal heart size. On room air, her arterial blood gas values were pH—7.39, Pa_{CO_2}—39 mm Hg, HCO_3^-—24 mEq/L, and Pa_{O_2}—93 mm Hg. The patient was discharged on day 5.

DISCUSSION

This case illustrates the adverse effects of poor blood circulation on the function of the kidneys and lungs. Essentially, all of the clinical manifestations in this case can be traced back to the patient's left ventricular failure (a prerenal abnormality). As pointed out in this chapter, prerenal problems are the most common and generally are reversible if identified and treated early. One of the early clinical manifestations of prerenal failure is a sharp reduction in urine output. On admission, the patient had no urine output. With the decline in renal function, the kidney's ability to secrete hydrogen ions (H^+) and to conserve bicarbonate (HCO_3^-) progressively decreases. Furthermore, during the more advanced stages of renal failure, hyperkalemia (increased K^+) is a frequent finding. Thus, because of the increased H^+ and K^+ ion levels and the loss of HCO_3^-, *metabolic acidosis* is an inevitable clinical manifestation in severe renal failure.

Because of the left ventricular failure, fluid progressively accumulated in the patient's lungs and extremities. The fluid accumulation, in turn, increased the density of the alveolar-capillary membranes, causing the white fluffy patches visible on the patient's chest x-ray. In addition, as the fluid accumulation in her lungs worsened, the oxygen diffusion across the alveolar-capillary membrane decreased (see Figure 3–6). This pathologic process was verified by the Pa_{O_2} of 64 mm Hg on admission. Moreover, because the blood flow through the pulmonary system was impeded (because of the left ventricular failure), blood accumulated throughout the patient's extremities, thus causing swelling in the ankles, hands, and eyelids. Fortunately, the patient received aggressive treatment in a timely manner to reverse all of these potentially fatal pathologic processes.

2 CLINICAL APPLICATION CASE

A 42-year-old male firefighter was found unconscious in a smoke-filled room on the fourth floor of a burning office building. He had second- and third-degree burns over portions of his left shoulder, left arm, and left hand, and over the anterior portion of his chest and abdominal region. His pulse was rapid and his respiration was slow and gasping. He was quickly carried out of the building and placed in a waiting ambulance. It was later estimated that the patient had been unconscious in the smoke-filled room for more than 10 minutes. En route to the hospital, the patient was manually ventilated with 100 percent oxygen. An intravenous infusion was started and Ringer's lactated solution was administered. The patient's clothing was cut away and the burn wounds were covered to prevent shock, fluid loss, and heat loss.

When the patient arrived in the emergency department, the skin that was not burned appeared cherry red. His vital signs were blood pressure—96/55 mm Hg and heart rate—124 beats/min. He was still being manually ventilated with 100 percent oxygen. Bilateral bronchospasm and crackles were heard when his lungs were auscultated. The patient was then intubated. Black, frothy secretions were suctioned from his lungs. A chest x-ray showed white fluffy densities throughout both lung fields. Arterial blood gas values were pH—7.52, Pa_{CO_2}—28 mm Hg, HCO_3^-—22 mEq/L, Pa_{O_2}—47 mm Hg. His *carboxyhemoglobin* (CO_{Hb}) level was 47 percent. The emergency department physician felt the patient was hypovolemic and going into shock.

The patient was transferred to the intensive care unit and placed on a mechanical ventilator. His progress was stormy during the first 24 hours. The respiratory-care team had to make several

Parameter*	Profile No. 1	Profile No. 2
BP	63/39 mm Hg	125/83 mm Hg
CVP	12 mm Hg	3 mm Hg
RAP	13 mm Hg	3 mm Hg
$\overline{PA}$	25 mm Hg	14 mm Hg
CO	2.7 L/min	5.8 L/min
Urine Output	0 mL/hr	54 mL/hr

Hemodynamic Profile

*BP = blood pressure; CVP = central venous pressure; RAP = right atrial pressure; $\overline{PA}$ = mean pulmonary artery pressure; CO = cardiac output.

ventilator adjustments. The patient's hemodynamic profile was classified as critical (see Hemodynamic Profile No. 1). His cardiopulmonary status, however, was finally stabilized on the second day. At this time, the patient's ventilator settings were a ventilatory rate of 12 breaths/min, an inspired oxygen concentration (FI_{O_2}) of 1.0, and a positive end-expiratory pressure (PEEP) of +15 cm H_2O. Arterial blood gas values were pH—7.38, Pa_{CO_2}—37 mm Hg, HCO_3^-—24 mEq/L, Pa_{O_2}—78 mm Hg, and Sa_{O_2}—93 percent.

Two days later, the patient's cardiopulmonary status was upgraded to fair. His ventilator settings at this time were 6 breaths/min, FI_{O_2}—0.5, and PEEP—+8 cm H_2O. Arterial blood gas values were pH—7.41, Pa_{CO_2}—38 mm Hg, HCO_3^-—24 mEq/L, Pa_{O_2}—84 mm Hg, and Sa_{O_2}—93 percent. His carboxyhemoglobin (CO_{Hb}) level was 11 percent. His hemodynamic status had significantly improved and he was producing urine (see Hemodynamic Profile No. 2). The patient progressively improved and was discharged 2 weeks later.

(continues)

DISCUSSION

Similar to Case 1, this case illustrates a prerenal abnormality. The patient's burns caused fluid sequestration, which in turn lead to *hypovolemia* (see Table 16–3). As a result of the hypovolemia, the blood flow though the patient's kidneys decreased. Again, one of the early clinical manifestations of prerenal failure is a sharp reduction in urine output. Note the low cardiac output and no urine output charted on Hemodynamic Profile No. 1. Fortunately, the patient responded favorably to therapy and his hemodynamic status and urine output returned to normal (see Hemodynamic Profile No. 2).

Note also that the patient's pulmonary status, unrelated to the poor kidney function, was very serious on admission. The patient's pathologic lung changes in the distal airways and alveoli were most likely caused by the irritant and toxic gases and suspended soot particles associated with incomplete combustion and smoke. Many of the substances found in smoke are extremely caustic to the tracheobronchial tree and poisonous to the body. The injuries that develop from smoke inhalation include inflammation of the tracheobronchial tree, bronchospasm, excessive bronchial secretions and mucus plugging, decreased mucosal ciliary transport mechanism, atelectasis, alveolar edema, and frothy secretions. Evidence of this condition was documented by the white, fluffy densities found throughout both lung fields and the low Pa_{O_2} (47 mm Hg) at admission. Finally, the patient's carbon monoxide level (CO_{Hb}—47%) was dangerously high in the emergency department. Although the patient initially responded slowly to respiratory care, the above pathologic processes were ultimately reversed and the cardiopulmonary status was normal at the time of discharge.

REVIEW QUESTIONS

1. The outer one-third of the kidney is called the
   - A. medulla
   - B. minor calyces
   - C. renal pyramid
   - D. cortex

2. Glomerular filtration is directly proportional to
   - A. blood cell size
   - B. hydrostatic pressure
   - C. osmotic pressure
   - D. the patient's fluid intake

3. Tubular reabsorption occurs primarily in the
   - A. renal corpuscle
   - B. proximal convoluted tubule
   - C. loop of Henle
   - D. distal convoluted tubule

4. The major substance(s) transported by means of tubular secretion is (are)
   - I. H^+
   - II. Cl^-

    III. K^+
    IV. HCO_3^-
    V. Na^+
       A. I only
       B. II and IV only
       C. IV and V only
       D. I and III only

5. The urine produced by the healthy kidney has a specific gravity of about
    A. 1.000–1.001
    B. 1.006–1.020
    C. 1.003–1.030
    D. 1.060–1.080

6. Which of the following can be classified as a prerenal condition?
    I. Heart failure
    II. Intratubular obstruction
    III. Bladder outlet obstruction
    IV. Hypovolemia
       A. II only
       B. IV only
       C. II and III only
       D. I and IV only

7. Which of the following are the functional units of the kidneys?
    A. Collecting ducts
    B. Major calyces
    C. Peritubular capillaries
    D. Nephrons

8. Which of the following empties urine into the bladder?
    A. Collecting ducts
    B. Ureters
    C. Distal convoluted tubules
    D. Urethra

9. Normally, the net glomerular filtration pressure is about
    A. 5 mm Hg
    B. 10 mm Hg
    C. 15 mm Hg
    D. 20 mm Hg

10. Which of the following is(are) part of the nephron?
    I. Proximal convoluted tubules
    II. Loop of Henle
    III. Glomerulus
    IV. Distal convoluted tubules
       A. III only
       B. II, III, and IV only
       C. I, II, and III only
       D. All of these

CLINICAL APPLICATION QUESTIONS

CASE 1

1. In this case, all of the clinical manifestations can be traced back to the patient's _____

   _____

   _____

2. What was the early clinical manifestation of prerenal failure presented?

   _____

   _____

3. Why did metabolic acidosis develop?

   _____

   _____

4. What clinical manifestations developed as a result of left ventricular failure?

   _____

   _____

   _____

   _____

CASE 2

1. What was the cause of the prerenal abnormality in this case?

   _____

   _____

2. What lung injuries developed as a result of smoke inhalation?

   _____

   _____

3. What was the clinical evidence that the lung injuries listed in question 2 were present?

   _____

   _____

CHAPTER 17

Sleep Physiology and Its Relationship to the Cardiopulmonary System

OBJECTIVES

By the end of this chapter, the student should be able to:

1. Differentiate sleep from a coma.
2. Define polysomography.
3. Define polysomnogram (epoch).
4. Describe the purpose of the following monitiors:
   —Electroencephalogram (EEG)
   —Electrooculogram (EOG)
   —Electromyogram (EMG)
5. Differentiate between the following EEG waveforms:
   —Beta waves
   —Alpha waves
   —Theta waves
   —Delta waves
   —K complexes
   —Sleep spindles
   —Sawtooth waves
   —Vertex waves
6. Identify the major epoch physiologic components for the following:
   —Eyes open—wake
   —Eyes closed—wake
   —Stage 1, non-REM sleep
   —Stage 2, non-REM sleep
   —Stage 3, non-REM sleep
   —Stage 4, non-REM sleep
   —REM sleep
7. Outline the normal sleep cycle.

8. Describe the following two most widely accepted theories regarding the purpose of sleep:
   —Restoration
   —Energy conservation
9. Describe circadian rhythms.
10. Describe the normal sleep patterns for the following groups:
    —Newborn and infants
    —Toddler and preschooler
    —Child and adolescent
    —Young adult and older adult
11. List factors that affect sleep.
12. Describe the following common sleep disorders:
    —Insomnia
    —Hypersomnia
    —Narcolepsy
    —Sleep apnea
      • Obstructive sleep apnea
      • Central sleep apnea
      • Mixed sleep apnea
    —Periodic limb movement disorder
    —Restless legs syndrome
13. Describe the physiologic changes that occur during sleep for the following:
    —Autonomic nervous system
    —Musculoskeletal system
    —Thermal regulation

(continues)

—Renal function
—Genital function
—Gastrointestinal function
—Endocrine function
—Cardiovascular function

—Sleep-related arrhymias
—Cerebral blood flow
—Respiratory physiology

14. Complete the review questions at the end of this chapter.

Sleep is a naturally occurring state of partial unconsciousness, diminished activity of the skeletal muscles, and depressed metabolism from which a person can be awakened by stimulation. Because sleep is readily reversible, it is distinguished from a *coma,* which is a state of unconsciousness from which a person cannot be awakened—even by the most forceful stimuli. Interestingly, an individual's environmental monitoring often continues to function during sleep, as illustrated by the fact that a strong stimulus—like a baby's cry—can immediately awaken a parent. In fact, it is well documented that individuals who sleepwalk can actually navigate around objects or climb stairs while truly asleep.

All mammals and birds sleep. Body size appears to play an important role in determining the amount of sleep a species needs. In general, large mammals need less sleep than small mammals. For example, a giraffe or elephant sleeps about 3 to 4 hours a day, whereas a cat or ferret needs about 12 to 14 hours of sleep a day. Bats, opossums, and armadillos sleep 18 or more hours a day. The newborn requires about 17 hours of sleep a day, whereas the adult needs about 6 to 8 hours a day.

During the past several years, there has been a tremendous increase in the demand for sleep medicine care services—driven, in part, by (1) the heightened appreciation of sleep disorders in the general population and (2) the increased scientific research now available concerning sleep and sleep disorders. In response to the increased need for sleep care services, many specialized sleep centers and laboratories are now available throughout the health care industry. These sleep centers offer **polysomography** (sleep study) with qualified sleep technologists who provide many diagnostic and therapeutic services. A **polysomnogram**, or **epoch**, is a recorded measurement of time during a sleep study of multiple physiologic variables that can be used to identify the different phases of sleep and, importantly, sleep disorders. For example, several sleep-related disorders, such as *obstructive sleep apnea,* are now known to adversely impact the cardiopulmonary system in numerous ways, and they are commonly treated by the respiratory care practitioner.

The major physiologic variables provided on an epoch include (1) an **electroencephalogram** (EEG), which measures the electrophysiologic changes in the brain; (2) an **electrooculogram** (EOG), which monitors the movements of the eyes; and (3) an **electromyogram** (EMG), which measures muscle activity. Table 17–1 provides an overview of common

TABLE 17-1
Common EEG Waveforms

An **electroencephalogram** (EEG) measures the electrophysiologic changes in the brain. The EEG electrical activity is characterized by frequency in cycles per second or hertz (Hz), amplitude (voltage), and the direction of major defection (polarity). The following are the most common frequency ranges.

Beta Waves
(>13 Hz)

One of the four brain waves, characterized by relatively low voltage or amplitude and a frequency greater than 13 Hz. Beta waves are known as the "busy waves" of the brain. They are recorded when the patient is awake and alert with eyes open. They are also seen during Stage 1 sleep.

Alpha Waves
(8–13 Hz)

One of the four brain waves, characterized by a relatively high voltage or amplitude and a frequency of 8–13 Hz. Alpha waves are known as the "relaxed waves" of the brain. They are commonly recorded when the individual is awake, but in a drowsy state and when the eyes are closed. Alpha waves are commonly seen during Stage 1 sleep. Bursts of Alpha waves are also seen during brief awakenings from sleep-called arousals. Alpha waves may also be seen during REM sleep.

Theta Waves
(4–7 Hz)

One of the four types of brain waves, characterized by a relatively low frequency of 4–7 Hz and low amplitude of 10 microvolts (μV). Theta waves are known as the "drowsy waves" of the brain. They are seen when the individual is awake, but relaxed and sleepy. They are also recorded in Stage 1 sleep, REM sleep, and as background waves during Stage 2 sleep.

Delta Waves
(<4 Hz)

The slowest of the four types of brain waves. Delta waves are characterized by a frequency of less than 4 Hz and high amplitude (>75 μV) broad waves. Although delta EEG activity is usually defined as <4 Hz, in human sleep scoring, the slow-wave activity used for staging is defined as EEG activity < 2 Hz (> 0.5 second duration) and a peak-to-peak amplitude of >75 μV. Delta waves are called the "deep-sleep waves." They are associated with a dreamless state from which an individual is not easily aroused. Delta waves are seen primarily during Stage 3 and 4 sleep.

K Complexes

K complexes are intermittent high-amplitude, biphasic waves of at least 0.5 second duration that signal the start of Stage 2 sleep (green bars). A K complex consists of a sharp negative wave (upward deflection), followed immediately by a slower positive wave (downward deflection), that is >0.5 second. K complexes are usually seen during Stage 2 sleep. They are sometimes seen in Stage 3. Sleep spindles are often superimposed on K complexes.

Sleep Spindles

Sleep spindles are sudden bursts of EEG activity in the 12–14 Hz frequency (6 or more distinct waves) and duration of 0.5 to 1.5 seconds (pink bars). Sleep spindles mark the onset of Stage 2. They may be seen in Stage 3 and 4, but usually do not occur in REM sleep.

Sawtooth Waves

Sawtooth waves are notched-jagged waves of frequency in the theta range (3–7 Hz) (brown bars). They are commonly seen during REM sleep. Although sawtooth waves are not part of the criteria for REM sleep, their presence is a clue that REM sleep is present.

Vertex Waves

Vertex waves are sharp negative (upward deflection) EEG waves, often in conjunction with high amplitude and short (2–7 Hz) activity (yellow bar). The amplitude of many of the vertex sharp waves are greater than 20 μV and, occasionally, they may be as high as 200 μV. Vertex waves are usually seen at the end of Stage 1.

Figure 17–1

Eyes open—wake. As shown in the yellow bar, the EEG records beta waves with high-frequency, low-amplitude activity, and sawtooth waves. EOG is low frequency and variable, and the EMG activity is relatively high. The epoch appears similar to REM sleep.

EEG waveforms. Other physiologic features typically monitored during a sleep study include (1) the presence or absence of snoring, (2) nasal and oral airflow, (3) chest movement, (4) abdomen movement, (5) Sa_{O_2}, and (6) an electrocardiogram (ECG).

Figure 17–1 provides a representative sleep study epoch of a patient with "eyes open and awake." Most sleep study epochs are 30 seconds in duration. Thus, between 720 and 960 separate epoch recordings are generated over a 6- to 8-hour sleep study period.

TYPES OF SLEEP

Non-rapid-eye-movement sleep (non-REM sleep or NREM sleep) and **rapid-eye-movement sleep** (REM sleep) are the two major types of sleep. The following subsections provide a more in-depth discussion of the two major types of sleep, and the physiologic changes commonly observed during a full sleep cycle.

Eyes Open—Wake

The **eyes open—wake** state appears very similar to REM sleep. The EEG shows **beta waves** with high-frequency, low-amplitude activity, and **sawtooth waves**. The EOG is low frequency and variable, and the EMG activity is relatively high (see Figure 17–1).

Eyes Closed—Wake

The EEG during the **eyes closed—wake** (drowsy) period is characterized by prominent **alpha waves** (>50 percent). The EOG tracing usually shows slow, rolling eye movements, and the EMG activity is relatively high (Figure 17–2).

Figure 17–2
Eyes closed—wake. As shown in the purple bar, the EEG records prominent alpha waves (>50 percent). The EOG tracing often shows slow, rolling eye movements, and the EMG activity is relatively high.

Non-Rem Sleep

Non-REM sleep consists of four stages of sleep. In general, *Stages 1* and *2* are described as *light sleep stages*, and *Stages 3* and *4* are referred to as *deep sleep* or *slow-wave sleep stages*. Non-REM sleep accounts for about 75 to 80 percent of sleep time in the average adult. During the first 30 to 45 minutes of sleep, an individual passes through all four stages of non-REM sleep; progressively moving toward slow-wave sleep, Stages 3 and 4. In the average young adult, Stage 1 comprises about 3 to 8 percent of sleep time; Stage 2 about 45 to 55 percent; and Stage 3 and Stage 4 make up about 15 to 20 percent of total sleep time. The following is a general overview of the four stages of non-REM sleep.

Stage 1

Stage 1 is the transitional stage between drowsiness and sleep. The person feels sleepy and often experiences a drifting or floating sensation. The sleeper may experience sudden muscle contractions called **hypnic myoclonia**. These contractions are frequently preceded by a sensation of starting to fall. These sudden muscle movements are similar to the "jump" one elicits when startled. Under normal conditions, Stage 1 lasts between 10 to 12 minutes and is very light sleep. A person can be easily awakened during this period.

As the person moves into Stage 1, the EEG shows light sleep comprised of low-voltage, mixed-frequency activity, with **alpha waves** (8–12 Hz*; <50 percent) and **theta waves**. Alpha waves indicate that the brain is in a calm and relaxed state of wakefulness. Some **beta waves** (>13 Hz) may also appear. **Vertex waves** commonly appear toward the end of Stage 1. The EOG shows slow, rolling eye movements. The EMG reveals decreased activity and muscle relaxation. Respirations become regular and the heart rate and blood pressure decrease slightly. Snoring may occur. If awakened, persons may state that they were not asleep (Figure 17–3).

Stage 2

Stage 2 is still a relatively light sleep stage, although arousal is a bit more difficult. The EEG becomes more irregular and is comprised predominantly of **theta waves** (4–7 Hz), intermixed with sudden bursts of **sleep spindles** (12–18 Hz), and one or more **K complexes**. **Vertex waves** may also be seen during this stage. The EOG shows either slow eye movements or absence of slow eye movements. The EMG has low electrical activity. The heart rate, blood pressure, respiratory rate, and temperature decrease slightly. Snoring may occur. Stage 2 occupies the greatest proportion of the total sleep time and accounts for about 40 to 50 percent of

Hz = cycles per second.

Figure 17–3
Stage 1 non-REM sleep. EEG records low-voltage, mixed-frequency activity, with alpha waves (8–12 Hz, <50 percent) (purple bar) and theta waves (blue bar). Some beta waves (>13 Hz) (yellow bar) may also appear. Vertex waves commonly appear toward the end of Stage 1 (orange bar). The EOG shows slow, rolling eye movements. The EMG reveals decreased activity and muscle relaxation. Respirations become regular and the heart rate and blood pressure decrease slightly. Snoring may occur.

sleep. The duration of Stage 2 NREM sleep is between 10 and 15 minutes. If awakened, the person may say he or she was thinking or daydreaming (Figure 17–4).

Stage 3

Stage 3 (medium deep sleep) is present when 20 to 50 percent of the EEG activity consists of high-amplitude (>75 μV), slow-frequency (2 Hz or slower) **delta waves**. Both **sleep spindles** and **K complexes** may be present during Stage 3. There is little or no eye movement on the EOG, and the EMG activity is low. The skeletal muscles are very relaxed, but tone is maintained. There is a continued decrease in the heart rate, blood pressure, respiratory rate, body temperature, and oxygen consumption. Snoring may occur. Dreaming may occur, but is less dramatic, more realistic, and

Figure 17–4
Stage 2 non-REM sleep. The EEG becomes more irregular and is comprised mostly of theta waves (4–7 Hz) (blue bar), intermixed with sudden bursts of sleep spindles (12–18 Hz) (pink bar), and one or more K complexes (green bars). Vertex waves may also be seen during this stage (yellow bar). The EOG shows either slow eye movements or absence of slow eye movements. The EMG has low electrical activity. The heart rate, blood pressure, respiratory rate, and temperature decrease slightly. Snoring may occur.

may lack plot. The sleeper becomes more difficult to arouse. Stage 3 is usually reached about 20 to 25 minutes after the onset of Stage 1 (Figure 17–5).

Stage 4

Stage 4 (deep slow-wave sleep) is present when more than 50 percent of the EEG activity consist of **delta waves** (amplitude >75 μV, and frequency 2 Hz or less). The EOG shows no eye movements, and the EMG has little or no electrical activity. The sleeper is very relaxed and seldom moves. The vital signs reach their lowest, normal level. In fact, the sleeper's heart and respiratory rate are generally decreased 20 to 30 percent below his or her normal waking hour levels. Oxygen consumption is low. The patient is very difficult to awaken. Stage 4 is thought to be important for mental and physical restoration. This is the stage in which bed-wetting, night terrors, and sleepwalking are most likely to occur (Figure 17–6).

Figure 17–5
Stage 3 non-REM sleep. EEG records 20 to 50 percent activity of high-amplitude (>75 μV), slow-frequency (2 Hz or slower) delta waves (orange bar). Sleep spindles (pink bar) and K complexes (green bar) may be present during Stage 3. The EOG records little or no eye movement, and the EMG activity is low. There is a continued decrease in the heart rate, blood pressure, respiratory rate, body temperature, and oxygen consumption. Snoring may occur.

REM Sleep

REM sleep resembles the eyes open—wake state. The EEG reveals low-voltage, mixed EEG activity, and frequent **sawtooth waves**. **Alpha waves** may be present. The EOG shows REM. The EMG recording shows low electrical activity, and a temporary paralysis of most of the skeletal muscles (e.g., arms, legs) is present. During REM sleep, brain metabolism may increase as much as 20 percent. The breathing rate increases and decreases irregularly. The heart rate becomes inconsistent with episodes of increased and decreased rates. Snoring may or may not present. When the sleeper is very tired, the duration of each REM is very short or even absent. As the person becomes more rested through the sleep period, the length of the REM sleep increases.

Figure 17–6

Stage 4 non-REM sleep. EEG records more than 50 percent activity of delta waves (amplitude >75 µV, and frequency 2 Hz or less) (orange bar). The EOG shows no eye movements, and the EMG has little or no electrical activity. The sleeper's heart and respiratory rate are generally decreased 20 to 30 percent below normal waking hour levels.

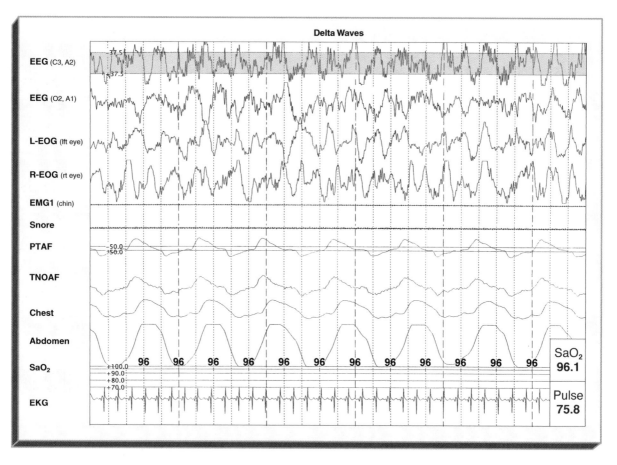

About 25 percent of the sleep of the young normal adult consists of REM sleep. The first REM sleep period usually occurs about 70 to 90 minutes after one falls asleep, and lasts 5 to 30 minutes. REM is not as restful as NREM sleep. In fact, REM sleep is also known as **paradoxic sleep**, since the EEG pattern is similar to the normal awake pattern. Most dreams occur during REM sleep. They are frequently remembered during the wakeful state, and are often described as having vivid content, full color, sounds, implausible or bizarre settings, and a sense of paralysis (Figure 17–7).

Table 17–2 summarizes the types of sleep.

Figure 17–7
REM sleep. Resembles the eyes open—wake epoch. The EEG records low-voltage, mixed EEG activity, and frequent sawtooth waves (brown bar). Alpha waves may be present (purple bar). The EOG records rapid eye movement (REM). The EMG records low electrical activity and documents a temporary paralysis of most of the skeletal muscles (e.g., arms, legs). The breathing rate increases and decreases irregularly. During REM sleep, the heart rate becomes inconsistent with episodes of increased and decreased rates. Snoring may or may not be present. REM is not as restful as NREM sleep. REM is also known as paradoxic sleep. Most dreams occur during REM sleep.

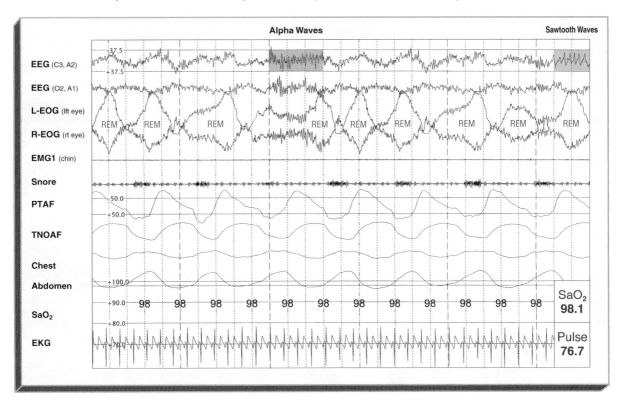

NORMAL SLEEP CYCLES

Under normal circumstances, most people require 10 to 30 minutes to fall asleep. The time needed to fall asleep is called **sleep latency**. A sleep latency period of less than 5 minutes indicates excessive sleepiness; a sleep latency period of longer than 30 minutes is associated with the lack of sleepiness, emotional stress, environmental disturbances, medication, illness, or pain.

One full sleep cycle begins with Stage 1. The sleeper then progresses through Stages 2, 3, and 4; followed by a return to Stage 3 and then Stage 2. From Stage 2, the sleeper slips into REM sleep. The end of REM sleep is the conclusion of the first sleep cycle.

From REM sleep, the individual moves back to Stage 2 and a new sleep cycle begins (Figure 17–8). The duration of each sleep cycle is about 90 to

TABLE 17-2
Types of Sleep

STAGE	EEG	CHARACTERISTICS
Eyes Open— Wake		The EEG shows **beta waves**, and high-frequency, low-amplitude activity. The EOG look very similar to REM sleep waves—low amplitude, mixed frequency, and sawtooth waves. EMG activity is relatively high
Eyes Closed— Wake (drowsy)		The EEG is characterized by prominent **alpha waves** (>50%). The EOG shows slow, rolling eye movements, and the EMG activity is relatively high.
NON-RAPID EYE MOVEMENT (NON-REM SLEEP)		
Stage 1 (light sleep)		The EEG shows low-voltage, mixed-frequency activity, **alpha waves** (8–12 Hz, <50%), and **theta waves**. Some **beta waves** (>13 Hz) may also appear. **Vertex waves** commonly appear toward the end of Stage 1. The EOG shows slow, rolling eye movements. The EMG reveals decreased activity and muscle relaxation. Respirations become regular and the heart rate and blood pressure decrease slightly. Snoring may occur. If awakened, the person may state that they were not asleep.
Stage 2 (light sleep)		The EEG becomes more irregular and is comprised predominantly with **theta waves** (4–7 Hz), intermixed with sudden bursts of **sleep spindles** (12–18 Hz), and one or more **K complexes**. **Vertex waves** may also be seen during this stage. The EOG shows either slow eye movements or absence of slow eye movements. The EMG has low electrical activity. The heart rate, blood pressure, respiratory rate, and temperature decrease slightly. Snoring may occur. If awakened, the person may say they were thinking or daydreaming.
Stage 3 (medium deep sleep)		EEG shows 20%–50% **delta waves**. Both **sleep spindles** and **K complexes** may be present. EOG shows little or no eye movement and the EMG activity is low. Continued decrease in the heart rate, blood pressure, respiratory rate, body temperature, and oxygen consumption. Snoring may occur and there is no eye movement. Dreaming may occur and the sleeper becomes more difficult to arouse.
Stage 4 (deep sleep)		EEG shows more than 50% **delta waves**. The EOG shows no eye movements, and the EMG has little or no electrical activity. The sleeper is very relaxed and seldom moves. The vital signs reach their lowest, normal level. Oxygen consumption is low. The patient is very difficult to awaken. Bed-wetting, night terrors, and sleepwalking may occur.
RAPID EYE MOVEMENT (REM)		
		About 90 minutes into the sleep cycle, there is an abrupt EEG pattern change. The EEG pattern resembles the wakeful state with low voltage, mixed EEG activity. **Sawtooth waves** are frequently seen. **Alpha waves** may be seen. The respiratory rate increases and is irregular and shallow. The heart rate and blood pressure increase. Rapid eye movement occurs and there is paralysis of most skeletal muscles. Most dreams occur during REM.

Figure 17–8
Normal sleep cycle. The sleeper progresses through Stages 1, 2, 3, and 4; followed by a return to Stages 3 and 2. From Stage 2 the sleeper moves into REM sleep. The end of REM sleep ends the first sleep cycle. From REM sleep, the sleeper moves back to stage 2 and a new sleep cycle begins.

110 minutes. The sleep cycles become longer as the sleeper becomes rested. Between four to six full cycles of sleep occur during a normal night's sleep.

The normal young adult moves from Stages 1 to 4 in about 30 minutes. The sleeper usually remains in Stage 4 for about 20 or 30 minutes. During the next 20 or 30 minutes, the sleeper moves back to Stage 3, and then Stage 2. The first REM sleep lasts for about 5 to 30 minutes. As the night progresses, REM sleep periods increase in duration and deep sleep (Stages 3 and 4) decreases. If awakened during any stage, the sleeper must return to stage 1 sleep and proceed through all the stages. By morning, the majority of sleep is spent in Stages 1, 2, and REM.

Older sleeping adults, in either Stage 2 or 3 non-REM sleep, often bypass REM sleep altogether and awaken. Except for the older adult, changes in body position during sleep usually occur 20 to 40 times during the night. One or two awakenings are normal for the young adult. The number and duration of nocturnal awakenings tend to increase with age. The duration of non-REM and REM sleep varies with age. Figure 17–9 illustrates the normal sleep cycles of children, young adults, and older adults.

Figure 17–9

Normal sleep cycles of children, young adults, and older adults.

FUNCTIONS OF SLEEP

In spite of the fact that sleep is essential for survival—right alongside food and water—the precise function of sleep is still unknown. Once considered a passive, dormant part of our daily lives, it is now known that the brain is very active during sleep. For example, during sleep the cortical activity is depressed, but the brainstem continues to control such functions as respiration, heart rate, and blood pressure.

In addition, the lack of sleep has adverse affects on our physical and mental health in numerous ways that are just now beginning to be understood. For example, too little sleep leaves the individual drowsy and unable to concentrate. It also leads to impaired memory and physical performance and reduced ability to carry out basic mental functions. Extreme sleep deprivation can lead to depression, paranoia, hallucinations, and mood swings.

The two most widely accepted theories regarding the purpose of sleep are *restoration* and *energy conservation.*

Restoration

The most widely accepted theory of sleep function is that it provides the body with a period for **restoration** and recuperation. It is thought that non-REM, slow-wave sleep promotes physical growth and healing. This theory is further supported by the fact that slow-wave sleep coincides with the release of growth hormone in children and young adults. Furthermore, many of the body's cells also show increased production and reduced breakdown of proteins during deep sleep. REM sleep appears to play an important role in the restoration of the brain processes, such as attention span, learning and memory, emotional healing, and performing basic social skills.

Energy Conservation

Some suggest that sleep is an extension of homeostasis. In other words, the increased energy used during wakeful hours must be offset by the decreased energy consumed while asleep. This is based, in part, by the fact that the metabolic rate decreases 5 to 25 percent during non-REM, slow-wave sleep. The **energy conservation** theory is further supported by the fact that slow-wave sleep declines with age; that is, as the energy requirements decrease with age, the need to conserve energy also decreases. It is believed that the decreased need to conserve energy is directly reflected in the decreased slow-wave sleep seen in the older adult.

CIRCADIAN RHYTHMS

Biologic rhythms that occur at regular intervals of about 24 hours are called **circadian rhythms**. Examples of biorhythms include the sleep–wake cycles, changes in cortisol levels, and body temperature fluctuations.

When an individual's biologic clock corresponds to a good sleep–wake pattern, the person is said to be in **circadian synchronization**. In other words, the person is asleep when his or her physiologic and psychologic rhythms are at their lowest level, and awake when his or her physiologic and psychologic rhythms are at their highest level.

In fact, current publications that deal with many public policy and safety issues involving sleep, sleep deprivation, and sleep disorders strongly suggest that the number one sleep-related problem affecting most people today is **sleep debt**. Sleep debt is based on the assumption that each person has a specific sleep requirement, an amount that must be obtained each night to maintain constant functioning. All amounts less than this specific sleep requirement constitute lost sleep, and the size of an individual's sleep debt is the total of all nights of lost sleep. A discussion of the relationship of circadian synchronization and normal sleep patterns throughout the average life span follows.

NORMAL SLEEP PATTERNS

Sleep patterns are well established in the first few months of life and continue throughout life. With advancing age, regular sleep patterns gradually decrease. In general, the well-rested person awakens feeling refreshed, mentally alert, energized, and ready to meet the daily challenges of life. However, the normal sleep–wake pattern (circadian rhythm) varies significantly throughout life.

Newborn and Infant

The **newborn** sleeps about 16 to 17 hours a day. However, this total sleep time is usually divided into about seven fairly equal sleep periods throughout the day and night. Initially, the infant usually awakens every 3 or 4 hours, eats, and then goes back to sleep. About 50 percent of the sleep period is spent in non-REM (Stages 3 and 4), and about 50 percent is spent in REM. During the REM periods, the infant commonly exhibits a lot of activity; such as twitching movements, gurgles, and coughing. By 4 months, most infants sleep through the night and take short naps throughout the day. At the end of 1 year, most infants sleep about 14 hours a day and take one or two naps during daylight hours.

Toddler and Preschooler

Total sleep time declines from about 14 hours a day at age 2 to about 12 hours a day by the fifth year—primarily due to the elimination of the afternoon nap. Most **preschoolers** still need an afternoon nap. Getting the child to sleep, however, is a frequently reported problem. REM sleep decreases to about 30 percent. Slow-wave sleep is also high.

Child and Adolescent

School-age children sleep between 8 and 12 hours a day. As the child approaches 12 years of age, less sleep is usually required. About 20 percent is spent in REM sleep. Most **adolescents** need between 8 and 10 hours of sleep. About 20 percent is spent in REM sleep.

Young Adult and Older Adult

The **young adult** usually requires between 6 and 8 hours of sleep a day. About 20 percent is spent in REM sleep. Stage 3 and 4 progressively decrease during this age, and the number of arousals from sleep increases. The **older adult** needs about 6 hours of sleep a day. About 20 to 25 percent is spent in REM sleep. Stage 3 and 4 are significantly reduced or absent. Older adults frequently require longer periods of time to fall asleep, awaken more frequently, take longer to fall back to sleep, often feel drowsy during the daytime, and take longer to adjust to changes in schedules.

FACTORS AFFECTING SLEEP

A number of factors affect both the quality (i.e., appropriate amounts of REM and non-REM sleep) and the total time an individual sleeps. Table 17–3 provides an overview of factors affecting sleep.

COMMON SLEEP DISORDERS

A basic understanding of common sleep disorders helps the health care practitioner gather and assess important clinical information. Sleep-related problems play an important role in a number of human disorders. For example, problems like an asthma attack tend to occur more often during the night and early morning, perhaps because of changes in hormones, heart rate, and other characteristics observed during sleep. The most common sleep disorders include insomnia, hypersomnia, narcolepsy, sleep apnea, periodic limb movement disorder (PLMD), and restless legs syndrome (RLS).

Insomnia

Insomnia is the most common sleep disorder. It is characterized by the inability to fall asleep or to remain asleep. Insomnia is the most common sleep disorder. Insomnia is classified as **transient insomnia** (lasting less than a week), **short-term insomnia** (lasting 1 to 3 weeks), or **chronic insomnia** (lasting longer than 3 weeks). Almost everyone suffers from transient insomnia at one time or another. Common causes of insomnia include changes in sleep environment, unpleasant room temperature,

TABLE 17-3
Factors Affecting Sleep

Age	Age is one of the most important factors affecting sleep.
Illness	Illnesses that cause pain and physical stress can disrupt sleep. Respiratory problems can disrupt a person's sleep. Elevated temperatures can cause reduction in Stages 3 and 4 sleep and REM sleep.
Environment	The environment can either enhance or hinder sleep. For example, a sudden noise change or light change in the environment can disrupt sleep. Too much or too little ventilation can affect sleep. Too warm or too cold environments can also affect sleep.
Fatigue	Moderate fatigue promotes restful sleep. The more fatigued an individual is, the shorter the first periods of REM sleep. As the sleeper becomes more rested, the REM sleep increases in duration.
Lifestyle	Frequent work shift changes (e.g., nights vs. days) disrupt sleep. Moderate exercise enhances sleep, whereas excessive exercise can delay sleep.
Emotional stress	Anxiety and depression can disrupt sleep.
Alcohol and stimulants	Excessive alcohol often disrupts sleep and may cause nightmares. Caffeine beverages stimulate the central nervous system and, thus, can interfere with sleep.
Diet	Both weight loss and weight gain are felt to affect sleep. Weight loss is usually associated with decreased sleep time, more arousals, and earlier awakenings. Weight gain is associated with an increased total sleep time, fewer arousals, and later awakenings.
Smoking	Smokers usually have more difficulty falling asleep, are easily aroused and often describe themselves as light sleepers. This is thought to be due to the stimulating effects of nicotine.
Motivation	Fatigue can often be overcome when a person desires to remain awake (e.g., a tired person watching a basketball game). However, when an individual is bored and unmotivated to stay awake, sleep usually rapidly ensues.
Medications	Hypnotics disrupt Stage 3 and 4 NREM sleep and suppress REM sleep. Beta-blockers may cause insomnia and nightmares. Narcotics suppress REM sleep and cause frequent arousals and drowsiness. Tranquilizers disrupt REM sleep.

excessive noise, stressful events, jet lag, acute medical or surgical illnesses, ingestion of stimulant medications, and diet. Current research indicates that many insomniacs are hypermetabolic. Insomnia tends to increase with age and affects more women than men.

Hypersomnia

Hypersomnia is defined as periods of deep, long sleep, or sleep of excessive depth or abnormal duration. It is commonly caused by psychologic rather than physical factors. The individual with hypersomnia is often described as being in a state of confusion on awakening, or having extreme drowsiness associated with lethargy.

Narcolepsy

Narcolepsy is characterized by sudden "sleep attacks" that often occur several times a day. The attacks last from several seconds to more than 30 minutes. Narcolepsy is classified as a hypersomnia. Individuals with narcolepsy may also experience *cataplexy* (loss of muscle tone and paralysis of voluntary muscles triggered by emotion), temporary paralysis when they awaken, and visual or auditory hallucinations at the onset or offset of sleep. Its cause is unknown. The symptoms of narcolepsy begin in adolescence or young adulthood and persist throughout life.

Sleep Apnea

Sleep apnea is a sleep disorder characterized by the temporary cessation or absence of breathing during sleep. Based on the analyses of breathing patterns, the following three types of sleep apnea have been identified: obstructive sleep apnea, central sleep apnea, and mixed sleep apnea.

Obstructive sleep apnea is defined as the cessation of airflow through the nose and mouth with the persistence of the diaphragmatic and intercostal muscle activities. Obstructive sleep apnea is the most common. During an episode of obstructive sleep apnea, the sleeper attempts to inhale during a period in which the upper airway muscle tone is momentarily absent. The negative pressure generated during inspiration causes the throat to narrow and the tongue to be sucked back into the oropharygeal area.

The obstructive sleep apnea episode is characterized by loud snoring, followed by silence, during which the sleeper struggles to breathe against an obstructed airway. As the oxygen level falls, the sleeper works even harder to inhale, which, in turn, increases the upper airway negative pressure and further augments the airway obstruction. Often the apneic episode ends only after an intense struggle, followed by a loud snorting. The sleeper then resumes snoring. In severe cases, the sleeper may suddenly awaken, sit up in bed, and gasp for air. This cycle may be repeated hundreds of times a night.

The frequent and intense struggles to breathe leave the person sleepy, irritable, or depressed during the day. In addition, because of the low oxygen concentrations associated with each apnea episode, the patient with sleep apnea is more likely to have morning headaches, a loss of interest in sex, a decline in mental function, high blood pressure, irregular heart rhythms, heart attacks, and strokes. The obstructive sleep apnea patient is two to three times more likely to have an automobile accident that the general population. In severe cases, obstructive sleep apnea may even lead to sudden death from respiratory failure during sleep.

Central sleep apnea is characterized by the cessation of airflow with *no* respiratory efforts, that is, both the diaphragmatic and intercostals muscle activities are absent. **Mixed sleep apnea** is characterized by an initial cessation of airflow with no respiratory effort (central apnea), followed by a period of upper airway obstruction (obstructive apnea).

It is estimated that approximately 18 million people in the United States have sleep apnea. However, most have not had the problem diagnosed. Common characteristics of sleep apnea include loud snoring, obesity, and excessive daytime sleepiness and fatigue. The disorder can easily be diagnosed at a specialized sleep center that performs polysomnography. If sleep apnea is diagnosed, several treatments are available based on the type of sleep apnea the patient demonstrates.

Periodic Limb Movement Disorder

Periodic limb movement disorder (PLMD) is characterized by repetitive stereotyped movements of the leg muscle during sleep with a rhythmic pattern occurring about 30 seconds apart. PLMD occurs during non-REM sleep and usually stops when the patient awakens. Because the patient is not aware of the problem, the disorder is usually first reported by a family member. The incidence of PLMD increases with age. PLMD is often seen in patients with *restless legs syndrome.*

Restless Legs Syndrome

Restless legs syndrome (RLS) is characterized as intense unpleasant feelings described as crawling, prickling, tingling, burning, painful, aching, cramping, knifelike, or itching sensations. These crawling sensations occur mostly between the knees and ankles, causing a strong urge to move the legs to relieve the feelings. Motor restlessness in noted mostly in the legs, but occasionally it is reported in the arms.

RLS is emerging as one of the most common sleep disorders. Although it may occur at any age, it is most common among the elderly. The disorder causes a constant leg movement during the day and insomnia during the night. RLS may be exacerbated during pregnancy or by caffeine, iron deficiency, diabetes, or renal insufficiency.

NORMAL CARDIOPULMONARY PHYSIOLOGY DURING SLEEP

In spite of the fact that the complete purpose of sleep is not known, a significant amount of scientific knowledge is known about the physiologic differences between wakefulness periods and sleep periods. The following provides an overview of important physiologic changes that normally occur during sleep.

Autonomic Nervous System

In general, at sleep onset parasympathetic activity increases and continues throughout non-REM sleep. The parasympathetic tone continues to increase during the transition to REM sleep. This increased parasympathetic activity causes a number of autonomic nervous systems changes throughout several areas of the body, including the musculoskeletal system, thermal regulation, renal function, genital function, gastrointestinal function, endocrine function, cardiovascular function, sleep-related arrhythmias, cerebral blood flow, and respiratory physiology.

Musculoskeletal System

The somatic skeletal muscles usually have their highest muscle tone during the wakeful state. The muscle tone decreases with sleep onset and throughout non-REM sleep. Muscle tone is at its lowest level during REM sleep. During REM sleep, neural impulses to most skeletal muscles stop and a lack of muscle tone ensues. In essence, the sleeper is temporarily paralyzed. This is especially true for the muscles of the back, neck, arms, legs, and the posterior muscles of the pharynx, including the **genioglossus muscle** (which normally pulls the tongue down and forward), the **infrahyoid muscle group**, and the **palatal muscle group**. The partial paralysis may allow the tongue to fall back into the oral pharyngeal area during inspiration (i.e., negative pressure phase). In severe cases, this condition can lead to obstructive sleep apnea.

Less affected are the muscles that move the eyes and the diaphragm. This explains, in part, why the sleeper does not physically act out a vivid dream during REM sleep—such as running from someone or swinging at a baseball. Instead the sleeper only twitches or makes small movements. Sleepers with a malfunctioning REM system, on the other hand, thrash around in their sleep, oftentimes hitting their spouse or hurting themselves as they act out a dream (the so-called REM behavior disorder).

Thermal Regulation

The body temperature usually falls by 1°C to 2°C during non-REM sleep. During REM sleep, the body temperature tends to increase with cyclic variability.

Renal Function

Renal perfusion is decreased during non-REM sleep, resulting in decreased urine production. In addition, water reabsorption increases during non-REM sleep, causing a decrease in urine production. Urine production decreases even more during REM sleep.

Genital Function

There are few or no changes in the genital function during non-REM sleep. In men, REM sleep is associated with penile tumescence (erection). The erection usually occurs at the start of REM sleep and continues throughout the REM sleep phase. In most cases, the erection is lost at the end of REM sleep. Similar genital changes occur in the erectile tissue of women during REM sleep. The sleep-related erections develop as a result of the increased parasympathetic activity and local vasodilation that normally occurs during REM sleep.

Gastrointestinal Function

The effects of sleep on the gastrointestinal system are mainly caused by an increased parasympathetic activity, circadian rhythm factors, and central nervous system activity. During sleep, salivation and esophageal motility (swallowing) are markedly decreased. Gastric acid secretion follows a circadian rhythm, with the peak acid production occurring between 10:00 P.M. and 2:00 A.M. This circadian pattern is mediated by the vagus nerve. During sleep colonic function is also decreased, which, in turn, results in a reduced colonic motility. When awakened in the morning, the colonic motility increases significantly.

Endocrine Function

Plasma growth hormone concentrations usually peak about 90 minutes after the onset of sleep, typically during Stages 3 and 4. Patients with obstructive sleep apnea or narcolepsy commonly have a decreased correlation between sleep and growth hormone concentration. Adrenocorticotropic hormone (ACTH) and cortisol secretions follow a circadian pattern, which typically peaks during delta sleep (Stages 3 and 4) between 4:00 A.M. and 8:00 A.M.

Cardiovascular Function

During non-REM sleep, the vagal nerve function provides relative autonomic stability. The heart rate variations during non-REM sleep follow a sinusoidal pattern. That is, during a normal inspiration, the heart rate increases briefly in order to accommodate venous return and increased cardiac output. During expiration, the heart rate gradually decreases. This normal cardiac rhythm unevenness is a positive marker for good cardiac health. Its absence is associated with increased age, abnormal vagus nerve function, or heart pathology. During REM sleep, the heart rate becomes inconsistent with episodes of increased and decreased rates. The heart rate may increase as much as 35 percent during REM sleep.

Sleep-Related Arrhythmias

The increased activity of the vagal nerve during non-REM sleep results in a decreased heart rate, blood pressure, and cardiac metabolism. Collectively, these activities reduce the sleeper's risk for cardiac arrhythmia. However, the decreased blood pressure during non-REM sleep may lead to myocardial hypoperfusion. On the other hand, the surge of autonomic activity during REM sleep increases the heart rate and blood pressure and increases the risk for heart arrhythmias. In addition, the increased sympathetic activity during REM sleep results in a reduced oxygen supply-to-demand ratio, coronary vasoconstriction, and variation of both cardiac ventricular preload and afterload.

Cerebral Blood Flow

During non-REM sleep, cerebral blood flow decreases. During REM sleep, cerebral blood flow increases. Spinal cord blood flow also increases during REM sleep. In addition, the cerebral blood flow is decreased during post-sleep wakefulness when compared to pre-sleep wakefulness. The cerebral metabolic rate increases during REM sleep.

Respiratory Physiology

As discussed in Chapter 9, the intrinsic rhythmicity of ventilation is coordinated by the medulla oblongata, which responds to neural impulses generated from the oxygen (P_{O_2}) sensitive peripheral chemoreceptors (located in the aorta and carotid arteries) and the carbon dioxide (P_{CO_2}) or H^+ sensitive central chemoreceptors (located in the medulla). The primary function of ventilation, therefore, is to maintain the P_{O_2} and P_{CO_2} within normal physiologic boundaries.

Although the precise mechanism is not known, the medulla's ability to respond to P_{O_2} and P_{CO_2} changes is reduced during non-REM sleep. This is especially true in regard to the medulla's ability to react to sudden changes in the P_{CO_2} level. In non-REM sleep, the respiratory rate decreases, causing the minute ventilation to fall as much as 0.5 to 1.5 L/min. It is suggested that the reduced minute ventilation is caused, in part, by (1) the decreased metabolic rate that occurs during sleep, (2) the reduced ability for the medulla to respond to ventilatory signals during sleep, (3) the decreased sensitivity of the P_{O_2} and P_{CO_2} chemoreceptors to send signals to the medulla during sleep, and (4) the increased airway resistance caused by reduced muscle tone in the upper airway. Figure 17-10 illustrates the normal ventilatory response to changing P_{CO_2} levels during non-REM and REM sleep. During REM sleep, the respiratory rate increases and decreases irregularly. This irregular respiratory pattern is thought to be secondary to brainstem respiratory neuron activity.

CHAPTER SUMMARY

Sleep is a naturally occurring state of partial unconsciousness. The two major types of sleep are non-rapid-eye-movement sleep (non-REM sleep or NREM sleep) and rapid-eye-movement sleep (REM sleep). Non-REM sleep consists of Stages 1 and 2, which are described as light-sleep stages, and Stages 3 and 4 are referred to as deep sleep or slow-wave sleep stages. REM sleep resembles wakefulness on the EEG and is the period in which most dreaming occurs and when there is temporary paralysis of

Figure 17–10
Normal ventilatory response to changing P_{CO_2} level during non-REM and REM sleep.

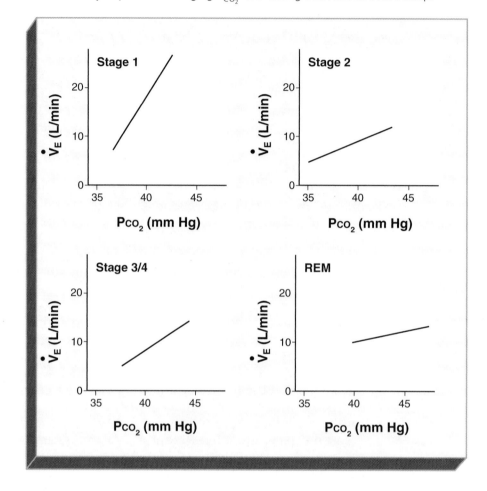

most of the skeletal muscles. One full sleep cycle begins with Stage 1 and progresses through Stages 2, 3, and 4; followed by a return to Stages 3 and 2. From Stage 2, the sleeper moves into REM sleep. The conclusion of REM sleep ends the first sleep cycle. Between four and six full sleep cycles occur during a normal night's sleep.

The two most accepted theories regarding the purpose of sleep are restoration and energy conservation. Biologic rhythms that occur at regular intervals of 24 hours are called circadian rhythms. When an individual's biologic clock corresponds to a good sleep–wake pattern, the person is said be in circadian synchronization. Sleep patterns are well established in the first few months of life and continue throughout life. With advancing age, regular sleep patterns gradually decrease.

Numerous facts affect both the quality of and the total time an individual sleeps. Such factors include age, illness, environment, fatigue, lifestyle, emotional stress, alcohol and stimulants, diet, smoking, motivation, and medications. Common sleep disorders include insomnia, hypersomnia, narcolepsy, sleep apnea, periodic limb movement disorder, and restless legs syndrome. Although not fully understood, a considerable amount of information is known regarding the differences in physiology during wakefulness and sleep. Such differences include those affecting the autonomic nervous system, musculoskeletal system, thermal regulation, renal function, genital function, gastrointestinal function, endocrine function, cardiovascular function, sleep-related arrhythmias, cerebral blood flow, and respiratory physiology.

REVIEW QUESTIONS

1. Which of the following is also known as paradoxic sleep?
   A. Stage 1 non-REM sleep
   B. Stage 2 non-REM sleep
   C. Stage 3 non-REM sleep
   D. Stage 4 non-REM sleep
   E. REM sleep

2. Most sleep study epochs are
   A. 10 seconds in duration
   B. 20 seconds in duration
   C. 30 seconds in duration
   D. 60 seconds in duration

3. K complexes first appear in which of the following stages during one full sleep cycle?
   A. Stage 1
   B. Stage 2
   C. Stage 3
   D. Stage 4

4. The newborn sleeps about how many total hours during a 24-hour period?
   A. 6 to 8 hours
   B. 8 to 12 hours
   C. 13 to 15 hours
   D. 16 to 17 hours

5. Which of the following is the most common sleep disorder?
   A. Insomnia
   B. Narcolepsy
   C. Sleep apnea
   D. Restless legs syndrome

6. Which of the following is characterized by prominent alpha waves (>50 percent)?
   A.   Eyes open—wake
   B.   Eyes closed—wake
   C.   Stage 2 non-REM sleep
   D.   REM sleep

7. Which of the following occupies the greatest proportion of the total sleep time?
   A.   Stage 2 non-REM sleep
   B.   Stage 3 non-REM sleep
   C.   Stage 4 non-REM sleep
   D.   REM sleep

8. Sleep spindles first appear in which of the following?
   A.   Stage 1 non-REM sleep
   B.   Stage 2 non-REM sleep
   C.   Stage 3 non-REM sleep
   D.   REM sleep

9. Vertex shape waves often appear toward the end of which of the following sleep stages?
   A.   Stage 1 non-REM sleep
   B.   Stage 2 non-REM sleep
   C.   Stage 4 non-REM sleep
   D.   REM sleep

10. Delta waves are associated with which of the following stages?
   I.   Stage 1 non-REM sleep
   II.   Stage 2 non-REM sleep
   III.   Stage 3 non-REM sleep
   IV.   Stage 4 non-REM sleep
   V.   REM sleep
      A. V only
      B. I and II only
      C. II and IV only
      D. III and IV only

DIRECTIONS: Match the type of waveform listed under Column A to the graphic appearance of the waveform shown under Column B.

COLUMN A

1. _____ Delta waves

2. _____ Alpha waves

3. _____ K complex

4. _____ Sleep spindles

5. _____ Beta waves

COLUMN B

A.

B.

C.

D.

E.

SECTION THREE

THE CARDIOPULMONARY SYSTEM DURING UNUSUAL ENVIRONMENTAL CONDITIONS

CHAPTER 18

Exercise and Its Effects on the Cardiopulmonary System

OBJECTIVES

By the end of this chapter, the student should be able to:

1. Describe the effects of exercise on the following components of the cardiopulmonary system:
   —Ventilation
   —Oxygen consumption
   —Arterial blood gases
   —Oxygen diffusion capacity
   —Alveolar-arterial oxygen tension difference
   —Circulation
   • Sympathetic discharge
   • Cardiac output
   • Arterial blood pressure
   • Pulmonary vascular pressures
   • Muscle capillaries

2. Describe the interrelationships between muscle work, oxygen consumption, and cardiac output.

3. Describe the effect of training on the heart and on cardiac output.

4. Differentiate between stroke volume and heart rate in increasing the cardiac output.

5. Describe how body temperature and cutaneous blood flow relate to a number of symptoms collectively referred to as heat stroke.

6. List the benefits of cardiopulmonary rehabilitation.

7. Complete the review questions at the end of this chapter.

During heavy exercise, components of the cardiopulmonary system may be stressed close to their limit. Alveolar ventilation may increase as much as 20-fold, oxygen diffusion capacity as much as 3-fold, cardiac output as much as 6-fold, muscle blood flow as much as 25-fold, oxygen consumption as much as 20-fold, and heat production as much as 20-fold.

Muscle training can increase muscle size and strength 30 to 60 percent. The efficiency of intracellular metabolism may increase by 30 to 50 percent. The size of the heart chambers and the heart mass in elite athletes, such as marathon runners, may be increased by 40 percent. When the level of exercise is greater, however, than the ability of the cardiopulmonary system to provide a sufficient supply of oxygen to the muscles, anaerobic metabolism ensues. The point at which anaerobic metabolism develops is called the **anaerobic threshold**.

VENTILATION

Control of Ventilation

The precise mechanism responsible for increased alveolar ventilation during exercise is not well understood. Exercise causes the body to consume a large amount of oxygen and, simultaneously, to produce a large amount of carbon dioxide. Alveolar ventilation increases so much, however, that the concentration of these gases in the body does not change significantly. In addition, no oxygen or carbon dioxide chemoreceptors have been identified on the venous side of circulation, or in the lungs, that could account for the increased alveolar ventilation during exercise. Thus, it is unlikely that the increased ventilation seen in exercise is caused by either of these gases.

It has been suggested that the increased ventilation is caused by neural impulses sent to the medulla by way of the following pathways (Figure 18–1):

1. The cerebral cortex sending signals to the exercising muscles may also send collateral signals to the medulla oblongata to increase the rate and depth of breathing.

Figure 18–1
Mechanisms by which exercise stimulates ventilation. (1) Collateral fibers from the motor neurons travel to the medulla; (2) sensory signals from the exercising limbs are sent to the medulla; (3) the increase in body temperature during exercise may also increase ventilation.

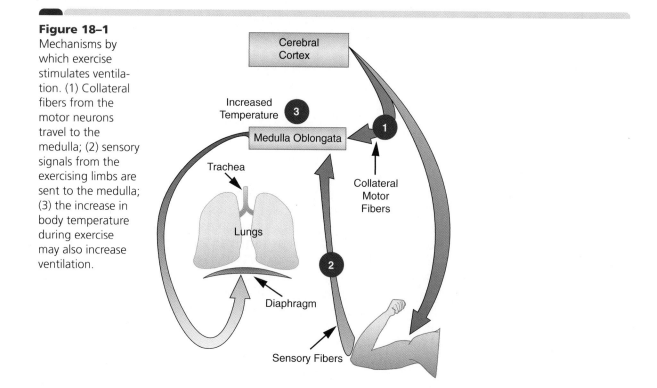

2. Proprioceptors in the moving muscles, tendons, and joints transmit sensory signals via the spinal cord to the respiratory centers of the medulla.

3. The increase in body temperature during exercise also may contribute to increased ventilation.

Alveolar Ventilation

During normal quiet breathing, an adult exchanges about 6 L of air per minute. During strenuous exercise, this can increase to 120 L/min, a 20-fold increase. Depending on the intensity and duration of the exercise, alveolar ventilation must increase to (1) supply sufficient oxygen to the blood and (2) eliminate the excess carbon dioxide produced by the skeletal muscles. The increased alveolar ventilation is produced mainly by an increased depth of ventilation (increased tidal volume), rather than by an increased rate of ventilation. During very heavy exercise, however, both an increased depth and frequency of ventilation are seen. The tidal volume is usually about 60 percent of the vital capacity, and the respiratory rate may be as high as 30 breaths/min.

Three distinct consecutive breathing patterns are seen during mild and moderate exercise. The **first stage** is characterized by an increase in alveolar ventilation, within seconds after the onset of exercise. The **second stage** is typified by a slow, gradual further increase in alveolar ventilation developing during approximately the first 3 minutes of exercise. Alveolar ventilation during this period increases almost linearly with the amount of work performed. During the **third stage**, alveolar ventilation stabilizes. When an individual stops exercising, alveolar ventilation decreases abruptly (Figure 18–2).

Figure 18–2
The relationship of exercise and ventilation. Note the abrupt increase in ventilation at the outset of exercise (A) and the even larger, abrupt decrease in ventilation at the end of exercise (B).

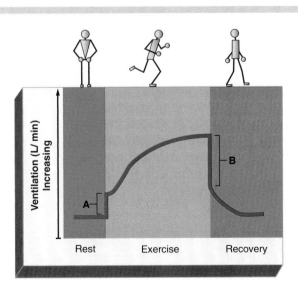

During very heavy exercise, the steady-state third stage may not be seen. In fact, when approximately 60 to 70 percent of the maximal exercise level is reached during the linear second stage, alveolar ventilation increases proportionately more than the oxygen uptake. The additional stimulation is thought to be caused primarily by the accumulation of lactic acids in the blood after the anaerobic threshold has been reached. It is suggested that the H^+ ions generated by the lactic acids stimulate the peripheral chemoreceptors, which in turn send neural impulses to the medulla oblongata to increase alveolar ventilation (see Figure 9–8).

The maximum alveolar ventilation generated during heavy exercise under normal conditions is only about 50 to 65 percent of the maximum voluntary ventilation (also called maximum breathing capacity). This provides the athlete with an important reserve of alveolar ventilation, which may be required in such conditions as short bursts of increased exercise, exercise at high altitudes, or exercise during very hot and humid conditions. Because there is normally a large alveolar ventilatory reserve during exercise, it is not the limiting factor in the delivery of oxygen to the muscles during maximal muscular aerobic metabolism. As discussed later, the inability of the heart to pump sufficient blood to the working muscles is the major limiting factor.

Oxygen Consumption

At rest, normal oxygen consumption ($\dot{V}_{O_2}$) is about 250 mL/min. The skeletal muscles account for approximately 35 to 40 percent of the total $\dot{V}_{O_2}$. During exercise, the skeletal muscles may account for more than 95 percent of the $\dot{V}_{O_2}$. During heavy exercise, the $\dot{V}_{O_2}$ of an untrained person may be more than 3500 mL of O_2/min. The $\dot{V}_{O_2}$ of an elite athlete while running a marathon may be over 5000 mL O_2/min. Figure 18–3 shows the linear relationship between $\dot{V}_{O_2}$ and alveolar ventilation exercise intensity increases.

Arterial Blood Gas Levels During Exercise

No significant Pa_{O_2}, Pa_{CO_2}, or pH changes are seen between rest and approximately 60 to 70 percent of maximal $\dot{V}_{O_2}$. During very heavy exercise, however, when lactic acidosis is present, both the pH and Pa_{CO_2} decline. Although controversy exists, it is believed that arterial acidosis stimulates the carotid chemoreceptors, causing increased alveolar ventilation and promoting respiratory acid-base compensation. The Pa_{O_2} remains constant during mild, moderate, and heavy exercise (Figure 18–4).

Oxygen Diffusion Capacity

The oxygen diffusion capacity increases linearly in response to the increased oxygen consumption ($\dot{V}_{O_2}$), during exercise (Figure 18–5). The

Figure 18–3

There is a linear relationship between oxygen consumption ($\dot{V}_{O_2}$) and alveolar ventilation as the intensity of exercise increases. Note that when the anaerobic threshold is reached during strenuous exercise, the linear relationship between $\dot{V}_{O_2}$ and alveolar ventilation will no longer exist. When the anaerobic threshold is reached, there will be an abrupt increase in alveolar ventilation with little or no increase in $\dot{V}_{O_2}$.

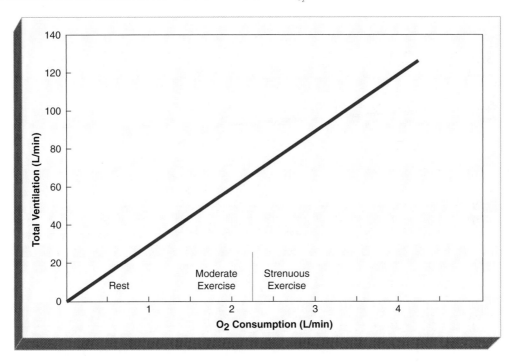

oxygen diffusion capacity may increase as much as threefold during maximum exercise. It has been shown that the increased oxygen diffusion capacity results from the increased cardiac output during exercise. The increased cardiac output causes the intravascular pressure in the pulmonary artery and left atrium to increase, which in turn serves to (1) distend the pulmonary capillaries that are not fully dilated and (2) open, or recruit, closed pulmonary capillaries (see Figure 5–21). As more blood flows through the lungs, more alveolar-capillary units become available for gas exchange. This provides a greater surface area through which oxygen can diffuse into the pulmonary capillary blood.

Alveolar-Arterial P_{O_2} Difference

Normally, there is a mean alveolar-arterial oxygen tension difference $P_{(A-a)O_2}$ of about 10 mm Hg because of (1) mismatching of ventilation and perfusion and (2) right-to-left pulmonary shunting of blood. Despite increases in oxygen consumption ($\dot{V}_{O_2}$), alveolar ventilation, and cardiac

Figure 18–4

The effect of oxygen consumption on Pa_{O_2} and Pa_{CO_2} as the intensity of exercise increases.

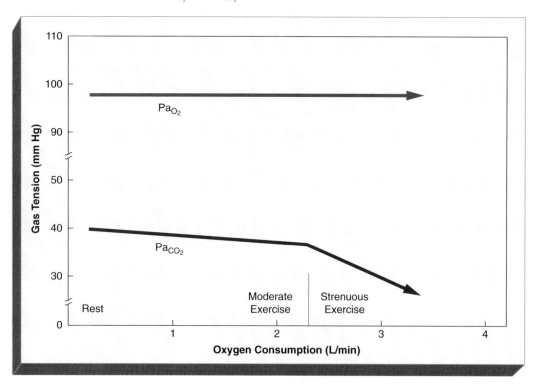

Figure 18–5

Oxygen diffusion capacity increases linearly in response to increased oxygen consumption as the intensity of exercise increases.

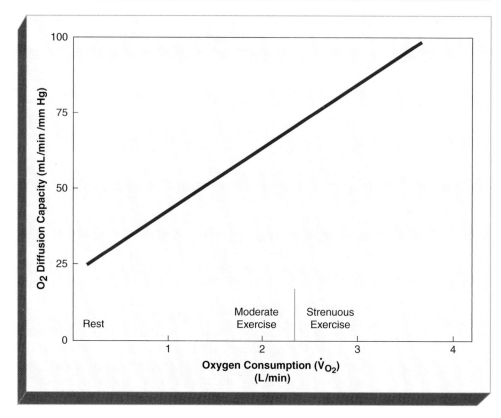

Figure 18–6

The alveolar-arterial oxygen tension difference $P_{(A-a)O_2}$ begins to increase when approximately 40 percent of the maximal $\dot{V}_{O_2}$ is exceeded.

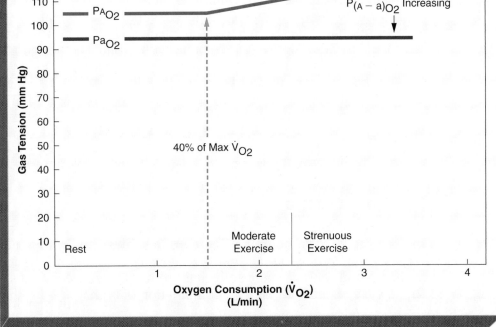

output, the $P_{(A-a)O_2}$ remains essentially constant until 40 percent of the maximal $\dot{V}_{O_2}$ is reached, beyond this point, the $P_{(A-a)O_2}$ begins to increase (Figure 18–6). An average $P_{(A-a)O_2}$ of 33 mm Hg has been reported for endurance runners exercising at their maximal $\dot{V}_{O_2}$.

CIRCULATION

Heavy exercise is one of the most stressful conditions the circulatory system encounters. Blood flow to the working muscles may increase as much as 25-fold and the total cardiac output may increase as much as 8-fold.

The ability of an individual to increase cardiac output to the muscles is the major determinant of how long and to what intensity the exercise can be sustained. In fact, the speed of a marathon runner or swimmer is almost directly proportional to the athlete's ability to increase his or her cardiac output. Thus, the circulatory system is as important as the muscles themselves in setting the limits for exercise.

During exercise, three essential physiologic responses must occur in order for the circulatory system to supply the working muscles with an adequate amount of blood: (1) sympathetic discharge, (2) increase in cardiac output, and (3) increase in arterial blood pressure.

Sympathetic Discharge

At the onset of exercise, the brain transmits signals to the vasomotor center in the medulla oblongata to trigger a sympathetic discharge. This sympathetic discharge has two circulatory effects: (1) the heart is stimulated to increase its rate and strength of contraction, and (2) the blood vessels of the peripheral vascular system constrict, except for the blood vessels of the working muscles, which strongly dilate in response to local vasodilators in the muscles themselves. The net result is an increased blood supply to the working muscles while the blood flow to nonworking muscles is reduced. Note that vasoconstriction in the heart and brain does not occur during exercise, because both the heart and the brain are as important to exercise as the working muscles themselves.

Cardiac Output

The increased oxygen demands during exercise are met almost entirely by an increased cardiac output. Figure 18–7 shows the linear relationship between the cardiac output and the intensity of exercise. The increased cardiac output during exercise results from (1) increased stroke volume, (2) increased heart rate, or (3) a combination of both.

Increased Stroke Volume

The increased stroke volume during exercise is primarily due to vasodilation in the working muscles; that is, the vasodilation in the working muscles increases the venous return to the heart. The heart, in turn, pumps more oxygenated blood back to the working muscles. Thus, the degree of vasodilation in the working muscles directly influences the stroke volume and, therefore, the greater the vasodilation in the working muscles, the greater the stroke volume and cardiac output. Another factor that facilitates an increased venous return during exercise is the sympathetic discharge. This causes a constriction of all venous blood reservoirs and forces more blood out of the veins and toward the heart.

As discussed in Chapter 5, the ability of the heart to accommodate the increased venous return and, subsequently, increase the cardiac output is due to the Frank-Starling curve (see Figure 5–19). When more venous blood returns to the heart, the heart chambers increase in size to accommodate the increased volume. As the heart chambers increase in size, the force of the heart muscle contractions increase, which in turn increases the stroke volume.

In addition to the Frank-Starling curve, the heart is also strongly stimulated by the sympathetic discharge. Increased sympathetic stimulation

Figure 18–7
A linear relationship exists between cardiac output and the intensity of exercise.

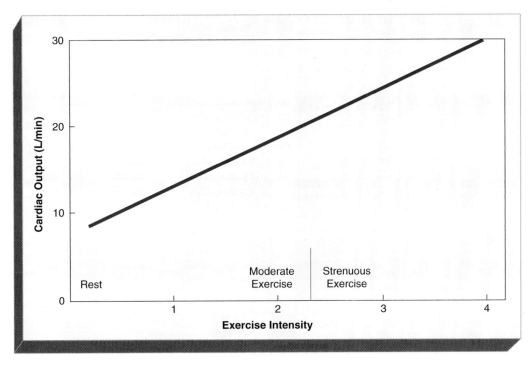

causes (1) increased heart rate (as high as 200 bpm) and (2) increased strength of contraction. The combined effect of these two mechanisms greatly increases the heart's ability to pump blood beyond what could be accomplished by the Frank-Starling curve alone.

Increased Heart Rate

An individual's maximum heart rate is estimated by the following formula:

maximum heart rate = 220 − age (years)

Thus, the maximum heart rate for a 45-year-old person is about 175 (220 − 45 = 175).

Although the heart rate increases linearly with oxygen consumption, the magnitude of the change is influenced by the size of the stroke volume; that is, when the stroke volume decreases, the heart rate increases, and when the stroke volume increases, the heart rate decreases. The stroke volume, in turn, is influenced by (1) the individual's physical condition, (2) the specific muscles that are working, and (3) the distribution of blood flow. The body's ability to increase the heart rate and stroke volume during exercise progressively declines with age.

Arterial Blood Pressure

There is an increase in arterial blood pressure during exercise because of the (1) sympathetic discharge, (2) increased cardiac output, and (3) vasoconstriction of the blood vessels in the nonworking muscle areas. Depending on the physical condition of the individual, as well as the intensity and duration of the exercise, the systolic arterial blood pressure may increase as little as 20 mm Hg or as much as 80 mm Hg.

Pulmonary Vascular Pressures

As oxygen consumption and cardiac output increase during exercise, the systolic, diastolic, and mean pulmonary arterial and wedge pressures also increase linearly (Figure 18–8). As discussed earlier, this mechanism enhances oxygen uptake by (1) distending the pulmonary capillaries and (2) opening closed pulmonary capillaries.

Figure 18–8

The systolic, diastolic, and mean pulmonary arterial and wedge pressures increase linearly as oxygen consumption and cardiac output increase.

Muscle Capillaries

At rest, approximately only 20 to 25 percent of the muscle capillaries are dilated. During heavy exercise, all these capillaries dilate to facilitate the distribution of blood. This reduces the distance that oxygen and other nutrients must travel from the capillaries to the muscle fiber. At the same time, the blood vessels of the viscera and nonworking muscles constrict.

The dilation of the blood vessels in the working muscles is caused primarily by local vasodilators acting directly on the arterioles. The most important local vasodilator effect is the reduction of oxygen in the working muscles. It is suggested that a diminished oxygen concentration in the muscles causes vasodilation because either (1) the vessels are unable to maintain contraction at low oxygen levels or (2) low oxygen levels cause the release of vasodilator substances. The most likely vasodilator substance is *adenosine*. Other vasodilator substances include potassium ions, acetylcholine, adenosine triphosphate, lactic acids, and carbon dioxide. The precise role of each of these substances in increasing blood flow to working muscles is not known.

Finally, because the vasodilation of the major working muscle groups is greater than the vasoconstriction of the nonworking muscle groups, the overall peripheral vascular resistance decreases. This is why elite athletes can substantially increase their cardiac output with only a slight increase in their mean systemic arterial blood pressure. Untrained individuals have a high peripheral vascular resistance and, therefore, high arterial blood pressure in response to modest increases in cardiac output during exercise.

INTERRELATIONSHIPS BETWEEN MUSCLE WORK, OXYGEN CONSUMPTION, AND CARDIAC OUTPUT

Figure 18–9 shows that muscle work, oxygen consumption, and cardiac output are all related to each other. Increased muscle work increases oxygen consumption and the increased oxygen consumption, in turn, dilates the intramuscular blood vessels. As the intramuscular blood vessels dilate, venous return increases, causing the cardiac output to rise. Marathon runners can have a cardiac output as great as 40 L/min. The maximum cardiac output of a young, untrained individual is less than 25 L/min.

THE INFLUENCE OF TRAINING ON THE HEART AND CARDIAC OUTPUT

The increased cardiac output seen in marathon runners results mainly from the fact that the heart chambers and heart mass increase as much as 40 percent. Cardiac enlargement and increased pumping ability occur

Figure 18–9

Relationship between muscle work, oxygen consumption, and cardiac output.

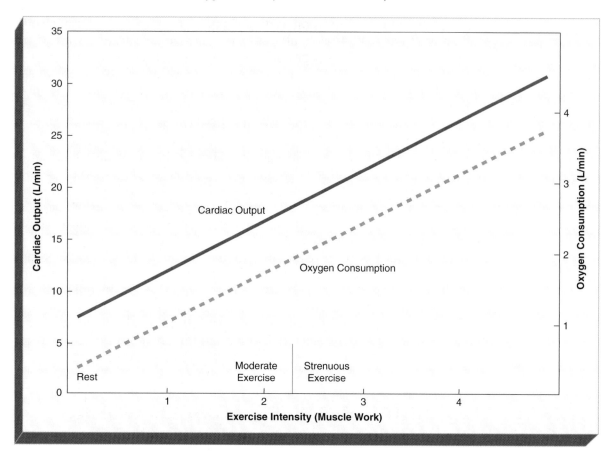

only in the endurance type of athletic training and not in the sprint type of activity. The "athlete's heart" is an effective and physiologically sound heart. It should not be considered a pathologic heart. At rest, the cardiac output of the elite athlete is almost the same as that of the average untrained individual. The former, however, has a greater stroke volume and a reduced heart rate.

STROKE VOLUME VERSUS HEART RATE IN INCREASING CARDIAC OUTPUT

Figure 18–10 shows the approximate changes that occur in stroke volume and heart rate as the cardiac output increases from about 5 to 30 L/min in a marathon runner. The stroke volume increases from about 100 mL to

Figure 18–10

Approximate changes in stroke volume and heart rate that occur when the cardiac output increases from about 5 to 30 L/min in a marathon runner.

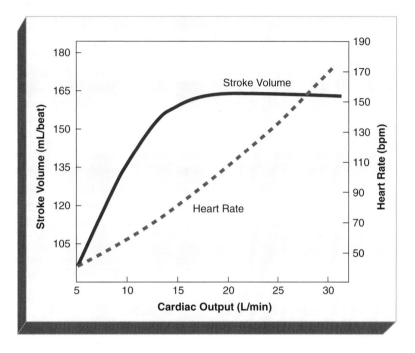

about 150 mL, an increase of about 50 percent. The heart rate increases from 50 to 180 beats/min, an increase of 260 percent. Thus, during very strenuous exercise the increase in heart rate accounts for a much greater proportion of the increased cardiac output than the increase in stroke volume. In fact, the stroke volume reaches its maximum when the maximum cardiac output is at only approximately 50 percent. Thus, any further increase in cardiac output beyond the midway point is due solely to the increased heart rate.

At maximum exercise, cardiac output reaches about 90 percent of the maximum than can be achieved. Because maximum exercise taxes the respiratory system only about 65 percent of maximum, it can be seen that normally the cardiovascular system is a greater limiting factor on maximal exercise than the respiratory system. Thus, the maximum performance that a marathon runner can achieve is directly related to the condition of the cardiovascular system. Any type of heart disease that reduces the heart's ability to pump blood will also decrease an individual's muscle power. This explains in part why a patient with congestive heart failure may have difficulty in generating enough muscle power to climb out of bed or to walk short distances.

BODY TEMPERATURE/CUTANEOUS BLOOD FLOW RELATIONSHIP

During exercise, the body generates a tremendous amount of heat and heat production may increase as much as 20-fold. Although some of the heat is stored in the body during exercise, most of the heat is dissipated through the skin. This requires a substantial increase in blood flow to the body surface. Nevertheless, even during normal temperature and humidity conditions the body temperature may rise from its normal 98.6°F to 102° to 103°F (37°C to 40°C) during endurance athletics.

When exercise is performed during very hot and humid conditions, or without adequately ventilated clothing, heat loss may be impaired and an unusually large amount of blood may be distributed to the skin. During these conditions the body temperature can easily rise to 106°F to 108°F (41°C to 42°C). As much as 5 to 10 lb of body fluid can be lost in 1 hour. When this happens, a number of signs and symptoms may appear, which collectively are referred to as **heat stroke**. These signs and symptoms include:

- Profuse sweating, followed by no sweating
- Extreme weakness
- Muscle cramping
- Exhaustion
- Nausea
- Headache
- Dizziness
- Confusion
- Staggering gait
- Altered level of consciousness
- Unconsciousness
- Circulatory collapse.

Heat stroke can be fatal if not treated immediately. Even when the individual stops exercising, the temperature does not readily return to normal, because (1) the temperature-regulating mechanism often fails at a very high temperature, and (2) the intracellular metabolism is much faster at higher temperatures, which in turn generates still more heat.

The primary treatment of heat stroke is to reduce the victim's body temperature as fast as possible. This is done by (1) spraying cool water on the victim's body, (2) continually sponging the victim with cool water, (3) blowing air over the body with a strong fan, or (4) a combination of all three measures.

CARDIOPULMONARY REHABILITATION

Cardiopulmonary rehabilitation is now a well-accepted, multidisciplinary health care service. It provides patients with a process of developing and maintaining a desirable level of physical, social, and psychologic well-being. The typical cardiopulmonary rehabilitation team consists of a physician, nurse, respiratory therapist, physical therapist, psychologist or social worker, and dietitian. The primary goal of the program is to achieve and maintain the patient's maximum level of independence and functioning in the community. Cardiopulmonary rehabilitation programs are commonly divided into the following three phases:

Phase I

This phase is the pretesting portion of the program. The patient performs a variety of tests such as pulmonary function studies, stress tests, and 6- to 12-minute walking tests. During this phase the patient is also evaluated for any nutritional, psychologic, lifestyle, and vocational needs.

Phase II

This phase also consists of patient and family education, group and individual counseling, and group discussion sessions. Educational topics include basic cardiopulmonary anatomy and physiology, breathing techniques, pulmonary hygiene, nutritional guidelines, medications, respiratory therapy equipment, and the importance of exercise. During this phase, the patient begins active range-of-motion exercises. Such exercises include work on the treadmill, air-dyne bike, arm ergometer, rowing machine, chest pulleys, and steps. The primary objective during this phase is the conditioning of the cardiovascular system (aerobic) and skeletal muscles. During the last portion of this phase, long-term graded exercises are emphasized, such as walking, walking/jogging, stationary bicycling, and/or swimming.

Phase III

This phase consists of follow-up care and long-term maintenance. Components of this phase include efforts to modify risk factors (e.g., control of blood lipids, hypertension, obesity, smoking cessation) and the establishment of a routine program of physical activity. This phase should continue indefinitely. The patient commonly undergoes yearly evaluation, which includes graded exercise testing. Some patients may require more frequent evaluations.

The benefits of cardiopulmonary rehabilitation include improved exercise capacity and decreased angina pectoris, dyspnea, and fatigue. Cardiopulmonary rehabilitation may improve oxygen transport, reduce the myocardial oxygen requirements during work, and reduce myocardial ischemia during physical activity. Finally, the efforts to modify risk factors during cardiopulmonary rehabilitation have clearly shown a reduction in the progression of coronary artery disease, morbidity, and mortality.

CHAPTER SUMMARY

A basic knowledge of the effects of exercise on the cardiopulmonary systems is helpful to the respiratory care practitioner. Important topics regarding ventilation during exercise include the control of ventilation, alveolar ventilation, oxygen consumption, arterial blood gas values, increased oxygen diffusion capacity, and alveolar-arterial difference. In addition, exercise has a significant effect on circulation. Topics in this area include sympathetic discharge, cardiac output, arterial blood pressure, pulmonary vascular pressure, and the dilation of muscle capillaries. In addition, a basic understanding of the following should be mastered: the interrelationship between muscle work, oxygen consumption, and cardiac output; the influence of training on the heart and on cardiac output; and the relationship between body temperature and cutaneous blood flow. Finally, the respiratory care practitioner should know the primary components of the three phases of a cardiopulmonary rehabilitative program.

REVIEW QUESTIONS

1. During strenuous exercise, an adult's alveolar ventilation can increase as much as
   A. 10-fold
   B. 20-fold
   C. 30-fold
   D. 40-fold

2. The maximum alveolar ventilation generated during heavy exercise under normal conditions is about what percent of the maximum voluntary ventilation?
   A. 20–35 percent
   B. 30–45 percent
   C. 40–55 percent
   D. 50–65 percent

3. During heavy exercise, the total cardiac output may increase as much as
   A. 2-fold
   B. 4-fold
   C. 6-fold
   D. 8-fold

4. At the onset of exercise, sympathetic discharge causes the
   I. heart rate to decrease
   II. peripheral vascular system to constrict

    III.   heart to increase its strength of contraction
    IV.   blood vessels of the working muscles to dilate
        A. III only
        B. II and IV only
        C. I and II only
        D. II, III, and IV only

5. During exercise, the stroke volume reaches its peak when the cardiac output is at about what percent of its maximum?
    A.   30 percent
    B.   40 percent
    C.   50 percent
    D.   60 percent

6. During exercise, heat production may increase as much as
    A.   10-fold
    B.   20-fold
    C.   30-fold
    D.   40-fold

7. During exercise, the oxygen consumption ($\dot{V}_{O_2}$) of the skeletal muscles may account for more than
    A.   65 percent of the total $\dot{V}_{O_2}$
    B.   75 percent of the total $\dot{V}_{O_2}$
    C.   85 percent of the total $\dot{V}_{O_2}$
    D.   95 percent of the total $\dot{V}_{O_2}$

8. During very heavy exercise, the
    I.   pH increases
    II. Pa_{CO_2} decreases
    III. Pa_{O_2} remains constant
    IV.   pH decreases
    V. Pa_{CO_2} increases
        A. I and II only
        B. IV and V only
        C. II and IV only
        D. II, III, and IV only

9. During maximum exercise, the oxygen diffusion capacity may increase as much as
    A.   3-fold
    B.   6-fold
    C.   9-fold
    D.   12-fold

10. During exercise, the $P_{(A-a)O_2}$ begins to increase when the oxygen consumption reaches about what percent of its maximum?
    A.   10 percent
    B.   20 percent
    C.   30 percent
    D.   40 percent

CHAPTER 19

High Altitude and Its Effects on the Cardiopulmonary System

O B J E C T I V E S

By the end of this chapter, the student should be able to:

1. Describe the effects of high altitude on the following components of the cardiopulmonary system:
   —Ventilation
   —Red blood cell production (polycythemia)
   —Acid-base status
   —Oxygen diffusion capacity
   —Alveolar-arterial oxygen tension difference
   —Ventilation-perfusion relationships
   —Cardiac output
   —Pulmonary vascular system

2. Describe other physiologic changes caused by high altitude, including:
   —Sleep disorders
   —Myoglobin concentration
   —Acute mountain sickness
   —High-altitude pulmonary edema
   —High-altitude cerebral edema
   —Chronic mountain sickness

3. Complete the review questions at the end of this chapter.

HIGH ALTITUDE

The effects of high altitude on the cardiopulmonary system are of interest because better understanding of long-term oxygen deprivation can be applied to the treatment of chronic hypoxia caused by lung disease.

The barometric pressure progressively decreases with altitude (Figure 19–1). At an altitude of 18,000 to 19,000 ft, the barometric pressure is about half the sea level value of 760 mm Hg (380 mm Hg). The barometric pressure on the summit of Mount Everest (altitude: 29,028 ft) is about 250 mm Hg (the atmospheric P_{O_2} is about 43 mm Hg). At an altitude of about 65,000 ft, the barometric pressure falls below the pressure of water vapor and tissue fluids begin to "boil" or "vaporize."

When an individual who normally lives near sea level spends a period of time at high altitudes, a number of compensatory responses

Figure 19–1

The barometric pressure and the atmospheric P_{O_2} decrease linearly as altitude increases.

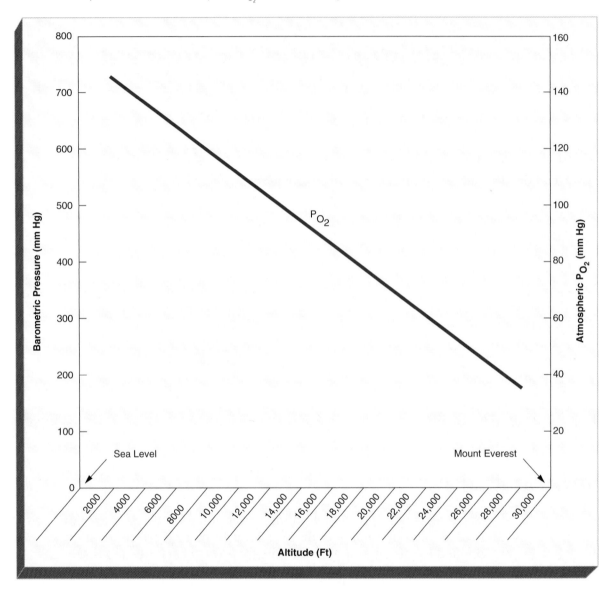

develop—a process known as acclimatization. For example, it is an interesting fact that after a period of acclimatization, an individual may reach the summit of Mount Everest without supplemental oxygen. However, when an individual is suddenly exposed to the oxygen tension found at the summit of Mount Everest, a loss of consciousness occurs within minutes.

The following are some of the primary cardiopulmonary changes seen after a period of acclimatization at high altitude.

Ventilation

One of the most prominent features of acclimatization is increased alveolar ventilation. As already mentioned, when an individual ascends above the earth's surface, the barometric pressure progressively decreases and the atmospheric P_{O_2} declines. As the atmospheric P_{O_2} decreases, the individual's arterial oxygen pressure (Pa_{O_2}) also decreases. Eventually, the Pa_{O_2} will fall low enough (to about 60 mm Hg) to stimulate the carotid and aortic bodies, known collectively as the **peripheral chemoreceptors** (see Figure 9–4). When the peripheral chemoreceptors are stimulated, they transmit signals to the medulla to increase ventilation (see Figure 9–5). Because the peripheral chemoreceptors do not acclimate to a decreased oxygen concentration, increased alveolar ventilation will continue for the entire time the individual remains at the high altitude.

Polycythemia

When an individual is subjected to a low concentration of oxygen for a prolonged period of time, the hormone *erythropoietin* from the kidneys stimulates the bone marrow to increase red blood cell (RBC) production. The increased hemoglobin available in polycythemia is an adaptive mechanism that increases the oxygen-carrying capacity of the blood. In fact, people who live at high altitudes often have a normal, or even above-normal, oxygen-carrying capacity, despite a chronically low Pa_{O_2} and oxygen saturation.

In lowlanders who ascend to high altitudes, the RBCs increase for about 6 weeks before the production rate levels off. As the level of RBCs increases the plasma volume decreases. Thus, there is no significant change in the total circulating blood volume. After 6 weeks, an average hemoglobin concentration of 20.5 g/dL has been observed in mountain climbers who climbed to altitudes greater than 18,000 ft.

Acid-Base Status

Because of the increased ventilation generated by the peripheral chemoreceptors at high altitudes, the Pa_{CO_2} decreases, causing a secondary respiratory alkalosis. Over a 24- to 48-hour period, the renal system tries to offset the respiratory alkalosis by eliminating some of the excess bicarbonate. In spite of this mechanism, however, a mild respiratory alkalosis usually persists. In fact, even natives who have been at high altitudes for generations commonly have a mild respiratory alkalosis.

It is assumed that respiratory alkalosis may be advantageous for the transfer of oxygen across the alveolar-capillary membrane because alkalosis increases the affinity of hemoglobin for oxygen. In other words, the alkalosis enhances the loading of oxygen to the hemoglobin as desaturated blood passes through the alveolar-capillary system (see Figure 6–9). It is also argued, however, that the increased affinity interferes with the unloading of oxygen at the cells (see Figure 6–10).

There is both experimental and theoretical evidence that the increased oxygen affinity at high altitude is beneficial. This is further supported by the fact that a mild respiratory alkalosis usually persists in mountain climbers, high-altitude natives, and even in animals who live in low-oxygen environments. The alkalosis persists even after the kidneys should have had more than enough time to fully eliminate the excess bicarbonate.

Oxygen Diffusion Capacity

There is no significant change in the oxygen diffusion capacity of lowlanders who are acclimatized to high altitude. High-altitude natives, however, have been shown to have an oxygen diffusion capacity that is about 20 to 25 percent greater than predicted, both during rest and exercise. The increased oxygen diffusion may be explained, in part, by the polycythemia that often develops at high altitudes. Increased numbers of red blood cells increase the diffusion capacity of oxygen (see Table 3–4).

The increased oxygen diffusion may be explained by the larger lung volumes or capacities seen in high-altitude natives. It is suggested that the larger lungs provide an increased alveolar surface area and a larger capillary blood volume. This is further supported by studies that demonstrate that when animals are exposed to low-oxygen partial pressures during their active growth period, they develop larger lungs and greater diffusion capacity. On the other hand, animals exposed to high concentrations of oxygen during their active growth period develop smaller lungs than expected.

Alveolar-Arterial P_{O_2} Difference

At high altitude, oxygen diffusion across the alveolar-capillary membrane is limited and this results in an increased **alveolar-arterial oxygen tension difference** ($P_{(A-a)O_2}$) Figure 19–2 shows that under normal circumstances there is ample time for oxygen to equilibrate between the alveoli and the end-capillary blood. In contrast, Figure 19–3 shows the estimated time necessary for oxygen to equilibrate for a climber at rest on the summit of Mount Everest. Note that the pulmonary blood enters the alveolar-capillary system with a P_{O_2} of about 21 mm Hg and slowly rises to about 28 mm Hg. Thus, as the blood leaves the alveolar-capillary system, there is a large $P_{(A-a)O_2}$ characteristic of oxygen diffusion-limitations. At high altitude, the $P_{(A-a)O_2}$ is further increased (1) during exercise—because of the increased cardiac output—and (2) in individuals with alveolar thickening caused by interstitial lung disease.

Figure 19–2

Under normal resting conditions, blood moves through the alveolar-capillary membrane in about 0.75 second. The oxygen pressure P_{O_2} reaches equilibrium in about 0.25 second—one-third of the time available.

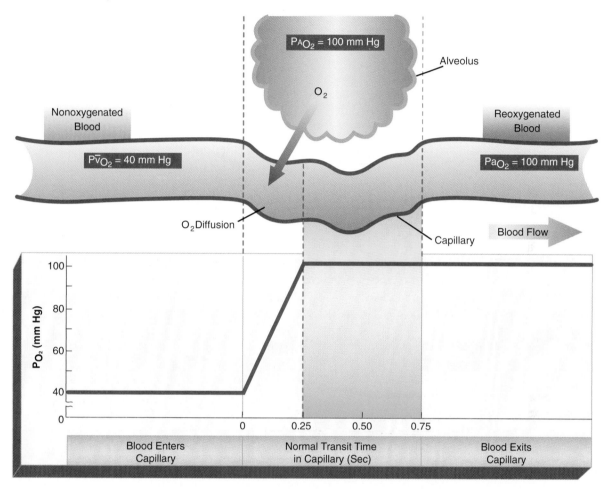

Ventilation-Perfusion Relationships

At high altitude, the overall ventilation-perfusion ratio improves as a result of the more uniform distribution of blood flow that develops in response to the increased pulmonary arterial blood pressure. Under normal circumstances the better gas exchange that results from the improved ventilation-perfusion ratio is relatively insignificant.

Cardiac Output

During acute exposure to a hypoxic environment, the cardiac output during both rest and exercise increases, which, in turn, increases the oxygen

Figure 19–3

Estimated time necessary for oxygen diffusion for a climber at rest on the summit of Mount Everest. As the blood leaves the alveolar-capillary system, there is a large alveolar-arterial oxygen tension difference $P_{(A-a)O_2}$.

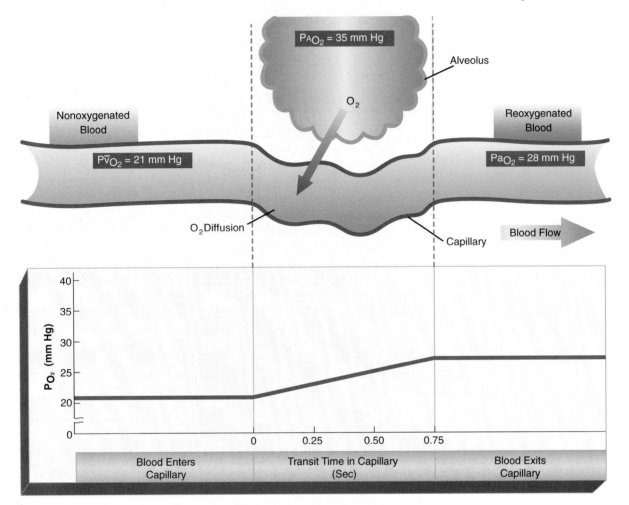

delivery to the peripheral cells. In individuals who have acclimatized to high altitude, however, and in high-altitude natives, increased cardiac output is not seen. Cardiac output and oxygen uptake are the same as at sea level. The precise reason for the return of the cardiac output and oxygen uptake to sea level values is unknown. It has been suggested that the polycythemia that develops in well-acclimatized subjects may play a role.

Pulmonary Vascular System

As an individual ascends from the earth's surface, pulmonary hypertension progressively increases as a result of hypoxic pulmonary vasoconstriction.

Figure 19–4
Pulmonary hypertension increases linearly as altitude increases.

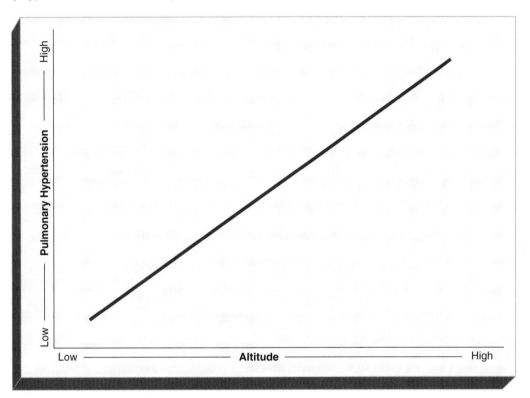

A linear relationship exists between the degree of ascent and the degree of pulmonary vasoconstriction and hypertension (Figure 19–4). The exact mechanism of this phenomenon is unclear. It is known, however, that it is the partial pressure of oxygen in the alveoli, not the partial pressure of arterial oxygen, that chiefly controls this response.

OTHER PHYSIOLOGIC CHANGES

Sleep Disorders

During the first few days at high altitude, lowlanders frequently awaken during the night and complain that they do not feel refreshed when they awake in the morning. When sleeping, they commonly demonstrate breathing that waxes and wanes with apneic periods of 10 to 15 seconds duration (Cheyne-Stokes respiration). The arterial oxygen saturation (Sa_{O_2}) fluctuates accordingly.

Myoglobin Concentration

The concentration of myoglobin in skeletal muscles is increased in high-altitude natives, and studies of this group have shown a high concentration of myoglobin in the diaphragm, the adductor muscles of the leg, the pectoral muscles, and the myocardium. Myoglobin enhances the transfer of oxygen between the capillary blood and peripheral cells, buffers regional P_{O_2} differences, and provides an oxygen storage compartment for short periods of very severe oxygen deprivation.

Acute Mountain Sickness

Newcomers to high altitude frequently experience what is known as **acute mountain sickness**, which is characterized by headache, fatigue, dizziness, palpitation, nausea, loss of appetite, and insomnia. Symptoms usually do not occur until 6 to 12 hours after an individual ascends to a high altitude. The symptoms generally are most severe on the second or third day after ascent. Acclimatization is usually complete by the fourth or fifth day.

The precise cause of acute mountain sickness is not known. It is suggested that the primary cause is hypoxia, complicated by the hypocapnia and respiratory alkalosis associated with high altitude. It may also be linked to a fluid imbalance, because pulmonary edema, cerebral edema, and peripheral edema are commonly associated with acute and chronic mountain sickness.

Sensitivity to acute mountain sickness varies greatly among individuals. Being physically fit is no guarantee of immunity. Younger people appear to be more at risk. In some cases, descent to a lower altitude may be the only way to reduce the symptoms.

High-Altitude Pulmonary Edema

High-altitude pulmonary edema is sometimes seen in individuals with acute mountain sickness. A typical scenario is as follows: A lowlander rapidly ascends to a high altitude and is very active during the trip or upon arrival. Initially, the lowlander demonstrates shortness of breath, fatigue, and a dry cough. Physical signs include tachypnea, tachycardia, and crackles at the lung bases. Orthopnea (see page 115) is commonly present at this time. In severe cases, the lowlander may cough up large amounts of pink, frothy sputum. Death may occur.

The exact cause of high-altitude pulmonary edema is not fully understood. It may be associated with the pulmonary vasoconstriction that occurs in response to the alveolar hypoxia. It may also be associated with an increased permeability of the pulmonary capillaries. The best treatment of high-altitude pulmonary edema is rapid descent. Oxygen therapy should be administered.

High-Altitude Cerebral Edema

High-altitude cerebral edema is a serious complication of acute mountain sickness. It is characterized by photophobia, ataxia, hallucinations, clouding of consciousness, coma, and possibly death. The precise cause of high-altitude cerebral edema is unclear. It is suggested that it may be linked to the increased cerebral vasodilation and blood flow that result from hypoxia. Oxygen therapy should be administered if available.

Chronic Mountain Sickness

Chronic mountain sickness (also known as Monge's disease) is sometimes seen in long-term residents at high altitude. It is characterized by fatigue, reduced exercise tolerance, headache, dizziness, somnolence, loss of mental acuity, marked polycythemia, and severe hypoxemia. The severe oxygen desaturation and polycythemia cause a cyanotic appearance. A hematocrit of 83 percent and hemoglobin concentrations as high as 28 g/dL have been reported. As a result of the high hematocrit, the viscosity of the blood is significantly increased. Right ventricular hypertrophy is common.

CHAPTER SUMMARY

A basic knowledge of the effects of high altitude on the cardiopulmonary system can enhance the respiratory care practitioner's understanding of how chronic oxygen deprivation can be applied to the treatment of chronic hypoxia caused by lung disease. Major cardiopulmonary changes seen after a period of acclimatization at high altitude include increased ventilation, polycythemia, acid-base balance changes, an increased oxygen diffusion capacity, an increased alveolar-arterial P_{O_2} difference, and an overall improved ventilation-perfusion ratio. Long-term exposure to high altitude does not change an individual's cardiac output but does cause pulmonary hypertension. Finally, high altitudes disrupt normal sleep patterns, and increase myoglobin in the skeletal muscles, and can cause acute or chronic mountain sickness, pulmonary edema, and cerebral edema.

REVIEW QUESTIONS

1. The barometric pressure is about half the sea level value of 760 mm Hg at an altitude of
   A. 4,000–5,000 ft
   B. 9,000–10,000 ft
   C. 14,000–15,000 ft
   D. 18,000–19,000 ft

2. The oxygen diffusion capacity of high-altitude natives is about
   A. 5–10 percent greater than predicted
   B. 10–15 percent greater than predicted
   C. 15–20 percent greater than predicted
   D. 20–25 percent greater than predicted

3. Acute mountain sickness is characterized by
   I. sleep disorders
   II. headache
   III. dizziness
   IV. palpitation
   V. loss of appetite
      A. I and III only
      B. II and IV only
      C. III, IV, and V only
      D. I, II, III, IV, and V

4. The symptoms of acute mountain sickness are generally most severe on the
   A. first or second day after ascent
   B. second or third day after ascent
   C. third or fourth day after ascent
   D. fourth or fifth day after ascent

5. When an individual is subjected to a high altitude for a prolonged period of time, which of the following is(are) seen?
   I. An increased red blood cell production
   II. A decreased Pa_{CO_2}
   III. An increased $P_{(A-a)O_2}$
   IV. A decreased alveolar ventilation
      A. I and III only
      B. II and IV only
      C. III and IV only
      D. I, II, and III only

6. At high altitude, the overall ventilation-perfusion ratio improves.   True _____ False _____

7. In individuals who have acclimatized to a high altitude, an increased cardiac output is seen.   True _____ False _____

8. There is a linear relationship between the degree of ascent and the degree of pulmonary vasoconstriction and hypertension.   True _____ False _____

9. Natives who have been at high altitudes for generations commonly demonstrate a mild respiratory alkalosis.   True _____ False _____

10. The concentration of myoglobin in skeletal muscles is decreased in high-altitude natives.   True _____ False _____

CHAPTER 20

High-Pressure Environments and Their Effects on the Cardiopulmonary System

OBJECTIVES

By the end of this chapter, the student should be able to:

1. Describe the following effects of a high-pressure environment on the cardiopulmonary system:
   —Breath-hold diving
   —The CO_2–O_2 paradox

   —The mammalian diving reflex
   —Decompression sickness
   —Hyperbaric medicine

2. Complete the review questions at the end of this chapter.

High-pressure environments have a profound effect on the cardiopulmonary system. Such environments are encountered in recreational scuba diving, deep sea diving, and hyperbaric medicine. The effects of high-pressure environments on the cardiopulmonary system are typically studied in (1) actual dives in the sea, (2) hyperbaric chambers where the subject is exposed to mixtures of compressed gases (known as "simulated dry dives"), and (3) a water-filled hyperbaric chamber that can simulate any depth by adjusting the gas pressure above the water (known as "simulated wet dives").

DIVING

Because water is incompressible, the pressure increases linearly with depth. For every 33 feet (10 m) below the surface, the pressure increases 1.0 atmosphere (760 mm Hg). Thus, the total pressure at a depth of 33 feet is 2 atmospheres (1520 mm Hg)—1.0 atmosphere (1 atm) owing to the water column and 1.0 atmosphere pressure owing to the gaseous atmosphere above the water. At 66 feet (20 m) below the surface, the pressure is 3.0 atmospheres (2280 mm Hg) (Figure 20–1).

553

Figure 20–1

Pressure increases linearly with depth. For every 33 feet (10 m) below sea level, the pressure increases 1.0 atmosphere. The depth in feet below sea water is referred as *feet of sea water* (FSW).

As an individual descends into water, the lung is compressed according to Boyle's law:

$$P_1 \times V_1 = P_2 \times V_2$$

where P_1 = the pressure prior to the dive, V_1 = the lung volume prior to the dive, P_2 = the pressure generated at a specific water depth, and V_2 = the lung volume at that water depth.

Thus, if an individual fully inhales to a total lung capacity of 6 L at sea level, and dives to a depth of 33 feet, the lungs will be compressed to about 3 L:

$$V_2 = \frac{P_1 \times V_1}{P_2}$$

$$= \frac{1 \times 6}{2}$$

$$= 3 \text{ L}$$

At 66 feet, the lungs would be compressed to about 2 L. At 99 feet, the lungs would be compressed to about 1.5 L.

Boyle's law can also be used to calculate the pressure within a diver's lungs at a specific depth. For example, when the previously mentioned diver descends from sea level to a depth of 33 feet (compressing the lung volume from 6 to 3 L), the pressure within the diver's lungs will increase from 760 mm Hg to about 1520 mm Hg:

$$P_2 = \frac{P_1 \times V_1}{V_2}$$

$$= \frac{760 \times 6}{3}$$

$$= 1520 \text{ mm Hg}$$

At 66 feet, the pressure within a diver's lungs will be about 2280 mm Hg. At 99 feet, the pressure will be about 3040 mm Hg.

Breath-Hold Diving

Breath-hold diving is the simplest and most popular form of diving. The maximum duration of a breath-hold dive is a function of (1) the diver's metabolic rate, and (2) the diver's ability to store and transport O_2 and CO_2. A delicate balance exists between the diver's O_2 and CO_2 levels during a breath-hold dive. For example, the P_{CO_2} must not rise too rapidly and reach the so-called respiratory drive **breaking point** (generally about 55 mm Hg) before the diver returns to the surface. On the other hand, the diver's P_{CO_2} must rise fast enough (relative to the decrease in O_2) to alert the diver of the need to return to the surface before hypoxia-induced loss of consciousness occurs.

Voluntary hyperventilation can prolong the duration of a breath-hold dive. Hyperventilation reduces the diver's CO_2 stores and, therefore increases the time before the CO_2 stores are replenished and the breaking point is reached. Note, however, that hyperventilation prior to a breath-hold dive can be dangerous. The diver's oxygen stores may fall to a critically low level before the CO_2 breaking point is reached. Should this happen, the diver could lose consciousness before reaching the surface and drown.

The CO_2–O_2 Paradox

When an individual breath-hold dives to a great depth, a so-called paradoxical reversal occurs in the flow of CO_2 and O_2 between the alveoli and the pulmonary capillary blood. This **CO_2–O_2 paradox** is caused by the pressure changes that develop around the diver's body during the dive. The CO_2 paradox occurs as the diver descends, and the O_2 paradox occurs as the diver ascends.

The reason for the CO_2 paradox is as follows: As the diver descends, the lungs are compressed and the pressure in the lungs increases. In fact, the gas pressure in the lungs is about doubled when the diver reaches a depth of 33 feet (2 atm). Thus, assuming a normal $P_{A_{O_2}}$ of about 100 mm Hg and $P_{A_{CO_2}}$ of about 40 mm Hg, at a depth of 33 feet the $P_{A_{O_2}}$ will be about 200 mm Hg and the $P_{A_{CO_2}}$ will be about 80 mm Hg.

In view of these pressure increases, it can be seen that as a diver progressively descends, a CO_2 paradox will occur when the $P_{A_{CO_2}}$ becomes greater than the $P_{v_{CO_2}}$ of the pulmonary capillary blood (normally about 46 mm Hg). In other words, the CO_2 in the alveoli will move into the pulmonary capillary blood. As the diver returns to the surface, the alveolar air expands, causing the $P_{A_{CO_2}}$ to decrease. When this happens, the CO_2 from the pulmonary capillary blood will again move into the alveoli. It is suggested that this mechanism might work to relieve the respiratory CO_2 drive (breaking point) as the diver moves toward the surface.

The reason for the O_2 paradox is as follows: Like the $P_{A_{CO_2}}$, the $P_{A_{O_2}}$ increases as the diver descends, causing more O_2 to move from the alveoli into the pulmonary capillary blood. This mechanism provides more dissolved O_2 for tissue metabolism. However, this physiologic advantage is lost as the diver returns to the surface and the lungs expand and the $P_{A_{O_2}}$ decreases. If a good portion of the O_2 is taken up from the lungs during descent, the $P_{A_{O_2}}$ decline during ascent may be significant. In fact, the $P_{A_{O_2}}$ can fall below the $P_{v_{O_2}}$ of the pulmonary capillary blood. When this happens, the O_2 paradox occurs. That is, the O_2 in the pulmonary capillary blood moves into the alveoli. The fall in $P_{A_{O_2}}$ as a diver returns to the surface is also known as the **hypoxia of ascent**.

The Mammalian Diving Reflex

The **mammalian diving reflex** (also known as *diving reflex* or *diving response*) consists of bradycardia, decreased cardiac output, lactate accumulation in underperfused muscles, and peripheral vasoconstriction elicited during a breath-hold deep dive. The mammalian diving reflex is a set of physiologic reflexes that acts as the first line of defense against hypoxia. The diving reflex may partially explain the survival of numerous near-drowning cases in cold water after submersion lasting more than 40 minutes. It is suggested that the peripheral vasoconstriction elicited during a deep dive conserves oxygen for the heart and central nervous system by shunting blood away from less vital tissues.

Decompression Sickness

During a deep dive, the dissolved nitrogen in the diver's blood will move into body tissues. The amount of dissolved gas that enters the tissues is a function of (1) the solubility of the gas in the tissues, (2) the partial pressure of the gas, and (3) the hydrostatic pressure in the tissue.

During ascent (decompression) the pressure around the diver's body falls, reducing the hydrostatic pressure in the tissues and, therefore, the ability of the tissues to hold inert gases. When the decompression is performed at an appropriately slow rate, the gases leaving the tissues will be transported (in their dissolved state) by the venous blood to the lungs and exhaled. When the decompression is conducted too rapidly, the gases will be released from the tissue as bubbles. Depending on the size, number, and location of the bubbles, they can cause a number of signs and symptoms, collectively referred to as **decompression sickness**. Decompression sickness includes, but is not limited to, joint pains (the bends), chest pain and coughing (the chokes), paresthesia and paralysis (spinal cord involvement), circulatory failure and, in severe cases, death.

HYPERBARIC MEDICINE

The administration of oxygen at increased ambient pressures is now being used routinely to treat a variety of pathologic conditions. Clinically, this therapy is referred to as **hyperbaric medicine** and is accomplished by means of a compression chamber (also called a hyperbaric chamber). Most of the therapeutic benefits of hyperbaric oxygenation are associated with the increased oxygen delivery to the tissues.

As discussed in Chapter 6, hemoglobin is about 97 percent saturated with oxygen at a normal arterial P_{O_2} of 80 to 100 mm Hg. Very little additional O_2 can combine with hemoglobin once this saturation level is reached. However, the quantity of dissolved O_2 will continue to rise linearly as the Pa_{O_2} increases. Approximately 0.3 mL of O_2 physically dissolves in each 100 mL of blood for every Pa_{O_2} increase of 100 mm Hg (Figure 20–2).

Indications for Hyperbaric Oxygenation

As shown in Table 20–1, the administration of hyperbaric oxygen is now indicated for a number of clinical conditions. Hyperbaric oxygen has long been useful in the treatment of diseases such as decompression sickness

Figure 20–2

The quantity of dissolved O_2 increases linearly as the Pa_{O_2} increases. About 0.3 mL of O_2 physically dissolves in each 100 mL of blood for every 100 mm Hg increase in Pa_{O_2}.

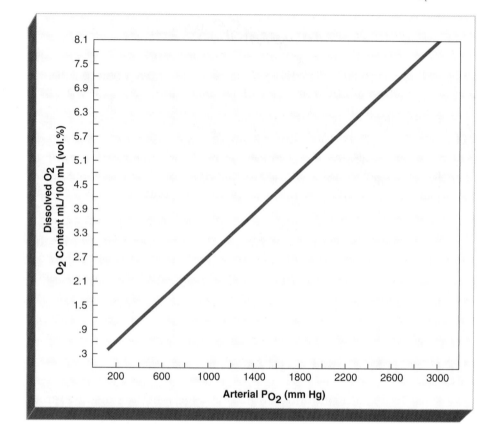

and gas embolism. Regardless of the cause of the bubbles, hyperbaric oxygen is effective in reducing bubble size, accelerating bubble resolution, and maintaining tissue oxygenation.

Hyperbaric oxygen is used empirically to enhance wound healing in conditions associated with ischemic hypoxia. Clinically, such conditions include radiation necrosis of bone or soft tissue, diabetic microangiopathy, compromised skin grafts, crush wounds, acute traumatic ischemias, and thermal burns. It appears that hyperbaric oxygen not only increases tissue oxygenation in these conditions but increases capillary density as well.

Clinical evidence supports the use of hyperbaric oxygen for the treatment of anaerobic infections, including clostridial myonecrosis (gas gangrene), a variety of necrotizing soft-tissue infections, and chronic refractory

---

TABLE 20–1
Indications for Hyperbaric Oxygenation

Gas Diseases
- Decompression sickness
- Gas embolism

Vascular Insufficiency States
- Radiation necrosis of bone or soft tissue
- Diabetic microangiopathy
- Compromised skin grafts
- Crush wounds
- Acute traumatic ischemias
- Thermal burns

Infections
- Clostridial myonecrosis
- Necrotizing soft-tissue infections
- Chronic refractory osteomyelitis

Defects in Oxygen Transport
- Carbon monoxide poisoning

---

osteomyelitis. Hyperbaric oxygen added to surgery and antibiotics in the treatment of clostridial myonecrosis increases tissue salvage and decreases mortality.

Hyperbaric oxygen is effective in the treatment of carbon monoxide poisoning. Carbon monoxide poisoning, which is caused by all sources of combustion, such as defective indoor heaters, automobile exhaust systems, or smoke inhalation, is the leading cause of death by poisoning in the United States. The severity of intoxication is a function of both the level and duration of carbon monoxide exposure. The administration of hyperbaric oxygen (1) increases the physically dissolved O_2 in the arterial blood by as much as 5 vol% O_2, (2) increases the pressure gradient for driving oxygen into ischemic tissues, and (3) reduces the half-life of **carboxyhemoglobin** (CO_{Hb}). The CO_{Hb} half-life when a victim is breathing room air at 1 atm is approximately 5 hours. That is, a CO_{Hb} of 20 percent will decrease to about 10 percent in 5 hours and 5 percent after another 5 hours. Breathing 100 percent oxygen at 1 atm reduces the CO_{Hb} half-life to less than 1 hour.

CHAPTER SUMMARY

High-pressure environments have a profound effect on the cardiopulmonary system. Important topics in this area include scuba diving, breath-hold diving, the CO_2–O_2 paradox, the mammalian diving reflex, and decompression sickness. Currently, the administration of hyperbaric oxygen is being used routinely to treat a variety of pathologic conditions, including gas diseases (e.g., decompression sickness), vascular insufficiency states (e.g., compromised skin grafts, thermal burns), infections (e.g., clostridial myonecrosis), and defects in oxygen transport (e.g., carbon monoxide poisoning).

REVIEW QUESTIONS

1. At what depth below the water surface does the pressure increase to 3.0 atmospheres?
   A. 33 feet
   B. 66 feet
   C. 99 feet
   D. 132 feet

2. If an individual fully inhales to a total lung capacity of 4.5 L at sea level (760 mm Hg) and dives to a depth of 66 feet, the lungs will be compressed to about
   A. 1.0 L
   B. 1.5 L
   C. 2.0 L
   D. 2.5 L

3. At sea level, a diver has the following:

   • Lung volume: 6 L
   • Pressure within the lungs: 755 mm Hg

   If the above individual dives to a depth of 99 feet and compresses the lung volume to 2 L, what will be the pressure within the diver's lungs?
   A. 960 mm Hg
   B. 1420 mm Hg
   C. 1765 mm Hg
   D. 2265 mm Hg

4. The diving reflex consists of
   I. tachycardia
   II. decreased cardiac output
   III. bradycardia
   IV. peripheral vasoconstriction

    A. II only
    B. III and IV only
    C. I and III only
    D. II, III, and IV only

5. The half-life of carboxyhemoglobin (CO_{Hb}) when a victim is breathing room air at 1 atmosphere is approximately
    A.   2 hours
    B.   3 hours
    C.   4 hours
    D.   5 hours

6. Hyperventilation prior to a breath-hold dive can be dangerous.   True _____ False _____

7. The fall in $P_{A_{O_2}}$ as a diver returns to the surface is known as the hypoxia of ascent.   True _____ False _____

8. Chest pain and coughing caused by decompression sickness is known as the bends.   True _____ False _____

9. The so-called P_{CO_2} respiratory drive breaking point during a dive is about 55 mm Hg.   True _____ False _____

10. Approximately 0.3 mL of O_2 is physically dissolved in each 100 mL of blood for every Pa_{O_2} increase of 100 mm Hg.   True _____ False _____

GLOSSARY

Abduct to draw away from the median plane of the body or from one of its parts.

Absolute shunt the sum of the anatomic and capillary shunts is referred to as *true* or *absolute shunt.* Absolute shunting is refractory to oxygen therapy.

Acclimatization physiologic or psychologic adjustment to a new environment.

Acetylcholine a chemical found in most organs and tissues. Acetylcholine plays an important role in the transmission of parasympathetic nerve impulses at the synapses.

Acid a compound that yields hydrogen ions when dissociated in aqueous solution (Arrhenius definition) or acts as a hydrogen ion donor (Brønsted definition) or acts as an electron pair acceptor (Lewis definition). Acids turn blue litmus red, have a sour taste, and react with bases to form salts. Acids have chemical properties essentially the opposite to those of bases.

Acidemia a decrease in the arterial blood pH below 7.35. The hydrogen ion concentration of the blood increases as reflected by a lowering of serum pH values.

Acidosis (*adj. acidotic*) an abnormal increase in hydrogen ion concentration in the body, resulting from an accumulation of an acid or the loss of a base. It is indicated by a blood pH below the normal range (7.35 to 7.45). The various forms of acidosis are named for their cause; for example, renal tubular acidosis results from failure of the kidney to secrete hydrogen ions or reabsorb bicarbonate ions, respiratory acidosis results from respiratory retention of CO_2, and diabetic acidosis results from an accumulation of ketones associated with lack of insulin. Treatment depends on diagnosis of the underlying abnormality and concurrent correction of the acid-base imbalance. Compare **alkalosis**.

Acinus (*pl. acini*) any small saclike structure, particularly one found in a gland. A subdivision of the lung consisting of the tissue distal to a terminal bronchiole. Also called **alveolus**.

Acromion process lateral portion of the spine of the scapula that forms the point of the shoulder. It articulates with the clavicle and gives attachment to the deltoid and trapezius muscles.

Action potential an electrical impulse consisting of a self-propagating series of polarizations and depolarizations, transmitted across the plasma membranes of a nerve fiber during the transmission of a nerve impulse and across the plasma membranes of a muscle cell during contraction or other activity. In the absence of an impulse, the inside is electrically negative and the outside is positive (the resting potential). During the passage of an impulse at any point on the nerve fiber, the inside becomes positive and the outside, negative. Also called *action current.*

Acute beginning abruptly with marked intensity or sharpness, then subsiding after a relatively short period. Compare **chronic**.

Acute epiglottitis a severe, rapidly progressing bacterial infection of the upper respiratory tract that occurs in young children, primarily between 2 and 7 years of age. It is characterized by sore throat, croupy stridor, and inflamed epiglottis, which may cause sudden respiratory obstruction and possibly death. The infection is generally caused by *Haemophilus influenzae*, type B, although streptococci may occasionally be the causative agent. Transmission occurs by infection with airborne particles or contact with infected secretions. The diagnosis is made by bacteriologic identification of *H. influenzae*, type B, in a specimen taken from the upper respiratory tract or in the blood. A lateral x-ray film of the neck shows an enlarged epiglottis and distention of the hypopharynx, which distinguishes the condition from croup. Direct visualization of the inflamed, cherry-red epiglottis by depression of the tongue or indirect laryngoscopy is also diagnostic but may produce total acute obstruction and should be attempted only by trained personnel with equipment to establish an airway or to provide respiratory resuscitation, if necessary. Compare **croup**.

Adrenergic nerve fibers that, when stimulated, release epinephrine at their endings. Adrenergic fibers include nearly all sympathetic postganglionic fibers except those innervating sweat glands.

Afferent carrying impulses toward a center.

Afferent nerves nerves that carry impulses from the periphery to the central nervous system.

Affinity attraction between two substances that, when united, form new substances (i.e., oxygen and hemoglobin form oxyhemoglobin).

Agranulocyte any leukocyte that does not contain predominant cytoplasmic granules, such as a monocyte or lymphocyte.

Air trapping the prevention of gas from leaving the alveoli during exhalation. This is usually caused by airway closure during exhalation.

Airway resistance a measure of the impedance to airflow through the bronchopulmonary system. Calculated by the pressure difference between the mouth and alveoli divided by flow rate.

Alkalemia an increase in the arterial blood pH above 7.45 due to a decrease in the hydrogen ion concentration or an increase in hydroxyl ions.

Alkalosis an abnormal condition of body fluids, characterized by a tendency toward a blood pH level greater than 7.45, for example, from an excess of alkaline bicarbonate or a deficiency of acid. Respiratory alkalosis may be caused by hyperventilation, resulting from an excess loss of carbon dioxide and a carbonic acid deficit. Metabolic alkalosis may result from an excess intake or retention of bicarbonate, loss of gastric acid in vomiting, potassium depletion, or any stimulus that increases the rate of sodium-hydrogen exchange. When a buffer system, such as carbon dioxide retention or bicarbonate excretion, prevents a shift in pH, it is labeled compensating alkalosis. Treatment of uncompensated alkalosis involves correction of dehydration and various ionic deficits to restore the normal acid-base balance in which the ratio of carbonic acid to bicarbonate is 20:1. Compare **acidosis**.

Allergen any substance that causes an allergic reaction. It may or may not be a protein.

Allergy a hypersensitive reaction to common, often intrinsically harmless substances, most of which are environmental.

Alpha receptor any of the postulated adrenergic components of receptor tissues that respond to norepinephrine and to various blocking agents. The activation of the alpha receptors causes such physiologic responses as increased peripheral vascular resistance, dilation of the pupils, and contraction of pilomotor muscles. Also called *alpha-adrenergic receptor*. Compare **beta receptor**.

Alveolar sac an air sac at one of the terminal cavities of lung tissue.

Alveolus a small outpouching of walls of alveolar space through which gas exchange between alveolar air and pulmonary capillary blood takes place. The term is often used interchangeably with acinus. See also **alveolar sac**, **pulmonary alveolus**.

Amniotic fluid liquid produced by the fetal membranes and the fetus; it surrounds the fetus throughout pregnancy, usually totaling about 1000 mL at term.

Anaerobic threshold the point at which the level of exercise is greater than the ability of the cardiopulmonary system to provide a sufficient supply of oxygen to the muscles, causing anaerobic metabolism to ensue.

Analogous similar in function but having a different origin or structure.

Anastomosis joining of vessels, either naturally or surgically, to allow flow to other structures.

Anatomic shunt an anatomic shunt (also called a *true shunt*) exists when blood flows from the right side of the heart to the left side without coming in contact with an alveolus for gas exchange. In the healthy lung, there is a normal anatomic shunt of about 3 percent of the cardiac output. This normal shunting is caused by nonoxygenated blood completely bypassing the alveoli and entering (1) the pulmonary vascular system by means of the bronchial venous drainage and (2) the left atrium by way of the thebesian veins. Common abnormalities that cause anatomic shunting include congenital heart disease, intrapulmonary fistula, and vacular lung tumors.

Anemia disorder characterized by a decrease in hemoglobin in the blood to levels below the normal range.

Anemic hypoxia a type of hypoxia in which the oxygen tension in the arterial blood is normal, but the oxygen-carrying capacity of the blood is inadequate. This form of hypoxia may develop from (1) a low amount of hemoglobin in the blood or (2) a deficiency in the ability of hemoglobin to carry oxygen, such as carbon monoxide poisoning.

Anoxia an abnormal condition characterized by a local or systemic lack of oxygen in body tissues. It may result from an inadequate supply of oxygen to the respiratory system, an inability of the blood to carry oxygen to the tissues, or a failure of the tissues to absorb the oxygen from the blood.

Anterior indicating the front of a structure or body surface relative to other body parts.

Antibody protein substance that develops in response to and interacts with an antigen. The antigen-antibody reaction forms the basis of immunity.

Antigen substance that induces the formation of antibodies that interact specifically with it.

The antigen-antibody reaction forms the basis for immunity.

Antitrypsin inhibitor of trypsin; may be deficient in persons with emphysema.

Aorta the main trunk of the systemic arterial circulation, comprising four parts: the ascending aorta, the arch of the aorta, the thoracic portion of the descending aorta, and the abdominal portion of the descending aorta.

Aperture opening or hole in an object or anatomic structure.

Apex top end or tip of a structure.

Apnea complete absence of spontaneous ventilation.

Apneustic center a portion of the pontine respiratory centers that influences the respiratory components of the medulla. If unrestrained, the apneustic center continually sends neural impulses to the ventral respiratory group and dorsal respiratory group in the medulla.

Arrhythmia any deviation from the normal pattern of the heartbeat.

Arterial pertaining to one artery or a network of arteries.

Arteriole the smallest of the arteries. Blood flowing from the heart is pumped through the arteries, to the arterioles, to the capillaries, into the veins, and retuned to the heart. The muscular walls of the arterioles constrict and dilate in response to both local factors and neurochemical stimuli; thus, arterioles play a significant role in peripheral vascular resistance and in regulation of blood pressure.

Arteriosclerosis a common arterial disorder characterized by thickening, loss of elasticity, and calcification of arterial walls, resulting in a decreased blood supply.

Arteriovenous shunt a passageway, artificial or natural, that allows blood to flow from an artery to a vein without going through a capillary network.

Artery one of the large blood vessels carrying blood in a direction away from the heart.

Asphyxia severe hypoxia leading to hypoxemia and hypercapnia, loss of consciousness, and, if not corrected, death. Some of the more common causes of asphyxia are drowning, electrical shock, aspiration of vomitus, lodging of a foreign body in the respiratory tract, inhalation of toxic gas or smoke, and poisoning. Oxygen and artificial ventilation are promptly administered to prevent damage to the brain. The underlying cause is then treated.

Aspiration (1) drawing in or out by suction. (2) the act of withdrawing a fluid, such as mucus or serum, from the body by a suction device. See also **aspiration pneumonia**.

Aspiration pneumonia an inflammatory condition of the lungs and bronchi caused by the inhalation of foreign material or acidic vomitus.

Asthma a respiratory disorder characterized by recurring episodes of paroxysmal dyspnea, wheezing on expiration and/or inspiration caused by construction of the bronchi, coughing, and viscous mucoid bronchial secretions. The episodes may be precipitated by inhalation of allergens or pollutants, infection, cold air, vigorous exercise, or emotional stress. Treatment may include elimination of the causative agent, hyposensitization, aerosol or oral bronchodilators, beta-adrenergic drugs, methylxanthines, cromolyn, leukotriene inhibitors, and short- or long-term use of corticosteroids.

Ataxia an abnormal condition characterized by impaired ability to coordinate movement.

Atelectasis an abnormal condition characterized by the collapse of alveoli, preventing the respiratory exchange of carbon dioxide and oxygen in a part of the lungs. Symptoms may include diminished breath sounds or aspiratory crackles, a mediastinal shift toward the side of the collapse, fever, and increasing dyspnea. The condition may be caused by obstruction of the major airways and bronchioles, by compression of the lungs as a result of fluid or air in the pleural space, or by pressure from a tumor outside the lung. Loss of functional lung tissue may secondarily cause increased heart rate, blood pressure, and respiratory rate. Secretions retained in the collapsed alveoli are rich in nutrients for bacterial growth, a condition often leading to stasis pneumonia in critically ill patients.

Atherosclerosis a common arterial disorder characterized by yellowish plaques of cholesterol, lipids, and cellular debris in the medial layer of the walls of the large and medium-sized arteries.

Atmospheric pressure pressure of the air on the earth at mean sea level; approximately 760 mm Hg (14.7 pounds per square inch).

Atrium (*pl. atria*) a chamber or cavity, such as the right and left atria of the heart or the nasal cavity.

Augment to enlarge or increase in size, amount, or degree; make bigger.

Automaticity the unique ability of the cells in the sinoatrial node of the heart to generate an action potential without being stimulated.

B

Bacteriuria the presence of bacteria in the urine.

Baroreceptor one of the pressure-sensitive nerve endings in the walls of the atria of the heart, the aortic arch, and the carotid sinuses. Baroreceptors stimulate central reflex mechanisms that allow physiologic adjustment and adaptation to changes in blood pressure via changes in heart rate, vasodilation, or vasoconstriction. Baroreceptors are essential for homeostasis. Also called *pressoreceptor*.

Basal pertaining to the fundamental or the basic, as basal anesthesia, which produces the first stage of unconsciousness, and the basal metabolic rate, which indicates the lowest metabolic rate; basal membrane.

Base a chemical compound that increases the concentration of hydroxide ions in aqueous solution.

Basophil a type of white blood cell that has a granular nucleus stained with basic dyes. These cells represent 1 percent or less of the total white blood cell count. Normal range: 0 to 0.75 percent of leukocyte differential.

Beta receptor any one of the postulated adrenergic (sympathetic fibers of autonomic nervous system) components of receptor tissues that respond to epinephrine and such blocking agents as propranolol. Activation of beta receptors causes various physiologic reactions such as relaxation of the bronchial muscles and an increase in the rate and force of cardiac contraction. Also called *beta-adrenergic receptor*. Compare **alpha receptor**.

Bicarbonate (HCO_3^-) an anion of carbonic acid in which only one of the hydrogen atoms has been removed, as in sodium bicarbonate ($NaHCO_3$).

Bicuspid valve the bicuspid valve is situated between the left atrium and the left ventricle and is the only valve with two rather than three cusps. The bicuspid valve allows blood to flow from the left atrium into the left ventricle but prevents blood from flowing back into the atrium. Ventricular contractions in systole forces the blood against the valve, closing the two cusps and assuring the flow of blood from the ventricle into the aorta. Also called the *mitral valve*.

Bifurcation a separation into two branches; the point of forking.

Biot's breathing short episodes of rapid, uniformly deep inspirations, followed by 10 to 30 seconds of apnea.

Blood-brain barrier membrane between the circulating blood and the brain that prevents or slows the passage of some drugs and other chemical compounds, radioactive ions, and disease-causing organisms such as viruses from the blood into the central nervous system.

Bohr effect as the PCO_2 level increases (increased H^+ concentration), the oxyhemoglobin saturation decreases, shifting the oxyhemoglobin dissociation curve to the right, whereas decreasing PCO_2 levels (decreased H^+ concentration) shift the curve to the left. The effect of PCO_2 and pH on the oxyhemoglobin curve is known as the Bohr effect.

Bradycardia a slow heartbeat marked by a pulse rate below 60 beats per minute in an adult.

Bradykinin a peptide produced by activation of the kinin system in a variety of inflammatory conditions. It is an extremely potent vasodilator; it also increases vascular permeability, stimulates pain receptors, and causes contraction of a variety of extravascular smooth muscles.

Bronchoconstriction a narrowing of the lumen of the bronchi restricting airflow to and from the lungs. See also **bronchospasm**.

Bronchodilator a substance, especially a drug, that relaxes contractions of the smooth muscle of the bronchioles to improve ventilation to the lungs. Pharmacologic bronchodilators are prescribed to improve aeration in asthma, bronchiectasis, bronchitis, and emphysema. Commonly used bronchodilators include albuterol, terbutaline, and various derivatives and combinations of these drugs. The adverse effects vary, depending on the particular class of bronchodilating drug. In general, bronchodilators are given with caution to people with impaired cardiac function. Nervousness, irritability, gastritis, or palpitations of the heart may occur.

Bronchospasm an excessive and prolonged contraction of the smooth muscle of the bronchi and bronchioles, resulting in an acute narrowing and obstruction of the respiratory airway. The contractions may be localized or general and may be cased by irritation or injury to the respiratory mucosa, infections, or allergies. A cough with generalized wheezing usually indicates the condition. Bronchospasm is a chief characteristic of asthma and bronchitis. Treatment includes the use of active bronchodilators, catecholamines, corticosteroids, or methylxanthines and preventive drugs such as cromolyn sodium. Also called **bronchoconstriction**.

Buffer a substance or group of substances that tends to control the hydrogen ion concentration in a solution by reacting with hydrogen ions of an acid added to the system and releasing hydrogen ions to a base added to the system. Buffers minimize significant changes of pH in a chemical system. Among the functions carried out by buffer systems in the body is maintenance of the acid-base balance of the blood and of the proper pH in kidney tubules.

Calcification process in which organic tissue becomes hardened by the deposition of lime salts in the tissue.

Calculus a pathologic stone formed of mineral salts. Calculi are usually found within hollow organs or ducts.

Caliber the inside diameter of a tube, commonly given in millimeters and fractions of an inch.

Canalicular pertaining to a small channel or canal.

Capacitance vessels the veins differ from the arteries in that they are capable of holding a large amount of blood with very little pressure change. Because of this unique feature, the veins are called capacitance vessels.

Capillary shunt a capillary shunt exists when blood flows from the right side of the heart to the left side without coming in contact with ventilated alveoli for gas exchange. Capillary shunting is commonly caused by (1) alveolar collapse or atelectasis, (2) alveolar fluid accumulation, or (3) alveolar consolidation.

Capillary stasis stagnation of normal flow of fluids or blood in capillaries.

Carbon dioxide (CO_2) colorless, odorless, incombustible gas formed during respiration and combustion.

Cardiac output (CO) the total volume of blood discharged from the ventricles per minute.

Cartilage dense, firm, compact connective tissue capable of withstanding considerable pressure and tension. Located in the tracheobronchial tree, all true joints, the outer ear, and the movable sections of the ribs.

Catecholamines biologically active amines that behave as epinephrine and norepinephrine.

Central venous pressure (CVP) pressure within the superior vena cava, which reflects the pressure under which the blood is returned to the right atrium.

Cerebrospinal fluid (CSF) fluid cushion that protects the brain and spinal cord from shock.

C-fibers an extensive network of free nerve endings located in the small conducting airways, blood vessels, and interstitial tissues between the pulmonary capillaries and alveolar walls. The C-fibers near the alveolar capillaries are called juxtapulmonary-capillary receptors, or J-receptors. These receptors react to certain chemicals and to mechanical stimulation. When stimulated, a reflex response triggers a rapid, shallow breathing pattern.

Chemoreceptor sense organ or sensory nerve ending, located outside the central nervous system, which is stimulated by and reacts to chemical stimuli.

Cheyne-Stokes respiration 10 to 30 seconds of apnea, followed by a gradual increase in the volume and frequency of breathing, followed by a gradual decrease in the volume of breathing until another period of apnea occurs.

Chloride shift during carbon dioxide transport, as HCO_3^- moves out of the red blood cells, the Cl^- (which has been liberated from the NaCl compound) moves into the red blood to maintain electric neutrality. This movement is known as the chloride shift or the *Hamburger phenomenon*.

Chordae tendineae the strands of tendon that anchor the cusps of the mitral and tricuspid valves to the papillary muscles of the ventricles of the heart, preventing prolapse of the valves into the atria during ventricular contraction.

Chronic persisting for a long period, often for the remainder of a person's lifetime. Compare **acute**.

Chronic bronchitis a very common, debilitating pulmonary disease, characterized by greatly increased production of mucus by the glands of the trachea and bronchi and resulting in a cough with expectoration for at least 3 months of the year for more than 2 consecutive years.

Cilia small, hairlike projections on the surface of epithelial cells. In the bronchi they propel mucus and foreign particles in a whiplike movement toward the throat.

Circulatory hypoxia a form of hypoxia in which the arterial blood reaching the tissue cells has a normal oxygen tension and content, but the amount of blood—and, therefore, the amount of oxygen—is not adequate to meet tissue needs.

Clinical manifestations symptoms or signs demonstrated by a patient.

Colloid a state of matter composed of single large molecules or aggregations of smaller molecules of solids, liquids, or gases, in a continuous medium (dispersal medium), which also may be a solid, liquid, or gas.

Composition makeup; what something is made of.

Compromise a blending of the qualities of two different things; an unfavorable change.

Concave a hollow surface, like the inside of a bowl.

Conception the union of sperm and ovum.

Conductivity the ability of the heart cells to transmit electrical current from cell to cell throughout the entire conductive system.

Congenital existing at and usually before birth; referring to conditions that are present at birth, regardless of their cause.

Congestion an abnormal accumulation of fluid in an organ or body area. The fluid is often mucus, but it may be bile or blood.

Congestive heart failure (CHF) an abnormal condition that reflects impaired cardiac pumping. Its causes include myocardial infarction, ischemic heart disease, and cardiomyopathy. Failure of the ventricles to eject blood efficiently results in volume overload, ventricular dilation, and elevated intracardiac pressure. Increased pressure in the left side of the heart causes pulmonary congestion; increased pressure in the right side causes systemic venous congestion and peripheral edema.

Consolidation the combining of separate parts into a single whole; a state of solidification; (in medicine) the process of becoming solid, as when lungs become firm and inelastic in pneumonia.

Constriction an abnormal closing or reduction in the size of an opening or passage of the body, as in vasoconstriction of a blood vessel.

Contiguous being in actual contact; touching along a boundary or at a point.

Contractility the ability of muscle tissue to contract when its thick (myosin) and thin (actin) filaments slide past each other.

Contusion injury in which the skin is not broken; a bruise.

Convex having a rounded, somewhat elevated surface, resembling a segment of the external surface of a sphere.

Cor pulmonale failure of the right ventricle resulting from disorders of the lungs or pulmonary vessels.

Coronary sinus the wide venous channel, about 2.25 cm long, situated in the coronary sulcus and covered by muscular fibers from the left atrium. Through a single semilunar valve it drains five coronary veins: the great cardiac vein, the small cardiac vein, the middle cardiac vein, the posterior vein of the left ventricle, and the oblique vein of the left atrium.

Corpuscle any small, rounded body; an encapsulated sensory nerve ending.

Cortex the outer layer of an organ.

Cotyledons the visible segments on the maternal surface of the placenta. A typical placenta may have 15 to 28 cotyledons, each consisting of fetal vessels, chorionic villi, and intervillous space.

Crackle a common, abnormal respiratory sound consisting of discontinuous bubbling noises heard on auscultation of the chest during inspiration. Fine crackles have a popping sound produced by air entering distal bronchioles or alveoli that contain serous secretions, as in congestive heart failure, pneumonia, or early tuberculosis. Coarse crackles may originate in the larger bronchi have a lower pitch. Crackles are not cleared by coughing. Formerly called *rales*. Compare **rhonchus**, **wheeze**.

Creatinine a substance formed from the metabolism of creatine, commonly found in blood, urine, and muscle tissue.

Croup an acute viral infection of the upper and lower respiratory tract that occurs primarily in infants and young children 3 months to 3 years of age after an upper respiratory tract infection. It is characterized by hoarseness; irritability; fever; a distinctive harsh, brassy cough; persistent stridor during inspiration; and dyspnea and tachypnea, resulting from obstruction of the larynx. Cyanosis or pallor occurs in severe cases. The most common causative agents are the parainfluenza viruses, especially type 1, followed by the respiratory syncytial viruses and influenza A and B viruses. Also called *angina trachealis, exudative angina, laryngostasis.* Compare **acute epiglottitis**.

Cystic fibrosis an inherited autosomal-recessive disorder of the exocrine glands, causing those glands to produce abnormally thick secretions of mucus, elevation of sweat electrolytes, increased organic and enzymatic constituents of saliva, and overactivity of the autonomic nervous system. The glands most affected are those in the pancreas and respiratory system and the sweat glands. Cystic fibrosis is usually recognized in infancy or early childhood, chiefly among Caucasians. The earliest manifestation is meconium ileus, an obstruction of the small bowel by viscid stool. Other early signs are a chronic cough; frequent, foul-smelling stools; and persistent upper respiratory infections. The most reliable diagnostic tool is the sweat test, which shows elevations of levels of both sodium and chloride. Because there is no known cure, treatment is directed at prevention of respiratory infections, which are the most frequent cause of death. Mucolytic agents and bronchodilators are used to help liquefy the thick, tenacious mucus. Physical therapy measures, such as postural drainage and breathing exercises, can also dislodge secretions. Broad-spectrum antibiotics may be used prophylactically.

Dead space ventilation volume of gas that is ventilated, but not physiologically effective. There are three types of dead space ventilation: *Anatomic dead space*—the volume of gas in the conducting airways: the nose, mouth, pharynx, larynx, and lower airways down to, but not including, the respiratory bronchioles. *Alveolar dead space*—alveoli that are ventilated, but not perfused with blood. *Physiologic dead space*—the sum of the anatomic dead space and alveolar dead space.

Defensin a peptide with natural antibiotic activity found within human neutrophils. Three types of defensins have been identified, each consisting of a chain of about 30 amino acids. Similar molecules occur in white blood cells of other animal species. They show activity toward viruses and fungi, in addition to bacteria.

Density mass of a substance per unit of volume (g/cm^3).

Deoxyhemoglobin hemoglobin not bound with oxygen. Also called *reduced hemoglobin.*

Deoxyribonucleic acid (DNA) a large, double-stranded, helical molecule that is the carrier of genetic information. In eukaryotic cells, it is found principally in the chromosomes of the nucleus. DNA is composed of four kinds of serially repeating nucleotide bases: adenine, cytosine, guanine, and thymine. Genetic information is coded in the sequence of the nucleotides. Also called *desoxyribonucleic acid.*

Depolarize to reduce to a nonpolarized condition; to reduce the amount of electrical charge between oppositely charged particles (ions).

Desquamation the process in which the cornified layer of the epidermis is sloughed in fine scales.

Determinant an element that identifies or determines the nature of something or that fixes or conditions an outcome.

Diabetes a general term referring to a variety of disorders characterized by excessive urination (polyuria), as in diabetes mellitus and diabetes insipidus.

Diagnostic pertaining to the use of scientific and skillful methods to establish the cause and nature of a sick person's disease.

Diapedesis the passage of red or white blood corpuscles through the walls of the vessels that contain them without damage to the vessels.

Diastole normal period in the heart cycle during which the muscle fibers lengthen, the heart dilates, and the chambers fill with blood.

Differentiate to separate according to differences.

Diffusion the movement of gas molecules from an area of relatively high concentration of gas to one of low concentration. Different gases each move according to their own individual partial pressure gradients. Diffusion continues until all the gases in the two areas are in equilibrium.

Digitation a finger-like projection.

Distal away from or being the farthest from any point of reference.

Dorsal pertaining to the back or to the posterior portion of a body.

Driving pressure pressure difference between two areas in any vessel or airway.

Ductus arteriosus vessel between the left pulmonary artery and the aorta that bypasses the lungs in the fetus.

Dyspnea difficulty in breathing, of which the individual is aware.

Ectopic foci an area of the heart that produces abnormal beats. Ectopic foci may occur in both healthy and diseased hearts and are usually associated with irritation of a small area of myocardial tissue. They are produced in association with myocardial ischemia, drug (catecholamine) effects, emotional stress, and stimulation by foreign objects, including pacemaker catheters.

Edema a local or generalized condition in which the body tissues contain an excessive amount of extracellular fluid.

Efferent carrying away from a central organ or section.

Efferent nerves nerves that carry impulses from the brain or spinal cord to the periphery.

Elastance the natural ability of matter to respond directly to force and to return to its original resting position or shape after the external force no longer exists. In pulmonary physiology, elastance is defined as the change in pressure per change in volume.

Electrocardiogram (ECG) record of the electrical activity of the heart.

Electrolyte an element or compound that, when melted or dissolved in water or other solvent, dissociates into ions and is able to conduct an electric current.

Elongation the condition or process of being extended.

Embryonic pertaining to the early stages (i.e., first 3 months) of fetal development.

Emphysema an abnormal condition of the pulmonary system, characterized by overinflation and destructive changes in alveolar walls. It results in a loss of lung elasticity and decreased gas exchange. See also **pulmonary emphysema**.

End-expiration the portion of a ventilatory cycle at which expiration stops.

End-inspiration the portion of a ventilatory cycle at which inspiration stops .

Endocardium the lining of the heart chambers, containing small blood vessels and a few bundles of smooth muscle. It is continuous with the endothelium of the great blood vessels.

Endothelium the layer of epithelial cells, originating from the mesoderm, that lines the cavities of the heart, the blood and lymph vessels, and the serous cavities of the body.

Endotracheal within or through the trachea.

Endotracheal intubation the management of the patient with an airway catheter inserted through the mouth or nose into the trachea. An endotracheal tube may be used to maintain a patent airway, to prevent aspiration or material from the digestive tract in the unconscious or paralyzed patient, to permit suctioning of tracheobronchial secretions, or to administer positive-pressure ventilation that cannot be given effectively by a mask. Endotracheal tubes may be made of rubber or plastic and usually have an inflatable cuff to maintain a closed system with the ventilator.

Endotracheal tube a large-bore catheter inserted through the mouth or nose and into the trachea to a point above the bifurcation of the trachea. It is used for delivering oxygen under pressure when ventilation must be totally controlled and in general anesthetic procedures. See also **endotracheal intubation**.

Eosinophil a cell or cellular structure that stains readily with the acid stain eosin; specifically, a granular leukocyte. Normal range: 1 to 4 percent of leukocyte differential.

Epicardium one of the three layers of tissue that form the heart wall. It is composed of a single sheet of squamous epithelial cells overlying delicate connective tissue. Epicardium is the visceral portion (visceral layer) of the serous pericardium and folds back on itself to form the parietal portion of the serous pericardium.

Epinephrine one of two active hormones (the other is norepinephrine) secreted by the adrenal medulla.

Epistaxis bleeding from the nose. Also called *nosebleed*.

Equilibrium condition in which one or more forces are evenly balanced by opposite forces.

Erythrocyte a mature red blood cell (RBC).

Erythropoiesis the process of erythrocyte production involving the maturation of a nucleated precursor into a hemoglobin-filled nucleus-free erythrocyte that is regulated by erythropoietin, a hormone produced by the kidney.

Etiology study of the cause of disease.

Eupnea normal, spontaneous breathing.

Excitability the ability of a cell to reach its threshold potential and respond to a stimulus or irritation. The lower the stimulus needed to activate a cell, the more excitable the cell; conversely, the greater the stimulus needed, the less excitable the cell.

Excretion elimination of waste products from the body.

Excursion the extent of movement from a central position or axis.

Expectoration clearing the lungs by coughing up and spitting out matter.

External respiration gas exchange between the pulmonary capillaries and the alveoli.

Extra-alveolar pertaining to the area outside of the alveoli.

Extracellular outside a cell or in the cavities or spaces between cell layers or groups of cells.

Extravascular outside a vessel.

Fascia the fibrous connective membrane of the body that may be separated from other specifically organized structures, such as the tendons, the aponeuroses, and the ligaments, and that covers, supports, and separates muscles.

Fertilization the union of sperm and ovum.

Fetus the developing human *in utero* from the third month to birth.

Fibrin whitish, filamentous protein formed by the action of thrombin on fibrinogen.

Fibroelastic composed of fibrous and elastic tissue.

Fibrosis the repair and replacement of inflamed tissues or organs by connective tissues. The process results in the replacement of normal cells by fibroblasts (and eventually, the replacement of normal organ tissue by scar tissue).

Fissure cleft or groove on the surface of an organ, often marking the division of the organ into parts, such as the lobes of the lung.

Fistula abnormal passage or communication, usually between two internal organs or leading from an internal organ to the surface of the body.

Flail chest a thorax in which multiple rib fractures cause instability in part of the chest wall and paradoxical breathing, with the lung underlying the injured areas moving in on inspiration and bulging on expiration. If it is uncorrected, hypoxia will result.

Flex to contract, as a muscle; to increase the angle of a joint.

Foramen ovale an opening in the septum between the right and the left atria in the fetal heart. This opening provides a bypass for blood that would otherwise flow to the fetal lungs. After birth the foramen ovale functionally closes when the newborn takes the first breath and full circulation through the lungs begins.

Forced vital capacity the maximum volume of gas that can be forcibly and rapidly exhaled after a full inspiration.

Frank-Starling curve a graphic illustration that shows the relationship between the degree of myocardial stretch and cardiac output.

Functional residual capacity the volume of air remaining in the lungs after a normal exhalation.

Functionally according to its proper use or action; working as it should.

Gastrointestinal tract the route taken by food from the stomach to the rectum.

Generation the process of forming a new organism or part of an organism.

Gestation the period of time from the fertilization of the ovum until birth.

Glomerulonephritis inflammation of the glomerulus in the nephron of the kidney.

Glomerulus a tuft or cluster; a structure composed of blood vessels or nerve fibers, such as a *renal glomerulus.*

Glossopharyngeal nerve the ninth cranial nerve.

Glycoprotein any of a class of conjugated proteins consisting of a compound of a protein with a carbohydrate group.

Goblet cell one of many specialized epithelial cells that secrete mucus and form glands of the epithelium of the stomach, the intestine, and parts of the respiratory tract.

Gradient a slope or grade; a difference in values between two points.

Granulocyte a type of leukocyte characterized by the presence of cytoplasmic granules.

Gravity dependent a phrase used to describe the natural tendency of blood, which is a relatively heavy substance, to move to the portion of the body, or portion of the organ, that is closest to the ground.

Haldane effect the phenomenon in which deoxygenated blood enhances the loading of carbon dioxide and the oxygenation of blood enhances the unloading of carbon dioxide during carbon dioxide transport.

Hamburger phenomenon see **chloride shift**.

Heart the muscular cone-shaped hollow organ, about the size of a clenched fist, that pumps blood throughout the body and beats normally about 70 times per minute by coordinated nerve impulses and muscular contractions.

Hematocrit volume of erythrocytes packed by centrifugation in a given volume of blood; is expressed as the percentage of total blood volume that consists of erythrocytes.

Hemodynamics the study of the physical aspects of blood circulation, including cardiac function and peripheral vascular physiologic characteristics.

Hemoglobin a complex protein-iron compound in the blood that carries oxygen to the cells from the lungs and carbon dioxide away from the cells to the lungs. Each erythrocyte contains 200 to 300 molecules of hemoglobin.

Hemolysis the breakdown of red blood cells and the release of hemoglobin.

Heparin a polysaccharide produced by the mast cells of the liver and by basophil leukocytes that inhibits coagulation by preventing conversion of prothrombin to thrombin. It also inhibits coagulation by preventing

liberation of thromboplastin from blood platelets.

Histamine a substance that is normally present in the body and exerts a pharmacologic action when released from injured cells. It is produced from the amino acid *histidine*.

Histotoxic hypoxia a type of hypoxia that develops in any condition that impairs the ability of tissue cells to utilize oxygen.

Homeostasis a physiologic state resulting from a dynamic equilibrium maintained by monitoring processes and altered effector activity, incorporating negative feedback pathways.

Hormone a substance originating in an organ or gland that is conveyed through the body to another part of the body, which it stimulates by chemical action to increased functional activity and/or increased secretion.

Hydrostatic pertaining to the pressure of liquids in equilibrium and the pressure exerted on liquids.

Hydrous containing water, usually chemically combined.

Hypercapnia greater than normal amount of carbon dioxide in the blood. Also called *hypercarbia*.

Hyperchloremia an excessive level of chloride in the blood that results in acidosis.

Hyperinflation distention by air, gas, or liquid, as in the hyperinflation of the alveoli.

Hyperkalemia increased amount of potassium in the blood.

Hyperpnea increased depth (volume) of breathing, with or without an increased frequency.

Hypersecretion substance or fluid produced by cells or glands in an excessive amount or more than normal.

Hypersensitivity an abnormal condition characterized by an exaggerated response of the immune system to an antigen.

Hypertension higher than normal blood pressure.

Hyperthermia higher than normal body temperature.

Hyperventilation pulmonary ventilation rate greater than that metabolically necessary for gas exchange, resulting in a Pa_{CO_2} below 35 mm Hg. It is the result of an increased respiratory rate, an increased tidal volume, or both.

Hypochloremia a decreased amount of chloride in the blood.

Hypokalemia a decreased amount of potassium in the blood.

Hypoperfusion deficiency of blood coursing through the vessels of the circulatory system.

Hypothalamus portion of the brain that controls certain metabolic activities.

Hypoventilation pulmonary ventilation rate less than that metabolically necessary for gas exchange, resulting in a Pa_{CO_2} greater than 45 mm Hg. It is the result of a decreased respiratory rate, a decreased tidal volume, or both.

Hypoxemia an abnormal deficiency in the concentration of oxygen in arterial blood. Symptoms of acute hypoxemia are cyanosis, restlessness, stupor, coma, Cheyne-Stokes respiration, apnea, increased blood pressure, tachycardia, and an initial increase in cardiac output that later falls, producing hypotension and ventricular fibrillation or asystole.

Hypoxia inadequate oxygen tension at the cellular level, characterized by tachycardia, hypertension, peripheral vasoconstriction, dizziness, and mental confusion.

Iliac crest long curved upper margin of the hip bone.

Immaturity the state of being not fully developed or ripened.

Immunoglobulin one of a family of closely related but not identical proteins that are capable of acting as antibodies.

Immunologic mechanism reaction of the body to substances that are foreign or are interpreted by the body as foreign.

Impede to slow down; to stand in the way of; to fight against.

Inferior vena cava (IVC) venous trunk for the lower extremities and the pelvic and abdominal viscera.

Inflammation the protective response of body tissues to irritation or injury. Inflammation may be acute or chronic; its cardinal signs are redness, heat, swelling, and pain, often accompanied by loss of function. The process begins with a transitory vasoconstriction, then is followed by a brief increase in vascular permeability. The second stage is prolonged and consists of sustained increase in vascular permeability, exudation of fluids from the vessels, clustering of leukocytes along the vessels walls, phagocytosis of microorganisms, deposition of fibrin in the vessel, disposal of the accumulated debris by macrophages, and finally migration of fibroblast to the area and development of new, normal cells. The severity, timing, and local character of any particular inflammatory response depend on the cause, the area affected, and the condition of the host. Histamine, kinins, and various other substances mediate the inflammatory process.

Inguinal ligament a fibrous band formed by the inferior border of the aponeurosis of the external oblique that extends from the anterior superior iliac spine to the pubic tubercle.

Inhibitory repressive; tending to restrain a function.

Innervation the distribution or supply of nerve fibers or nerve impulses to a body part.

Inspiratory capacity the volume of air that can be inhaled after a normal exhalation.

Interatrial septum the partition or wall that separates the right and left atrium of the heart.

Internal respiration gas exchange between the systemic capillaries and the cells.

Interstitial placed or lying between; pertaining to the interstices or spaces within an organ or tissue.

Interventricular septum the partition or wall that separates the right and left ventricles of the heart.

Intra prefix meaning within.

Intra-alveolar within the alveoli.

Intrapleural within the pleura.

Intrapulmonary within the lungs.

Intrarenal within the kidneys.

Intratubular within a tube.

Intubation passage of a tube into a body aperture; specifically, the insertion of a breathing tube through the mouth or nose or into the trachea to ensure a patent airway for the delivery of anesthetic gases and oxygen or both. Kinds of intubation include **endotracheal intubation** and *nasotracheal intubation*.

Inverse opposite in order, nature, or effect; as one variable increases, the other decreases.

Ion atom, group of atoms, or molecule that has acquired a net electrical charge by gaining or losing electrons.

Ischemia decreased blood supply to a body organ or part.

Isobar a line on a map, chart, or nomogram connecting areas of equal pressure.

Ketoacidosis acidosis accompanied by an accumulation of ketones in the body, resulting from extensive breakdown of fats because of faulty carbohydrate metabolism. It occurs primarily as a complication of diabetes mellitus and is characterized by a fruity odor of acetone on the breath, mental confusion, dyspnea, nausea, vomiting, dehydration, weight loss, and, if untreated, coma.

Kussmaul breathing abnormally deep, very rapid sighing respirations characteristic of diabetic ketoacidosis.

Lactic acid acid formed in muscles during activity by the breakdown of sugar without oxygen.

Leukocyte a white blood cell, one of the formed elements of the circulating blood system. Five types of leukocytes are classified by the presence or absence of granules in the cytoplasm of the cell. Normal range: 5000 to 10,000/mm³. The agranulocytes are lymphocytes and monocytes. The granulocytes are neutrophils, basophils, and eosinophils. Also called *leucocyte, white blood cell*, and *white corpuscle*.

Leukocytosis an abnormal increase in the number of circulating white blood cells. An increase often accompanies bacterial, but not usually viral, infections. The normal range is 5000 to 10,000/mm³. Leukemia may be associated with a white blood cell count as high as 500,000 to 1 million per cubic millimeter of blood, the increase being either equally or disproportionately distributed among all types. Kinds of leukocytosis include *basophilia, eosinophilia,* and *neutrophilia.*

Ligamentum nuchae upward continuation of the supraspinous ligament, extending from the seventh cervical vertebra to the occipital bone.

Linea alba "white line" of connective tissue in the middle of the abdomen from sternum to pubis.

Linear response a response or output that is directly proportional to the input.

Lipid any of numerous fats generally insoluble in water that constitute one of the principal structural materials of cells.

Lobar pertaining to a lobe, such as the lobes of the lung.

Lumen inner open space of a tubular organ, such as a blood vessel or intestine.

Lung compliance a measure of the ease of expansion of the lungs and thorax. It is determined by pulmonary volume and elasticity. A high degree of compliance indicates a loss of elastic recoil of the lungs, as in old age or emphysema. Decreased compliance means a greater change in pressure is needed for a given change in volume, as in atelectasis, edema, fibrosis, pneumonia, or absence of surfactant. Dyspnea on exertion is the main symptom of diminished lung compliance.

Lymphocyte small agranulocytic leukocytes originating from fetal stem cells and developing in the bone marrow. Lymphocytes normally comprise 25 percent of the total white blood cell count but increase in number in response to infection. Two forms occur: B cells and T cells. B cells circulate in an immature form and synthesize antibodies for insertion into their own cytoplasmic membranes. T cells are lymphocytes that have circulated through the thymus gland and have differentiated to become thymocytes. When exposed to an antigen, they divide rapidly and produce large numbers of new T cells sensitized to that antigen.

Macrophage any phagocytic cell of the reticuloendothelial system, including specialized Kupffer's cells in the liver, lungs, spleen, and histocyte in loose connective tissue.

Magnitude pertaining to size.

Malar pertaining to the cheek or cheekbones.

Malformation deformity; abnormal shape or structure, especially congenital.

Mastoid process projection of the posterior portion of the temporal bone; gives attachment to the sternocleidomastoid, splenius capitis, and longissimus capitis muscles.

Mean occupying a middle position; being near the average.

Mechanical relating to physical properties.

Mechanoreceptor receptor that receives mechanical stimuli such as pressure from sound or touch.

Medial pertaining to the middle.

Mediastinum a part of the thoracic cavity in the middle of the thorax, between the pleural sacs containing the two lungs. It extends from the sternum to the vertebral column and contains all the thoracic viscera except the lungs. It is enclosed in a thick extension of the thoracic subserous fascia and is divided into the cranial part and the caudal part.

Mediated between two parts or sides.

Medulla oblongata a bulbous continuation of the spinal cord just above the foramen magnum and separated from the pons by a horizontal groove. It is one of three parts of the brainstem and mainly contains white substance with some mixture of gray substance. The medulla contains the cardiac, vasomotor, and respiratory centers of the brain; medullary injury or disease often proves fatal.

Mesoderm the middle of the three cell layers of the developing embryo, which lies between the ectoderm and endoderm.

Metabolism sum of all physical and chemical changes that take place within an organism; all energy and material transformations that occur within living cells.

Microvilli minute cylindrical processes on the free surface of a cell (especially cells of the proximal convoluted renal tubule and those of the intestinal epithelium), which increase the surface area of the cell.

Mitral valve see **bicuspid valve**.

Molecular weight weight of a molecule attained by adding the atomic weight of its constituent atoms.

Monocyte a large, mononuclear leukocyte normally found in lymph nodes, spleen, bone marrow, and loose connective tissue. Normal range: 3 to 7 percent of leukocyte differential.

Motor nerve a nerve consisting of efferent fibers that conduct impulses from the brain or the spinal cord to one of the muscles or organs.

Mucous pertaining to or resembling mucus; secreting mucus.

Mucus the viscous, slippery secretions of mucous membranes and glands, containing mucin, white blood cells, water, inorganic salts, and exfoliated cells.

Myelin a lipoproteinaceous substance constituting the sheaths of various nerve fibers throughout the body and enveloping the axis of myelinated nerves. It is largely composed of phospholipids and protein, which gives the fibers a white, creamy color. the substance that constitutes the sheaths of various nerve fibers throughout the body. It is largely composed of fat, giving the fibers a white, creamy color.

Myoepithelial cells spindle-shaped cells found around sweat, mammary, and salivary glands. The myoepithelial cells are contractile and resemble smooth muscle cells.

Myoglobin a ferrous globin complex consisting of one heme group and one globin polypeptide chain. It is responsible for the red pigment seen in skeletal muscle.

Necrosis localized tissue death that occurs in groups of cells in response to disease or injury.

Neoplasm any abnormal growth of new tissue, benign or malignant. Also called *tumor*.

Neuropathy any abnormal condition characterized by inflammation and degeneration of the peripheral nerves.

Neutrophil a polymorphonuclear, granular leukocyte that stains easily with neutral dyes. The nucleus stains dark blue and contains three to five lobes connected by slender threads of chromatin. The cytoplasm contains fine, inconspicuous granules. Neutrophils are the circulating white blood cells essential for phagocytosis and proteolysis by which bacteria, cellular debris, and solid particles are removed and destroyed. Normal range: 57 to 67 percent of leukocyte differential.

Nomogram a graph consisting of several lines or curves (usually parallel) graduated for different variables in such a way that a straight line cutting the three lines gives the related values of the three variables.

Nonlinear having or being a response or output that is not directly proportional to the input.

Norepinephrine one of two active hormones (the other is epinephrine) secreted by the adrenal medulla. It is chiefly a vasoconstrictor and has little effect on cardiac output.

Occipital referring to the back part or bone of the head.

Occlude to close, obstruct, or join together.

Olfactory pertaining to the sense of smell.

Oncotic pressure the osmotic pressure of a colloid in solution, such as when there is a higher concentration of protein in the plasma on one side of a cell membrane than in the neighboring interstitial fluid.

Orthopnea a condition in which an individual is able to breathe most comfortably only in the upright position.

Osmosis the movement of a pure solvent such as water through a differentially permeable membrane from a solution that has a lower solute concentration to one that has a higher solute concentration. The membrane is impermeable to the solute but is permeable to the solvent. The rate of osmosis depends on the concentration of solute, the temperature of the solution, the electrical charge of the solute, and the difference between the osmotic pressures exerted by the solutions. Movement across the membrane continues until the concentrations of the solutions equalize.

Osmotic pressure pressure that develops when two solutions with different concentrations of solutes are separated by a semipermeable membrane.

Oxygen consumption the amount of oxygen in milliliters per minute that the body requires for normal aerobic metabolism; normally about 250 mL/min.

Oxygen content total amount of oxygen in the blood.

Oxygen extraction ratio the amount of oxygen extracted by the peripheral tissues divided by the amount of oxygen delivered to the peripheral cells. Normally, about 25 percent. Also known as *oxygen coefficient ratio* or *oxygen utilization ratio*.

Oxyhemoglobin the product of combining hemoglobin with oxygen. The loosely bound complex dissociates easily when the concentration of oxygen is low.

Pallor an unnatural paleness or absence of color in the skin.

Papillitis an abnormal condition characterized by the inflammation of a papilla.

Paradoxic pertaining to a person, situation, statement, or act that may appear to have inconsistent or contradictory qualities or that may be true but appears to be absurd or unbelievable. Also *paradoxical*.

Parasympathetic nervous system a division of the autonomic nervous system that is mediated by the release of acetylcholine and primarily involves the protection, conservation, and restoration of body resources.

Parenchyma essential parts of an organ that are concerned with its function.

Parietal layer pertaining to the outer wall of a cavity or organ.

Paroxysmal concerning the sudden, periodic attack or recurrence of symptoms of a disease.

Parturition the action or process of giving birth to offspring.

Pathogen any agent causing disease, especially a microorganism.

Perfusion passing of blood or fluid through a vascular bed.

Peribronchial located around the bronchi.

Pericardium a fibroserous sac that surrounds the heart and the roots of the great vessels.

Peripheral airways small bronchioles on the outer sections of the lung.

Peristalsis a progressive wave movement that occurs involuntarily in hollow tubes of the body, especially the intestines.

Perivascular located around a vessel, especially a blood vessel.

Permeable capable of allowing the passage of fluids or substances in solution.

Persistent pulmonary hypertension of the neonate (PPHN) an elevated pulmonary vascular resistance in the newborn caused by a low P_{O_2} level. The infant's ductus arteriosus remains open as a result of this condition.

pH symbol for the logarithm of the reciprocal of the hydrogen ion concentration. The abbreviation for potential hydrogen, a scale representing the relative acidity of a solution in which a value of 7.0 is neutral, below 7.0 is acid, and above 7.0 is alkaline.

Phalanges the bones of the fingers and toes.

Phosphate a salt of phosphoric acid. Phosphates are extremely important in living cells, particularly in the storage and use of energy and the transmission of genetic information within a cell and from one cell to another.

Photophobia abnormal sensitivity of the eyes to light.

Pituitary gland an endocrine gland suspended beneath the brain in the pituitary fossa of the sphenoid bone, supplying numerous hormones that govern many vital processes.

Plasma the watery straw-colored fluid part of the lymph and the blood in which the leukocytes, erythrocytes, and platelets are suspended. Plasma is made up of water, electrolytes, proteins, glucose, fats, bilirubin, and gases and is essential for carrying the cellular elements of the blood through the circulation, transporting nutrients, maintaining the acid-base balance of the body, and transporting wastes from the tissues. Plasma and interstitial fluid correspond closely in content and concentration of proteins; therefore, plasma is important in maintaining the osmotic pressure and the exchange of fluids and electrolytes between the capillaries and the tissues.

Platelet the smallest cells in the blood. They are formed in the red bone marrow and some are stored in the spleen. Platelets are disk shaped, contain no hemoglobin, and are essential for the coagulation of blood and in maintenance of hemostasis. Normally, between 140,000 and 340,000/mm^3.

Pleura (*pl. pleurae*) a delicate serous membrane enclosing the lung, composed of a single layer of flattened mesothelial cells resting on a delicate membrane of connective tissue. Beneath the membrane is a stroma of collagenous tissue containing yellow elastic fibers. The pleura divides into the visceral pleura, which covers the lungs, dipping into the fissures between the lobes, and the parietal pleura, which lines the chest wall, covers the diaphragm, and reflects over the structures of the mediastinum. The parietal and visceral pleurae are separated from each other by a small amount of fluid that acts as a lubricant as the lungs expand and contract during respiration. See also **pleural space**.

Pleural space the potential space between the visceral and parietal layers of the pleurae. The space contains a small amount of fluid that acts as a lubricant, allowing the pleurae to slide smoothly over each other as the lungs expand and contract with respiration.

Pneumotaxic center a portion of the pontine respiratory centers that influences the respiratory components of the medulla. Neural impulses from the pneumotaxic center simultaneously cause (1) the depth of breathing to decrease and (2) the rate of breathing to increase by almost an equal amount. Some investigators believe the pneumotaxic center is closely related to the so-called panting center in animals such as dogs.

Pneumothorax a collection of air or gas in the pleural space, causing the lung to collapse.

Point of maximal intensity (PMI) the place where the apical pulse is palpated as strongest, often in the fifth intercostal space of the thorax, just medial to the left midclavicular line.

Polycythemia an increase in the number of erythrocytes in the blood caused by chronic hypoxemia secondary to pulmonary disease, heart disease, or prolonged exposure to high altitudes, or it may be idiopathic.

Polymer a compound formed by combining or linking a number of monomers, or small molecules. A polymer may be composed of many units of more than one type of monomer (a copolymer) or of many units of the same monomer (homopolymer).

Posterior back part of something; toward the back.

Premature ventricular complex (PVC) an arrhythmia characterized by ventricular depolarization occurring earlier than expected. It appears on the electrocardiogram as an early wide QRS complex without a preceding related P wave. PVCs may occur occasionally in a regular pattern or as several in sequence. They may be idiopathic or caused by stress, electrolyte imbalance, ischemia, hypoxemia, hypercapnia, ventricular enlargement, or a toxic reaction to drugs. Isolated PVCs are not clinically significant in healthy individuals, but they may produce decreased cardiac output in people with heart disease, and frequent PVCs may be a precursor of ventricular tachycardia or fibrillation.

Prerenal pertaining to the area in front of the kidney; pertaining to events occurring before reaching the kidney.

Pressoreceptor see **baroreceptor**.

Pressure a force, or stress, applied to a surface by a fluid or an object, usually measured in units of mass per unit of area, such as pounds per square inch.

Prognosis a prediction of the probable outcome of a disease based on the conditions of the person and the usual course of the disease as observed in similar situations.

Proliferate increasing or spreading at a rapid rate; the process or result of rapid reproduction.

Prostaglandins a group of fatty acid derivatives present in many organs that affect the cardiovascular system and smooth muscle and stimulate the uterus to contract.

Prostate a gland in males that surrounds the neck of the bladder and the deepest part of the urethra and produces a fluid that becomes part of semen.

Prostatic hypertrophy enlargement of the prostate gland.

Proximal nearest the point of attachment, center of the body, or point of reference.

Pubic symphysis junction of the pubic bones, composed of fibrocartilage.

Pulmonary pertaining to the lungs or the respiratory system.

Pulmonary alveolus one of the numerous terminal air sacs in the lungs where oxygen and carbon dioxide are exchanged.

Pulmonary congestion an excessive accumulation of fluid in the lungs, usually associated with either an inflammation or congestive heart failure.

Pulmonary edema the accumulation of extravascular fluid in lung tissues and alveoli, caused most commonly by congestive heart failure. Serous fluid is pushed through the pulmonary capillaries into alveoli and quickly enters bronchioles and bronchi. The condition also may occur in barbiturate and opiate poisoning, diffuse infections, hemorrhagic pancreatitis, and renal failure or after a stroke, skull fracture, near-drowning, inhalation of irritating gases, and rapid administration of whole blood, plasma, serum albumin, or IV fluids.

Pulmonary emphysema a chronic obstructive disease of the lungs, marked by an overdistention of the alveoli and destruction of the supporting alveolar structure. See also **emphysema**.

Pulmonary shunting that portion of the cardiac output that enters the left side of the heart without exchanging gases with alveolar gases.

Pulmonary surfactant see **surfactant**.

Pulmonary vascular resistance (PVR) pressure loss, per unit of blood flow, from the pulmonary artery to the left ventricle. The resistance in the pulmonary vascular bed against which the right ventricle must eject blood.

Pyelonephritis a diffuse pyogenic infection of the pelvis and parenchyma of the kidney.

Rales see **crackle**.

Reflex an involuntary response to a stimulus.

Relative shunt see **shunt-like effect**.

Renal pertaining to the kidneys.

Renal dysplasia abnormal development of tissue in the kidneys.

Resonance quality of the sound heard on percussion of a hollow structure such as the chest or abdomen.

Respiration the molecular exchange of oxygen and carbon dioxide within the body's tissue. Compare **ventilation**.

Resting membrane potential (RMP) the transmembrane voltage that exists when the heart muscle is at rest.

Rhonchus (*pl. rhonchi*) an abnormal sound heard on auscultation of an airway obstructed by thick secretions, muscular spasm, neoplasm, or external pressure. The continuous rumbling sound is more pronounced during expiration and characteristically clears on coughing, whereas gurgles do not.

Semipermeable permitting diffusion or flow of some liquids or solutes but preventing the transmission of others, usually in reference to a membrane.

Septic pertaining to infection or contamination.

Septicemia systemic infection in which pathogens are present in the circulating blood, having spread from an infection in any part of the body. It is diagnosed by culture of the blood and is vigorously treated with antibiotics. Characteristically septicemia causes fever, chill, hypotension, prostration, pain, headache, nausea, or diarrhea. Also called *blood poisoning*.

Septum wall dividing two cavities.

Serotonin a potent vasoconstrictor that is present in platelets, gastrointestinal mucosa, mast cells, and carcinoid tumors.

Serum clear watery fluid, especially that moistening surfaces of serous membranes or exuded inflammation of any of those membranes; the fluid portion of the blood obtained after removal of the fibrin clot and blood cells; sometimes used as a synonym for antiserum.

Shunt to turn away from; to divert; an abnormal passage to divert flow from one route to another.

Shunt-like effect pulmonary capillary perfusion in excess of alveolar ventilation; commonly seen in patients with chronic obstructive lung disorders and alveolar-capillary diffusion defects. Also called *relative shunt*.

Sign an objective finding as perceived by an examiner, such as fever, a rash, or the whisper heard over the chest in pleural effusion. Many signs accompany symptoms; for example, erythema and a maculopapular rash are often seen with pruritus. Compare **symptom**.

Smooth muscle muscle tissue that lacks cross-striations on its fibers, is involuntary in action, and is found principally in visceral organs.

Somatic nerve nerve that innervates somatic structures, that is, those constituting the body wall and extremities.

Somnolence the condition of being sleepy or drowsy.

Spasm involuntary sudden movement or convulsive muscular contraction.

Sputum substance expelled by coughing or clearing the throat that may contain a variety of materials from the respiratory tract, including one or more of the following: cellular debris, mucus, blood, pus, caseous material, and microorganisms.

Stasis stagnation of normal flow of fluids, as of the blood, urine, or intestinal mechanism. A disorder in which the normal flow of a fluid through a vessel of the body is slowed or halted.

Stroke volume amount of blood ejected by the ventricle at each beat.

Subcutaneous under the skin.

Sulfonamide one of a large group of synthetic, bacteriostatic drugs that are effective in treating infections caused by many gram-negative and gram-positive microorganisms.

Superior vena cava venous trunk draining blood from the head, neck, upper extremities, and chest.

Surfactant an agent, such as soap or detergent, dissolved in water to reduce its surface tension or the tension at the interface between the water and another liquid. Certain lipoproteins reduce the surface tension of pulmonary fluids, allowing the exchange of gases in the alveoli of the lungs and contributing to the elasticity of the pulmonary tissue. Also called *pulmonary surfactant*.

Sympathetic nervous system a division of the autonomic nervous system that accelerates the heart rate, constricts blood vessels, and raises blood pressure.

Sympathomimetic producing effects resembling those resulting from stimulation of the sympathetic nervous system.

Symptom a subjective indication of a disease or a change in condition as perceived by the patient. For example, the halo symptom of glaucoma is seen by the patient as colored rings around a single light source. Many symptoms are accompanied by objective signs, such as pruritus, which is often reported with erythema and a maculopapular eruption on the skin. Some symptoms may be objectively confirmed, such as numbness of the body part, which may be confirmed by absence of response to a pin prick. Compare **sign**.

Systemic pertaining to the whole body rather than to one of its parts.

Systemic reaction whole body response to a stimulus.

Systole that part of the heart cycle in which the heart is in contraction.

Systolic pressure maximum blood pressure; occurs during contraction of the ventricle.

Tachycardia an abnormal circulatory condition in which the myocardium contracts regularly but at a rate of greater than 100 beats per minute.

Tachypnea a rapid rate of breathing.

Thoracolumbar relating to the thoracic and lumbar portions of the vertebral column.

Thrombocyte combining form meaning "platelet": *thrombocytopenia, thrombocytosis*.

Tidal volume the volume of air that normally moves into and out of the lungs in one quiet breath.

Tone that state of a body or any of its organs or parts in which the functions are healthy and normal.

Total lung capacity the maximum amount of air that the lung can accommodate.

Transairway pressure the barometric pressure difference between the mouth pressure and the alveolar pressure.

Transient passing especially quickly into and out of existence; passing through or by a place with only a brief stay.

Transpulmonary pressure the difference between the alveolar pressure and the pleural pressure.

Transthoracic pressure the difference between the alveolar pressure and the body surface pressure.

Tricuspid valve a valve with three main cusps situated between the right atrium and right ventricle of the heart. The tricuspid valve includes the ventral, dorsal, and medial cusps. The cusps are composed of strong fibrous tissue and are anchored to the papillary muscles of the right ventricle by several tendons. As the right and left ventricles relax during the diastolic phase of the heartbeat, the tricuspid valve opens, allowing blood to flow into the ventricle. In the systolic phase of the heartbeat, both blood-filled ventricles contract, pumping out their contents, while the tricuspid and mitral valves close to prevent any backflow.

Trimester one of the three periods of approximately 3 months into which pregnancy is divided.

True shunt see **absolute shunt**.

Unilateral renal agenesis failure of one of the kidneys to develop.

Vagus nerve the 10th cranial nerve. It is a mixed nerve, having motor and sensory functions and a wider distribution than any of the other cranial nerves.

Vascular relating to or containing blood vessels.

Vascular system the circulatory network composed of two major subdivisions: the systemic system and the pulmonary system.

Vasoconstriction decrease in the caliber of blood vessels.

Vasodilation widening of blood vessels, especially the small arteries and arterioles.

Vasomotor tone the state of vascular contraction.

Vein any one of the many vessels that convey blood from the capillaries as part of the pulmonary venous system, the systemic venous network, and the portal venous complex. Most of the veins of the body are systemic veins that convey blood from the whole body (except the lungs) to the right atrium of the heart. Each vein is a macroscopic structure enclosed in three layers of different kinds of tissue homologous with the layers of the heart. The outer tunica adventitia of each vein is homologous with the epicardium, the tunica media with the myocardium, and the tunica intima with the endocardium. Deep veins course through the more internal parts of the body, and superficial veins lie near the surface, where many of them are visible through the skin. Veins have thinner coatings and are less elastic than arteries and collapse when cut. They also contain semilunar valves at various intervals to control the direction of the blood flow back to the heart.

Venous pertaining to a vein or veins.

Venous admixture the mixing of shunted, non-reoxygenated blood with reoxygenated blood distal to the alveoli.

Venous return the amount of blood returning to the atria of the heart.

Ventilation the mechanical movement of air into and out of the lungs in a cyclic fashion. It is the mechanism by which oxygen is carried from the atmosphere to the alveoli and by which carbon dioxide is carried from the lungs to the atmosphere. Compare **respiration**.

Ventilation-perfusion ratio the relationship of the overall alveolar ventilation (L/min) to the overall pulmonary blood flow (L/min). The normal ventilation-perfusion ratio is 4:5, or 0.8.

Ventral pertaining to the anterior portion or front of the body.

Ventricle either of two lower chambers of the heart.

Venule any one of the small blood vessels that gather blood from the capillary plexuses and anastomose to form the veins.

Viscera (*sing. viscus*) the internal organs enclosed within a body cavity, including the abdominal, thoracic, pelvic, and endocrine organs.

Viscosity stickiness or gumminess; internal friction resistance offered by a fluid to change of form or relative position of its particles due to attraction of molecules to each other.

Viscous sticky; gummy; gelatinous.

Vital capacity the maximum volume of air that can be exhaled after a maximal inspiration.

Volume percent (vol%) the number of milliliters (mL) of a substance contained in 100 mL of another substance. For example, under normal conditions there are about 20 mL of oxygen in every 100 mL of arterial blood—or 20 vol% oxygen.

Wenckebach phenomenon named for Karel F. Wenckebach, Dutch-Austrian physician (1864–1940), a form of second-degree atrioventricular block with a progressive beat-to-beat prolongation of the PR interval, finally resulting in a nonconducting P wave. At this point the sequence recurs and is referred to as Wenckebach periodicity. Also called *Mobitz I* and *type I AV block.*

Wheeze a form of rhonchi characterized by a high-pitched or low-pitched musical quality. It is caused by a high-velocity flow of air passing through a narrowed airway and is heard during both inspiration and expiration. It may be caused by bronchospasm, inflammation, or obstruction of the airway by a tumor or foreign body. Wheezes are associated with asthma and chronic bronchitis. Unilateral wheezes are characteristic of bronchogenic carcinoma, foreign bodies, and inflammatory lesions. In asthma expiratory wheezing is more common, although inspiratory and expiratory wheezes are heard. Compare **crackle, rhonchus**.

Symbols and Abbreviations

The symbols and abbreviations listed below are commonly used in respiratory physiology.

PRIMARY SYMBOLS

Gas Symbols		Blood Symbols	
P	Pressure	Q	Blood volume
V	Gas volume	$\dot{Q}$	Blood flow
$\dot{V}$	Gas volume per unit of time, or flow	C	Content in blood
F	Fractional concentration of gas	S	Saturation

SECONDARY SYMBOLS

Gas Symbols		Blood Symbols	
I	Inspired	a	Arterial
E	Expired	c	Capillary
A	Alveolar	v	Venous
T	Tidal	$\bar{v}$	Mixed venous
D	Dead space		

ABBREVIATIONS

Lung Volume	
VC	Vital capacity
IC	Inspiratory capacity
IRV	Inspiratory reserve volume
ERV	Expiratory reserve volume
FRC	Functional residual capacity

(continues)

Lung Volume (continued)

RV	Residual volume
TLC	Total lung capacity
RV/TLC(%)	Residual volume to total lung capacity ratio, expressed as a percentage
V_T	Tidal volume
$\dot{V}_A$	Alveolar ventilation
V_D	Dead space ventilation
V_L	Actual lung volume

Spirometry

FVC	Forced vital capacity with maximally forced expiratory effort
FEV_T	Forced expiratory volume timed
$FEF_{200-1200}$	Average rate of airflow between 200–1200 mL of the FVC
$FEF_{25\%-75\%}$	Forced expiratory flow during the middle half of the FVC (formerly called the maximal midexpiratory flow or MMF)
PEFR	Maximum flow rate that can be achieved
$\dot{V}_{max\,x}$	Forced expiratory flow related to the actual volume of the lungs as denoted by subscript x, which refers to the amount of lung volume remaining when measurement is made
MVV	Maximal voluntary ventilation as the volume of air expired in a specified interval

Mechanics

C_L	Lung compliance; volume change per unit of pressure change
R_{aw}	Airway resistance; pressure per unit of flow

Diffusion

DL_{CO}	Diffusing capacity of carbon monoxide (CO)

Blood Gases

PA_{O_2}	Alveolar oxygen tension
Pc_{O_2}	Pulmonary capillary oxygen tension
Pa_{O_2}	Arterial oxygen tension
$P\bar{v}_{O_2}$	Mixed venous oxygen tension
PA_{CO_2}	Alveolar carbon dioxide tension
Pc_{CO_2}	Pulmonary capillary carbon dioxide tension
Pa_{CO_2}	Arterial carbon dioxide tension
Sa_{O_2}	Arterial oxygen saturation

Blood Gases (continued)

$S\bar{v}_{O_2}$	Mixed venous oxygen saturation
pH	Negative logarithm of the H^+ concentration used as a positive number
HCO_3^-	Plasma bicarbonate concentration
mEq/L	The number of grams of solute dissolved in a normal solution
Ca_{O_2}	Oxygen content of arterial blood
Cc_{O_2}	Oxygen content of capillary blood
$C\bar{v}_{O_2}$	Oxygen content of mixed venous blood
$\dot{V}/\dot{Q}$	Ventilation-perfusion ratio
$\dot{Q}_S/\dot{Q}_T$	Shunt fraction
$\dot{Q}_T$	Total cardiac output

Oxygen Transport Studies

$C(a - \bar{v})_{O_2}$	Arterial-venous oxygen content difference
$\dot{V}_{O_2}$	Oxygen consumption (oxygen uptake)
O_2ER	Oxygen extraction ratio
D_{O_2}	Total oxygen delivery

HEMODYNAMIC MEASUREMENT ABBREVIATIONS

Direct Measurements

CVP	Central venous pressure
RAP	Right atrial pressure
$\overline{PA}$	Mean pulmonary artery pressure
PCWP	Pulmonary capillary wedge pressure
PAW	Pulmonary artery wedge
PAO	Pulmonary artery occlusion
CO	Cardiac output

Indirect Measurements

SV	Stroke volume
SVI	Stroke volume index
CI	Cardiac index
RVSWI	Right ventricular stroke work index
LVSWI	Left ventricular stroke work index
PVR	Pulmonary vascular resistance
SVR	Systemic vascular resistance

METRIC MEASUREMENT ABBREVIATIONS

Linear Measurements

m	meter
cm	centimeter (m $\times$ 10^{-2})
mm	millimeter (m $\times$ 10^{-3})
μm	micrometer (m $\times$ 10^{-6})

Volume Measurements

L	liter
dL	deciliter (1 $\times$ 10^{-1})
mL	milliliter (1 $\times$ 10^{-3})
μL	microliter (1 $\times$ 10^{-6})
nL	nanoliter (1 $\times$ 10^{-9})

Weight Measurements

g	gram
mg	milligram (g $\times$ 10^{-3})
μg	microgram (g $\times$ 10^{-6})
ng	nanogram (g $\times$ 10^{-9})

Units of Measurement

METRIC LENGTH

Meter	Centimeter	Millimeter	Micrometer	Nanometer
1	100	1000	1,000,000	1,000,000,000
.01	1	10	10,000	10,000,000
.001	.1	1	1000	1,000,000
.000001	.0001	.001	1	1000
.000000001	.0000001	.000001	.001	1

METRIC VOLUMES

Liter	Centiliter	Milliliter	Microliter	Nanoliter
1	100	1000	1,000,000	1,000,000,000
.01	1	10	10,000	10,000,000
.001	.1	1	1000	1,000,000
.000001	.0001	.001	1	1000
.000000001	.0000001	.000001	.001	1

METRIC WEIGHT

Grams	Centigrams	Milligrams	Micrograms	Nanograms
1	100	1000	1,000,000	1,000,000,000
.01	1	10	10,000	10,000,000
.001	.1	1	1000	1,000,000
.000001	.0001	.001	1	1000
.000000001	.0000001	.000001	.001	1

WEIGHT CONVERSIONS (METRIC AND AVOIRDUPOIS)

Grams	Kilograms	Ounces	Pounds
1	.001	.0353	.0022
1000	1	35.3	2.2
28.35	.02835	1	$\frac{1}{16}$
454.5	.4545	16	1

WEIGHT CONVERSIONS (METRIC AND APOTHECARY)

Grams	Milligrams	Grains	Drams	Ounces	Pounds
1	1000	15.4	.2577	.0322	.00268
.001	1	.0154	.00026	.0000322	.00000268
.0648	64.8	1	$\frac{1}{60}$	$\frac{1}{480}$	$\frac{1}{5760}$
3.888	3888	60	1	$\frac{1}{8}$	$\frac{1}{96}$
31.1	31104	480	8	1	$\frac{1}{12}$
373.25	373248	5760	96	12	1

APPROXIMATE HOUSEHOLD MEASUREMENT EQUIVALENTS (VOLUME)

1 tsp =	5 mL
1 tbsp = 3 tsp =	15 mL
1 fl oz = 2 tbsp = 6 tsp =	30 mL
1 cup = 8 fl oz	= 240 mL
1 pt = 2 cups = 16 fl oz	= 480 mL
1 qt = 2 pt = 4 cups = 32 fl oz	= 960 mL
1 gal = 4 qt = 8 pt = 16 cups = 128 fl oz	= 3840 mL

Courtesy of Des Jardins, *Clinical Manifestations of Respiratory Disease* (2nd ed.). © 1990 by Mosby Year Book Medical Publishers, Inc., Chicago.

WEIGHT

Metric	Approximate Apothecary Equivalents
Grams	Grains
.0002	$\frac{1}{300}$
.0003	$\frac{1}{200}$
.0004	$\frac{1}{150}$
.0005	$\frac{1}{120}$
.0006	$\frac{1}{100}$
.001	$\frac{1}{60}$
.002	$\frac{1}{30}$
.005	$\frac{1}{12}$
.010	$\frac{1}{6}$
.015	$\frac{1}{4}$
.025	$\frac{3}{8}$
.030	$\frac{1}{2}$
.050	$\frac{3}{4}$
.060	1
.100	$1\frac{1}{2}$
.120	2
.200	3
.300	5
.500	$7\frac{1}{2}$
.600	10
1	15
2	30
4	60

LIQUID MEASURE

Metric	Approximate Apothecary Equivalents
Milliliters	
1000	1 quart
750	$1\frac{1}{2}$ pints
500	1 pint
250	8 fluid ounces
200	7 fluid ounces
100	$3\frac{1}{2}$ fluid ounces
50	$1\frac{3}{4}$ fluid ounces

(continues)

LIQUID MEASURE (Continued)

Metric	Approximate Apothecary Equivalents
Milliliters	
30	1 fluid ounce
15	4 fluid drams
10	$2\frac{1}{2}$ fluid drams
8	2 fluid drams
5	$1\frac{1}{4}$ fluid drams
4	1 fluid dram
3	45 minims
2	30 minims
1	15 minims
0.75	12 minims
0.6	10 minims
0.5	8 minims
0.3	5 minims
0.25	4 minims
0.2	3 minims
0.1	$1\frac{1}{2}$ minims
0.06	1 minim
0.05	$\frac{3}{4}$ minim
0.03	$\frac{1}{2}$ minim

VOLUME CONVERSIONS (METRIC AND APOTHECARY)

Milliliters	Minims	Fluid Drams	Fluid Ounces	Pints
1	16.2	.27	.0333	.0021
.0616	1	$\frac{1}{60}$	$\frac{1}{480}$	$\frac{1}{7680}$
3.697	60	1	$\frac{1}{8}$	$\frac{1}{128}$
29.58	480	8	1	$\frac{1}{16}$
473.2	7680	128	16	1

Liters	Gallons	Quarts	Fluid Ounces	Pints
1	.2642	1.057	33.824	2.114
3.785	1	4	128	8
.946	$\frac{1}{4}$	1	32	2
.473	$\frac{1}{8}$	$\frac{1}{2}$	16	1
.0296	$\frac{1}{128}$	$\frac{1}{32}$	1	$\frac{1}{16}$

LENGTH CONVERSIONS (METRIC AND ENGLISH SYSTEM)

Unit	Millimeters	Centimeters	Inches	Feet	Yards	Meters
1 Å =	$\frac{1}{10,000,000}$	$\frac{1}{100,000,000}$	$\frac{1}{254,000,000,000}$	$\frac{1}{3,050,000,000}$	$\frac{1}{9,140,000,000}$	$\frac{1}{10,000,000,000}$
1 nm =	$\frac{1}{1,000,000}$	$\frac{1}{10,000,000}$	$\frac{1}{25,400,000}$	$\frac{1}{305,000,000}$	$\frac{1}{914,000,000}$	$\frac{1}{1,000,000,000}$
1 μm =	$\frac{1}{1000}$	$\frac{1}{10,000}$	$\frac{1}{25,400}$	$\frac{1}{305,000}$	$\frac{1}{914,000}$	$\frac{1}{1,000,000}$
1 mm =	1.0	0.1	0.03937	0.00328	0.0011	0.001
1 cm =	10.0	1.0	0.3937	0.03281	0.0109	0.01
1 in. =	25.4	2.54	1.0	0.0833	0.0278	0.0254
1 ft =	304.8	30.48	12.0	1.0	0.333	0.3048
1 yd =	914.40	91.44	36.0	3.0	1.0	0.9144
1 m =	1000.0	100.0	39.37	3.2808	1.0936	1.0

Poiseuille's Law

POISEUILLE'S LAW FOR FLOW REARRANGED TO A SIMPLE PROPORTIONALITY

$$\dot{V} \simeq \Delta P r^{4,} \text{ or rewritten as } \frac{\dot{V}}{r^4} \simeq \Delta P.$$

When ΔP remains constant, then

$$\frac{\dot{V}_1}{r_1^{\,4}} \simeq \frac{\dot{V}_2}{r_2^{\,4}}$$

Example 1. If the radius (r_1) is decreased to one-half its previous radius $(r_2 = \frac{1}{2} r_1)$, then

$$\frac{\dot{V}_1}{r_1^{\,4}} \simeq \frac{\dot{V}_2}{(\frac{1}{2}r_1)^4}$$

$$\frac{\dot{V}_1}{r_1^{\,4}} \simeq \frac{\dot{V}_2}{(\frac{1}{16}r_1)^4}$$

$$(r_1^{\,4})\frac{\dot{V}_1}{r_1^{\,4}} \simeq (r_1^{\,4})\frac{\dot{V}_2}{(\frac{1}{16})r_1^{\,4}}$$

$$\dot{V}_1 \simeq \frac{\dot{V}_2}{\frac{1}{16}}$$

$$(\tfrac{1}{16})\dot{V}_1 \simeq (\tfrac{1}{16})\frac{\dot{V}_2}{\frac{1}{16}}$$

$$(\tfrac{1}{16})\dot{V}_1 \simeq \dot{V}_2$$

and gas flow $(\dot{V}_1)$ is reduced to $\frac{1}{16}$ its original flow rate $[\dot{V}_2 \simeq (\frac{1}{16})\dot{V}_1]$.

Example 2. If the radius (r_1) is decreased by 16% ($r_2 = r_1 - 0.16\ r_1 = 0.84r_1$), then

$$\frac{\dot{V}_1}{r_1^{\,4}} \simeq \frac{\dot{V}_2}{r_2^{\,4}}$$

$$\frac{\dot{V}_1}{r_1^{\,4}} \simeq \frac{\dot{V}_2}{(0.84r_1)^4}$$

$$\dot{V}_2 \simeq \frac{(0.84r_1)^4\dot{V}_1}{r_1^{\,4}}$$

$$\dot{V}_2 \simeq \frac{0.4979\ \cancel{r_1^{\,4}}\ \dot{V}_1}{\cancel{r_1^{\,4}}}$$

$$\dot{V}_2 \simeq \tfrac{1}{2}\,\dot{V}_1$$

and the flow rate ($\dot{V}_1$) would decrease to one-half the original flow rate ($\dot{V}_2 \simeq \tfrac{1}{2}\dot{V}_1$).

POISEUILLE'S LAW FOR PRESSURE REARRANGED TO A SIMPLE PROPORTIONALITY

$$P \simeq \frac{\dot{V}}{r^4}, \text{ or rewritten as } P \cdot r^4 \simeq \dot{V}$$

when $\dot{V}$ remains constant, then

$$P_1 \cdot r_1^{\,4} \simeq P_2 \cdot r_2^{\,4}$$

Example 1. If the radius (r_1) is reduced to one-half its original radius [$r_2 = (\tfrac{1}{2})\ r_1$], then

$$P_1 \cdot r_1^{\,4} \simeq P_2 \cdot r_2^{\,4}$$

$$P_1 \cdot r_1^{\,4} \simeq P_2[(\tfrac{1}{2})r_1]^4$$

$$P_1 \cdot r_1^{\,4} \simeq P_2 \cdot (\tfrac{1}{16})r_1^{\,4}$$

$$\frac{P_1 \cdot \cancel{r_1^{\,4}}}{\cancel{r_1^{\,4}}} \simeq \frac{P_2 \cdot (\tfrac{1}{16})\cancel{r_1^{\,4}}}{\cancel{r_1^{\,4}}}$$

$$P_1 \simeq P_2 \cdot (\tfrac{1}{16})$$

$$16\,P_1 \simeq \cancel{16} \cdot P_2 \cdot \cancel{(\tfrac{1}{16})}$$

$$16\,P_1 \simeq P_2$$

and the pressure (P_1) will increase to 16 times its original level ($P_2 \simeq 16 \cdot P_1$).

Example 2. If the radius (r_1) is decreased by 16% $(r_2 = r_1 - 0.16\ r_1 = 0.84r_1)$, then

$$P_1 \cdot r_1{}^4 \simeq P_2 \cdot r_2{}^4$$

$$P_1 \cdot r_1{}^4 \simeq P_2(0.4979)r_1{}^4$$

$$\frac{P_1 r_1{}^4}{(0.4979)r_1{}^4} = P_2$$

$$2\ P_1 = P_2$$

and the pressure (P_1) would increase to twice its original pressure $(P_2 \simeq 2 \cdot P_1)$.

DuBois Body Surface Chart

Directions

To find body surface of a patient, locate the height in inches (or centimeters) on Scale I and the weight in pounds (or kilograms) on Scale II and place a straightedge (ruler) between these two points which will intersect Scale III at the patient's surface area.

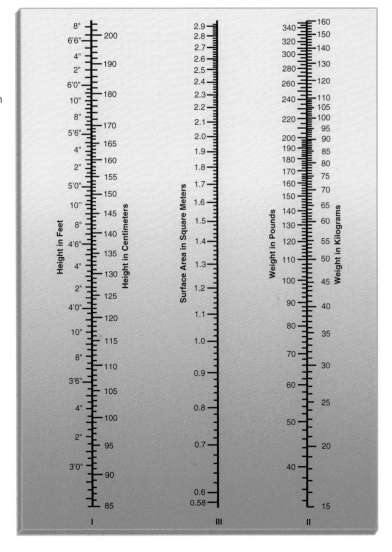

Adapted from DuBois and Eugene F. *Basal Metabolism in Health and Disease*. Philadelphia: Lea and Febiger, 1924.

Cardiopulmonary Profile

A representative example of a cardiopulmonary profile sheet used to monitor the critically ill patient. See Chapters 5, 6, and 7 for explanations of the various components presented in this sample cardiopulmonary profile. Areas shaded in pink represent normal ranges.

Quadrant 1: Hypovolemia
Quadrant 2: Optimal Function
Quadrant 3: Hypervolemia
Quadrant 4: Cardiac Failure

Temperature: _____

Heart Rate: _____

Cardiac Output: _____

Medications: _____

_____

Shaded areas represent normal ranges.

Patient's Name _____

Date _____

Time _____

$P_{CO_2}/HCO_3^-/pH$ Nomogram

Nomogram — Slide 1

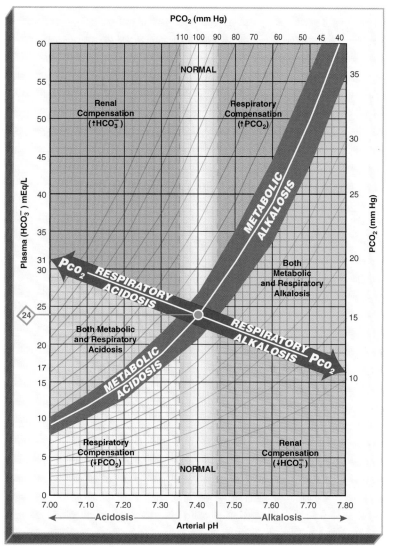

Cut out the above two-sided nomogram and have it laminated for use as a handy, pocket-sized reference tool.

See Chapter 7 on how to use the nomogram in the clinical setting.

Nomogram — Slide 2

pH, PCO$_2$, HCO$_3$ RELATIONSHIP

PaCO$_2$		pH	HCO$_3$
100	$\approx$	7.10	30
80	$\approx$	7.20	28
60	$\approx$	7.30	26
40	$\approx$	7.40	24
30	$\approx$	7.50	22
20	$\approx$	7.60	20
10	$\approx$	7.70	18

EX: ACUTE CHANGES ON CVF

AVF on CVF		CVF Baseline		AAH on CVF
		pH		
7.21	$\leftarrow$	7.39	$\rightarrow$	7.53
		PaCO$_2$		
110	$\leftarrow$	76	$\rightarrow$	51
		HCO$_3$		
43	$\leftarrow$	41	$\rightarrow$	37
		PaO$_2$		
34	$\leftarrow$	61	$\rightarrow$	46

CVF: Chronic ventilatory failure
AVF: Acute ventilatory failure
AAH: Acute alveolar hyperventilation

PaO$_2$ & SaO$_2$ RELATIONSHIP

	PaO$_2$	SaO$_2$
Normal	97	97
Range	>80–100	>95
Hypoxemia	<80	<95
Mild	60–80	90–95
Moderate	40–60	75–90
Severe	<40	<75

PaO$_2$ & SaO$_2$ RELATIONSHIP

PO$_2$ 30 $\approx$ 60% saturated
PO$_2$ 40 $\approx$ 75% saturated
PO$_2$ 50 $\approx$ 85% saturated
PO$_2$ 60 $\approx$ 90% saturated

FIO$_2$ & PaO$_2$ RELATIONSHIP

FIO$_2$		PaO$_2$
0.30	$\approx$	150
0.40	$\approx$	200
0.50	$\approx$	250
0.80	$\approx$	400
1.00	$\approx$	500

O$_2$ TRANSPORT

	Normal Values
DO$_2$	1000 ml O$_2$/min
$\dot{V}$O$_2$	250 ml O$_2$/min
C(a–$\bar{v}$)O$_2$	5 vol%
O$_2$ER	25%
S$\bar{v}$O$_2$	75%

Calculating Heart Rate by Counting the Number of Large ECG Squares

Distance Between Two QRS Complexes (no. of large squares)	Estimated Heart Rate (per min)
1	300
1½	200
2	150
2½	125
3	100
3½	85
4	75
4½	65
5	60
5½	55
6	50
6½	45

THE ANATOMY AND PHYSIOLOGY OF THE RESPIRATORY SYSTEM

Chapter 1

1. A	8. D	15. D
2. D	9. D	16. A
3. A	10. B	17. B
4. B	11. C	18. C
5. A	12. C	19. B
6. D	13. C	20. A
7. A	14. A	

VENTILATION

Chapter 2

1. A	12. D
2. A	13. D
3. D	14. 6375 mL
4. D	15. Part I: 79 mL/cm H_2O
5. C	Part II: 70 mL/cm H_2O
6. C	Part III: decreasing
7. B	16. D
8. B	17. C
9. D	18. A
10. B	19. D
11. A	20. A

CLINICAL APPLICATION QUESTIONS

Case 1

1. Low
2. Large; little or no
3. Tracheobronchial tree constriction; excessive airway secretions
4. Longer; long
5. Decreases

Case 2

1. Caved inward
2. Partially collapsed; decreased
3. Positive pressure; moved outward; resting level

THE DIFFUSION OF PULMONARY GASES

Chapter 3

1. C	5. B	9. A
2. B	6. C	10. B
3. A	7. C	
4. E	8. D	

CLINICAL APPLICATION QUESTIONS

Case 1

1. Also increase
2. Decreased
3. Pa_{O_2}; P_1
4. Pressure at the level of the alveoli; Fi_{O_2} to 0.4

Case 2

1. Thickness
2. P_A (P_1)
3. T (thickness)
4. Increased oxygen concentration (P_1)

PULMONARY FUNCTION MEASUREMENTS

Chapter 4

1. D	5. C	9. B
2. B	6. B	10. B
3. D	7. D	11. A
4. D	8. B	

CLINICAL APPLICATION QUESTIONS

Case 1

1. Personal best PEFR
2. Effort-independent flow; dynamic compression; equal pressure point
3. Closer to the alveoli

Case 2

1. FVC; FEV_1; $FEF_{200-1200}$; PEFR
2. VC; RV; FRC
3. Increased; increased

THE ANATOMY AND PHYSIOLOGY OF THE CIRCULATORY SYSTEM

Chapter 5

1. D	6. D	11. B
2. C	7. B	12. D
3. B	8. B	13. D
4. C	9. B	14. D
5. A	10. A	15. A

CLINICAL APPLICATION QUESTIONS

Case 1

1. Baroreceptors; decreased
2. Blood pressure (78/42 mm Hg)
3. Decreases
4. (1) Lowering the patient's head and elevating her legs, which used the effects of gravity to move blood to the patient's lungs; (2) replacing the volume of blood lost by administering Ringer's lactated solution through the patient's intravenous tube

Case 2

1. High blood pressure of 214/106 mm Hg
2. Rales; rhonchi
3. Decreased Pa_{O_2} of 48 mm Hg
4. Distended neck veins and peripheral edema
5. Afterloads

OXYGEN TRANSPORT

Chapter 6

1. A	5. B	9. D
2. C	6. D	10. D
3. C	7. D	
4. B	8. C	

11. Case Study: Automobile Collision Victim

Based on the questions asked and the information provided, the patient's $P_{A_{O_2}}$, Cc_{O_2}, and $C\bar{v}_{O_2}$ should first be calculated.

$$
\begin{aligned}
P_{A_{O_2}} &= (BP - P_{H_2O})\, F_{I_{O_2}} - Pa_{CO_2}\,(1.25) \\
&= (745 - 47)\, 0.50 - 38\,(1.25) \\
&= (698)\, 0.50 - 47.5 \\
&= 349 - 47.5
\end{aligned}
$$

Answer = 301.5 mm Hg

$$
\begin{aligned}
Cc_{O_2} &= (Hb \times 1.34) + P_{A_{O_2}} \times 0.003 \\
&= (11 \times 1.34) + 301.5 \times 0.003 \\
&= 14.74 + 0.904
\end{aligned}
$$

Answer = 15.64 vol% O_2

$$
\begin{aligned}
Ca_{O_2} &= (Hb \times 1.34 \times Sa_{O_2}) + (Pa_{O_2} \times 0.003) \\
&= (11 \times 1.34 \times 0.90) + (60 \times 0.003) \\
&= 13.266 + 0.18
\end{aligned}
$$

Answer = 13.446 vol% O_2

$$
\begin{aligned}
C\bar{v}_{O_2} &= (Hb \times 1.34 \times S\bar{v}_{O_2}) + (P\bar{v}_{O_2} \times 0.003) \\
&= (11 \times 1.34 \times 0.65) + (35 \times 0.003) \\
&= 9.581 + 0.105
\end{aligned}
$$

Answer = 9.686 vol% O_2

With the above information and the data provided in the question, the following can now be calculated:

A. Total Oxygen = $\dot{Q}_T \times Ca_{O_2} \times 10$

$$
\begin{aligned}
\text{Delivery} &= 6\,L \times 13.446\ \text{vol\%} \times 10 \\
&= 806.76\ \text{mL}\ O_2/\text{min}
\end{aligned}
$$

Answer: 806.76 mL O_2/min

B. Arterial-Venous Oxygen Content Difference
$C(a - \bar{v})_{O_2}$

$$
\begin{aligned}
C(a - \bar{v})_{O_2} &= Ca_{O_2} - C\bar{v}_{O_2} \\
&= 13.446 - 9.686 \\
&= 3.760\ \text{vol\%}\ O_2
\end{aligned}
$$

Answer: 3.76 vol% O_2

C. Intrapulmonary Shunting ($\dot{Q}_S/\dot{Q}_T$)

$$
\begin{aligned}
(\dot{Q}_S/\dot{Q}_T) &= \frac{Cc_{O_2} - Ca_{O_2}}{Cc_{O_2} - C\bar{v}_{O_2}} \\
&= \frac{15.644 - 13.446}{15.664 - 9.686} \\
&= \frac{2.198}{5.958} \\
&= 0.368\%
\end{aligned}
$$

Answer: 36.8%

D. Oxygen Consumption ($\dot{V}_{O_2}$)

$$
\begin{aligned}
\dot{V}_{O_2} &= \dot{Q}_T\,[C(a - \bar{v})_{O_2} \times 10] \\
&= 6L \times 3.760 \times 10 \\
&= 225.6\ \text{mL}\ O_2/\text{min}
\end{aligned}
$$

Answer: 225.6 mL O_2/min

E. Oxygen Extraction Ratio $= \dfrac{Ca_{O_2} - C\bar{v}_{O_2}}{Ca_{O_2}}$

$$
\begin{aligned}
&= \frac{13.446 - 9.686}{13.446} \\
&= \frac{3.760}{13.446} \\
&= 0.279
\end{aligned}
$$

Answer: 27.9%

CLINICAL APPLICATION QUESTIONS

Case 1

1. Unconscious, cyanotic, and hypotensive, and her skin was cool and damp to the touch
2. D_{O_2}, O_2ER
3. 68%

Case 2

1. Decreased; increased
2. Increased; increased; decreased
3. Right
4. Lower

CARBON DIOXIDE TRANSPORT AND ACID-BASE BALANCE

Chapter 7

1. D
2. B
3. A
4. C
5. D
6. D
7. D
8. D
9. D
10. B
11. A
12. B
13. 9 mEq/L
14. Both metabolic and respiratory acidosis
15. Acute alveolar hyperventilation with partial renal compensation, or partially compensated respiratory alkalosis

CLINICAL APPLICATION QUESTIONS

Case 1

1. Impaired
2. Left
3. Cherry red
4. Increased the total oxygen delivery
5. (1) Low Pa_{CO_2}; (2) loss of stomach acid
6. Decreased Pa_{CO_2}

Case 2

1. Acids
2. Low Pa_{O_2} (38 mm Hg), which produces lactic acids
3. Aggressive ventilation
4. Higher

VENTILATION-PERFUSION RELATIONSHIPS

Chapter 8

1. D	3. D	5. B
2. C	4. D	

CLINICAL APPLICATION QUESTIONS

Case 1

1. Ineffective
2. Wasted or dead space
3. Decreased; decreased

Case 2

1. Low
2. Fall
3. A. decreased; B. increased; C. decreased; D. increased; E. decreased

CONTROL OF VENTILATION

Chapter 9

1. C	3. D	5. D
2. B	4. A	6. D

7. D	9. D
8. C	10. B

CLINICAL APPLICATION QUESTIONS

Case 1

1. True
2. False
3. Peripheral chemoreceptors
4. Decreases
5. An increased Pa_{CO_2} level, the formation of H^+, and the stimulation of the central chemoreceptors, which, in turn, increases the individual's ventilatory rate

Case 2

1. Ketone acids
2. Peripheral chemoreceptors
3. No
4. The decreased Pa_{CO_2} worked to offset the patient's acidic pH level caused by the increased ketone acids.

FETAL DEVELOPMENT AND THE CARDIOPULMONARY SYSTEM

Chapter 10

1. B	5. A	9. D
2. B	6. B	10. D
3. A	7. D	
4. D	8. D	

CLINICAL APPLICATION QUESTIONS

Case 1

1. 28th
2. Infant respiratory distress syndrome (IRDS)
3. Interstitial edema; intra-alveolar edema; intra-alveolar hemorrhage; alveolar consolidation; intra-alveolar hyaline membrane formation; atelectasis

4. All the conditions listed in answer No. 3 cause the alveolar-capillary membrane's thickness to increase.

5. Cyanosis, increased respiratory rate and heart rate, and decreased Pa_{O_2}; nasal flaring, intercostal retractions, exhalation grunting, bilateral crackles, and ground-glass appearance and air bronchogram on the chest x-ray

6. Because the baby's Pa_{O_2} was less than 45 mm Hg shortly after he was born, the ductus arteriosus remained patent. As the infant's Pa_{O_2} increased, the ductus arteriosus closed and the signs and symptoms associated with PPHN disappeared.

Case 2

1. The ability of the fetus to absorb oxygen, nutrients, and other substances and excrete carbon dioxide and other wastes was interrupted. Complete separation brings about immediate death of the fetus.

2. Abdominal pain, uterine tenderness, uterine contraction, and hemorrhage

3. Shock and death can occur in minutes; cesarean section

AGING AND THE CARDIOPULMONARY SYSTEM

Chapter 11

1. D	5. D	9. D
2. D	6. C	10. C
3. D	7. D	
4. B	8. D	

ELECTROPHYSIOLOGY OF THE HEART

Chapter 12

1. I	5. H	9. A
2. J	6. F	10. B
3. G	7. C	
4. D	8. E	

THE STANDARD 12-ECG SYSTEM

Chapter 13

1. D	5. B	9. A
2. A	6. B	10. D
3. D	7. C	
4. D	8. C	

ECG INTERPRETATION

Chapter 14

1. QRS duration: *0.6 second* QT duration: *0.40 second*

   Ventricular rate & rhythm: *86/min*

   Atrial rate & rhythm: *86/min*

   PR interval: *0.16 second*

   Interpretation: *sinus rhythm 86/min with one PAC (6th complex)*

2. QRS duration: *0.08 second* QT duration: *cannot determine*

   Ventricular rate & rhythm: *75–150/min*

   Atrial rate & rhythm: *cannot determine*

   PR interval: *none*

   Interpretation: *atrial fibrillation, ventricular rate 75–150/min*

3. QRS duration: *0.10 second* QT duration: *0.44 second*

   Ventricular rate & rhythm: *50/min regular*

   Atrial rate & rhythm: *50/min regular*

   PR interval: *0.16–0.20 second*

   Interpretation: *sinus bradycardia at 40/min*

4. QRS duration: *0.40–0.10 second* QT duration: *cannot determine*

   Ventricular rate & rhythm: *86–100/min*

   Atrial rate & rhythm: *300*

   PR interval: *none*

   Interpretation: *atrial flutter, ventricular rate 86–100/min*

5. QRS duration: *0.08 second* QT duration: *0.36 second*

   Ventricular rate & rhythm: *86/min*

   Atrial rate & rhythm: *75/min*

PR interval: *0.24 second*

Interpretation: *first-degree AV block*

6. QRS duration: *0.12 second* QT duration: *0.32 second*

Ventricular rate & rhythm: *168/min regular*

Atrial rate & rhythm: *cannot determine*

PR interval: *cannot determine*

Interpretation: *ventricular tachycardia at 168/min*

7. QRS duration: *0.08 second* QT duration: *0.28 second*

Ventricular rate & rhythm: *150/min regular*

Atrial rate & rhythm: *150/min regular*

PR interval: *0.16 second*

Interpretation: *sinus tachycardia at 150/min*

8. QRS duration: *cannot determine* QT duration: *cannot determine*

Ventricular rate & rhythm: *cannot determine*

Atrial rate & rhythm: *cannot determine*

PR interval: *cannot determine*

Interpretation: *ventricular fibrillation*

9. QRS duration: *0.08 second* QT duration: *0.38 second*

Ventricular rate & rhythm: *60/min*

Atrial rate & rhythm: *60/min*

PR interval: *0.16 second*

Interpretation: *sinus ventricular rate at 60/min with a PAC (last complex)*

10. QRS duration: *0.06 second* QT duration: *0.32 second*

Ventricular rate & rhythm: *125/regular*

Atrial rate & rhythm: *125/regular*

PR interval: *0.16 second*

Interpretation: *sinus tachycardia at 125/min with frequent uniform PVCs*

HEMODYNAMIC MEASUREMENTS

Chapter 15

1. F	6. G	11. D
2. E	7. J	12. D
3. A	8. B	13. D
4. K	9. D	14. D
5. D	10. I	15. A

CLINICAL APPLICATION QUESTIONS

Case 1

1. The SVR (peripheral vascular resistance) to increase

2. Nitroprusside is a vasodilator. It was used to reduce the patient's afterload.

3. As the patient's SVR decreased in response to the nitroprusside, the left ventricular afterload also decreased. This action in turn allowed blood to be more readily ejected from the left ventricle.

Case 2

1. 5 cm H_2O was the PEEP level that produced the least depression of cardiac output and the maximum total oxygen delivery.

2. Profile 1:
$$
\begin{aligned}
Ca_{O_2} &= (Hb \times 1.34 \times Sa_{O_2}) + (Pa_{O_2} \times 0.003) \\
&= (15 \times 1.35 \times 0.91) + (57 \times 0.003) \\
&= (20.1 \times 0.91) = 0.17 \\
&= 18.29 + 0.17 \\
&= 18.46
\end{aligned}
$$

Profile 2:
$$
\begin{aligned}
Ca_{O_2} &= (Hb \times 1.34 \times Sa_{O_2}) + (Pa_{O_2} \times 0.003) \\
&= (15 \times 1.35 \times 0.9) + (61 \times 0.003) \\
&= (20.1 \times 0.91) = 0.18 \\
&= 18.09 + 0.18 \\
&= 18.27
\end{aligned}
$$

Profile 1:
$$
\begin{aligned}
D_{O_2} &= \dot{Q}T \times (Ca_{O_2} \times 10) \\
&= 3.83 \times (18.46 \times 10) \\
&= 3.83 \times 184.6 \\
&= 707 \text{ mL } O_2/min
\end{aligned}
$$

Profile 2:
$$
\begin{aligned}
D_{O_2} &= \dot{Q}T \times (Ca_{O_2} \times 10) \\
&= 3.1 \times (18.27 \times 10) \\
&= 3.1 \times 182.7 \\
&= 566 \text{ mL } O_2/min
\end{aligned}
$$

A PEEP of 5 cm H_2O resulted in a D_{O_2} of 707 mm O_2/min. A PEEP of 10 cm H_2O resulted in a D_{O_2} of 566 mL O_2/min. The "best PEEP" in this case was 5 cm H_2O, which resulted in a D_{O_2} that was 141 mL O_2/min more than the PEEP of 10 cm H_2O.

RENAL FAILURE AND ITS EFFECTS ON THE CARDIOPULMONARY SYSTEM

Chapter 16

1. D	5. C	9. B
2. B	6. D	10. D
3. B	7. D	
4. D	8. B	

CLINICAL APPLICATION QUESTIONS

Case 1

1. The patient's left ventricular failure (a prerenal abnormality)
2. A sharp reduction in urine output
3. Because of increased H^+ and K^+ ion levels and the loss of HCO_3
4. Fluid accumulation in the patient's lungs and extremities, causing swelling in the patient's ankles, hands, and eyelids; white fluffy patches visible on the patient's chest x-ray; Pa_{O_2} of 64 mm Hg

Case 2

1. Hypovolemia
2. Inflammation of the tracheobronchial tree, bronchospasm, excessive bronchial secretions and mucous plugging, decreased mucosal ciliary transport mechanism, atelectasis, alveolar edema, and frothy secretions
3. White fluffy densities throughout both fields (x-ray), and the low Pa_{O_2} of 47 mm Hg

SLEEP PHYSIOLOGY AND ITS RELATIONSHIP TO THE CARDIOPULMONARY SYSTEM

Chapter 17

1. E	3. B	5. A
2. C	4. D	6. B

7. A	9. A
8. B	10. D

Matching

1. D	3. A	5. C
2. E	4. B	

EXERCISE AND ITS EFFECTS ON THE CARDIOPULMONARY SYSTEM

Chapter 18

1. B	5. C	9. A
2. D	6. B	10. D
3. D	7. D	
4. D	8. D	

HIGH ALTITUDE AND ITS EFFECTS ON THE CARDIOPULMONARY SYSTEM

Chapter 19

1. D	5. D	9. True
2. D	6. True	10. False
3. D	7. False	
4. B	8. True	

HIGH-PRESSURE ENVIRONMENTS AND THEIR EFFECTS ON THE CARDIOPULMONARY SYSTEM

Chapter 20

1. C	5. D	9. True
2. B	6. True	10. True
3. D	7. True	
4. D	8. False	

BIBLIOGRAPHY

GENERAL ANATOMY AND PHYSIOLOGY

Colbert BJ, Ankney J, Lee KT (2006). *Anatomy and Physiology for Health Professionals.* Upper Saddle River, NJ: Prentice Hall.

Marieb EN, Hoehn K (2003). *Human Anatomy and Physiology* (7th ed.). Redwood City, CA: Pearson-Benjamin Cummings.

Martini FH (2005). *Fundamentals of Anatomy and Physiology* (7th ed.). Redwood City, CA: Pearson-Benjamin Cummings.

Saladin KS (2007). *Anatomy and Physiology: The Unity of Form and Function* (4th ed.). New York: McGraw-Hill.

Seeley RR, Stephens TD, Tate P (2004). *Anatomy and Physiology* (7th ed.). New York: McGraw-Hill.

Shier DN, Butler JL, Lewis R (2006). *Hole's Human Anatomy Physiology* (11th ed.). New York: McGraw-Hill.

Solomon EP (2003). *Introduction to Human Anatomy and Physiology* (2nd ed.). Philadelphia: WB Saunders.

Thibodeau GA, Patton KT (2003). *Anatomy and Physiology* (5th ed.). St. Louis: Mosby.

Tortora GJ, Derrickson BH (2005). *Principles of Anatomy and Physiology* (11th ed.). New York: John Wiley Sons.

CARDIOPULMONARY ANATOMY AND PHYSIOLOGY

Comroe JH (1974). *Physiology of Respiration* (2nd ed.). Chicago: Year Book Medical Publishers.

Conover MH, Zalis EG (2003). *Understanding Electrocardiography* (8th ed.). St. Louis: Mosby.

Cottrell, GP (2001). *Cardiopulmonary Anatomy and Physiology for Respiratory Care Practitioners.* Philadelphia: FA Davis.

Hicks GH (2000). *Cardiopulmonary Anatomy and Physiology.* Philadelphia: WB Saunders.

Levitzky MG (1999). *Pulmonary Physiology* (5th ed.). New York: McGraw-Hill Health Professions.

Murray JF (1986). *The Normal Lung* (2nd ed.). Philadelphia: WB Saunders.

Murray JG, Nadel JA (2005). *Textbook of Respiratory Medicine* (4th ed.). Philadelphia: WB Saunders.

Slonim NB, Hamilton LH (1987). *Respiratory Physiology* (5th ed.). St. Louis: Mosby.

West JB (2000). *Respiratory Physiology: The Essentials* (6th ed.). Philadelphia: Lippincott Williams and Wilkins.

SELECTED OXYGENATION TOPICS

Cane RD et al. (1988). Unreliability of oxygen tension-based indices in reflecting intrapulmonary shunting in critically ill patients. *Crit Care Med* 16:1243.

Hess D, Kacmarek RM (1993). Techniques and devices for monitoring oxygenation. *Respir Care* 38(6):646.

Kandel G, Aberman A (1993). Mixed venous oxygen saturation: Its role in the assessment of the critically ill patient. *Arch Intern Med* 143:1400.

Nelson LD (1993). Assessment of oxygenation: Oxygenation indices. *Respir Care* 38(6):631.

Nelson LD, Rutherford EJ (1992). Monitoring mixed venous oxygen. *Respir Care* 37(2):154.

Rasanen J et al. (1987). Oxygen tension and oxyhemoglobin saturations in the assessment of pulmonary gas exchange. *Crit Care Med* 15:1058.

SELECTED HYPOXIC-DRIVE TOPICS

Aubier M et al. (1980). Effects of the administration of oxygen on ventilation and blood gases in patients with chronic obstructive pulmonary disease during acute respiratory failure. *Am Rev Respir Dis* 122:747.

Dunn WF, Nelson SB, Hubmayr RD (1991). Oxygen-induced hypercapnia in obstructive pulmonary disease. *Am Rev Respir Dis* 144:526.

French W (2000, February/March). Hypoxic-drive theory revisited. *J Respir Care Practitioners*, pp. 84–85.

Sassoon CS, Hassell KT, Mahutte CK (1987). Hyperoxic-induced hypercapnia in stable chronic obstructive pulmonary disease. *Am Rev Respir Dis* 135:907.

HEMODYNAMICS

Darovic GO (2002). *Hemodynamic Monitoring: Invasive and Noninvasive Clinical Applications* (3rd ed.). Philadelphia: WB Saunders.

Darovic GO (2004). *Handbook of Hemodynamic Monitoring* (2nd ed.). Philadelphia: WB Saunders.

Hodges RK, Garrett K, Chernecky CC, Schumacher L (2005). *Real World Nursing Survival Guide: Hemodynamic Monitoring.* Philadelphia: WB Saunders.

PULMONARY FUNCTION TESTING

Ferguson GT et al. (2000). Office spirometry for lung health assessment in adults: A consensus statement from the National Lung Health Education Program. *Chest* 117(4):1146.

Hyatt RE, Scanlon PD (2002). *Interpretation of pulmonary function tests: A practical guide* (2nd ed.). Philadelphia: JB Lippincott.

Madama VC (1998). *Pulmonary Function Testing and Cardiopulmonary Stress Testing* (2nd ed.). Albany, NY: Delmar Publishers.

Ruppel GL (2004). *Manual of Pulmonary Function Testing* (8th ed.). St. Louis: Mosby.

ARTERIAL BLOOD GASES

Malley WJ (2005). *Clinical Blood Gases: Applications and Interventions* (2nd ed.). Philadelphia: WB Saunders.

Martin L (1999). *All You Really Need to Know to Interpret Arterial Blood Gases* (2nd ed.). Baltimore: Williams and Wilkins.

Shapiro BA, Peruzzi WT, Kozlowska-Templin R (1994). *Clinical Application of Blood Gases* (5th ed.). St. Louis: Mosby.

SLEEP PHYSIOLOGY

Aldrich MS (1999). *Sleep Medicine* (pp. 3–26). New York: Oxford University Press.

Allen R, Hening W, Montplaisir J, et al. (2003). Restless legs syndrome: Diagnostic criteria, special considerations, and epidemiology workshop at the National Institute of Health. *Sleep Med* 4(2):101–119.

American Sleep Disorders Association (2001). *International Classification of Sleep Disorders, Revised: Diagnostic and Coding Manual.* Rochester, NY: Author.

American Thoracic Society (1996). Standards and indication for cardiopulmonary sleep studies in children. *Am J Respir Crit Care Med* 159:866–878.

American Thoracic Society (1999). Cardio-respiratory studies in children: Establishment of normative data and polysomnographic predictors of morbidity. *Am J Resp Crit Care Med* 160:1381–1387.

Berry RB (2002). Nasal esophageal pressure monitoring. In Lee-Chiong TL, Sateia MJ, Caraskadon MA (Eds.), *Sleep Medicine* (pp. 661–671). Philadelphia: Hanley and Belfus.

Berry RB (2003). *Sleep Medicine Pearls* (2nd ed.). Philadelphia: Hanley and Belfus.

Bliwise DL (1997). Sleep and aging. In Pressman MR, Orr WC (Eds.), *Understanding Sleep: The Evaluation and Treatment of Sleep Disorders* (pp. 441–464). Washington, DC: American Psychological Association.

Bliwise DL (2000). Normal aging. In Kryger MH, Roth T, Dement WC (Eds.), *Principles and Practice of Sleep Medicine* (3rd ed., pp. 26–42). Philadelphia: WB Saunders.

Borbely A, Achermann P (2000). Sleep homeostasis and models of sleep regulation. In Kryger M, Roth T, Dement WC (Eds.), *Principles and Practice of Sleep Medicine* (pp. 377–390). Philadelphia: WB Saunders.

Butkov N. (2003). Polysomnography. In Lee-Chiong TL, Sateia MJ, Carskadon MA (Eds.), *Sleep Medicine.* Philadelphia: Hanley and Belfus.

Caraskadon MA, Rechschaffen A. (2000). Monitoring and staging human sleep. In Kryger MH, Roth T, Dement WC (Eds.), *Principles and Practice of Sleep Medicine* (pp. 1197–1215). Philadelphia: WB Saunders.

Carney PR, Berry RB, Geyer JD (2005). *Clinical Sleep Disorders.* Philadelphia: Lippincott Williams and Wilkins.

Chokroverty S (1999). An overview of sleep. In Chokroverty S (Ed.), *Sleep Disorders Medicine: Basic Science, Technical Considerations and Clinical Aspects* (2nd ed., pp. 7–20). Boston: Butterworth-Henemann.

Hening W, Allen RP, Thanner S, et al. (2003). The Johns Hopkins Telephone diagnostic interview for the restless legs syndrome: Preliminary investigation for validation in a multi-center patient and control population. *Sleep Med* 4(2):137–141.

Hening WA, Walters AS, Wagner M, et al. (1999). Circadian rhythm of motor restlessness and sensory symptoms in the idiopathic restless leg syndrome. *Sleep* 22(7):901–912.

International Restless Legs Syndrome Study Group (2003). Validation of the International Restless Legs Syndrome Study Group rating scale for restless legs syndrome. *Sleep Med* 4(2)121–132.

Jones B (2000). Basic mechanisms of sleep–wake states. In Kryger M, Roth T, Dement WC (Eds.), *Principles and Practice of Sleep Medicine* (pp. 134–154). Philadelphia: WB Saunders.

Keenan SA (1999). Polysomnographic techniques: An overview. In Chokroverty S (Ed.), *Sleep Disorders Medicine* (pp. 151–169). Boston: Butterworth-Heinemann.

Kryger MH (2000). Monitoring respiratory and cardiac function. In Kryger MH, Roth T, Dement WC (Eds.), *Principles and Practice of Sleep Medicine* (pp. 1217–1230). Philadelphia: WB Saunders.

Marcus CL. (2001). Sleep-disordered breathing in children: State of the art. *Am J Resp Crit Care Med* 164:16–30.

Michaud M, Paquet J, Lavigne G, et al. (2002). Sleep laboratory diagnosis of restless legs syndrome. *Eur Neurol* 48(2):108–113.

Radtke R. (2003). Sleep disorders: Laboratory evaluation. In Ebersole JS, Pedley TA (Eds.), *Current Practice of Clinical Electroencephalography* (pp. 803–832). Philadelphia: Lippincott Williams and Wilkins.

Redline S, Kapur VK, Sanders MH, et al. (2000). Effects of varying approaches for identifying respiratory disturbances on sleep apnea assessment. *Am J Respir Crit Care Med* 161:369–374.

Redline S, Kirchner HL, Quan SF, et al. (2004). The effects of age, sex, ethnicity and sleep-disordered breathing on sleep architecture. *Arch Intern Med* 164:406–418.

Sheldon SH, Riter S, Detrojan M (1999). *Atlas of Sleep Medicine in Infants and Children.* Armonk, NY: Futura.

Siegel J (2002). *The Neural Control of Sleep and Waking.* New York: Springer-Verlag.

Taheri S, Bloom S. (2001). Orexins/hypocretins: Waking up the scientific world. *Clin Endocrinol* 54:421–429.

Tassi P, Muzet A (2000). Sleep inertia. *Sleep Med Rev* 4:341–353.

Van Dongen HP, Maislin G, Mullington JM, et al. (2003). The cumulative cost of additional wakefulness: Dose–response effects on neurobehavioral functions and sleep physiology from chronic sleep restriction and total sleep deprivation. *Sleep* 26:117–126.

PATHOPHYSIOLOGY

Cotran R, Kumar V, Collins T (1999). *Robbins' Pathologic Basis of Disease* (6th ed.). Philadelphia: WB Saunders.

Gould BE (2002). *Pathophysiology for the Health Professions.* Philadelphia: WB Saunders.

McCance KL, Huether SE (1998). *Pathophysiology: The Biologic Basis for Disease in Adults and Children* (3rd ed.). St. Louis: Mosby.

Porth CM (2003). *Essentials of Pathophysiology: Concepts of Altered Health States.* Philadelphia: JB Lippincott.

Price SA, Wilson LM (2003). *Pathophysiology: Clinical Concepts of Disease Processes* (6th ed.). St. Louis: Mosby.

PULMONARY DISORDERS

Albert RK, Spiro SG, Jett JR (2004). *Clinical Respiratory Medicine* (2nd ed.). St. Louis: Mosby.

Crapo JD, Glassroth JL, Karlinsky JB, King TE (2003). *Baum's Textbook of Pulmonary Diseases* (7th ed.). Philadelphia: JB Lippincott.

Fishman AP, Elias JA (Eds.) (1998). *Fishman's Pulmonary Diseases and Disorders* (3rd ed.). New York, 1998, New York: McGraw-Hill.

Fraser RS, Colman NC, Nestor ML, Pare PD (2005). *Synopsis of Diseases of the Chest* (3rd ed.). Philadelphia: WB Saunders.

George RB, Light RW, Matthay MA, Matthay RA (2005). *Chest Medicine—Essentials of Pulmonary and Critical Care Medicine* (4th ed.). Philadelphia: JB Lippincott.

Gibson J, Geddes D, Costabel U, Sterk P, Corrin B (2003). *Respiratory Medicine* (3rd ed.). Philadelphia: WB Saunders.

McCane KL, Huether SE (2002). Pathophysiology: *The Biologic Basis for Disease in Adults and Children* (4th ed.). St. Louis: Mosby.

Murray JF, Nadel JA (2005). *Textbook of Respiratory Medicine* (4th ed.). Philadelphia: WB Saunders.

Weinberger SE (2003). *Principles of Pulmonary Medicine* (4th ed.). Philadelphia: WB Saunders.

West JB (1998). *Pulmonary Pathophysiology: The Essentials* (5th ed.). Baltimore: Williams and Wilkins.

Wilkins RL, Dexter JR (1993). *Respiratory Disease: Principles of Patient Care.* Philadelphia: FA Davis.

CARDIOPULMONARY ANATOMY AND PHYSIOLOGY OF THE FETUS AND THE NEWBORN

Aloan CA, Hill TV (1997). *Respiratory Care of the Newborn and Child* (2nd ed.). Philadelphia: JB Lippincott.

Avory A, Martin R, Martin R (2001). *Neonatal-Perinatal Medicine* (7th ed.). St. Louis: Mosby.

Barnhart SL, Czervinske MP (2003). *Perinatal and Pediatric Respiratory Care* (2nd ed.). Philadelphia: WB Saunders.

Behrman RE, Kliegman RM, Arvin AM (2000). *Nelson Textbook of Pediatrics* (16th ed.). Philadelphia: WB Saunders.

Feischer GR, Ludwig S (2000). *Textbook of Pediatric Emergency Medicine* (4th ed.). Baltimore: Williams and Wilkins.

MacDonald M, Mullett M, Seshia M (2005). *Avery's Neonatology Pathophysiology and Management of the Newborn* (6th ed.). Philadelphia: JB Lippincott.

Taussig LM, Landau LI (1999). *Pediatric Respiratory Medicine*. St. Louis: Mosby.

Whitaker K (2001). *Comprehensive Perinatal and Pediatric Respiratory Care* (3rd ed.). Albany, NY: Delmar Publishers.

AGING AND THE CARDIOPULMONARY SYSTEM

Beers MH, Jones TV, et al. (Eds.) (2005). *The Merck Manual of Geriatrics*. Whitehouse Station, NJ: Merck Company.

Cardus J, Burgos R, et al. (1997). Increase in pulmonary ventilation-perfusion inequality with age in healthy individuals. *Am J Resp Crit Care Med* 56(2):648–653.

Cerveri I, Zoia MC, et al. (1995). Reference values of arterial oxygen tension in the middle aged and elderly. *Am J Resp Crit Care Med* 152(3):934–941

Cristian A (2005). *Aging with a Disability, An Issue of Physical Medicine and Rehabilitation Clinics*. Philadelphia: WB Saunders

Cristian A (2006). *Geriatric Rehabilitation, An Issue of Clinics in Geriatric Medicine*. Philadelphia: WB Saunders

Derstine JB, Drayton Hargrove S (2001). *Comprehensive Rehabilitation Nursing*. Philadelphia: WB Saunders

Frownfelter D, Dean E (2006). *Cardiovascular and Pulmonary Physical Therapy* (4th ed.). St. Louis: Mosby

Hazzard WR et al. (Eds.). (2003). *Principles of Geriatric Medicine and Gerontology*. New York: McGraw-Hill.

Malley WJ (2005). *Clinical Blood Gases: Applications and Intervention* (2nd ed.). Philadelphia: WB Saunders.

Martinson IM, Widmer AG, Portillo C (2002). *Home Health Care Nursing* (2nd ed.). Philadelphia: WB Saunders

Novelli, WD (2005). *The Merck Manual of Health and Aging*. Whitehouse Station, NJ: Merck Company.

Oxyenham H, Sharpe N (2003). Cardiovascular aging and heart failure. *Euro J Heart Failure* 5:427–434.

EXERCISE AND ITS EFFECTS ON THE CARDIOPULMONARY SYSTEM

Buckley J, Homes J, Mapp G (1998). *Exercise on Prescription—Activity for Cardiovascular Health*. Boston: Butterworth-Heinemann

Costill DL, Wilmore JH (2005). *Physiology of Sport and Exercise* (3rd ed.). Champaign, IL: Human Kinetics Publishers.

Cuppert M, Walsh K (2005). *General Medical Conditions in the Athlete*. St. Louis: Mosby

Froelicher VF, Myers JN (2006). *Exercise and the Heart* (5th ed.). Philadelphia: WB Saunders.

Katch FI, Katch VL, Mcardle W (2006). *Essentials of Exercise Physiology*. Philadelphia: Lippincott Williams and Wilkins

Myers JN (1996). *Essentials of Cardiopulmonary Exercise Testing.*; Champaign, IL: Human Kinetics Publishers.

Reilly T, Waterhouse J (2005). *Sport Exercise and Environmental Physiology.* New York: Churchill Livingstone

Robergs RA, Keteyian SJ (2002). *Fundamentals of Exercise Physiology.* New York: McGraw-Hill College.

Whyte G, Spurway N, MacLaren D (2006). *The Physiology of Training.* New York: Churchill Livingstone.

HIGH ALTITUDE AND ITS EFFECTS ON THE CARDIOPULMONARY SYSTEM

Auerbach P (2001). *Wilderness Medicine: Management of Wilderness and Environmental Emergencies* (4th ed.). St. Louis: Mosby

Hornbein TF, Schoene RB (Eds.) (2001). *High Altitude: An Exploration of Human Adaptation* (*Lung Biology in Health and Disease,* Vol. 161). New York: Marcel Dekker.

Hultgren H (1997). *High Altitude Medicine.* Stanford, CA: Hultgren Publications

Murray JG, Nadel JA (2005). *Textbook of Respiratory Medicine* (4th ed.). Philadelphia: WB Saunders.

Pollard AJ, Murdock DR (1998). *The High Altitude Medicine Handbook* (2nd ed.). Abingdon, UK: Radcliffe Publishing.

Ward MP, Milledge JS, West JB (2000). *High Altitude Medicine and Physiology* (3rd ed.). London: Arnold.

HIGH-PRESSURE ENVIRONMENTS AND THEIR EFFECT ON THE CARDIOPULMONARY SYSTEM

Bove AA, Davis JC (2004). *Diving Medicine* (4th ed.). Philadelphia: WB Saunders

Kindwall E, Whelan H (1999). *Hyperbaric Medicine Practice* (2nd ed.). Flagstaff, AZ: Best Publishing Company.

Neubauer RA (2004). *Textbook of Hyperbaric Medicine.* Göttingen, Germany: Hogrefe Huber Pub.

FUNDAMENTALS OF RESPIRATORY CARE

Hess DR, MacIntyre NR, Galvin WF, Adams AB, Saposnick AB (2002). *Respiratory Care—Principles and Practice.* Philadelphia: WB Saunders.

Kacmarek RM, Dimas S (2005). *Essentials of Respiratory Care* (4th ed.). St. Louis, Mosby.

Wilkins RL, Stoller JK, Scanlan CL (2003). *Egan's Fundamentals of Respiratory Care* (8th ed.). St. Louis: Mosby.

MEDICAL DICTIONARIES

Anderson KN, Anderson LE, Walter GD (2006). *Mosby's Medical, Nursing, and Allied Health Dictionary* (7th ed.). St. Louis: Mosby.

Dorland's Illustrated Medical Dictionary (30th ed.). (2003). Philadelphia: WB Saunders.

INDEX

IMPORTANT! READ CAREFULLY: This End User License Agreement ("Agreement") sets forth the conditions by which Thomson Delmar Learning, a division of Thomson Learning Inc. ("Thomson") will make electronic access to the Thomson Delmar Learning-owned licensed content and associated media, software, documentation, printed materials, and electronic documentation contained in this package and/or made available to you via this product (the "Licensed Content"), available to you (the "End User"). BY CLICKING THE "I ACCEPT" BUTTON AND/OR OPENING THIS PACKAGE, YOU ACKNOWLEDGE THAT YOU HAVE READ ALL OF THE TERMS AND CONDITIONS, AND THAT YOU AGREE TO BE BOUND BY ITS TERMS, CONDITIONS, AND ALL APPLICABLE LAWS AND REGULATIONS GOVERNING THE USE OF THE LICENSED CONTENT.

1.0 SCOPE OF LICENSE

1.1 <u>Licensed Content</u>. The Licensed Content may contain portions of modifiable content ("Modifiable Content") and content which may not be modified or otherwise altered by the End User ("Non-Modifiable Content"). For purposes of this Agreement, Modifiable Content and Non-Modifiable Content may be collectively referred to herein as the "Licensed Content." All Licensed Content shall be considered Non-Modifiable Content, unless such Licensed Content is presented to the End User in a modifiable format and it is clearly indicated that modification of the Licensed Content is permitted.

1.2 Subject to the End User's compliance with the terms and conditions of this Agreement, Thomson Delmar Learning hereby grants the End User, a nontransferable, nonexclusive, limited right to access and view a single copy of the Licensed Content on a single personal computer system for noncommercial, internal, personal use only. The End User shall not (i) reproduce, copy, modify (except in the case of Modifiable Content), distribute, display, transfer, sublicense, prepare derivative work(s) based on, sell, exchange, barter or transfer, rent, lease, loan, resell, or in any other manner exploit the Licensed Content; (ii) remove, obscure, or alter any notice of Thomson Delmar Learning's intellectual property rights present on or in the Licensed Content, including, but not limited to, copyright, trademark, and/or patent notices; or (iii) disassemble, decompile, translate, reverse engineer, or otherwise reduce the Licensed Content.

2.0 TERMINATION

2.1 Thomson Delmar Learning may at any time (without prejudice to its other rights or remedies) immediately terminate this Agreement and/or suspend access to some or all of the Licensed Content, in the event that the End User does not comply with any of the terms and conditions of this Agreement. In the event of such termination by Thomson Delmar Learning, the End User shall immediately return any and all copies of the Licensed Content to Thomson Delmar Learning.

3.0 PROPRIETARY RIGHTS

3.1 The End User acknowledges that Thomson Delmar Learning owns all rights, title and interest, including, but not limited to all copyright rights therein, in and to the Licensed Content, and that the End User shall not take any action inconsistent with such ownership. The Licensed Content is protected by U.S., Canadian and other applicable copyright laws and by international treaties, including the Berne Convention and the Universal Copyright Convention. Nothing contained in this Agreement shall be construed as granting the End User any ownership rights in or to the Licensed Content.

3.2 Thomson Delmar Learning reserves the right at any time to withdraw from the Licensed Content any item or part of an item for which it no longer retains the right to publish, or which it has reasonable grounds to believe infringes copyright or is defamatory, unlawful, or otherwise objectionable.

4.0 PROTECTION AND SECURITY

4.1 The End User shall use its best efforts and take all reasonable steps to safeguard its copy of the Licensed Content to ensure that no unauthorized reproduction, publication, disclosure, modification, or distribution of the Licensed Content, in whole or in part, is made. To the extent that the End User becomes aware of any such unauthorized use of the Licensed Content, the End User shall immediately notify Thomson Delmar Learning. Notification of such violations may be made by sending an e-mail to delmarhelp@thomson.com.

5.0 MISUSE OF THE LICENSED PRODUCT

5.1 In the event that the End User uses the Licensed Content in violation of this Agreement, Thomson Delmar Learning shall have the option of electing liquidated damages, which shall include all profits generated by the End User's use of the Licensed Content plus interest computed at the maximum rate permitted by law and all legal fees and other expenses incurred by Thomson Delmar Learning in enforcing its rights, plus penalties.

6.0 FEDERAL GOVERNMENT CLIENTS

6.1 Except as expressly authorized by Thomson Delmar Learning, Federal Government clients obtain only the rights specified in this Agreement and no other rights. The Government acknowledges that (i) all software and related documentation incorporated in the Licensed Content is existing commercial computer software within the meaning of FAR 27.405(b)(2); and (2) all other data delivered in whatever form, is limited rights data within the meaning of FAR 27.401. The restrictions in this section are acceptable as consistent with the Government's need for software and other data under this Agreement.

7.0 DISCLAIMER OF WARRANTIES AND LIABILITIES

7.1 Although Thomson Delmar Learning believes the Licensed Content to be reliable, Thomson Delmar Learning does not guarantee or warrant (i) any information or materials contained in or produced by the Licensed Content, (ii) the accuracy, completeness or reliability of the Licensed Content, or (iii) that the Licensed Content is free from errors or other material defects. THE LICENSED PRODUCT IS PROVIDED "AS IS," WITHOUT ANY WARRANTY OF ANY KIND AND THOMSON DELMAR LEARNING DISCLAIMS ANY AND ALL WARRANTIES, EXPRESSED OR IMPLIED, INCLUDING, WITHOUT LIMITATION, WARRANTIES OF MERCHANTABILITY OR FITNESS FOR A PARTICULAR PURPOSE. IN NO EVENT SHALL THOMSON DELMAR LEARNING BE LIABLE FOR: INDIRECT, SPECIAL, PUNITIVE OR CONSEQUENTIAL DAMAGES INCLUDING FOR LOST PROFITS, LOST DATA, OR OTHERWISE. IN NO EVENT SHALL THOMSON DELMAR LEARNING'S AGGREGATE LIABILITY HEREUNDER, WHETHER ARISING IN CONTRACT, TORT, STRICT LIABILITY OR OTHERWISE, EXCEED THE AMOUNT OF FEES PAID BY THE END USER HEREUNDER FOR THE LICENSE OF THE LICENSED CONTENT.

8.0 GENERAL

8.1 <u>Entire Agreement</u>. This Agreement shall constitute the entire Agreement between the Parties and supercedes all prior Agreements and understandings oral or written relating to the subject matter hereof.

8.2 <u>Enhancements/Modifications of Licensed Content</u>. From time to time, and in Thomson Delmar Learning's sole discretion, Thomson Delmar Learning may advise the End User of updates, upgrades, enhancements and/or improvements to the Licensed Content, and may permit the End User to access and use, subject to the terms and conditions of this Agreement, such modifications, upon payment of prices as may be established by Thomson Delmar Learning.

8.3 <u>No Export</u>. The End User shall use the Licensed Content solely in the United States and shall not transfer or export, directly or indirectly, the Licensed Content outside the United States.

8.4 <u>Severability</u>. If any provision of this Agreement is invalid, illegal, or unenforceable under any applicable statute or rule of law, the provision shall be deemed omitted to the extent that it is invalid, illegal, or unenforceable. In such a case, the remainder of the Agreement shall be construed in a manner as to give greatest effect to the original intention of the parties hereto.

8.5 <u>Waiver</u>. The waiver of any right or failure of either party to exercise in any respect any right provided in this Agreement in any instance shall not be deemed to be a waiver of such right in the future or a waiver of any other right under this Agreement.

8.6 <u>Choice of Law/Venue</u>. This Agreement shall be interpreted, construed, and governed by and in accordance with the laws of the State of New York, applicable to contracts executed and to be wholly preformed therein, without regard to its principles governing conflicts of law. Each party agrees that any proceeding arising out of or relating to this Agreement or the breach or threatened breach of this Agreement may be commenced and prosecuted in a court in the State and County of New York. Each party consents and submits to the nonexclusive personal jurisdiction of any court in the State and County of New York in respect of any such proceeding.

8.7 <u>Acknowledgment</u>. By opening this package and/or by accessing the Licensed Content on this Web site, THE END USER ACKNOWLEDGES THAT IT HAS READ THIS AGREEMENT, UNDERSTANDS IT, AND AGREES TO BE BOUND BY ITS TERMS AND CONDITIONS. IF YOU DO NOT ACCEPT THESE TERMS AND CONDITIONS, YOU MUST NOT ACCESS THE LICENSED CONTENT AND RETURN THE LICENSED PRODUCT TO DELMAR LEARNING (WITHIN 30 CALENDAR DAYS OF THE END USER'S PURCHASE) WITH PROOF OF PAYMENT ACCEPTABLE TO THOMSON DELMAR LEARNING, FOR A CREDIT OR A REFUND. Should the End User have any questions/comments regarding this Agreement, please contact Thomson Delmar Learning at delmarhelp@thomson.com.

StudyWare™ to Accompany Cardiopulmonary Anatomy & Physiology Fifth Edition

Minimum System Requirements

- Operating system: Microsoft Windows 2000, Windows XP, Windows Vista
- Processor: Pentium PC 500 MHz or higher (750 Mhz recommended)
- Memory: 64 MB of RAM (128 MB recommended)
- Screen resolution: 800 × 600 pixels
- Color depth: 16-bit color (thousands of colors)
- Macromedia Flash Player 9. The Macromedia Flash Player is free, and can be downloaded from http://www.adobe.com/products/flashplayer/

Installation Instructions

1. Insert disc into CD-ROM drive. The StudyWare™ installation program should start automatically. If it does not, go to step 2.
2. From My Computer, double-click the icon for the CD drive.
3. Double-click the *setup.exe* file to start the program.

Technical Support

Telephone: 1-800-648-7450, menu option 4, menu option 2; 8:30 A.M.–5:30 P.M. Eastern Time

Fax: 1-518-881-1247

E-mail: delmarhelp@thomson.com

StudyWare™ is a trademark used herein under license.

Microsoft® and Windows® are registered trademarks of the Microsoft Corporation.

Pentium® is a registered trademark of the Intel Corporation.

WF   Cardiopulmonary anatomy
101   & physiology
D441c
2008   Des Jardins, Terry R.
           08434

DATE LOANED	BORROWER'S NAME	DATE RETURNED

WF   Cardiopulmonary anatomy
101   & physiology
D441c
2008   Des Jardins, Terry R.

The CD-ROM to accompany this text is available at the circulation desk!